Behavioral Intervention Research: Designing, Evaluating, and Implementing

Laura N. Gitlin, PhD, is a professor in the Department of Community Public Health in the School of Nursing with joint appointments in the Department of Psychiatry and Division of Geriatrics and Gerontology, School of Medicine, Johns Hopkins University. She is the founding director of the Center for Innovative Care in Aging at Johns Hopkins University School of Nursing. The Center seeks to develop, test, and implement novel services, programs, and models that advance and support the well-being of diverse older adults, their families, and communities; enhance the yield of programs, policies, practices, and tools; and provide mentorship and research training in behavioral intervention research. Dr. Gitlin has been involved in behavioral intervention research for close to 30 years. Throughout these years, she has worked collaboratively with health and human service professionals and community agencies to develop and test a wide range of behavioral interventions. Her programs of research are multifold and include psychosocial, behavioral, and environmental approaches to address challenges of aging including physical disability, depressive symptoms, neuropsychiatric behaviors, and family caregiving. Dr. Gitlin is nationally and internationally recognized in these areas and a well-funded researcher, having received continuous funding from federal agencies and private foundations to test interventions. Some of these interventions have been translated for implementation in a variety of settings including home care, adult day care, hospitals, and senior centers. She has published extensively in peer-reviewed journals, and is a coauthor of a research text on quantitative and qualitative research methodologies, a book on the environmental skill–building intervention for family caregivers, a book on physical function in older adults, and a guide booklet for families challenged by behavioral symptoms common in persons with dementia.

She is a well-funded researcher, having received continuous research and training grants from federal agencies and private foundations for close to 28 years. A theme throughout her research is applying a social ecological perspective and a person-directed approach as well as collaborating with community organizations and health professionals to maximize the relevance and impact of intervention strategies. She is also involved in translating and implementing her team's proven interventions for delivery in different practice settings globally and in the United States.

Dr. Gitlin is a recipient of numerous awards including the 2009 Eastern Pennsylvania Geriatric Society Charles Ewing Presidential Award for outstanding contribution to geriatric care; the 2010 United Way Champion Impact Award for Healthy Aging at Home; the 2010 National Institute of Senior Centers Award with Center in the Park; the 2010 MetLife Award for translating the Skills$_2$Care Program (a dementia caregiver intervention program) with Fox Rehabilitation (a home health agency); the 2011 John Mackey Award for Excellence in Dementia Care from Johns Hopkins University; and the 2014 M. Powell Lawton Award from the Gerontological Society of America.

Sara J. Czaja, PhD, is a Leonard M. Miller Professor of the Psychiatry and Behavioral Sciences, with joint appointments in Psychology and Industrial Engineering at the University of Miami. She is also the scientific director of the Center on Aging at the University of Miami Miller School of Medicine and the director of the Center on Research and Education for Aging and Technology Enhancement (CREATE). CREATE is funded by the National Institute on Aging and involves collaboration with the Georgia Institute of Technology and Florida State University. The focus of CREATE is on older adults and their interactions with technology systems in work, health care, and everyday living domains. A particular emphasis is on how technology can be used as a mechanism for the delivery of interventions to foster independence among older people.

Dr. Czaja has extensive experience in aging research and a long commitment to developing intervention strategies to improve the quality of life for older adults and their families. She has been an active researcher in this area for more than 25 years. Her specific areas of research include aging and cognition; aging and health care informatics; family caregiving; older workers; training; and functional assessment. She brings a unique focus to these issues with her combined background in engineering and the behavioral sciences. She has broad experience with research methodologies in both laboratory and field settings and with translational research. She has received extensive funding from the National Institutes of Health as well as other federal agencies and foundations for her research. Dr. Czaja is very well published in the field of aging, and has written numerous book chapters and scientific articles. She has also collaborated with community organizations, health care providers, and with industry. She recently coauthored a book with other members of the CREATE team concerning the design of technology systems for older adult populations, and a book on training older adults. She is a fellow of the American Psychological Association, the Human Factors and Ergonomics Society, and the Gerontological Society of America. In addition, she is the current president of Division 20 (Adult Development and Aging) of the American Psychological Association. She is also a member of the National Academy of Science/National Research Council Board on Human Systems Integration.

Behavioral Intervention Research: Designing, Evaluating, and Implementing

Laura N. Gitlin, PhD

Sara J. Czaja, PhD

With Contributors

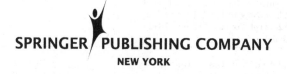

SPRINGER PUBLISHING COMPANY

NEW YORK

Springer Publishing Company, LLC
11 West 42nd Street
New York, NY 10036
www.springerpub.com

Acquisitions Editor: Sheri W. Sussman
Composition: S4Carlisle Publishing Services

ISBN: 978-0-8261-2658-0
e-book ISBN: 978-0-8261-2659-7

15 16 17 18 19 / 5 4 3 2 1

The author and the publisher of this Work have made every effort to use sources believed to be reliable to provide information that is accurate and compatible with the standards generally accepted at the time of publication. The author and publisher shall not be liable for any special, consequential, or exemplary damages resulting, in whole or in part, from the readers' use of, or reliance on, the information contained in this book. The publisher has no responsibility for the persistence or accuracy of URLs for external or third-party Internet websites referred to in this publication and does not guarantee that any content on such websites is, or will remain, accurate or appropriate.

Library of Congress Cataloging-in-Publication Data

Gitlin, Laura N., 1952- author. | Czaja, Sara J., author.
Behavioral intervention research : designing, evaluating, and implementing / Laura N. Gitlin and Sara J. Czaja.
New York : Springer Pub. Company, [2016] | Includes bibliographical references and index.
LCCN 2015034213 | ISBN 9780826126580
LCSH: Action research in public health—Methodology. | Behavior modification—Research. | Evidence based medicine—Research. | Evidence based social work—Research.
LCC RA440.85 .G58 2016 | DDC 362.1072—dc23

Special discounts on bulk quantities of our books are available to corporations, professional associations, pharmaceutical companies, health care organizations, and other qualifying groups. If you are interested in a custom book, including chapters from more than one of our titles, we can provide that service as well.

For details, please contact:
Special Sales Department, Springer Publishing Company, LLC
11 West 42nd Street, 15th Floor, New York, NY 10036-8002
Phone: 877-687-7476 or 212-431-4370; Fax: 212-941-7842
E-mail: sales@springerpub.com

Printed in the United States of America by Gasch Printing.

To Eduardo, Eric, Keith, and my family:
Como siempre. With love, gratitude, and honor—LNG

To my family, friends, and colleagues: Thank you for your continued support and inspiration—SJC

To our collaborators who share our passion;
To our study participants who drive our mission to find better ways.

CONTRIBUTORS

John Beilenson, MA, is Founder and President of Strategic Communications & Planning (SCP), a socially responsible communications consultancy in Wayne, Pennsylvania. Since 1987, he and his firm have worked with a wide range of foundations, nonprofit organizations, academic innovators, and associations to help them use communications to create social good. He is the author of 18 books, including *The Future Me: Authoring the Second Half of Your Life*, an interactive journal for people considering retirement and other transitions in later life.

Ronald W. Berkowsky, PhD, is a Postdoctoral Associate in the Department of Psychiatry and Behavioral Sciences at the University of Miami School of Medicine. He earned his doctorate in Medical Sociology at the University of Alabama at Birmingham in 2014. His research focuses primarily on older adults and their use of technology with emphasis on the impacts of technology use on mental health and well-being in old age. His research also examines the impacts of technology use on work–life balance and stress in the U.S. working population.

Joseph J. Gallo, MD, MPH, is Director of the Mixed Methods Research Training Program for the Health Sciences, a national program to develop the capacity to carry out mixed methods health research. He was a member of the 2011 panel convened by the Office of Behavioral and Social Sciences Research (OBSSR) to provide best practices for mixed methods research at the National Institutes of Health. He has published on risk factors, the course and epidemiology of depression, the form of depression in late life, health services research, comorbidity of depression and medical conditions, primary health care and mental health, cognitive impairment, and mixed methods.

Philip D. Harvey, PhD, is a Leonard M. Miller Professor of Psychiatry and Director of the Division of Psychology at the University of Miami Miller School of Medicine. He has authored over 900 scientific papers and abstracts and over 60 book chapters, edited six books, and written four books on topics of psychological assessment, schizophrenia, and aging. He was designated by Thompson-Reuters as being in the top 1% of researchers in citations in mental health research. Other awards include the Inaugural Schizophrenia International Research Society Clinical Scientist Distinguished Contributions award (2012), the 2014 Alexander Gralnick Schizophrenia Research award from the American Psychiatric Foundation, and the 2014 John Blair Barnwell award from the U.S. Department of Veterans Affairs.

Nancy A. Hodgson, PhD, RN, FAAN, is Assistant Professor at the Johns Hopkins University School of Nursing and Associate Director of Implementation Science at the Johns Hopkins University Center for Innovative Care in Aging. Her programs of research include the examination of factors associated with health-related quality of life in chronically ill older adults, the mechanism of action underlying nonpharmacological interventions for alleviating symptom distress in frail elders, and the translation and implementation of palliative models of care for older adults with complex health care needs and their caregivers.

Daniel E. Jimenez, PhD, is Assistant Professor in the Department of Psychiatry and Behavioral Sciences, and member of the Center on Aging at the University of Miami Miller School of Medicine. Dr. Jimenez has extensive experience in aging research, and has dedicated his career to improving access and engagement in mental health services among underserved populations. His research interests include geriatric mental health services research, health promotion, multicultural mental health, and mental illness prevention. He has combined these areas of research to design and implement culturally appropriate and novel approaches to preventing mental illness in racial/ethnic minority elderly.

Eric Jutkowitz is currently a doctoral candidate in the Division of Health Policy and Management in the University of Minnesota's School of Public Health. His research interests are in understanding the cost and value of care for older adults with dementia and other chronic diseases. He has participated as a research analyst in numerous grant-funded, cost-effectiveness studies conducted alongside nonpharmacological clinical trials, and has many publications in this area. His methodological interests include the economic evaluation of health technologies and decision analysis.

Su Yeon Lee, PhD, is associate research faculty at the Department of Mental Health at Johns Hopkins Bloomberg School of Public Health. Dr. Lee is also Policy Analyst at the Office for Research on Disparities and Global Mental Health at the National Institute of Mental Health. Her primary research interests are mental health disparities among Asian Americans, and the use of both quantitative and qualitative methods in mental health services research. She received a Doctor of Philosophy in Public Health at the Department of Mental Health at Johns Hopkins Bloomberg School of Public Health.

Bruce Leff, MD, is Professor of Medicine, with joint appointments in the Johns Hopkins Bloomberg School of Public Health and the Johns Hopkins School of Nursing. His principal areas of research concern the development, evaluation, and dissemination of novel models of care for older adults, including Hospital at Home, quality of care measurement and improvement for home-based medical care, and the care of people with multiple chronic conditions. He cares for patients in acute, ambulatory, and home settings. He is a member of the Board of Regents of the American College of Physicians, and immediate past-president of the American Academy of Home Care Medicine.

David L. Loewenstein, PhD, is Professor of Psychiatry and Behavioral Sciences at the University of Miami Miller School of Medicine and a board-certified neuropsychologist. He is the Director of Cognitive/Neuropsychological Laboratory and Psychological Services, Wien Center for Alzheimer's Disease and Related Disorders, Mount Sinai Medical Center, Miami Beach, Florida. Dr. Loewenstein's research is in aging and cognition; normative age–related cognitive changes and implications for assessments and treatments; and developing novel tests for assessment of early Alzheimer's disease, normal aging, and neurological and neuropsychiatric conditions. He has also conducted extensive work on the relationship between cognitive function and biomarkers of Alzheimer's.

John A. Nyman, PhD, is Professor of Health Economics in the University of Minnesota's School of Public Health. His research interests range from economic evaluations of new health technologies to the theory of demand for health insurance, and from long-term care policy analysis to the public health consequences of gambling. He has published over 100 research studies in top scholarly journals and has received almost 60 grants. The recipient of major awards for excellence in teaching at Minnesota and in his previous position at the University of Iowa, Dr. Nyman received his PhD in economics from the University of Wisconsin.

Marcia G. Ory, PhD, MPH, is Regents and Distinguished Professor, Department of Health Promotion and Community Health Sciences, School of Public Health (SPH) at The Texas A&M Health Science Center, College Station, Texas. Her primary administrative role is serving as Associate Dean for Research (since February 2015). She is also the Director of the SPH Program on Healthy Aging, chair of the Health and Wellness Committee, and the academic partner for the Community Research Center for Senior Health. She has been a principal investigator on multiple local, state, and federally funded grants to implement and evaluate evidence-based behavioral interventions for promoting healthy lifestyle changes in midlife and older ages. Co-directing a new SPH initiative on health technology and patient empowerment, she is working with an interdisciplinary cross-campus group to develop innovative research projects across public health, medicine, engineering, and computer sciences. In this vein, she has participated in the development and testing of several health behavioral interventions, especially concerning cancer survivorship.

Jeanine M. Parisi, PhD, is an Associate Scientist in the Department of Mental Health, Johns Hopkins Bloomberg School of Public Health, and holds a research position within the Center for Innovative Care in Aging, Johns Hopkins School of Nursing. Her interests are concerned with the identification of lifestyle factors (e.g., activity engagement, education, personality) that may serve as risk/protective mechanisms on cognition in adulthood; and the determination of how interventions may be designed, implemented, and improved in order to promote cognitive, physical, and mental health across the life span.

Laura T. Pizzi, PharmD, MPH, is Professor of Applied Health Economics at the Jefferson College of Pharmacy of Thomas Jefferson University. Dr. Pizzi's research foci include economic analysis of health care interventions and the impact of disease and treatments on productivity and quality of life. She has more than 60 peer-reviewed manuscripts and more than 90 scientific posters or podium presentations, is Deputy Editor of *American Health and Drug Benefits*, a member of the editorial boards for *PharmacoEconomics* and the *Jefferson Health Policy Newsletter*, and coeditor of the text *Economic Evaluation in U.S. Healthcare: Principles and Applications*.

George W. Rebok, PhD, is Professor in the Department of Mental Health in the Bloomberg School of Public Health at Johns Hopkins University, and holds joint faculty appointments in the Department of Psychiatry and Behavioral Sciences in the Johns Hopkins School of Medicine and in the Center on Aging and Health, Center for Innovative Care in Aging, and Center for Injury Research and Policy. He has over 35 years of experience in life-course developmental research, prevention science, and cognitive aging, and served as principal investigator of the NIA/NINR-funded ACTIVE trial and the NIA-funded Baltimore Experience Corps® trial.

Jyoti "Tina" Savla, PhD, is Associate Professor in the Department of Human Development and a Research Methodologist at the Center for Gerontology at Virginia Tech. Her research investigates how everyday life stress and daily hassles experienced by middle-aged and older adults get "under their skin" to affect their emotional and physical health. She has extensive experience in analyzing prospective longitudinal studies, missing data in longitudinal designs, and estimating statistical power; and has expertise on structural equation modeling, multilevel models, and time-series analysis. She serves as a biostatistician on several state and federal grants, including ones on obesity and diabetes from the National Institutes of Health.

CONTENTS

FOREWORD

Behavioral intervention research is coming of age, as evidenced by Gitlin and Czaja's book *Behavioral Intervention Research: Designing, Evaluating, and Implementing*. I applaud the book for providing a much needed overview of the entire "behavioral intervention pipeline." It fills a unique niche in its coverage of key theoretical and methodological aspects as well as its case examples and professional development considerations, which makes the content accessible and practical for a broad audience. The book reflects the current thinking that behavioral intervention research represents a growing science base whose history has unfolded over the past several decades based on the contributions of many researchers, practitioners, and consumers alike.

The importance of behavioral intervention research for improving the health and well-being of individuals, families, and communities cannot be overstated. There is a growing recognition that the application of evidence-based research can make a difference in health promotion and disease prevention efforts across the life course. The book's contributors recognize the challenges and complexities of behavioral intervention research, but also its many potential benefits. Behavioral intervention research is viewed comprehensively within a socioecological framework that values community-based participatory research perspectives and engagement of stakeholders in the construction of an intervention. The growing appreciation of the interplay between environmental, technological, and economic influences in designing and evaluating and then implementing interventions advances the frontiers of behavioral intervention research. Reflecting the long history of behavioral intervention research, the book appropriately sets its content alongside of and within the emerging field of implementation science, explaining the similarities and differences across these different but highly related fields of study.

I am most pleased to be asked to contribute an independent reflection on this book through its Foreword. It allows me to reflect on the activities that have helped spawn this growing field as well as my own small role in its development. Starting in the 1980s as a program director at the National Institute of Aging's Social Science Research on Aging Program, I had the distinct pleasure of helping to promote an aging, health, and behavior research agenda, and seeding the development of generations of stellar investigators who are now leaders in the behavioral intervention research field. This volume further emphasizes the importance of understanding and promoting translational research. Along with other colleagues, I am gratified to have been part of national research initiatives at the Robert Wood Johnson Foundation and federal agencies such as the Centers for Disease Control and Prevention and the Administration for Community Living that have pushed the application of research to practice into the forefront. This area is growing in practical importance, as new federal policies are tying reimbursement to evidence-based practices.

The lessons I learned resonate with those highlighted in the book. Our society faces complex public health problems calling for complex multilevel solutions. Behavioral intervention research as broadly viewed in this book offers one such promising solution. To meet the nation's public health goals, it is critical to have a better understanding of the design, evaluation, and implementation of a wide range of behavioral health interventions for addressing the multitude of health-related problems across diverse populations and settings. This book is a most welcome addition to helping us meet these research and public health goals, and offers us a much needed comprehensive framework for meeting these challenges and improving population health.

Marcia Ory, PhD
Regents and Distinguished Professor
Department of Health Promotion and Community Health Sciences
School of Public Health
The Texas A&M Health Science Center
College Station Texas

PREFACE

Behavioral interventions matter! Over the past 50 years, a wide range of novel and important behavioral (psychosocial, environmental, technology-based) or nonpharmacological interventions have been developed, evaluated, translated, and implemented in community and clinical settings. We have proven effective behavioral interventions that address a broad range of behavioral, physical, emotional, and cognitive health, as well as social issues across the life span. Exemplars include but are not limited to: reducing behavioral disturbances in young children (Chicago Parent Program, Gross et al., 2009); enhancing dementia caregiver well-being (REACH II, Belle et al., 2006; Skills$_2$Care^R, Gitlin, Jacobs, & Earland, 2010); reducing depression in older adults in primary care (IMPACT, Stewart, Perkins, & Callahan, 2014; Unützer et al., 2002) and the community (Get Busy Get Better: Helping Older Adults Beat the Blues, Gitlin et al., 2012); improving chronic disease self-management (CDSMP, Lorig et al., 1999) and its variants such as Harvest Health (Gitlin et al., 2008); reducing functional decline (ABLE, Gitlin et al., 2006), fall risk and fear of falling (LiFe Program, Clemson et al., 2012; Matter of Balance, Tennstedt et al., 1998); addressing delirium in hospital settings (HELP, Inouye et al., 1999); enhancing social connectedness (PRISM, Czaja et al., 2015); improving well-being through physical exercise (Fit and Strong, Hughes et al., 2004); addressing substance abuse in adolescence through the multidimensional family therapy intervention (MDFT, Liddle, Rowe, Dakoff, Ungaro, & Henderson, 2004); and enhancing cognitive status (ACTIVE, Rebok et al., 2014). These reflect only a very small fraction of the well-designed interventions that have been well tested using rigorous methodologies and that, in turn, have been shown to substantially improve the quality of life and health and well-being of the targeted individuals, families, and communities.

This book is intended to introduce the exciting, challenging, stimulating, and inspiring world of behavioral intervention research. It is about the science and state-of-the-art practices in designing, evaluating, and then translating, implementing, and disseminating novel behavioral interventions for maximum impact on the health and well-being of individuals, families, and their communities. Each chapter tackles critical considerations in behavioral intervention research. Our approach is to be as broad and inclusive as possible of the many nuances, intricacies, and issues in this form of inquiry. We cover a wide range of topics including examining the heart of the matter (Part I) or strategies for developing behavioral interventions including the pipeline for advancing interventions, the role of theory, intervention delivery characteristics, standardizing treatments, and use of technology. This is followed by evaluative considerations (Part II) including selecting control groups; identifying recruitment, retention, and fidelity strategies; using mixed methodologies; and ethical challenges. Then we examine outcome measures and analytic considerations (Part III) including economic evaluations for maximizing the yield of trial data, and, in Part IV, how implementation science can inform the development and advancement of behavioral interventions. Finally, in Part V, we explore a host of professional issues unique to this form of inquiry including challenges in staffing behavioral interventionist studies, how to obtain funding for developing and evaluating an intervention, and what, when, and where to publish.

Case examples from successful behavioral intervention trials are used throughout each chapter to illustrate key concepts. The primary goal of each chapter is to examine the science and best practices as well as to facilitate decision making related to the fundamental issues in conducting behavioral intervention research. The chapters also identify critical knowledge gaps in an effort to enhance scientific practices in each of the facets of behavioral intervention research.

Despite over 50 years of promising behavioral intervention research, the science of and best practices for behavioral intervention research are not well explicated, and common know-how remains largely undocumented or not systematically shared within the research community, especially across disciplines. Thus, there are lost opportunities for advancing the skills and abilities of the current and next generation of researchers in the state of the science (and art) of this form of inquiry. This book is intended to fill this gap. Whereas classical clinical trial texts provide foundational knowledge important to the conduct of behavioral intervention research, they favor methodologies specific to pharmacological and medical device development and testing. These sources tend to ignore fundamental considerations and challenges specific to behavioral intervention work such as fidelity monitoring, the role and important contributions of mixed methodologies, strategies for recruiting and retaining diverse populations, or approaches for embedding and evaluating interventions under field conditions such as in community and clinical settings. Thus, it is critical that the specifics related to behavioral intervention research be documented, discussed, and advanced.

We aspire to have this book positively impact the work of researchers interested in or actively engaged in behavioral intervention research. We also hope this book helps to advance a rich dialogue and to stimulate further research directed specifically at developing best practices in behavioral intervention research. Behavioral intervention research is a complex and challenging form of inquiry that takes time, occurs over many years, and can be daunting at times. Nevertheless, its potential for yielding evidence-based programs, protocols, strategies, and models of care that can make a real difference to real people in real settings makes it a most commendable scientific enterprise that is worthy of our careful attention and elevation.

Please join us in the conversation and the journey of designing, evaluating, translating, implementing, and disseminating novel, health-promoting, and valuable behavioral interventions that can make a difference in the lives of people, their families, and communities.

REFERENCES

Belle, S. H., Burgio, L., Burns, R., Coon, D., Czaja, S. J., Gallagher-Thompson, D., . . . Zhang, S. (2006). Enhancing the quality of life of dementia caregivers from different ethnic or racial groups: A randomized, controlled trial. *Annals of Internal Medicine, 145*(10), 727–738.

Clemson, L., Singh, M. A. F., Bundy, A., Cumming, R. G., Manollaras, K., O'Loughlin, P., & Black, D. (2012). Integration of balance and strength training into daily life activity to reduce rate of falls in older people (the LiFE study): Randomised parallel trial. *British Medical Journal, 345*, 1–15.

Czaja, S. J., Boot, W. R., Charness, N., Rogers, W. A., Sharit, J., Fisk, A. D., . . . Nair, S. N. (2015). The personalized reminder information and social management system (PRISM) trial: Rationale, methods and baseline characteristics. *Contemporary Clinical Trials, 40*, 35–46.

Gitlin, L. N., Chernett, N. L., Harris, L. F., Palmer, D., Hopkins, P., & Dennis, M. P. (2008). Harvest health: Translation of the chronic disease self-management program for older African Americans in a senior setting. *The Gerontologist: Practice Concepts, 48*(5), 698–705. doi:10.1093/geront/48.5.698

Gitlin, L. N., Harris, L. F., McCoy, M., Chernett, N. L., Jutkowitz, E., & Pizzi, L. T. (2012). A community-integrated home-based depression intervention for older African Americans: Description of the beat the blues randomized trial and intervention costs. *BMC Geriatrics, 12*(4), 1–11.

Gitlin, L. N., Jacobs, M., & Earland, T. V. (2010). Translation of a dementia caregiver intervention for delivery in homecare as a reimbursable Medicare service: Outcomes and lessons learned. *The Gerontologist, 50*(6), 847–854.

Gitlin, L. N., Winter, L., Dennis, M. P., Corcoran, M., Schinfeld, S., & Hauck, W. W. (2006). A randomized trial of a multicomponent home intervention to reduce functional difficulties in older adults. *Journal of the American Geriatrics Society, 54*(5), 809–816.

Gross, D., Garvey, C., Julion, W., Fogg, L., Tucker, S., & Mokros, H. (2009). Efficacy of the Chicago parent program with low-income African American and Latino parents of young children. *Prevention Science, 10*(1), 54–65.

Hughes, S. L., Seymour, R. B., Campbell, R., Pollak, N., Huber, G., & Sharma, L. (2004). Impact of the fit and strong intervention on older adults with osteoarthritis. *The Gerontologist, 44*(2), 217–228.

Inouye, S. K., Bogardus, S. T., Jr., Charpentier, P. A., Leo-Summers, L., Acampora, D., Holford, T. R., & Cooney, L. M., Jr. (1999). A multicomponent intervention to prevent delirium in hospitalized older patients. *New England Journal of Medicine, 340*(9), 669–676.

Liddle, H. A., Rowe, C. L., Dakof, G. A., Ungaro, R. A., & Henderson, C. E. (2004). Early intervention for adolescent substance abuse: Pretreatment to posttreatment outcomes of a randomized clinical trial comparing multidimensional family therapy and peer group treatment. *Journal of Psychoactive Drugs, 36*(1), 49–63.

Lorig, K. R., Sobel, D. S., Stewart, A. L., Brown, B. W., Jr., Bandura, A., Ritter, P., . . . Holman, H. R. (1999). Evidence suggesting that a chronic disease self-management program can improve health status while reducing hospitalization: A randomized trial. *Medical Care, 37*(1), 5–14.

Rebok, G. W., Ball, K., Guey, L. T., Jones, R. N., Kim, H. Y., King, J. W., . . . Willis, S. L. (2014). Ten-year effects of the advanced cognitive training for independent and vital elderly cognitive training trial on cognition and everyday functioning in older adults. *Journal of the American Geriatrics Society, 62*(1), 16–24.

Stewart, J. C., Perkins, A. J., & Callahan, C. M. (2014). Effect of collaborative care for depression on risk of cardiovascular events: data from the IMPACT randomized controlled trial. *Psychosomatic Medicine, 76*(1), 29–37.

Tennstedt, S., Howland, J., Lachman, M., Peterson, E., Kasten, L., & Jette, A. (1998). A randomized, controlled trial of a group intervention to reduce fear of falling and associated activity restriction in older adults. *The Journals of Gerontology Series B: Psychological Sciences and Social Sciences, 53*(6), P384–P392.

Unützer, J., Katon, W., Callahan, C. M., Williams, J. W., Jr., Hunkeler, E., Harpole, L., . . . Impact Investigators. (2002). Collaborative care management of late-life depression in the primary care setting: A randomized controlled trial. *JAMA, 288*(22), 2836–2845.

ACKNOWLEDGMENTS

We would like to express our sincere appreciation to numerous individuals who helped with the preparation of this book. In particular, we would like to recognize both Marissa Kobayashi, MHS, research assistant, who conducted various literature searches and reviewed chapters for reference accuracy, and Vincent A. Fields, Sr., MBA, Senior Administrator, for working on references and chapter formatting, both of the Center for Innovative Care in Aging, Johns Hopkins University School of Nursing. We would also like to thank Chin Chin Lee, MS, MPH, Senior Project Manager at the Center on Aging, University of Miami Miller School of Medicine, for her assistance with the literature review and references.

Our continued heartfelt gratitude to Sheri W. Sussman, our wonderful editor at Springer Publishing Company, LLC, for her long-held belief in the importance of this project, ongoing encouragement, and excellent suggestions for making this book the best it could be.

Although we did not have a grant to write this book, we would like to extend our gratefulness to the many federal and foundation sponsors who have supported and continue to support our behavioral intervention research. These include the National Institutes of Health, the Alzheimer's Association, the Retirement Research Foundation, the Hartford Foundation, the Administration on Aging, Langeloth Foundation, AT&T, and Cisco.

Finally, we are most grateful for the thoughtful and significant contributions of our colleagues who participated as authors or coauthors on select chapters in this book.

DEVELOPING INTERVENTIONS: HEART OF THE MATTER

The heart of the matter in behavioral intervention research is, obviously, the intervention. All other research-related considerations, such as the selection of outcome measures, study design, sampling, and recruitment processes, emanate from the purpose/goals of the intervention and the behavior, policy, and/or health care protocol that the intervention is intended to address.

Therefore, in Part I, we begin with a focus on the important and interrelated considerations in developing a behavioral intervention. This includes an examination of the: promises, challenges, and contexts of behavioral interventions (Chapter 1); pipelines for intervention advancement (Chapter 2); discovery period in which the anatomy of an intervention is developed (Chapter 3); role of theory as a driver of intervention development (and testing) (Chapter 4); selection of delivery characteristics of interventions (Chapter 5); ways to standardize protocols and practices (Chapter 6); and use of technology as a mechanism for delivering, monitoring, and analyzing interventions (Chapter 7).

The key "take home" points of Part I include the following:

- Interventions occur in a broad social ecological context that needs to be understood.
- A systems and user-centered design approach is essential for advancing novel interventions that are responsive to real-world contexts and needs of targeted populations.
- The evidence base for interventions is advanced through a series of iterative steps or phases.
- Interventions have a common etiology, referred to as "a period of discovery" in which the problem area, ways to ameliorate it, and targeted populations at risk are carefully identified.
- Theories or conceptual frameworks to understand why and how interventions work can maximize impact.
- Delivery characteristics of interventions need to be carefully chosen on the basis of theory; empirical evidence; and the specific goals, problem area, target population, context for delivery, and available resources.
- Standardization is critical to ensure treatment fidelity and internal validity, and to enable replication and wide-scale implementation.
- Technologies have an important role in the delivery, monitoring, and evaluation of interventions.

ONE

PROMISES AND CHALLENGES OF BEHAVIORAL INTERVENTION RESEARCH

An epidemiologist conducts a study showing a strong empirical link between caregiver physical strain and nursing home placement of frail older adults. He now wants to develop an intervention to help minimize the caregiver's physical strain and prevent residential relocation of the older adult.

A clinician scientist observes that her cancer survivor patients tend to have cognitive and functional complaints that are stressful to them. The literature provides evidence for these relationships and factors that contribute to them, but no interventions that address this distressful phenomenon. She seeks to develop an intervention that would help this growing clinical population.

A family member of a behavioral researcher has a life-altering health care event and experiences significant gaps when transitioning among care contexts, highlighting the critical need to develop and test strategies to improve care continuity.

A team consisting of academic and senior center directors implemented an evidence-based program in the senior center to improve chronic disease management. They find that it is less acceptable to and effective for their African American members and that it needs modification to improve its reach to and adoption by diverse groups.

A health care system seeks to adopt a proven health promotion intervention, but it is too costly to deliver to rural populations as originally designed. They partner with researchers to examine the effectiveness of using technology for its delivery.

These are real examples of the common pathways that lead practitioners, health and human service professionals, and novice and experienced researchers to embrace the need for and engage in behavioral intervention research. Behavioral interventions start with a specified problem and are designed to address pressing identifiable and documented public health issues or policy gaps, service delivery snafus, health disparities, or the need for better, more cost-efficient care approaches. Such interventions encompass a wide range of strategies that can involve manipulating cognitive, behavioral, physical, environmental, and/or psychosocial processes to improve outcomes for a targeted population or community. Interventions may be directed at individuals, families, communities, or organizations or their combination, and target cognitions (e.g., coping mechanisms, cognitive framing, problem solving), behaviors (e.g., communications, lifestyle choices, medication adherence), emotional or affective well-being, physical health and functioning, physical or social environments, policies, health care practices, or service delivery mechanisms and training. Behavioral interventions are relevant to and important for individuals of any age group, race or ethnicity, socioeconomic status, or culture, as well as families, communities, organizations, and societies at large.

WHY BEHAVIORAL INTERVENTION RESEARCH IS IMPORTANT

The growing recognition and increased acknowledgment of the value and importance of behavioral intervention research for improving the health and well-being of the public can be attributed to several critical trends. The first is the growing recognition that the most pressing contemporary health issues that impose high societal and individual costs primarily involve lifestyle and behavioral factors, such as obesity, smoking, addictions, chronic disease, comorbidities, and functional consequences of diseases, social isolation, depression, delirium, mental illness, family caregiving, and health disparities. Developing and testing behavioral, nonpharmacological interventions that tackle these serious, persistent public health challenges is a widely recognized imperative (Lovasi, Hutson, Guerra, & Neckerman, 2009; Milstein, Homer, Briss, Burton, & Pechacek, 2011; Jackson, Knight, & Rafferty, 2010).

Second, the existing research evidence consistently suggests that behavioral and environmental factors exert a powerful and large influence on health and well-being. This is particularly the case for aging-related processes in which social and environmental factors are intertwined with the medical care of older adults. Take, for example, functional decline associated with growing older. Microenvironmental (individual) and macroenvironmental (family and cultural) effects have been found to contribute to age-related changes in functioning and to account for increasing heterogeneity in abilities even more than genetic factors (Finkel, Ernsth-Bravell, & Pedersen, 2015). The contribution of genetics to the rate of change in functional abilities among older adults >75 years of age is estimated to be only about 16% for women and 9% for men (Christensen, Gaist, Vaupel, & McGue, 2002; Christensen, Holm, McGue, Corder, & Vaupel, 1999). Even for dementia, the genetic heritability is small, with most causes due to age itself and possibly environmental factors, although these are poorly understood (Gatz et al., 1997). Furthermore, although genetics may contribute in part to early onset of chronic diseases, environmental factors and behaviors overwhelmingly account for the wide variation in outcomes after age 75 (Svedberg, Lichtenstein, & Pedersen, 2001). Thus, enhancing health and well-being through behavioral, lifestyle, and environmental modifications is critical to improving the health of the public overall, and the promotion of "successful aging," in particular. The latter, in particular, is an issue of growing importance given the aging of the population, especially the increase in the "oldest old" cohort (85+ years.).

Third, despite an abundance of proven behavioral interventions, a gap of more than 17 years persists between the conduct of research and the production of evidence and the implementation of its yield. (Institute of Medicine [IOM], 2001). Only about 14% of evidence, including evidence-based intervention programs, is implemented in clinical and community settings, with Americans receiving only 50% of recommended preventive, acute, and long-term health care (McGlynn et al., 2003). Minority populations are at particular risk, receiving recommended evidence-informed programs less than an estimated 35% of the time (Balas & Boren, 2000; Brownson, Colditz, & Proctor, 2012; McGlynn et al., 2003; Riley, Glasgow, Etheredge, & Abernethy, 2013). This large gap appears to be due to system-level factors (e.g., policies that do not structurally and financially support the delivery of evidence-based programs), workforce-level factors (e.g., the lack of adequate preparation of health and human service professionals or others in using evidence-based programs), individual factors (e.g., the lack of awareness of available programs or inability to access programs), or mismatches between the needs of individuals, resources (financial and expertise) of service organizations, existing policies and practices, and the characteristics of tested and proven interventions.

It is unclear how to close the "chasm" between "knowing" versus "doing" that continues to haunt every part of health and human services for every age group and population. This chasm has led to the growing recognition of the need to reconsider traditional approaches to designing and testing behavioral interventions and to seek alternative approaches for developing interventions that have greater potentiality for being implemented more rapidly and sustained.

A fourth trend that heightens the importance of behavioral intervention research is the paradigm shift occurring in health care today. New approaches and expectations are emerging in health care to view patients and their families as active participants in the management of their own health (Bodenheimer, Lorig, Holman, & Grumbach, 2002). Health self-management may involve adherence to a diet, exercise or medication regimen, coordination of a care network, and use of medical technologies (e.g., activity monitor, blood glucose meter, blood pressure monitor). Self-management can be complex and involve the need for personal oversight of multiple wellness goals, chronic conditions, and medication regimes. Thus, there is growing recognition of the importance of behavioral interventions that can effectively instruct and support patients and their families in the practical skills for self-management. Furthermore, there is an increased awareness of the need for evidence-based approaches to foster adherence; promote engagement in wellness activities; facilitate care coordination, communications, and interactions with health care professionals; and manage transitions between health care practices, facilities, and professionals.

Finally, there is a societal push for the adoption of evidence-based practices in health service delivery settings and community agencies. Evidence-based practices are interventions that have been tested in high-quality research and that are unbiased, have strong internal validity, and in which the results are generalizable with a firm level of confidence in linking outcomes to interventions (Guyatt et al., 2000). Thus, behavioral intervention research is needed to uncover what treatment practices work best, for whom, and under what circumstances. At the same time, there is an emphasis on what is referred to as "translational research" or harnessing knowledge from science to inform treatments and ensure that evidence reaches the intended populations (Woolf, 2008). As a critical goal is to impact practice and health care, it has become imperative to understand how best to design interventions so that they can eventually be successfully applied to and adopted by individuals, clinical practices, services, organizations, and communities.

ADVANCEMENTS IN BEHAVIORAL INTERVENTION RESEARCH

Over the past 50 years, there has been a growing corpus of behavioral intervention research that has yielded well-tested programs and important advancements in the conduct of this form of inquiry. As in any research tradition, behavioral intervention research has an evolving language and specific techniques, methods, rules, and standards that are unique to this particular endeavor. Although it overlaps other forms of inquiry such as classic clinical trial methodologies, behavioral intervention research also has its own distinctive challenges and foci. In the chapters that follow, to the extent possible and where appropriate, we draw upon the most important lessons garnered from classic methodologies and approaches, but also discuss considerations specific to this type of inquiry.

Historically and broadly speaking, the initial wave of behavioral interventions had significant limitations. These included: misalignments between study samples, intervention intent, and measured outcomes; lack of theory-driven approaches and an understanding of underlying mechanism(s) of treatment effects; lack of inclusion of diverse populations; and simplistic approaches such as expecting and measuring behavioral change as an outcome from an intervention that provided only education materials and enhanced knowledge. Take, for example, initial caregiver intervention studies that sought to reduce depressive symptoms although study inclusion criteria did not specifically target depressed caregivers (Knight, Lutzky, & Macofsky-Urban, 1993). Not surprisingly, an initial wave of caregiver studies showed minimal to no treatment effects for depressive symptoms, as there was little to no room for improvement on this outcome (Callahan, Kales, Gitlin, & Lyketsos, 2013). Furthermore, many interventions were designed with little understanding of the context in which they might ultimately be implemented if they were proven to be effective. These missteps have led to a greater understanding and awareness that a translational phase is typically necessary to take an intervention and adapt it for delivery in specific service contexts (Gitlin, Marx, Stanley, & Hodgson, 2015).

Today, we have a much better understanding of best practices in the conduct of behavioral intervention research. Although there is no universal or agreed upon set of approaches, practices, designs, or strategies, the collective knowledge, experience, and empirical evidence as to what works and what does not work in conducting behavioral intervention research is being amassed. For example, we know how to align theory with intervention development, use epidemiologic findings to identify intervention targets, involve communities and stakeholders in developing and implementing interventions, evaluate who benefits the most from interventions, embed interventions in practice settings and evaluate effectiveness using sophisticated adaptive designs and analytic techniques, and monitor and measure the impact of treatment adherence on treatment outcomes. Further, we now have experience standardizing intervention protocols, developing treatment manuals and training protocols, and conducting multisite and pragmatic trial designs that can potentially accelerate knowledge generation and its transfer to broad real-world settings.

CASE EXEMPLARS

Currently, thousands of behavioral interventions have been developed, evaluated, and found to be effective for a very wide range of populations, purposes, public health issues, and outcomes. It is impossible to summarize this vast body of promising and proven behavioral interventions. Nevertheless, considered collectively, common characteristics can be discerned of effective interventions that are designed to address behavior change and complex health and social issues. These are shown in Table 1.1, although this list should not be construed as exhaustive. Effective approaches may differ by the specific purpose or intent of an intervention, its mode, and context of delivery.

However, one apparent shared characteristic of effective interventions for behavioral change is that most tend to involve multiple components each of which targets a different aspect of a presenting problem and pathway for effecting positive change. This is not surprising as most issues targeted by behavioral interventions are complex and multidimensional. For example, an intervention designed to prevent and treat delirium in hospital settings targets factors intrinsic to the person such as medication profile and pain, and extrinsic factors such as staff training and the physical environment (e.g., noise, lighting, cues for orientation) (Inouye et al., 1999). The Get Busy Get Better program to help African Americans address depressive symptoms seeks to improve mood by impacting various potential contributory factors including a person's anxiety, knowledge of depression, and ability to detect his/her symptoms; reducing stressors in the external environment including financial strain and unmet social, housing, and medical needs; and by helping people re-engage in activities that are meaningful to them (Gitlin, Roth, & Huang, 2014).

Effective interventions also appear to tailor or customize content and strategies to key risks, needs, or specific profiles of target populations and contexts (Richards et al., 2007). For example, the REACH II intervention for families caring for persons with dementia modified the intensity (time spent) and amount of exposure (dose) to each of its five treatment components based upon a caregiver's initial (baseline) risk profile (Belle et al., 2006; Czaja et al., 2009). More time was spent on one component versus the other, depending on the risk profile of the individual caregiver; a caregiver with a home safety risk received greater attention in this area than a caregiver without this risk, although both received a minimal dose of this treatment component. The Get Busy Get Better program for depressive symptoms included five treatment components (care management, referral and linkages, stress reduction, depression education and symptom recognition, and behavioral activation). Although all participants received all five treatment components at equivalent dosage and intensity, the content covered in each component was tailored to the participant's specific care needs; the person's preferred stress reduction techniques; housing, financial, and unmet medical needs; and self-identified preferred activity and behavioral goals (Gitlin et al., 2013).

Another shared element of many effective interventions is their flexible delivery schedule. Interventions that do not have rigid dosing requirements have a greater likelihood of being adopted by, and integrated into, clinical settings and by end users

TABLE 1.1 Characteristics of Effective and Ineffective Intervention Approaches

Effective Approaches	Ineffective Approaches
■ Intervention and its characteristics are grounded in theory	■ No theoretical basis for the design of the intervention
■ Multicomponent such that different strategies are used to address distinct factors contributing to the identified problem area	■ Focus on a singular aspect of a complex set of factors contributing to a particular problem area
■ Multimodal such that different pathways (e.g., physical exercise, cognitive stimulation) are targeted to impact the identified problem area	■ One pathway is targeted although multiple factors contribute to the identified problem area
■ Strategies are tailored to participant needs, characteristics, cultural preferences	■ Use of a "one size fits all" approach
■ Participant-centered in that it integrates the client perspective	■ Prescriptive, didactic, standard approach regardless of participant perspective
■ Participant-directed in that intervention addresses self-identified needs	■ Participant needs are assumed a priori
■ Use of active engagement of participants and/or problem solving	■ Use of didactic, prescriptive approach
■ Flexible delivery characteristics to accommodate differences in practice settings	■ Fixed dose and intensity
■ Outcomes are closely aligned with and reflect intervention intent	■ Outcomes are too distal from content or focus of intervention
■ Oriented toward building skills and problem solving to bring about behavior change	■ Providing education to enhance knowledge when goal is to change behavior
■ Criteria for participant inclusion reflect intent of intervention	■ Mismatch between intervention intent and participant inclusion criteria
■ Involving end users (participants) and/or stakeholders in the development of the intervention	■ Not considering the participant or stakeholder perspectives early on in designing an intervention

(e.g., interventionists and participants who may benefit). For example, the Adult Day Plus intervention provides care management, education, support, and skill building on an "as needed" basis for family caregivers who use adult day services for a relative for whom they provide care. Sessions initially occur biweekly for 3 months and at the time when a family member drops off or picks up their relative at the adult day service. Following this initial phase, ongoing contact is periodic and can be initiated by the service provider or family member (Reever, Mathieu, Dennis, & Gitlin, 2004).

In addition, repeated exposures to an intervention appear to yield better outcomes such as reducing nursing home placement or maintaining independence at home. For example, the Maximizing Independence at Home for persons with cognitive impairment provides ongoing care management for 18 months; pilot data with over 300 persons showed that this approach resulted in the reduction of some home safety risks and more days at home (versus nursing home placement or death) (Samus et al., 2014).

Finally, interventions that actively involve participants in the treatment process and the learning of new skills may be more effective than prescriptive, didactic approaches (Belle et al., 2003) when the intent is to change behavior and redesign lifestyles for healthier living. Self-paced programs, approaches in which participants have opportunity to practice and integrate behavioral change strategies, afford more positive outcomes than approaches that do not provide such opportunities. Similarly, if the goal is to improve self-management, certain strategies appear to be more effective than others. For example, using behavioral activation techniques (Hopko, Lejuez, Ruggiero, & Eifert, 2003) that involve individuals self-selecting personal life, health, or daily goals, or providing control-oriented strategies to help people achieve their daily activity goals, afford increased control over daily life events and result in better health outcomes (Heckhausen, Wrosch, & Schulz, 2010). Correspondingly, having participants codesign their own action plans for achieving healthier lifestyles (Lorig et al., 1999) are all strategies rooted in complementary theoretical frameworks that result in enhanced self-efficacy and health-related benefits. This is not to say that behavioral interventions must embrace each or all of these treatment elements to be effective. However, it does suggest that consideration be given to these characteristics in order to maximize the impact on certain types of behavioral change outcomes (Zarit & Femia, 2008). Each of these characteristics is rooted in various theories, best practices such as adult learning principles, and research evidence concerning what works and what does not in changing behavior and personal health practices.

We also have fairly good knowledge of what is ineffective when the goal is to change behavior and health care practices through an intervention. Although an implicit goal of an intervention is to have the biggest impact on the largest number of persons as possible, given the heterogeneity and diversity of populations, a "one size" approach typically does not work. For example, the REACH II intervention, overall, was more effective for Hispanic and White/Caucasian caregivers than for African Americans. However, further analyses showed that, within the African American sample, it was more effective for caregivers who were spouses and older. Devising ways of introducing choice and tailoring an intervention to preferences or situations is, in general, preferred (Belle et al., 2006).

Using prescriptive approaches or providing education alone when the goal is behavioral change has also been shown to be mostly ineffective. Fixed dosing requirements may be important, but this also limits the translation and implementation potential as clinical settings and other end users of an intervention may need greater flexibility in the delivery of such a program. Finally, developing interventions without fully understanding the context in which they will be implemented (see discussion below and Figure 1.2) limits its ultimate usability and acceptability. Involving immediate end users and stakeholders (e.g., interventionists, administrators, payors, participants themselves) early on in the intervention development process is emerging as a best practice. This systems-oriented approach integrates a usability testing and iterative process for developing interventions from the start, to optimize the fit between the intervention and the context in which it is designed for implementation if it is proven to be effective (see Chapter 2).

RELATIONSHIP OF BEHAVIORAL INTERVENTION RESEARCH TO IMPLEMENTATION SCIENCE

An emerging exciting, important, and unique area of inquiry is implementation science. As a complementary and synergistic relationship exists between behavioral intervention research and implementation science, it is important to clarify the scope and processes of each and their relationship to each other. Figure 1.1 maps this relationship and the connections to changing health, education, and/or human service practices, the ultimate goal of both of these domains of science.

Behavioral intervention research is directed at generating evidence in the form of tested and proven programs, protocols, interventions, and strategies. In contrast, implementation science has been variably defined, but basically examines the best strategies for implementing proven programs or evidence in specific practice and/ or service contexts (Brownson et al., 2012). It also aims to identify roadblocks (e.g., social, economic, organizational) that impede the implementation of a proven program or evidence base into practice. Specifically, implementation science represents an emerging, important, and dynamic field of inquiry that systematically examines how programs or interventions can be embedded or implemented and sustained in real-world settings and conditions.

Implementation science starts where behavioral intervention research has traditionally ended. It is based on the premise that there is a well-developed, tested, and proven program or intervention, and its goal is to systematically move "it" into community and/or clinical settings. In contrast, behavioral intervention research, and the focus of this book, is about the "it"—designing, evaluating, and building the evidence base for intervention protocols that have the potential for implementation in real-world settings.

Figure 1.1 also suggests that, to optimize the impact of behavioral intervention research on health and health care outcomes, we must begin with the end in mind or some idea of where our interventions will reside if effective. By understanding the downstream challenges and complexities of implementing evidence into a practice environment, we may be able to design and evaluate interventions upfront in more thoughtful, systematic ways that enhance their implementation and scalability potential once they are proven to be beneficial. In this way, knowledge gleaned from implementation science can help guide behavioral intervention research from the inception of an intervention idea through to its evaluation and translation for a practice setting. Starting with the end in mind requires a firm understanding of the characteristics of target populations, communities, organizations, work flow, and systems of care. For example, designing and implementing an Internet-based intervention requires some degree of technology literacy and computer/Internet access among the intervention recipients as well as broadband connectivity in the neighborhood/community. Understanding these challenges upfront is essential for

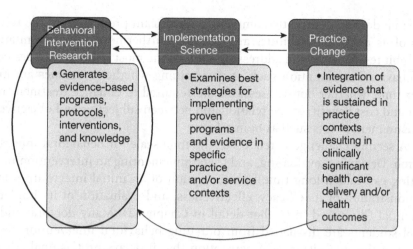

Figure 1.1   Relationship of behavioral intervention research to implementation science and practice change.

designing an intervention protocol, selecting the technology, identifying training requirements, and evaluating costs. Designing an intervention for delivery in a social service agency requires an understanding of the agency and, in particular, its staffing and work flow patterns to ensure compatibility with the delivery characteristics of the intervention.

In line with this way of thinking, many of the chapters in this book promote a new and necessary synergy between implementation science and the design and evaluation of behavioral intervention research. We discuss downstream challenges of implementation (e.g., readiness of individuals or organizations to change; workforce considerations for delivering an intervention) when appropriate to help inform the upstream work of behavioral intervention design and evaluation.

Our message is that changing behaviors and health and human service practices is complex. If we seek to have our interventions integrated in and used in real practice settings by health and human service professionals, and individuals and their families, then our interventions must be informed in part by implementation considerations and this emerging science.

CHALLENGES OF BEHAVIORAL INTERVENTION RESEARCH

There are numerous challenges in the conduct of behavioral intervention research. Foremost among them is that behavioral and health problems are complex and changing behaviors is tough; thus, this form of research can be as well. Advancing an intervention can be costly, recruitment is effortful and time consuming, the conduct of interventions (treatment and control groups) requires adequate staffing and standardization, follow-up assessments necessitate resources, and testing of protocols evolves over time. As grant dollars in most countries, including the National Institutes of Health in the United States, favor basic research and then moving findings to clinical applications (referred to as T2 research), behavioral intervention research does not currently command a significant proportion of the research dollars of its respective institutes and centers. Furthermore, budget limitations often prohibit researchers from addressing some of the most important issues concerning a behavioral intervention such as determining whether outcomes are maintained over time, whether booster sessions are required to enhance treatment receipt, its cost and cost benefit, or the relationship between subjective and objective outcome measurement points such as biomarkers.

A second challenge is related to the time scale for behavioral intervention research. Designing, evaluating, and then implementing an intervention in a practice setting can take a long time from inception of an initial intervention idea to the demonstration of its efficacy, effectiveness, and evaluation of its implementation potential (discussed in further detail in Chapter 2). Many doctoral and postdoctoral students are dissuaded from pursuing behavioral intervention research because of this complexity, the perception that it delays professional advancement, and that testing may need to evolve over a relatively long time frame, preventing productivity.

A third challenge is that owing to the complexity and multifaceted aspects of behavioral intervention research, developing effective intervention approaches typically requires multidisciplinary research teams in order to enable a complete understanding of the issues at hand. Such collaborations add another layer of complexity to this form of research as researchers from diverse disciplines typically have distinct languages, methodological approaches, and unique perspectives that may initially be challenging to understand and integrate. For example, the development of a technology-based intervention for family caregivers requires combining the expertise of scientists in behavioral sciences and family caregiving with the expertise in engineering and computer science. A team science approach still remains elusive to most researchers and is not fully celebrated and appropriately rewarded in academic institutions in the form of promotions, recognition, and time and space. This prevents moving forward with behavioral intervention work in novel and potentially more effective directions. This, combined with the need to involve end users and stakeholders, adds more complexities to the research endeavor and can also tax the expertise of the originator(s) of the intervention.

A related point is the need to bring individuals from diverse backgrounds together to derive a shared language and understanding of the issues and participate in joint problem solving in advancing a particular approach. Although this can be challenging, involvement of diverse disciplines and backgrounds is also exciting and can yield breakthroughs in approaches.

Another challenge is that the field is often stymied by the lack of adequate outlets for reporting the nuances of behavioral intervention studies. For example, the CONSORT guideline that is widely used in the reporting of trials does not address certain elements of high relevance to behavioral intervention research such as the theory base and fidelity plan used and how adherence affects outcomes (Schulz, Altman, & Moher, 2010). Many medical journals have significant word limitations and are typically uninterested in how theory drives the intervention and links to the outcomes. Few journals allow space for articles to fully detail an intervention and its delivery characteristics so that it can be adequately replicated. Similarly, access to treatment manuals may not be readily available or granted by investigators, and there are no agreed upon sets of criteria for developing such manuals. The focus on reporting positive outcomes in peer-reviewed journals is upheld to the exclusion of understanding why and how a particular outcome may or may not have been achieved. Knowing that an intervention is not effective for a targeted population can be as informative as understanding what does work, and can prevent the duplication of such unsuccessful intervention approaches.

One more challenge is that little is known about some of the fundamental practices of this form of research. There is limited empirical evidence, for example, as to: which blinding or masking techniques of research staff and study participants are most effective and for which types of interventions; what types of control groups are appropriate and when; what the best practices are for ethically consenting vulnerable populations; which recruitment/retention strategies and types of interventions work best for diverse populations; and which fidelity measures are most useful across different interventions. Documentation and evaluation of specific methodologies for use in each aspect of the conduct of behavioral intervention research is very much needed. Furthermore, there is significant conceptual confusion as to the steps or processes for advancing interventions. Funders, researchers, journals, editors, and reviewers all employ different terminology, definitions, and usages for concepts such as the pipeline, translation, implementation, diffusion, dissemination, fidelity, and so forth. Conceptual misuses and confusion cloud or muddy efforts and impede working toward general consensus as to key terms and methodologies for evaluating and advancing interventions.

Furthermore, the health care landscape and population demographics are changing dramatically. There is an unprecedented need for new research designs, methodologies, procedures, and intervention approaches. Treatments that work today may not be as effective in the future for aging cohorts. For example, the delivery of health care for many conditions is moving away from traditional clinical settings to nontraditional settings such as the home. Patients and caregivers are being asked to perform complex care tasks (e.g., attending to wound care or tube feeding) and use more medical technologies (e.g., infusion systems or blood pressure and heart rate monitoring devices) (Reinhard, Samis, & Levine, 2014). This, in turn, requires the development of intervention strategies to help ensure that patients and caregivers are able to deliver care protocols as intended and that are adhered to over time. Further, the increase in populations with special needs, such as the "oldest old," individuals aging with developmental and other forms of disability, long-distance caregivers, and individuals without family support, to name only a few, requires understanding the types of interventions that may benefit distinct and highly diverse groups and the approaches that are optimal.

CONCEPTUAL FRAMEWORK

This book is developed with these complexities and challenges in mind. It seeks to sort out and provide best practices and guide a thoughtful approach to designing, evaluating, and implementing behavioral interventions when the goal is to change current practices or address newly emerging problems or health care challenges with real-world solutions.

Our approach to understanding behavioral intervention research is guided by a socioecological systems framework. This framework, shown in Figure 1.2, conceptualizes interventions as being embedded within a complex system involving multiple and interacting components or levels of influence that also change over time. These interconnected levels include the personal or individual level (e.g., end user of an intervention), the physical environment or setting, the formal and informal social network, the community, neighborhood, organization, and the policy environment.

Consider a drug abuse prevention program whose overall objective is to reduce or prevent the use of illegal substances among high school students. The intervention includes video skill-building sessions that are delivered to both students and parents in the school and overseen by a trained facilitator. In this case, the personal and social levels include the students, teachers/school principal, and parents. The setting and community include the school and classroom where the sessions will be delivered and the surrounding neighborhood. The organizational and policy levels include the school district and school board as well as policies regarding training by outside sources, availability of classrooms for after-hours training, and so forth. Each level has varying and dynamic characteristics, and the interactions among the levels, in turn, can have a significant influence on the degree to which the goals and objectives of an intervention can be achieved and what its delivery characteristics ought to be to maximize benefits. For example, if most of the parents work, it would be difficult to schedule group sessions during the day; if the school policy is to forbid classroom use in the evening, then location could be an issue. Furthermore, the content of each session may need to be carefully reviewed and approved by the full school board prior to its implementation. Knowledge of the characteristics of these levels directly informs construction of an impactful intervention.

By means of our social ecological framework, several guiding principles for behavioral intervention research can be derived.

First, interventions must be understood as occurring within a context that includes multiple levels—the individual, the setting in which the intervention will be delivered (e.g., home, school, clinic, workplace), formal and informal networks and social support systems, the community, and the policy environment (Figure 1.2). Health and behavior, and hence intervention delivery characteristics, may be shaped by influences at each of these levels.

Second, as there are significant interactions among these levels, interventions are more likely to be successful and sustainable if they consider the characteristics of each level and the interactions among them. In other words, interventions cannot be designed in isolation or in a vacuum and focus solely on individual-level determinants of health and behaviors, as has typically been the practice. Rather, interventions must consider the independent and joint influences of determinants at all of the specified levels. Levels will be proximal and distal to the immediate outcomes sought (e.g., increasing physical activity among minority populations); however, at some point in the process of developing the intervention, each level will need to be actively considered.

Third, the levels and the interactions among them are dynamic, and determinants may change with time. Therefore, for interventions to be sustainable, their characteristics must be adaptable to potential changes and dynamic relationships over time.

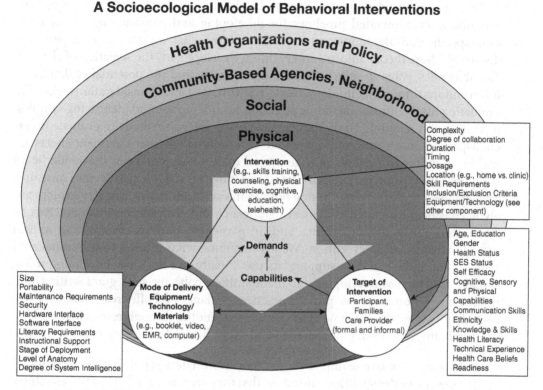

Figure 1.2 Social Ecological Systems Framework for Understanding Interventions.

Source: Adapted from: Czaja, S.J., Sharit, J., Charness, N., and Fisk, A.D. (2001). The Center for Research and Education on Aging and Technology Enhancement (CREATE): A program to enhance technology for older adults. Gerontechnology, 1, 50–59.

These principles are interwoven throughout this book and, taken as a whole, suggest that we need new ways of thinking about and acting upon the design, evaluation, and implementation of interventions.

ROADMAP

As we have suggested, behavioral intervention research can be exciting, yet it is complex and involves more than the simple design or singular test of an intervention. It requires consideration and understanding of a broad range of issues that may impact an intervention and its delivery (Figure 1.2). Thus, in this book, we cover a broad array of topics of high relevance to, and that impact on, the conduct of behavioral intervention research. We consider the entire "behavioral intervention pipeline" from conceptualization of an intervention through its implementation and sustainability in a practice setting, and examine how the context in which interventions are embedded affects their development and advancement. While our focus is not on implementation science directly, we draw upon it in terms of how it can help to inform the development and evaluation of an intervention. We emphasize the need for behavioral intervention researchers to consider the entire pipeline in their endeavors.

We start with what we consider to be the "heart of the matter" in Part I, by examining recommended pipelines for developing and constructing an intervention, specific considerations and steps that inform what we refer to as "a period of discovery," how theory informs intervention development, the selection of delivery characteristics, ways to standardize an intervention, and the potential of delivering interventions through technology. Next, in Part II, we tackle considerations related to evaluating interventions, including selecting control groups and identifying samples; recruiting and retaining study participants; using mixed methods to evaluate different aspects of intervention development; determining whether treatment effects are real by attending to fidelity; and the critical ethical considerations that underlie all study-design decision making. In Part III, we move on to look at outcomes measures and analytic considerations, linking both to intervention intent. We also explore analytic considerations such as clinical significance and economic evaluations. Part IV examines implementation science and, in particular, how its theories can inform ways to advance an intervention. We also examine what it takes to disseminate an intervention if the evidence supports its use. Finally, in Part V, we delve into professional issues such as developing and maintaining a cohesive staff, grant writing, and publishing. Throughout, we provide practical guidance and offer real exemplars. We also identify gray areas that need further understanding through research.

Implicitly, this book grapples with and raises big and critical queries:

- How do we move seamlessly from intervention design to full implementation?
- How do we design interventions so that they are more market ready if effective?
- How can we better identify, define, and standardize actions related to each phase of intervention development to enable the current and next generation of behavioral intervention researchers to succeed?

We seek to motivate the reader to participate in the behavioral intervention research arena, be more informed and better prepared to take on the exciting challenges that it presents, and enter into a dialogue about this form of research to derive consensus and empirically based answers to these big questions.

REFERENCES

Balas, E. A., & Boren, S. A. (2000). Managing clinical knowledge for health care improvement. In J. Bemmel & A. T. McCray (Eds.), *Yearbook of medical informatics 2000: Patient centered systems* (pp. 65–70). Stuttgart, Germany: Schattauer Verlagsgesellschaft GmbH.

Belle, S. H., Burgio, L., Burns, R., Coon, D., Czaja, S. J., Gallagher-Thompson, D., . . . Zhang, S. (2006). Enhancing the quality of life of dementia caregivers from different ethnic or racial groups: A randomized, controlled trial. *Annals of Internal Medicine, 145*(10), 727–738.

Belle, S. H., Czaja, S. J., Schulz, R., Burgio, L. D., Gitlin, L. N., Jones, R., . . . Ory, M. (2003). Using a new taxonomy to combine the uncombinable: Integrating results across diverse interventions. *Psychology and Aging, 18*(3), 396–405.

Bodenheimer, T., Lorig, K., Holman, H., & Grumbach, K. (2002). Patient self-management of chronic disease in primary care. *JAMA, 288*(19), 2469–2475.

Brownson, R. C., Colditz, G. A., & Proctor, E. K. (Eds.). (2012). *Dissemination and implementation research in health: Translating science to practice.* New York, NY: Oxford University Press.

Callahan, C. M., Kales, H. C., Gitlin, L. N., & Lyketsos, C. G. (2013). The historical development and state of the art approach to design and delivery of dementia care services. In H. de Waal, C. Lyketsos, D. Ames, & J. O'Brien (Eds.), *Designing and delivering dementia services* (pp. 17–30). West Sussex, UK: John Wiley & Sons. doi:10.1002/9781118378663.ch2

Christensen, K., Gaist, D., Vaupel, J. W., & McGue, M. (2002). Genetic contribution to rate of change in functional abilities among Danish twins aged 75 years or more. *American Journal of Epidemiology, 155*(2), 132–139.

Christensen, K., Holm, N. V., Mcgue, M., Corder, L., & Vaupel, J. W. (1999). A Danish population-based twin study on general health in the elderly. *Journal of Aging and Health, 11*(1), 49–64.

Czaja, S. J., Gitlin, L. N., Schulz, R., Zhang, S., Burgio, L. D., Stevens, A. B., . . . Gallagher Thompson, D. (2009). Development of the risk appraisal measure (RAM): A brief screen to identify risk areas and guide interventions for dementia caregivers. *Journal of the American Geriatrics Society, 57*(6), 1064–1072.

Finkel, D., Ernsth-Bravell, M., & Pedersen, N. L. (2015). Sex differences in genetic and environmental influences on longitudinal change in functional ability in late adulthood. *The Journals of Gerontology Series B: Psychological Sciences and Social Sciences, 1–9, 70*(5): 709–17. doi:10.1093/geronb/gbt134

Gatz, M., Pedersen, N. L., Berg, S., Johansson, B., Johansson, K., Mortimer, J. A., . . . Ahlbom, A. (1997). Heritability for Alzheimer's disease: The study of dementia in Swedish twins. *The Journals of Gerontology Series A: Biological Sciences and Medical Sciences, 52*(2), M117–M125.

Gitlin, L. N., Harris, L. F., McCoy, M. C., Chernett, N. L., Pizzi, L. T., Jutkowitz, E., . . . Hauck, W. W. (2013). A home-based intervention to reduce depressive symptoms and improve quality of life in older African Americans. *Annals of Internal Medicine, 159*(4), 243–252.

Gitlin, L. N., Marx, K., Stanley, I., & Hodgson, N. (2015). Translating evidence-based dementia caregiving interventions into practice: State-of-the-science and next steps. *The Gerontologist, 55* (2), 210–226. doi:10.1093/geront/gnu123

Gitlin, L. N., Roth, D. L., & Huang, J. (2014). Mediators of the impact of a home-based intervention (beat the blues) on depressive symptoms among older African Americans. *Psychology and Aging, 29*(3), 601–611.

Guyatt, G. H., Naylor, D., Richardson, W. S., Green, L., Haynes, R. B., Wilson, M. C., . . . Jaeschke, R. Z. (2000). What is the best evidence for making clinical decisions? (Reply). *JAMA, 284*(24), 3127–3128.

Heckhausen, J., Wrosch, C., & Schulz, R. (2010). A motivational theory of life-span development. *Psychological Review, 117*(1), 32–60. doi:10.1037/a0017668

Hopko, D. R., Lejuez, C. W., Ruggiero, K. J., & Eifert, G. H. (2003). Contemporary behavioral activation treatments for depression: Procedures, principles, and progress. *Clinical Psychology Review, 23*(5), 699–717.

Inouye, S. K., Bogardus, S. T., Charpentier, P. A., Leo-Summers, L., Acampora, D., Holford, T. R., & Cooney, L. M. (1999). A multi-component intervention to prevent delirium in hospitalized older patients. *New England Journal of Medicine, 340*, 668–676.

Institute of Medicine. (2001). *Crossing the quality chasm: A new health system for the 21st century*. Retrieved from http://www.nap.edu/catalog/10027.html

Jackson, J. S., Knight, K. M., & Rafferty, J. A. (2010). Race and unhealthy behaviors: Chronic stress, the HPA axis, and physical and mental health disparities over the life course. *American Journal of Public Health, 100*(5), 933–939.

Knight, B. G., Lutzky, S. M., & Macofsky-Urban, F. (1993). A meta-analytic review of interventions for caregiver distress: Recommendations for future research. *The Gerontologist, 33*(2), 240–248.

Lorig, K. R., Sobel, D. S., Stewart, A. L., Brown, B. W., Jr., Bandura, A., Ritter, P., . . . Holman, H. R. (1999). Evidence suggesting that a chronic disease self-management program can improve health status while reducing hospitalization: A randomized trial. *Medical Care, 37*(1), 5–14.

Lovasi, G. S., Hutson, M. A., Guerra, M., & Neckerman, K. M. (2009). Built environments and obesity in disadvantaged populations. *Epidemiologic Reviews, 31*(1), 7–20. doi:10.1093/epirev/mxp005

McGlynn, E. A., Asch, S. M., Adams, J., Keesey, J., Hicks, J., DeCristofaro, A., & Kerr, E. A. (2003). The quality of health care delivered to adults in the United States. *New England Journal of Medicine, 348*(26), 2635–2645.

Milstein, B., Homer, J., Briss, P., Burton, D., & Pechacek, T. (2011). Why behavioral and environmental interventions are needed to improve health at lower cost. *Health Affairs, 30*(5), 823–832.

Reever, K. E., Mathieu, E., Dennis, M. P., & Gitlin, L. N. (2004, October/December). Adult Day Services Plus: Augmenting adult day centers with systematic care management for family caregivers. *Alzheimer's Care Quarterly, 5*(4), 332–339.

Reinhard, S. C., Samis, S., & Levine, C. (2014). *Family caregivers providing complex chronic care to people with cognitive and behavioral health conditions.* Washington, DC: AARP Public Policy Institute. Retrieved from http://www.aarp.org/content/dam/aarp/research/public_policy_institute/health/2014/family-caregivers-cognitive-behavioral-AARP-ppi-health.pdf

Richards, K. C., Enderlin, C. A., Beck, C., McSweeney, J. C., Jones, T. C., & Roberson, P. K. (2007). Tailored biobehavioral interventions: A literature review and synthesis. *Research and Theory for Nursing Practice, 21*(4), 271–285.

Riley, W. T., Glasgow, R. E., Etheredge, L., & Abernethy, A. P. (2013). Rapid, responsive, relevant (R3) research: A call for a rapid learning health research enterprise. *Clinical and Translational Medicine, 2*(1), 1–6.

Samus, Q. M., Johnston, D. J., Black, B. S., Hess, E., Lyman, C., Vavilikolanu, . . . Lyketsos, C. G. (2014). A multidimensional home-based care coordination intervention for elders with memory disorders: The maximizing independence at home (MIND) pilot randomized trial. *American Journal of Geriatric Psychiatry, 22*(4), 398–414.

Schulz, K. F., Altman, D. G., & Moher, D. (2010). CONSORT 2010 statement: Updated guidelines for reporting parallel group randomised trials. *BMC Medicine, 8*(18), 1–9.

Svedberg, P., Lichtenstein, P., & Pedersen, N. L. (2001). Age and sex differences in genetic and environmental factors for self-rated health: A twin study. *The Journals of Gerontology Series B: Psychological Sciences and Social Sciences, 56*(3), S171–S178.

Woolf, S. H. (2008). The meaning of translational research and why it matters. *JAMA, 299*(2), 211–213.

Zarit, S., & Femia, E. (2008). Behavioral and psychosocial interventions for family caregivers. *The American Journal of Nursing, 108*(9), 47–53.

TWO

PIPELINES FOR DESIGNING, EVALUATING, AND IMPLEMENTING INTERVENTIONS

The gap between what we know and what we do in public health is lethal to Americans, if not the world.
—David Satcher, MD, PhD, Former U.S. Surgeon General

How does one build the evidence for a behavioral intervention? Whereas drug discovery and biomedical research follow a prescribed set of research steps moving from bench to bed to public health impact, for behavioral intervention research, there is no consensus, agreed upon approach, or recipe for advancing interventions and then implementing and sustaining them in real-world settings (Dougherty & Conway, 2008; Drolet & Lorenzi, 2011).

However, similar to biomedical research, there is no doubt that behavioral interventions develop over time and appear to follow an incremental pathway consisting of a set of activities that incrementally build the evidence for an intervention. This pathway, referred to as the "pipeline," is typically conceptualized as singular, linear, and methodical, occurring over a lengthy time frame projected as 17 years or upward (see Chapter 1; Craig et al., 2008; Kleinman & Mold, 2009; Westfall, Mold, & Fagnan, 2007).

Nevertheless, the specifics of this pipeline, such as its phases and associated activities, have been differentially conceptualized within the scientific community and among funding agencies. This chapter examines the pathways, both traditional and emerging, for advancing behavioral interventions. We begin by discussing the relative advantages of using the concept of a "pipeline" as a heuristic for understanding the level of development and evidence in support of an intervention and ways to proceed for building its evidence. We then describe two different "pipelines" that capture ways to conceptualize moving interventions forward: the classic or traditional four-phase linear pipeline, and a proposed elongated seven-phase trajectory that recognizes the need to attend to specific processes for moving an intervention from the randomized trial environment to communities or practice environments for public health impact. Finally, we propose a more iterative, dynamic portrayal of intervention development and identify various strategies that may shorten the time for generating behavioral interventions that are better aligned with real-world needs and practice contexts than what currently typically occur.

Our discussion is necessarily conceptual and abstract as it is intended to provide an overarching framework and foundational knowledge concerning the development of behavioral interventions. Each subsequent chapter will link specific intervention research processes to phases along the elongated pipeline and, when appropriate, refer to more dynamic strategies for advancing interventions.

PIPELINE AS A HEURISTIC

The pipeline concept is a traditional way of describing the scientific enterprise and how basic and human research makes its way through research processes to having an impact on the health of the public (Kleinman & Mold, 2009; U.S. National Library of Medicine, 2014). Applied to behavioral intervention research, it can be a useful heuristic for understanding intervention development for several reasons. First, it provides an organizing framework for categorizing interventions with regard to their level of development. Understanding where an intervention is along a pipeline helps to evaluate what has been done to date to develop the intervention and what still needs to happen to build a strong evidence base for the intervention. Each specified phase along a pipeline is associated, albeit loosely, with a set of goals, objectives, and actions for advancing an intervention. Thus, identifying and specifying phases along the pipeline structures the activities required for designing, evaluating, or implementing an intervention, and helps to identify what has been accomplished to date and what still needs to be accomplished in building the evidence for an intervention.

Referring to the pipeline is also helpful when seeking funding to support the development, evaluation, or implementation and dissemination of an intervention. Although funding agencies may define phases along the pipeline differentially, it helps to pinpoint the purpose of a proposal for agencies and reviewers by indicating the phase of an intervention's development along the pipeline (see Chapter 23 on grant writing). For example, when submitting a grant proposal, it is important to indicate whether the research is designed to definitively test the efficacy of an intervention, its effectiveness, or demonstrate proof of concept or feasibility. Reviewers will apply very different evaluative criteria to a proposal designed to evaluate feasibility and proof of concept compared with one that seeks to test efficacy. For the latter, the expectation is that there will be pilot data supporting proof of concept of the intervention and that clinical trial methodology including randomization, control groups, and other rigorous design elements to test the intervention will be proposed (Thabane et al., 2010). For a feasibility study, however, other design strategies including small sampled pre–post studies, focus groups, or use of mixed methods (see Chapter 11), to name a few, would be more appropriate to evaluate tolerability of a particular treatment or adherence to a protocol.

Furthermore, as a heuristic, the idea of a pipeline facilitates asking and answering the following fundamental questions:

- What is the level of development of the intervention?
- What type of evaluation is needed to move the intervention forward?
- Do the investigator and the investigative team have the requisite expertise to advance the intervention?

- Are the proposed activities in keeping with the phase of development of the intervention?
- Is there sufficient proof of concept to advance the intervention?
- Does the intervention have implementation potential? How would the intervention change practice (Craig et al., 2008)?

Finally, the concept of a pipeline itself reflects a particular approach or methodology for advancing an intervention. As an approach or methodology, it can be evaluated, critiqued, and hence modified and improved. That is, by specifying and delineating the phases and associated activities along a pipeline, we can scrutinize the process used for advancing behavioral interventions, experiment with ways to shorten or combine phases through novel methodologies, and adopt strategies for building and rolling out interventions more rapidly and efficiently. For example, we know that proceeding linearly from idea inception to prescribed testing phases may involve a journey of more than 17 years and that very few evidence-based interventions become available to the public or are effectively integrated into communities, clinics, and social service settings or result in change in health policy. Thus, ways to redesign the pipeline for behavioral intervention research to overcome these challenges has become an important topic and focus of attention in the scientific community and among funders.

TRADITIONAL PIPELINE

The traditional pipeline shown in Figure 2.1 was initially adapted from the steps followed for drug discovery and biomedical research and has subsequently been applied to behavioral intervention research (Medical Research Council, 2000). As mentioned earlier, it is based on the basic premise that research evidence is advanced in a linear, incremental, progressive fashion, and that, with adequate demonstration of evidence, uptake of the intervention and positive changes in a health care or human service environment will occur.

The traditional pipeline recognizes a discovery "prephase" in which the inception of an intervention idea and its theoretical basis emerge. As this discovery prephase is critical regardless of the pipeline followed, we discuss this in great depth in Chapter 3. Then the traditional pipeline involves four key phases, as illustrated in Figure 2.1. Although there is little consensus as to what constitutes the specific activities of each phase, the most common set of actions is described briefly here.

Phase I—Feasibility, Proof of Concept

Phase I typically involves one or more pilot-level studies to identify an appropriate theoretical base for an intervention (explored in Chapter 4), identifying and evaluating treatment components and determining their acceptability, feasibility, and safety. In this phase, a wide range of research design strategies can be used, such as case studies, pre–post study designs, focus groups, or a combination of them to define and refine the content of the intervention and derive delivery characteristics (dose, intensity, or treatment components—see Chapter 5 for a discussion

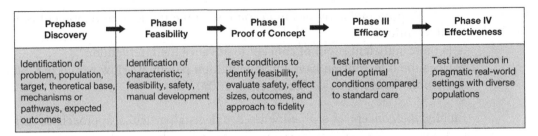

Figure 2.1 Traditional pipeline.

of delivery characteristics). The most common ones are listed in Table 2.1. Additionally, qualitative research and mixed methodologies that seek an integration of qualitative and quantitative strategies to derive comprehensive understandings of a phenomenon (see Chapter 11) can also be helpful in this phase to evaluate the acceptability and utility of intervention components and the potential barriers to adherence and behavioral change.

Phase II—Initial Comparison With a Control Group

Phase II involves an initial pilot test or series of pilot tests of the intervention that is conducted typically in comparison with an appropriate alternative. In this phase, a small pilot randomized trial (e.g., sample size of 20–60 participants) can be used to identify or refine appropriate outcomes and their measurement (see Chapters 14 and 15), evaluate whether measures are sensitive to expected changes from an intervention, determine the type of control group (see Chapter 8), and evaluate the potential treatment effects.

Also in Phase II, monitoring feasibility, acceptability, and safety may continue along with continued evaluation of whether and how the theoretical base informs observed changes. Another important task that can begin in Phases I or II is the evaluation of ways to evaluate treatment fidelity (see Chapter 12). Specifically, in these early phases, it is helpful to begin to think through a monitoring plan and identify measures to capture the extent to which intervention groups (e.g., treatment and control group conditions) are implemented as intended. Thus, pilot and feasibility studies in this phase can be used to evaluate a wide range of aspects for a larger study such as the feasibility of all procedures and design elements including recruitment, retention, and assessments or outcome measures, in addition to evaluating intervention components, dosing, and other delivery characteristics. This phase can yield: the preliminary evidence that the intervention has its desired effects; a clearer understanding of theoretical framework(s) that can inform the intervention; information about appropriate control groups; a well-defined treatment manual specifying delivery characteristics; the most appropriate outcome measures (see Chapters 14 and 15); and, finally, inform design considerations for a more definitive Phase III efficacy trial.

Although there is no doubt that conducting pilot and feasibility studies in both Phases I and II is critical for mapping larger scale studies of behavioral interventions, their methodological rigor and yield have come under increasing scrutiny. For example, whereas previously, pilot studies were often used to determine effect

TABLE 2.1 Basic Study Designs for Use Across the Pipeline

Design	Definition
Adaptive designs	Adaptive interventions, also known as "adaptive treatment strategies" or "dynamic treatment regimens," involve individually tailored treatments based on participants' characteristics or clinical presentations, and are adjusted over time in response to persons' needs. The approach reflects clinical practice in that dosages vary in response to participant needs. These designs used prespecified decision rules based on a set of key characteristics (referred to as "tailoring variables") (Collins et al., 2004; Lei et al., 2012; The Methodology Center, Penn State University, 2012).
Case-control designs	Case-control designs are typically retrospective. Individuals with an outcome of interest (e.g., some disease or condition) are selected and compared with individuals (matched on relevant characteristics) without the outcome or disease in an attempt to find the risk factors present in the cases but not in the controls. The goal is to understand the relative importance of a predictor variable in relation to the outcome (Kazdin, 1994; Mann, 2003).
Cohort/ longitudinal designs	These designs are often used to determine the incidence and history of a disease or condition, where a cohort is a group of people who have something in common and remain part of a group over an extended period of time (e.g., age group, people who have been exposed to some environmental condition or received a particular treatment). Cohort designs may be prospective or retrospective. In prospective designs, the individuals are followed for a certain period of time to determine whether they develop an outcome of interest. The investigator then measures variables that might be related to the outcome. For example, a cohort of individuals of the same age is followed longitudinally to determine whether they develop Alzheimer's disease. In retrospective designs, the cohort is examined retrospectively; the data already exist (Dawson & Trapp, 2004; Mann, 2003).
Cross-over designs	This design includes two groups—treatment and control. Initially, one group of individuals is assigned to the treatment group, and another group is assigned to the control (typically with random assignment). After a period of time, both groups of individuals are withdrawn from their original group for what is referred to as a "washout period," in which no treatments are administered. Following the "washout period," individuals initially assigned to the control group receive the treatment, and those who originally received the treatment are assigned to the control condition (Dawson & Trapp, 2004).
Cross-sectional designs	These designs are primarily used to understand the prevalence of an outcome (e.g., disease or condition). A group of individuals is selected at one point of time rather than over a time period, and data on these individuals relevant to a particular outcome are analyzed. All measurements on an individual are made at one point in time to determine whether he or she has the outcome of interest (Dawson & Trapp, 2004; Mann, 2003).

(Continued)

TABLE 2.1 Basic Study Designs for Use Across the Pipeline (*Continued*)

Design	Definition
Factorial designs	Factorial designs allow the investigation of the impact of more than one independent variable on an outcome measure(s) of interest. The independent variables are examined at different levels. An example of the 2 × 2 design is where there are two independent variables (e.g., intervention A and intervention B) each at two levels (e.g., dosage— high vs. low). In this case there are four groups, which represent each possible combination of the levels of the two factors. These designs allow for the assessment of the main effect of each variable and the interaction among the variables (Kazdin, 1994).
Hybrid designs	These study designs combine specific questions related to effectiveness and implementation, and reflect a dual testing approach determined a priori of implementing a study. Hybrid designs typically take one of three approaches: (a) testing effects of an intervention on outcomes while gathering information on implementation; (b) testing of clinical and implementation interventions/strategies; (c) testing of an implementation strategy while also evaluating impact on relevant outcomes (Bernet et al., 2013; Cully et al., 2012; Curran et al., 2012).
Meta-analysis	Meta-analysis is a quantitative synthesis of information from previous research studies to derive conclusions about a particular topic; it summarizes findings from a large number of studies. For example, several meta-analyses have been conducted of the caregiver intervention literature. By combining relevant evidence from many studies, statistical power is increased, and more precise estimates of treatment effects may be obtained (Trikalinos, Salanti, Zintzaras, & Ioannidis, 2008).
Pretest–posttest control group designs	Pretest–posttest control group designs are commonly used in intervention research, especially at the efficacy stage of the pipeline. This design consists of a minimum of two groups where participants are evaluated on outcome measures before and after the intervention. Thus, the impact of the intervention is reflected in the amount of change from pre- to postintervention assessment. Individuals are typically randomly assigned to groups (Kazdin, 1994).
Randomized control trial designs	Randomized control trials (RCTs) are considered to be the "gold standard" for evaluating the efficacy or the effectiveness of an intervention. In an RCT, after recruitment, screening, and baseline assessment, participants are randomly assigned to a condition (e.g., alternative interventions/treatments or intervention/treatment and control). Following randomization, the groups are treated and followed in the same way (e.g., assessment protocols)—the only difference is the treatment/intervention that they receive. Typically, a primary end point or outcome measure is identified prior to the beginning of the trial, and the trial is registered (e.g., clinical trials.gov) (Concato, Shah, & Horwitz, 2000).

(*Continued*)

TABLE 2.1 Basic Study Designs for Use Across the Pipeline (Continued)	
Design	**Definition**
Randomized block designs	The randomized block design, similar to stratified sampling is used to reduce variance in the data. Using this design, the sample is divided into homogeneous subgroups (e.g., gender), and then the individuals within the blocks are randomly assigned to a treatment/intervention condition or treatment/intervention and control condition (Bailey, 2004).
Single-case designs	In single-case design, an individual serves as his or her own control. In these cases, an individual is assessed prior to the treatment or intervention and then repeatedly over the course of the treatment. Repeated assessments are typically taken before the treatment is administered for a period of time, "the baseline phase," which allows the investigator to examine the stability of performance on some outcome. The treatment/intervention is then administered, and performance on the outcome is assessed during the course and after the treatment/intervention (Kazdin, 1994).
SMART designs	"Sequential Multiple Assignment Randomized Trials (SMART)" is an approach to inform the development of an adaptive intervention. A SMART enables an evaluation of the timing, sequencing, and adaptive selection of treatments in a systematic approach and use of randomized data. Participants may move through various stages of treatment, with each stage reflecting a documented decision or set of decision rules. Participants are randomized at each stage in which a treatment decision is made. Thus, participants move through multiple stages, which allows the investigator to make causal inferences concerning effectiveness of various intervention options (Almirall et al., 2012; Lei et al., 2012; Murphy, 2005).
Wait-list control designs	Using this design, participants are randomly assigned to either the treatment/intervention group or the wait-list group, which receives the treatment at a later date. The wait-list group is used as a control group. Typically, pre–post intervention data are gathered from both groups (Hart, Fann, & Novack, 2008).

sizes for a larger trial, research has shown that estimates may overestimate outcomes due to the inexactitude of data from small samples. Furthermore, feasibility results may not generalize beyond the inclusion and exclusion criteria of a pilot (Arain, Campbell, Cooper, & Lancaster, 2010). There is also confusion in the literature as to what constitutes a "pilot" versus a "feasibility" study, and what methodologies are most appropriate for each (Leon, Davis, & Kraemer, 2011; Thabane et al., 2010).

No guidelines have been agreed upon for pilot or feasibility studies or whether and how they should be distinguished. Arain and colleagues (2010) suggest that feasibility studies are typically conducted with more flexible methodologies and that results may not be generalizable beyond the sample inclusion criteria. Alternately, they suggest that pilot studies tend to incorporate more rigorous design elements and should be viewed as a necessary step prior to a larger scale test of an intervention. Regardless of conceptual confusion in the literature, at the very least, for feasibility studies, investigators should clearly state how feasibility will be defined and operationalized; and for pilots, the specific purpose(s) should be clearly articulated. There is also no doubt that feasibility and pilot tests are necessary endeavors prior to moving forward with larger scale evaluations of behavioral interventions.

Phase III—Efficacy

Phase III represents the definitive randomized controlled trial that compares a fully developed intervention with an appropriate alternative to show its efficacy. In other words, it is focused on evaluating the effects of the intervention on outcomes for individuals and a limited set of symptoms including psychosocial, biobehavioral, or clinical. This phase starts with the assumption that there is a well-crafted intervention based upon the preliminary evidence of benefit and feasibility garnered from Phases I and II.

In an efficacy trial, the primary concern is with enhancing the internal validity of the study design so that observed benefits can be attributed to the intervention rather than other potential confounding variables (e.g., access to or utilization of other services, spontaneous improvement). So, for example, samples tend to be homogeneous, interventionists tend to be "super" clinicians, and treatment exposure is tightly controlled. Thus, efficacy trials are designed to test interventions under controlled, ideal conditions. There are numerous evaluative designs that can be used in this study phase. As these are amply described in classic clinical trial texts, we highlight only the most common designs in Table 2.2 for ease of reference.

Phase IV—Effectiveness

In the traditional pipeline model, Phase IV is considered the final phase. Following a demonstration of efficacy in Phase III, Phase IV represents an effectiveness or replication trial to evaluate whether the intervention has an impact when delivered to a broader group of study participants than those included in the efficacy phase and/or within a particular practice or service context than those previously considered. Whereas Phase III methodological efforts are directed at ensuring internal validity, as already mentioned, the emphasis in Phase IV is on external validity or the extent to which the intervention can have a broader reach and be generalized to more heterogeneous samples and environmental contexts. Although internal validity remains important, external validity is the primary focus. As such, inclusion and exclusion criteria may be relaxed, or opened up, to include a broader mix of study participants reflecting real clinical populations. Similarly, small tweaks in intervention protocols such as the number or duration of sessions and/or who can deliver the intervention may occur in order to meet the expectations of different targeted populations and settings.

Balancing the need to maintain fidelity (refer to Chapter 12) yet accommodate an implementation context in an effectiveness phase can be challenging. If the intervention is changed too much, it may not result in the same level of benefits or type of outcomes achieved in the efficacy phase. However, if no adaptations are made, then there is the risk that the intervention will not be replicated in the designated setting (Washington et al., 2014). This is the essential challenge of this

TABLE 2.2 Examples of Trial Designs

Term	Definition
Comparative Effectiveness Research (CER)	CER is a rigorous evaluation of the effects of different treatments, interventions, or programs. The approach provides a comparison of the benefits and harms of alternative treatments. Its purpose is to inform decision making as to which treatments to use at the individual and population levels (Conway & Clancy, 2009; Congressional Budget Office, 2007; Sox & Greenfield, 2009).
Effectiveness trial	A Phase IV trial is concerned mostly with the external validity or generalizability of an intervention. In these trials, samples tend to be more heterogeneous than in efficacy trials to reflect real-world, clinical populations. Additionally, these trials usually include a broader range of outcomes such as quality of life and cost. The essential question that is being tested is whether a treatment or intervention does more good than harm when delivered under real-world conditions (Curran et al., 2012; Flay, 1986; Glasgow et al., 2003).
Efficacy trial	A Phase III trial (explanatory) determines whether an intervention has a desired outcome under ideal or optimum conditions. They are characterized by their standardization and strong methodological control features (Flay, 1986; Gartlehner et al., 2006; Glasgow et al., 2003).
Embedded trial	Also referred to as "practical trials," interventions are embedded in a setting or context in which they will be delivered in order to understand their effects in relation to other contextual factors that may or may not be manipulated (Allotey et al., 2008). This approach typically combines efficacy and effectiveness or effectiveness and implementation–type questions (Glasgow et al., 2005, 2007; Tunis et al., 2003;).
Equivalence trial	Equivalence trials, also referred to as "noninferiority trials," seek to determine whether a new intervention is similar (or not) to another, usually an existing treatment or standard of care. The aim may be to show the new intervention is equivalent to (or not inferior to) an established intervention or practice versus being better than that treatment (Christensen, 2007; Piaggio et al., 2006, 2012; Sedgwick, 2013).
Pragmatic trial	Pragmatic trials measure primarily the effectiveness or the benefit of a new intervention to routine care or clinical practice. It is similar to an embedded trial, described above, in that an intervention is rigorously tested in the context in which it will be delivered and is designed to inform decision making between a new and an existing treatment (Glasgow, 2013; Patsopoulos, 2011; Roland & Torgerson, 1998).
Superiority trial	A superiority trial is designed to show that a new intervention is statistically and clinically superior to an active control or an established therapy or a placebo (Christensen, 2007; D'Agostino et al., 2003; Landow, 2000).

phase. Determining whether changes result in a new intervention that needs further testing is critical yet subjective; there are no common metrics or approaches that can be uniformly applied. Traditionally, this decision has been in the hands of the originator of the intervention or investigative team.

Case Example: An example of the need for this balancing act when moving from efficacy to effectiveness is the National Institutes of Health REACH II (Resources for Enhancing Alzheimer's Caregiver Health) initiative. The REACH II intervention was tested in a Phase III efficacy trial involving five sites and 642 African American, Latino/Hispanic, and Caucasian caregivers of persons with dementia (Belle et al., 2006). The intervention that was tested involved 12 sessions (nine in-home and three telephone sessions, and five structured telephone support group sessions were provided). Participants received resource notebooks, educational materials, and telephones with display screens linked to a computer-integrated telephone system to provide information and facilitate group support conference calling. Fidelity was carefully maintained across all sites through various strategies and measurement approaches. Because of the positive outcomes of the trial, particularly for Hispanic/Latino caregivers, there has been considerable interest in evaluating whether this intervention can achieve similar benefits when integrated in different delivery contexts such as the Veterans Administration and social service agencies, as well as for other minority groups. However, moving the intervention from an efficacy trial to an effectiveness context has called for making various compromises. For example, it was not economically feasible to replicate the computer-integrated telephone system in other settings; it was also not feasible to conduct telephone support groups with families; nor was it feasible for busy social service practices to implement all 12 sessions (Burgio et al., 2009; Nichols, Martindale-Adams, Burns, Graney, & Zuber, 2011). The intervention as initially designed and tested in its efficacy phase could not easily fit with the work flow of existing social service agencies.

Determining Whether Further Testing Is Required

Thus, what is in question is whether modifications to the delivery of an intervention result in the need to retest the intervention in an efficacy trial. Whereas moving from Phase I to Phase IV is sometimes referred to as a "forward translational process," moving backward from effectiveness to efficacy is sometimes referred to as a "backward translational effort."

Although there are no clear metrics for determining how much change to an intervention is too much, several strategies can be employed. One strategy involves identifying a priori the core components and theoretically based principles (see Chapter 4) of an intervention that should be considered immutable or must remain intact. Similarly, it is helpful to identify a priori the aspects of an intervention that can be modified or delivered differently (Gitlin et al., 2000). Another strategy is to use analytical techniques such as mediation analyses, dose and response analyses (see Chapters 16), and fidelity assessments (e.g., analyses of the actual dose and intensity that was implemented) to inform decisions as to the aspects of the intervention that can and cannot be modified.

For example, in the randomized trial of the Get Busy Get Better intervention (Gitlin et al., 2013), an average of 8 of the 10 intended treatment sessions were found completed, which suggested that the number of visits could be reduced in future replication efforts. Importantly, using mediational analyses, it was also found that all of its five treatment components (care management, referral and linkage, instruction in stress reduction techniques, education about depression and symptom recognition, and behavioral activation) worked in concert and contributed similarly to reducing depressive symptoms (Gitlin, Huang, & Roth, 2014; Gitlin, Szanton, Huang & Roth, 2014). Thus, delivering all five components appears to be essential such that in its replication it would not be possible to eliminate one component or implement only select components. As these components can be delivered within 8 versus 10 home sessions, the intervention could be modified in this way, at least for most program participants.

National Institutes of Health Designation of Research Phases

This traditional pipeline has also been conceptualized in the National Institutes of Health (NIH) of the United States as involving three broad translational phases: research designed to bridge basic to human research, or T1 (translational) research; research to evaluate the efficacy and effectiveness of human research and moving it to the community, or T2 research; and research (dissemination, implementation, quality improvement) moving from community-based research to practice, referred to as T3 research (Kleinman & Mold, 2009). NIH funding favors T1 research with little monies offered for T2 or T3 (discussed in Chapter 23).

ELONGATED PIPELINE

An implicit premise of the traditional pipeline is that, if an intervention is shown to be efficacious and reaches the effectiveness phase, the intervention will be widely implemented. However, this reasoning has proven to be faulty (McCannon, Berwick, & Massoud, 2007). There is no empirical evidence to support the assumption that uptake of interventions occurs on the basis of the strength of the evidence that an efficacy trial may yield. Although a strong evidence base is an important prerequisite for knowledge translation or moving evidence from research to practice (Grimshaw, Eccles, Lavis, Hill, & Squires, 2012), the integration of evidence into practice does not happen magically or of its own accord (Wilson, Brady, & Lesesne, 2011). Furthermore, although the scientific reporting of trial outcomes is critical, publications alone do not lead to the adoption of evidence. A more systematic approach is necessary (see Chapter 21 on the dissemination process).

Hence, there is growing recognition that the road toward implementation of interventions in real settings is actually more challenging and nuanced, requiring time and enactment of purposeful actions, than previously considered (see Chapters 19 and 20 for further discussion of this point). This more recent way of thinking is reflected in an elongated pipeline shown in Figure 2.2. This alternative pipeline suggests that moving interventions forward into real-world settings requires additional phases and associated activities. As illustrated, this pipeline involves three additional phases reflecting the systematic processes that need to occur to move an intervention from effectiveness (Phase IV) to its integration within a practice environment (Gitlin, 2013). This elongated pipeline is referred to throughout this book.

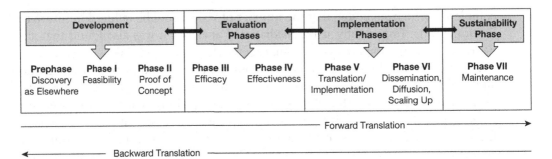

Figure 2.2 Elongated pipeline.

Phase V—Translation/Implementation

In this version of the pipeline, all previous phases discussed above are essentially similar. However, it recognizes a new Phase V that refers to a translation and/or implementation phase. As most interventions are tested outside of or independent of a particular setting in which it could eventually be implemented, its performance within a particular context is unknown. Thus, typically, a set of activities is necessary to "translate" the intervention from its testing phase for its implementation into a real setting. Also referred to as T3 research in the NIH environment, this translational phase seeks to interpret, convert, and adapt a proven intervention for consistent delivery ". . . to all patients in all settings of care and improve the health of individuals and populations" (Dougherty & Conway, 2008, p. 2319).

The issues related to Phase V are discussed in more detail in Chapters 19 and 20. Briefly, there is no consensus as to the specific steps involved in a translational phase, whether it is necessary in all cases when moving interventions forward, or whether it is a separate phase needed prior to an implementation study. Clearly, however, findings from implementation science are critical for informing Phase V.

It appears that when an intervention is tested external to a particular context in which it might be embedded, certain translational activities may be necessary prior to an implementation study (Gitlin, Jacobs, & Earland, 2010). Among these activities are: identifying immutable and mutable aspects of an intervention to refine efficiencies in its delivery and afford a better fit with a particular context (see our previous discussion above on this point as well); advancing manuals that standardize all aspects of delivery for use by agencies and interventionists; developing systematic training programs for instruction in the delivery of the intervention; identifying and evaluating referral mechanisms that enhance outreach to targeted populations; identifying the barriers and supports within a practice environment that support its implementation; identifying the resources and costs needed for implementation; and serving as a pilot test prior to scaling up for full implementation (Glasgow, 2010; Gitlin, Marx, Stanley, & Hodgson, 2015). Critical to this phase is ensuring that the active ingredient(s) identified as core to the effectiveness of an intervention remain intact and are not modified. These translational activities often serve as a pilot test prior to a full implementation study that evaluates, for example, the relative merits of different strategies for implementing an intervention or the rate of adoption by interventionists and participants. These activities may also compose what others

Case Example: As an example, the ABLE (Advancing Better Living for Elders) intervention was designed to help older adults ($\geq$70 years of age) carry out everyday activities of living with less functional challenges. Its essential active ingredient is that it is client-centered and client-directed. That is, ABLE addresses the areas of daily functioning that older adult participants themselves identify as most problematic to them (versus those identified by a health professional). In five home sessions, interventionists (occupational therapists) provide instruction in strategies such as using energy conservation techniques, assistive devices, and home modifications to support performance in those activities of value to a participant. A physical therapist also provided one visit to instruct in safe fall techniques and balance exercises (Gitlin et al., 2006). In its translation for delivery in a traditional home care agency, the intervention had to be simplified. The level of coordination between occupational therapy and physical therapy visits that was obtained in the efficacy trial proved challenging for a home care agency to replicate. Thus, the intervention was modified such that, during an occupational therapy session, an evaluation of fall risk was conducted with a future referral to physical therapy provided for those participants scoring in a range indicating fall risk. Also, certain home modifications (e.g., stair glides; improved lighting) were not possible to provide as they were too expensive or not available through the home care agency. Thus, referral was made to other programs for obtaining recommended home modifications. Finally, therapists had difficulty following a person-directed approach in which the functional areas addressed in the intervention were those identified by older adults themselves. Translating this intervention thus required creating a training program that reinforced its client-directed approach and evaluating whether such an approach had added value to a traditional functional assessment approach within the context of a busy home care practice (Gitlin, Earland, & Piersol, 2010). These modifications were identified in a small feasibility study to translate the intervention for delivery by therapists in home care practices.

have referred to as "pilot testing prior to implementation testing." Here, our earlier discussion of pilot tests and their definition and level of rigor would apply.

Methodologies

The preferred methodologies to use in a translational phase are also unclear. Translational studies tend to use a pre–post evaluative framework and focus on replicating positive outcomes from the original efficacy or effectiveness trials. Nevertheless, as noted above, there is no consensus as to what constitutes the specific activities as well as testing strategies that should be included in this phase, and this in turn has hindered an understanding of how a translational phase supports implementation (Gitlin et al., 2015). As suggested above, it may be helpful to consider translational activities, if necessary, as a pilot for a large-scale implementation study. Alternately, some study designs at the efficacy phase may enable investigators to avoid translational activities. For example, using a pragmatic trial study design (see Table 2.2 for its definition) in which an intervention is tested within the context in which it will ultimately be implemented may avoid the necessity of translation.

Thus, a translational study may serve as a pilot for a full-blown implementation study. An implementation study has multiple purposes, such as: evaluating different strategies for implementing an intervention; testing and standardizing mechanisms regarding how to identify the targeted populations and evaluate the feasibility of proposed referral and enrollment procedures; evaluating training approaches for interventionists; and identifying strategies to maintain fidelity. As for the latter, determining ways to monitor the quality of and the fidelity in delivery of the intervention is a primary focus of any translation and implementation study. The challenges of fidelity monitoring in this phase is doing so in real-world settings (see Chapter 12 for further discussion of this point).

Similar to the phases and pilot testing that need to occur prior to conducting an efficacy trial, there are various stages to implementation studies as well. Fixsen and colleagues identify these stages as exploration, installation, initial implementation, full implementation, innovation, and sustainability (Fixsen, Naoom, Blase, Friedman, & Wallace, 2005). However, there are no clear directives as to how to proceed with implementation testing. Furthermore, as discussed earlier, hybrid designs that combine effectiveness with implementation of scientific questions, or use of pragmatic trials, may provide an understanding of implementation such that a phase devoted to testing implementation approaches may not be necessary in all cases.

Phase VI—Dissemination

The relationship of translation, implementation, and dissemination is quite fluid and highly iterative, which is not necessarily captured in the linear graphic (Greenhalgh, 2005). However, for heuristic purposes, it is helpful to disentangle these activities and order them to understand them more fully. As such, following a phase in which the implementation potential of an intervention is demonstrated, a systematic plan for disseminating the intervention widely can be advanced (Phase VI). A dissemination phase (discussed more fully in Chapter 21) involves moving beyond simply publishing results to advancing a systematic strategy for reaching out to targeted practice settings to encourage adoption of an intervention on a wide scale. Similar to a marketing plan, clear "value propositions" need to be created that articulate the benefits of an intervention to different stakeholders such as administrators, practitioners, and individuals themselves or end beneficiaries of an intervention. Other aspects of a dissemination plan include ways to scale up activities such as training staff/interventionists in delivering the intervention, identifying communication channels, and a licensure structure for naming rights and use of the intervention.

Phase VII—Sustainability

Finally, Phase VII refers to processes related to maintaining or sustaining an intervention in a practice setting (Burke & Gitlin, 2012). The steps involved in and the challenges of sustainability are yet unknown. However, interventions may need to be supported in different ways to ensure continued fidelity to its implementation. Effective strategies for sustaining interventions may be dependent upon the type of intervention and setting. There may be no single approach that works for all behavioral interventions. Hand washing is an example of a proven intervention that has been integrated into hospital and other clinical settings, yet requires continued reinforcement of its use to sustain this basic proven practice. Various strategies have been tested and are in use, including signage or placement of hand-washing equipment such as liquid dispensers in patient rooms (Mayer et al., 2011).

As already discussed, moving an intervention from Phase I to Phase VII is referred to as a forward translation, in which each phase moves an intervention along for its ultimate implementation in a practice setting. However, new evidence may emerge from embedding an intervention into a practice setting or with implementation and sustainability experience. Dramatic modifications may call for new testing of the intervention in a Phase III or Phase IV context (backward translation).

Advantage of the Elongated Pipeline

The advantage of the elongated pipeline is that it recognizes the long haul and complex set of activities required to move an intervention from development to evaluation to implementation. These latter elongated phases, however, need more careful delineation and will benefit from the knowledge gleaned from implementation science (see Chapter 19).

As shown in Figure 2.2, these seven phases can be further classified into four overlapping and interactive larger domains of activities: development (discovery, Phases I and II); evaluation (Phases III and IV); implementation (Phases V and VI); and sustainability (Phase VII). This larger grouping of activities has the advantage of recognizing the interconnectedness of each of these phases.

STRATEGIES FOR ACCELERATING INTERVENTION DEVELOPMENT

Given the elongated time frame involved in building the evidence for behavioral interventions, recent efforts have been directed at identifying strategies for accelerating this process (Curran, Bauer, Mittman, Pyne, & Stetler, 2012; Glasgow, 2010; Riley, Glasgow, Etheredge, & Abernethy, 2013). To this end, we have identified six strategies that may result in more rapid intervention advancement as well as the generation of interventions that are more user-centric and flexible for implementation in different communities, practices, or service contexts. These strategies may be introduced at different points along the elongated pipeline and as early as in the discovery prephase (discussed in Chapter 3). Table 2.3 describes each strategy and the suggested phase in which it might best be considered.

Align Targets With Research Studies

The first strategy that can be considered is to better align intervention targets with findings from population-based or epidemiological studies when beginning to develop an intervention. Population-based studies may be helpful in identifying who is at high risk for the identified problem area, modifiable contributors, and who might benefit the most from an intervention. This may help to propel interventions forward with more efficiency and rapidity by ensuring relevance of intervention

TABLE 2.3 Strategies for Accelerating Intervention Development and Evaluation

Strategy	Phase to Use Strategy	Explanation of Strategy
Use epidemiological data to identify population need and potential targets for an intervention.	Discovery	Align intervention development with data from population-based epidemiological studies as it pertains to population needs and potential targets for intervention. This may result in interventions that are more responsive to public health issues.
Engage all stakeholders and end users (target population, interventionists, administrators).	Discovery and throughout all phases	Adopt a usability perspective. Involve key stakeholders (e.g., agency directors, administrators, representatives from health care organizations), including end users (e.g., representatives for the persons who will deliver the intervention and/or the targeted population or who will use the intervention). Their involvement may help ensure alignment of intervention delivery characteristics and testing strategies with the values, interests, and outcomes of most interest to targeted end users.
Identify and understand delivery context.	Starting in discovery and throughout pipeline	Identify context(s) in which the intervention can be integrated and the potential supports and barriers. This can inform the development of the intervention and delivery characteristics, training of interventionists, and preparation for implementation in early phases of intervention development.
Identify costs associated with intervention.	Phases I and II	Traditionally, cost analyses are performed after an efficacy phase in which an intervention is shown to be efficacious. However, at Phases I and II, the cost of each of the intervention components could be established. This could lead to an immediate understanding of whether the intervention is feasible, the resources needed for its implementation, and whether there are opportunities in Phase II or Phase III to curtail costs by altering the proposed delivery characteristics and evaluating impact.
Implement design efficiencies (technologies) to lower costs, scalability, and impact).	Phases I–IV	Knowledge of what aspects of the intervention are costly can inform changes to delivery characteristics to lower costs if necessary and improve scalability. For example, a home-based intervention may be too costly for a clinic to implement, whereas delivery of the content of the intervention via telephone videoconferencing or other technology may reduce costs, improve implementation potential, and widen reach of the intervention.

(Continued)

Strategy	Phase to Use Strategy	Explanation of Strategy
Use blended design strategies.	Phases II–VI	Design strategies such as a pragmatic trial, hybrid designs, and mixed methodologies efficiently combine research questions to optimize investigations testing interventions. This may minimize time between testing and full implementation.

TABLE 2.3 **Strategies for Accelerating Intervention Development and Evaluation** (*Continued*)

targets and appropriateness of identified populations and risk factors. Reviewing published epidemiological studies or conducting secondary analyses of population-based data sets are important ways to substantiate the basis for and importance of an intervention.

Identify Key Stakeholders

A second strategy is to involve key stakeholders and end users as one develops and evaluates an intervention throughout the elongated pipeline. Stakeholders may include decision makers, such as agency administrators, policy makers, or potential interventionists, who might adopt an intervention if it is found to be effective. End users, similarly, refer to those who will use and/or directly or indirectly benefit from an intervention including the individual, family member, or community that the intervention plans to target. Identifying and integrating the perspectives of key stakeholders and end users and/or using community-participatory strategies in the coconstruction of an intervention may maximize its relevance as it is being advanced. This user-centered perspective is widely used in technology development and innovative social designs and can be applied to the development of interventions as well (Brown & Wyatt, 2010; Czaja, et al., 2015; see also Chapter 1).

Identify Context

A third strategy is to identify early on in the developmental process of an intervention the location (e.g., community-based agency, home care, hospital, online platform) and context (reimbursement model, staffing, organizational considerations) in which an intervention may ultimately be delivered (Horner, & Blitz, 2014). Knowledge of location and context early on when developing an intervention can help to inform the selection of its delivery characteristics (e.g., dose and intensity, treatment components; see Chapter 5) and evaluation strategies (Jacobs, Weiner, & Bunger, 2014; Campbell et al., 2007). For example, the REACH II intervention that was tested as a 12-session intervention was unable to be implemented by community agencies whose care managers had limited time and interactions with clients (Burgio et al., 2009). If the intervention had been originally developed with a brief visit schedule or had been delivered through a community-based agency, it may have had a better fit with different service contexts and thus may not have required a translational set of activities.

Alternately, a targeted problem area may be complex (e.g., depression, addiction) and not amenable to brief sessions or delivery by, for example, telephone, although this could save an agency money. In this case, by knowing the preferences of an agency upfront (e.g., brief number of sessions), an investigator can be better prepared to demonstrate the added value of conducting home visits with regard to the benefits achieved and associated costs.

A related point is to carefully consider who can deliver an intervention early on if the intervention involves individuals (versus a technological platform) for implementation (this is further considered in Chapter 20). Interventions requiring highly skilled interventionists may be limited to those agencies and regions of a country that have access to such resources and thus influence its future scalability. Alternately, interventions that can be delivered by a broad array of individuals such as community health workers or the indigenous staff of a targeted context may have more opportunities for being widely adopted (Han et al., under review). Nevertheless, clearly, the choice of intervention characteristics must match the purpose of the intervention and targeted problem area and population (see Chapter 5 for discussion of delivery characteristics). Developing an intervention that can have a significant treatment effect yet also be scalable represents a delicate balance in decision making about intervention characteristics including who can deliver the intervention. This point is more fully explored in Chapter 19.

Cost the Intervention

A fourth strategy concerns identifying the costs associated with an intervention. Microcosting, or specifying the costs of each aspect of delivering an intervention (e.g., materials, travel, staff time, supervision), can be conducted once the characteristics of an intervention have been identified early on in the development process (Pizzi, Jutkowitz, Frick, Suh, Prioli, & Gitlin, 2014). An understanding of cost can inform whether the intervention will be economically viable. If it is too costly, then modifications may have to be carried out or a strong rationale provided for pursuing the approach. Formal economic evaluations of cost, benefit, and/or effectiveness from a societal or payor perspective can be conducted in a Phase III or Phase IV evaluation of the intervention. Economic evaluations are discussed in more detail in Chapter 18.

Improve Delivery Efficiencies

A fifth and related strategy involves identifying delivery efficiencies to lower costs, and to enhance scalability and impact. This may include using technology to deliver the intervention (see Chapter 7), delivering content in group versus one-on-one sessions, or employing community health workers or staff indigenous to a targeted setting versus more highly skilled or paid interventionists.

Enhance Design Efficiencies

A final consideration is to use innovative study design strategies that combine various phases along the pipeline; for example: hybrid designs that combine effectiveness and implementation research questions (Curran et al., 2012); embedded or pragmatic trial methodologies including stepped, wedge, or adaptive designs; mixed methodologies that are emerging as potential strategies for maximizing the yield of evidence that is generated when evaluating an intervention. Other hybrid models involve conducting implementation trials that secondarily evaluate treatment benefits (Curran et al., 2012) or embedding the test of dissemination strategies early on in the development process. Such approaches make the most of field testing and may move interventions forward more rapidly. However, whether these strategies result in shortening the 17-plus-year time frame for intervention development and the generation of interventions that are more relevant to end users and service contexts still remains an empirical question (see Table 2.2 for definitions of designs).

RECONSTRUCTING THE PIPELINE

Given that the processes for developing behavioral interventions are more complex and iterative than that portrayed by a linear conceptualization of a pipeline, recent efforts have been directed at its reconstruction. Various models are emerging suggesting spiral, iterative, interacting stages, social design, and nonsequential strategies for advancing interventions (Moore et al., 2015; Nieman et al., 2014; Onken, Carroll, Shoham, Cuthbert, & Riddle, 2014). In this respect, the field of behavioral intervention research is in fluidity. New conceptualizations need to be tested to evaluate whether they can lead to effective and efficient behavioral interventions more rapidly.

We suggest that the six strategies described above provide an opportunity to promote a more dynamic approach to generating interventions and one that connects development and evaluation phases with implementation and sustainability goals in an iterative fashion. As suggested in Figure 2.3, this iterative reconstruction of the pipeline highlights the interconnectivity of phases and suggests that keeping the end user and context in mind upfront when developing interventions may change the paradigm of this form of research.

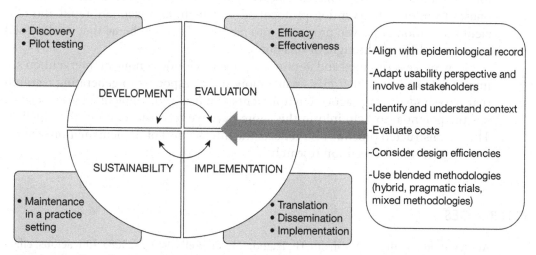

Figure 2.3 Iterative overlapping phase process for developing behavioral interventions.

CONCLUSION

Developing, evaluating, and then implementing and sustaining behavioral interventions in real settings is an important endeavor, but is not without its challenges. It takes many years of an investigator's and a team's effort to move an intervention from discovery to its efficacy testing, and then even more years for evaluation of its implementation and sustainability potential in practice settings.

Generally, interventions begin with a period of discovery or idea inception (discussed in Chapter 3), and move forward with formal evaluative processes, and then, if the intervention is efficacious, feasible, and responsive to community and/or individual needs, an evaluation of implementation and sustainability.

There is no single, agreed upon approach for advancing behavioral interventions. To understand the steps of and associated activities for intervention development, the pipeline concept is initially a useful heuristic. Although its assumptions of linearity and incremental progression are somewhat flawed, the research community at large and funding agencies and reviewers, in particular, continue to assess the adequacy of grant proposals for behavioral intervention research on the basis of how the evaluation of an intervention is described along a pipeline. Thus, understanding the assumed incremental steps in a linear pathway can still be useful, particularly in the grant application process.

The traditional pipeline for medical interventions and drug discovery has typically been applied to behavioral intervention work. Nevertheless, there is growing recognition that a traditional (Figure 2.1) pipeline is insufficient. Our elongated pipeline (Figure 2.2) is more responsive to the growing recognition that additional processes and steps are necessary for moving interventions beyond their initial testing phases. We refer to the elongated pipeline throughout this book.

However, new perspectives for intervention development are emerging. These include integrating a user perspective and identifying stakeholders early on when developing an intervention, among the other approaches we have discussed in this chapter. These strategies may provide the necessary knowledge of contextual factors and implementation challenges early on in the developmental and evaluation phases to inform intervention protocol advancement and facilitate rapid and efficient translation of proven programs into practice. This is a theme that is addressed in various chapters throughout this book.

New process-oriented and iterative approaches for designing an intervention are important to advance that may enable more rapid responses to generating research that is responsive to practice environments (Figure 2.3). Implementation science has the potential to help inform this more iterative reconstruction of the pipeline. This reconstructed pipeline also reflects the intersection of implementation science with behavioral intervention research.

REFERENCES

Allotey, P., Reidpath, D. D., Ghalib, H., Pagnoni, F., & Skelly, W. C. (2008). Efficacious, effective, and embedded interventions: Implementation research in infectious disease control. *BMC Public Health, 8*, 343. doi:10.1186/1471-2458-8-343

Almirall, D., Compton, S. N., Gunlicks-Stoessel, M., Duan, N., & Murphy, S. A. (2012). Designing a pilot sequential multiple assignment randomized trial for developing an adaptive treatment strategy. *Statistics in Medicine, 31*(17), 1887–1902. doi:10.1002/sim.4512

Arain, M., Campbell, M. J., Cooper, C. L., & Lancaster, G. A. (2010). What is a pilot or feasibility study? A review of current practice and editorial policy. *BMC Medical Research Methodology, 10,* 67. doi:10.1186/1471-2288-10-67

Bailey, R. (2004). *Association schemes: Designed experiments, algebra, and combinatorics.* Cambridge, UK: Cambridge University Press.

Belle, S. H., Burgio, L., Burns, R., Coon, D., Czaja, S. J., Gallagher-Thompson, D., . . . Zhang, S. (2006). Enhancing the quality of life of dementia caregivers from different ethnic or racial groups: A randomized, controlled trial. *Annals of Internal Medicine, 145*(10), 727–738.

Bernet, A. C., Willens, D. E., & Bauer, M. S. (2013). Effectiveness-implementation hybrid designs: Implications for quality improvement science. *Implementation Science, 8*(Suppl. 1), S2. doi:10.1186/1748-5908-8-s1-s2

Brown, T., & Wyatt, J. (2010). Design thinking for social innovation. *Development Outreach, 12*(1), 29–43. doi:10.1596/1020-797x_12_1_29

Burgio, L. D., Collins, I. B., Schmid, B., Wharton, T., McCallum, D., & Decoster, J. (2009). Translating the REACH caregiver intervention for use by area agency on aging personnel: The REACH OUT program. *Gerontologist, 49*(1), 103–116. doi:10.1093/geront/gnp012

Burke, J. P., & Gitlin, L. N. (2012). How do we change practice when we have the evidence? *American Journal Occupational Therapy, 66*(5), e85–e88. doi:10.5014/ajot.2012.004432

Campbell, N. C., Murray, E., Darbyshire, J., Emery, J., Farmer, A., Griffiths, F., . . . Kinmonth, A. L. (2007). Designing and evaluating complex interventions to improve health care. *British Medical Journal, 334*(7591), 455–459. doi:10.1136/bmj.39108.379965.BE

Christensen, E. (2007). Methodology of superiority vs. equivalence trials and non-inferiority trials. *Journal of Hepatology, 46*(5), 947–954. doi:10.1016/j.jhep.2007.02.015

Collins, L. M., Murphy, S. A., & Bierman, K. L. (2004). A conceptual framework for adaptive preventive interventions. *Prevention Science, 5*(3), 185–196.

Concato, J., Shah, N., & Horwitz, R. I. (2000). Randomized, controlled trials, observational studies, and the hierarchy of research designs. *New England Journal of Medicine, 342*(25), 1887–1892. doi:10.1056/nejm200006223422507

Congressional Budget Office. (2007). *Research on the comparative effectiveness of medical treatments: Issues and options for an expanded federal role.* Retrieved April 14, 2014, from www.cbo.gov/ftpdocs/88xx/doc8891/12-18-ComparativeEffectiveness.pdf

Conway, P. H., & Clancy, C. (2009). Comparative-effectiveness research—Implications of the Federal Coordinating Council's report. *New England Journal of Medicine, 361*(4), 328–330. doi:10.1056/NEJMp0905631

Craig, P., Dieppe, P., Macintyre, S., Michie, S., Nazareth, I., & Petticrew, M. (2008). Developing and evaluating complex interventions: The new Medical Research Council guidance. *British Medicine of Journal, 337,* a1655. doi:10.1136/bmj.a1655

Cully, J. A., Armento, M. E., Mott, J., Nadorff, M. R., Naik, A. D., Stanley, M. A., . . . Kauth, M. R. (2012). Brief cognitive behavioral therapy in primary care: A hybrid type 2 patient-randomized effectiveness-implementation design. *Implementation Science, 7,* 64. doi:10.1186/1748-5908-7-64

Curran, G. M., Bauer, M., Mittman, B., Pyne, J. M., & Stetler, C. (2012). Effectiveness-implementation hybrid designs: Combining elements of clinical effectiveness and implementation research to enhance public health impact. *Medical Care, 50*(3), 217–226. doi:10.1097/MLR.0b013e3182408812

Czaja, S. J., Boot, W. R., Charness, N., W, A. R., Sharit, J., Fisk, A. D., . . . Nair, S. N. (2015). The personalized reminder information and social management system (PRISM) trial: Rationale, methods and baseline characteristics. *Contemporary Clinical Trials, 40,* 35–46. doi:10.1016/j. cct.2014.11.004

D'Agostino, R. B., Sr., Massaro, J. M., & Sullivan, L. M. (2003). Non-inferiority trials: Design concepts and issues—The encounters of academic consultants in statistics. *Statistics in Medicine, 22*(2), 169–186. doi:10.1002/sim.1425

Dawson, B., & Trapp, R. G. (2004). *Basic & clinical biostatistics* (4th ed.). New York, NY: Lange Medical Books-McGraw-Hill, Medical Pub. Division.

Dougherty, D., & Conway, P. H. (2008). The "3T's" road map to transform US health care: The "how" of high-quality care. *JAMA, 299*(19), 2319–2321. doi:10.1001/jama.299.19. 2319

Drolet, B. C., & Lorenzi, N. M. (2011). Translational research: Understanding the continuum from bench to bedside. *Translation Research, 157*(1), 1–5. doi:10.1016/j.trsl.2010.10.002

Fixsen, D. L., Naoom, S. F., Blase, K. A., Friedman, R. M., & Wallace, F. (2005). *Implementation research: A synthesis of the literature* (FMHI Publication No. 231). Tampa, FL: University of South Florida, Louis de la Parte Florida Mental Health Institute, The National Implementation Research Network.

Flay, B. R. (1986). Efficacy and effectiveness trials (and other phases of research) in the development of health promotion programs. *Preventive Medicine, 15*(5), 451–474.

Gartlehner, G., Hansen, R. A., Nissman, D., Lohr, K. N., & Carey, T. S. (2006). *Criteria for distinguishing effectiveness from efficacy trials in systematic reviews.* Rockville, MD: Agency for Healthcare Research and Quality.

Gitlin, L. N. (2013). Introducing a new intervention: An overview of research phases and common challenges. *American Journal of Occupational Therapy, 67*(2), 177–184. doi:10.5014/ajot.2013.006742

Gitlin, L. N., Corcoran, M., Martindale-Adams, J., Malone, C., Stevens, A., & Winter, L. (2000). Identifying mechanisms of action: Why and how does intervention work? In R. Schulz (Ed.), *Handbook on dementia caregiving: Evidence-based interventions for family caregivers* (pp. 225–248). New York, NY: Springer Publishing.

Gitlin, L. N., Earland, T. E., & Piersol, C. V. (2010, Spring). Enhancing quality of life in functionally vulnerable older adults: From randomized trial to standard care [Special issue on translation of proven programs for older adults]. *Generations, 34*(1), 84–87.

Gitlin, L. N., Harris, L. F., McCoy, M. C., Chernett, N. L., Pizzi, L. T., Jutkowitz, E., . . . Hauck, W. W. (2013). A home-based intervention to reduce depressive symptoms and improve quality of life in older African Americans. *Annals of Internal Medicine, 159*(4), 243. doi:10.7326/0003-4819-159-4-201308200-00005

Gitlin, L. N., Harris, L. F., McCoy, M. C., Hess, E., & Hauck, W. (in press). Delivery characteristics and acceptability of a home-based depression intervention for older African Americans: The Get Busy Get Better Program. *The Gerontologist, Practice Concepts.*

Gitlin, L. N., Jacobs, M., & Earland, T. V. (2010). Translation of a dementia caregiver intervention for delivery in homecare as a reimbursable Medicare Service: Outcomes and lessons learned. *The Gerontologist, 50*(6), 847–854. doi:10.1093/geront/gnq057

Gitlin, L. N., Marx, K., Stanley, I. H., & Hodgson, N. (2015). Translating evidence-based dementia caregiving interventions into practice: State-of-the-science and next steps. *Gerontologist, 55*(2), 210–226. doi:10.1093/geront/gnu123

Gitlin, L. N., Reever, K., Dennis, M. P., Mathieu, E., & Hauck, W. W. (2006). Enhancing quality of life of families who use adult day services: Short and long-term effects of the Adult Day Services Plus program. *The Gerontologist, 46*(5), 630–639. doi:10.1093/ geront/46.5.630

Gitlin, L. N., Roth, D. L., & Huang, J. (2014). Mediators of the impact of a home-based intervention (beat the blues) on depressive symptoms among older African Americans. *Psychology and Aging, 29*(3), 601–611.

Gitlin, L. N., Szanton, S. L., Huang, J., & Roth, D. L. (2014). Factors mediating the effects of a depression intervention on functional disability in older African Americans. *Journal of the American Geriatrics Society, 62*(12), 2280–2287. doi:10.1111/jgs.13156

Gitlin, L. N., Winter, L., Dennis, M. P., Corcoran, M., Schinfeld, S., & Hauck, W. W. (2006). A randomized trial of a multicomponent home intervention to reduce functional difficulties in older adults. *Journal of the American Geriatrics Society, 54*(5), 809–816. doi: 10.1111/j.1532-5415.2006.00703.x

Glasgow, R. E. (2010). HMC research translation: Speculations about making it real and going to scale. *American Journal of Health Behavior, 34*(6), 833–840.

Glasgow, R. E. (2013). What does it mean to be pragmatic? Pragmatic methods, measures, and models to facilitate research translation. *Health Education & Behavior, 40*(3), 257–265. doi:10.1177/1090198113486805

Glasgow, R. E., Lichtenstein, E., & Marcus, A. C. (2003). Why don't we see more translation of health promotion research to practice? Rethinking the efficacy-to-effectiveness transition. *American Journal of Public Health, 93*(8), 1261–1267.

Glasgow, R. E., Magid, D. J., Beck, A., Ritzwoller, D., & Estabrooks, P. A. (2005). Practical clinical trials for translating research to practice: Design and measurement recommendations. *Medical Care, 43*(6), 551–557.

Glasgow, R. E., & Emmons, K. M. (2006). How can we increase translation of research into practice: Types of evidence needed. *Annual Review of Public Health, 2007. 28:* 413–33.

Greenhalgh, T. (2005). *Diffusion of innovations in health service organisations: A systematic literature review.* Malden, MA: Blackwell.

Grimshaw, J. M., Eccles, M. P., Lavis, J. N., Hill, S. J., & Squires, J. E. (2012). Knowledge translation of research findings. *Implementation Science, 7*, 50. doi:10.1186/1748-5908-7-50

Han, H., Kyounghae, K., Choi, J. S., Choi, E., Nieman, C. L., Joo, J. J., Lin, F. R., & Gitlin, L. N. (2015). Do community health worker interventions improve chronic disease management and care among vulnerable populations? A systematic review. *American Journal of Public Health.*

Hart, T., Fann, JR & Novack, TA (2008).The dilemma of the control condition in experience-based cognitive and behavioural treatment research. *Neuropsychol Rehabil. 18*(1): 1–21.

Horner, R., & Blitz, C. (2014, September). *The importance of contextual fit when implementing evidence-based interventions* (ASPE Issue Brief). Washington, DC: U.S. Department of Health and Human Services, Office of Human Services Policy, and Office of the Assistant Secretary for Planning and Evaluation.

Jacobs, S. R., Weiner, B. J., & Bunger, A. C. (2014). Context matters: Measuring implementation climate among individuals and groups. *Implementation Science, 9*, 46. doi:10.1186/1748-5908-9-46

Kazdin, A. E. (1994). Methodology, design, and evaluation in psychotherapy research. In A. E. Bergen & S. L. Garfield (Eds.), *Handbook of psychotherapy and behavior change* (4th ed.). New York, NY: John Wiley and Sons.

Kleinman, M. S., & Mold, J. W. (2009). Defining the components of the research pipeline. *Clinical and Translation Science, 2*(4), 312–314. doi:10.1111/j.1752-8062.2009.00119.x

Landow, L. (2000). Current issues in clinical trial design: Superiority versus equivalency studies. *Anesthesiology, 92*(6), 1814–1820.

Lei, H., Nahum-Shani, I., Lynch, K., Oslin, D., & Murphy, S. A. (2012). A "SMART" design for building individualized treatment sequences. *Annual Review of Clinical Psychology, 8*, 21–48. doi:10.1146/annurev-clinpsy-032511-143152

Leon, A. C., Davis, L. L., & Kraemer, H. C. (2011). The role and interpretation of pilot studies in clinical research. *Journal of Psychiatric Research, 45*(5), 626–629. doi:10.1016/j.jpsychires.2010.10.008

Mann, C. J. (2003). Observational research methods. Research design II: Cohort, cross sectional, and case-control studies. *Emergency Medical Journal, 20*(1), 54–60.

Mayer, J., Mooney, B., Gundlapalli, A., Harbarth, S., Stoddard, G. J., Rubin, M. A., . . . Samore, M. H. (2011). Dissemination and sustainability of a hospital-wide hand hygiene program emphasizing positive reinforcement. *Infection Control and Hospital Epidemiology, 32*(1), 59–66. doi:10.1086/657666

McCannon, C. J., Berwick, D. M., & Massoud, M. R. (2007). The science of large-scale change in global health. *JAMA, 298*(16), 1937–1939. doi:10.1001/jama.298.16.1937

Medical Research Council. (2000, April). *A framework for development and evaluation of RCTs for complex interventions to improve health.* Retrieved from http://www.mrc.ac.uk/...pdf/rcts-for-complex-interventions-to-improve-health/

The Methodology Center, Penn State University. (2012). *Adaptive interventions.* Retrieved April 14, 2014, from https://methodology.psu.edu/ra/adap-inter

Moore, G. F., Audrey, S., Barker, M., Bond, L., Bonell, C., Hardeman, W., . . . Baird, J. (2015). Process evaluation of complex interventions: Medical Research Council guidance. *British Medical Journal, 350*, h1258. doi:10.1136/bmj.h1258

Murphy, S. A. (2005). An experimental design for the development of adaptive treatment strategies. *Statistics in Medicine, 24*(10), 1455–1481. doi:10.1002/sim.2022

Nichols, L. O., Martindale-Adams, J., Burns, R., Graney, M. J., & Zuber, J. (2011). Translation of a dementia caregiver support program in a health care system—REACH VA. *Archives of Internal Medicine, 171*(4), 353–359. doi:10.1001/archinternmed .2010.548

Nieman, C. N., Mamo, S., Marrone, N., Szanton, S., Tanner, E., Thorpe, R., & Lin, F. (2014). *User-centered design and intervention development: The Baltimore HEARS pilot study.* Presentation at the Gerontological Society of America, Washington, DC

Onken, L. S., Carroll, K. M., Shoham, V., Cuthbert, B. N., & Riddle, M. (2014). Reenvisioning clinical science: Unifying the discipline to improve the public health. *Clinical Psychological Science, 2*(1), 22–34. doi:10.1177/2167702613497932

Patsopoulos, N. A. (2011). A pragmatic view on pragmatic trials. *Dialogues in Clinical Neuroscience, 13*(2), 217–224.

Piaggio, D., Elbourne, D. R., Altman, D. G., Pocock, S. J., Evans, S., J. W. for the CONSORT Group. (2006). Reporting of Noninferiority and Equivalence Randomized Trials An Extension of the CONSORT Statement. *Journal of the American Medical Association, 295*, 1152–1160.

Piaggio, G., Elbourne, D. R., Pocock, S. J., Evans, S. J., & Altman, D. G. (2012). Reporting of noninferiority and equivalence randomized trials: Extension of the CONSORT 2010 statement. *JAMA, 308*(24), 2594–2604. doi:10.1001/jama.2012.87802

Pizzi, L. T., Jutkowitz, E., Frick, K. D., Suh, D., Prioli, K. M., & Gitlin, L. N. (2014). Cost-effectiveness of a community-integrated home-based depression intervention in older African Americans. *Journal of the American Geriatrics Society, 62*(12), 2288–2295. doi:10.1111/jgs.13146

Riley, W. T., Glasgow, R. E., Etheredge, L., & Abernethy, A. P. (2013). Rapid, responsive, relevant (R3) research: A call for a rapid learning health research enterprise. *Clinical and Translational Medicine, 2*(1), 10. doi:10.1186/2001-1326-2-10

Roland, M., & Torgerson, D. (1998). Understanding controlled trials: What outcomes should be measured? *British Medical Journal, 317*(7165), 1075.

Sedgwick, P. (2013). What is a superiority trial? *British Medicine Journal, 347*, f5420.

Sox, H. C., & Greenfield, S. (2009). Comparative effectiveness research: A report from the Institute of Medicine. *Annual of Internal Medicine, 151*(3), 203–205.

Thabane, L., Ma, J., Chu, R., Cheng, J., Ismaila, A., Rios, L. P., . . . Goldsmith, C. H. (2010). A tutorial on pilot studies: The what, why and how. *BMC Medical Research Methodology, 10*, 1. doi:10.1186/1471-2288-10-1

Trikalinos, T. A., Salanti, G., Zintzaras, E., & Ioannidis, J. P. (2008). Meta-analysis methods. *Advances in Genetics, 60,* 311–334.

Tunis, S. R., Stryer, D. B., & Clancy, C. M. (2003). Practical clinical trials: Increasing the value of clinical research for decision making in clinical and health policy. *JAMA, 290*(12), 1624–1632. doi:10.1001/jama.290.12.1624

U. S. National Library of Medicine. (2014). *What are clinical trial phases?* Retrieved April 14, 2014, from http://www.nlm.nih.gov/services/ctphases.html

Washington, T., Zimmerman, S., Cagle, J., Reed, D., Cohen, L., Beeber, A. S., & Gwyther, L. P. (2014). Fidelity decision making in social and behavioral research: Alternative measures of dose and other considerations. *Social Work Research, 38*(3), 154–162. doi:10.1093/swr/svu021

Westfall, J. M., Mold, J., & Fagnan, L. (2007). Practice-based research—"Blue Highways" on the NIH roadmap. *JAMA, 297*(4), 403–406. doi:10.1001/jama.297.4.403

Wilson, K. M., Brady, T. J., & Lesesne, C. (2011). An organizing framework for translation in public health: The Knowledge to Action Framework. *Preventing Chronic Disease, 8*(2), A46.

THREE

GETTING STARTED—ANATOMY OF THE INTERVENTION

> *Innovation in health care includes important challenges: to find or create technologies and practices that are better able than the prevailing ones to reduce morbidity and mortality and to make those improvements ubiquitous quickly.*
> —McCannon, Berwick, and Massoud (2007, p. 1937)

How does one develop a behavioral intervention? Where does one begin? This is a common query and one for which there is no straightforward or simple response. Despite increased recognition of the importance of this form of inquiry, there is no consensus, agreed upon strategy, or recipe, as we discussed in Chapter 2, for getting started in developing an intervention.

However, all interventions have a common origin or etiology, the starting point of which is referred to as a period of "discovery" or a prephase to the pipelines discussed in Chapter 2. This prephase discovery period is one in which the fundamental idea for, or anatomy of, an intervention is conceptualized and fleshed out. It is the linchpin from which all subsequent decisions are made concerning the next steps to be taken to evaluate and advance an intervention. Although all succeeding steps, phases, pilot testing, and related research activities to advance an intervention are important, establishing the foundation of an intervention in this prephase of discovery is perhaps one of the most critical as it directs all subsequent thinking and action processes.

Therefore, the purpose of this chapter is to examine in depth this crucial period of "discovery" in which the basic concept for an intervention is initially conceptualized and defined. We provide a roadmap as to the essential decision making that needs to occur in the process of creating an intervention and some working tools to help map out this process.

GETTING STARTED

As noted, there is no consensus or uniformity as to the specific actions that compose this initial prephase of discovery. The Medical Research Council (MRC, 2000) suggests that a wide range of approaches may be used. Emphasized is the importance of drawing upon the best evidence and appropriate theories and then engaging in a series of pilot studies, which we have referred to in Chapter 2 as Phase I and Phase

II activities. The MRC has produced some of the most important documents on developing and evaluating complex interventions; still, specific initial actions are not well identified, and its initial approach emphasizes the traditional four-phase linear and incremental pipeline for advancing interventions (Craig et al., 2008).

Behavioral Intervention Mapping is another schema that offers a step-by-step approach for intervention development. As a planning model for developing theory- and evidence-informed programs, its purpose is "to provide planners with a framework for effective decision making at each step in the intervention development process" (Bartholomew, Parcel, & Kok, 1998, p. 545) and to link each step and related actions. It has been used to address a wide range of health behavior and education programs such as breast and cervical cancer screening for Hispanic farmworkers (Fernández, Gonzales, Tortolero-Luna, Partida, & Bartholomew, 2005), cervical cancer screening (Hou, Fernandez, & Chen, 2003), increasing effective illness behaviors in mental health patients (Koekkoek, van Meijel, Schene, & Hutschemaekers, 2010), or a worksite physical activity program (McEachan, Lawton, Jackson, Conner, & Lunt, 2008). Specifically, this approach involves highly iterative steps including identifying proximal program objects (e.g., who and what will change from an intervention); selecting a theory base for the methods and strategies employed; designing and organizing the intervention; and detailing implementation and evaluation plans.

Although Intervention Mapping is one of the few systematic approaches for intervention development that has also been formally evaluated (McEachan et al., 2008), it does not address some of the particulars concerning protocol development. On the basis of the MRC and intervention mapping approaches, we conceptualize the process of developing an intervention somewhat differently. We suggest that all interventions must start by fulfilling eight essential and interconnected thinking and action processes that need to be investigated, defined, or addressed prior to moving forward with a formal evaluation of an intervention. As described in Table 3.1, they include deriving a clear definition of the problem for which change is being sought; quantifying the problem that is being targeted for change; specifying the populations that may be at most risk; determining the pathways by which the problem occurs; identifying those pathways most amenable to change; identifying the outcomes of interest; quantifying the magnitude of change that may be possible; and identifying current practices or approaches to address the problem. Here we examine each consideration.

Define the Problem

As any intervention is designed to alter, modify, improve, or reduce a "problem" of public health importance, the first essential thinking and action process that needs to be accomplished is to clearly identify and define the specific problem area or focal point for an intervention. Problem areas can be identified from four primary sources and/or their combination: personal experience, clinical work, published research evidence including both qualitative and quantitative sources (e.g., needs assessments, focus groups, population-based studies), and/or existing or projected societal trends. In this period of discovery, a problem area must be clearly articulated and delineated; for example, parents of children with disability have more depression than those without a disabled child and this affects care provision; or, in an aging population, dementia is expected to increase exponentially and prevention strategies to reduce the risk of cognitive impairment must be identified and tested in middle-aged adults without cognitive impairment.

In the example shown in Table 3.1, clinical observations of older frail adults combined with evidence from epidemiological studies indicated that functional limitations were common, resulting in significant difficulties performing everyday activities (e.g., self-care and instrumental activities) at home. This in turn places older adults at risk for relocation to more restricted living environments, hospitalizations, social isolation, depression, poor quality of life, comorbidities, and mortality. Thus, a combination of observational and empirical data initially led to problem identification and substantiation of the need for an intervention to address functional concerns at home, subsequently referred to as the ABLE Program (Advancing Better Living for Elders; Gitlin et al., 2006).

Quantify the Problem

Once a problem area is defined, a related consideration is to quantify the scope of the problem. This involves identifying its prevalence and impact. The targeted problem area may affect a significant portion of a population such that it warrants intervention attention. Alternatively, the targeted problem area may affect only a small number of individuals; yet, it is the driver of significant personal and societal costs and thus important to address through intervention development.

The impact of the problem may include the number of persons affected; its associated sequelae on families, communities, or society at large; or its personal, community, or societal costs. The impact of the problem is one of the most important factors to consider when evaluating whether an investment of time and resources to develop and evaluate an intervention is warranted. The potential impact of an intervention proposed in a grant application will be heavily weighed by review committees of funding agencies. There are many clinical and/or localized concerns of interest to particular professional groups or practice settings for which an intervention could be developed. However, these important yet "small" clinical problems may not rise to the level of public health import necessary for obtaining funding to support intervention development, because they do not affect a significant number of persons, result in societal harm or costs, nor are associated with pernicious sequelae of events warranting investment in intervention development, or considered a public health priority.

Quantifying the prevalence and impact of the targeted issue using existing evidence is important for several reasons. First, it is important to build a strong case that the problem is a public health issue to secure funding from federal agencies and foundations (see Chapter 23 on grant writing). Second, quantifying the problem can provide a basis for understanding the potential impact of an intervention and resultant personal and societal cost savings. For the ABLE Program, it was documented that an estimated 38 million older adults by 2030 would be living in the community with significant functional limitations and that a greater portion of Medicare dollars compared to older adults without disabilities were being spent on this group. As this group is at high risk for falls and hospitalizations, the magnitude

TABLE 3.1 Key Considerations in Discovery Prephase

Key Consideration	Explanation	Exemplar—ABLE Program
Define problem	On the basis of epidemiological studies and/or needs assessments, identify problem and extent to which it represents a public health problem. Quantifying problem can demonstrate its impact.	Functional limitations place older adults at risk for relocation, health care utilization, hospitalizations, poor quality of life, social isolation, morbidity, and mortality.
Quantify problem	Determine prevalence of problem, cost of problem, or other indicators of its impact.	By 2030, 38 million older adults will have one or more functional limitations.
Specify populations at most risk	Within designated population, identify those most at risk who may need intervention.	Most at risk are minority and low-income, representing fastest growing segment of aging population. Also, older adults living in poor housing stock, those with multiple chronic comorbidities, the oldest old, those living alone and lacking resources are also at high risk.
Determine pathway(s)	Identify theoretical basis for an intervention that addresses the problem.	Disablement Model provides overarching framework for understanding pathways between functional limitations, disability, and poor outcomes. It suggests that a mismatch between capabilities (intrinsic) and home environments (extrinsic) heightens disability or ability to perform desired activities including self-care. Life-Span Theory of Control suggests that mismatch can be minimized through control-oriented strategies (e.g., compensatory techniques, seeking help and environmental adjustments).
Determine if pathways amenable to change	Evaluate whether hypothesized pathways are modifiable and what measures will be sensitive to change.	Although underlying impairment may not be amenable to change, it can mitigate disability caused from mismatch between capabilities and environments. Providing "control" enhancing strategies and modifying home environment may reduce impact of functional limitations, negative psychosocial consequences, and risk for relocation.
Specify potential outcomes	Identify potential proximal (immediate), primary (main), secondary, distal, and mediating outcomes and their measurement.	Proximal outcome was home safety and use of control-oriented strategies; primary outcomes included reduction in functional difficulties and improved self-efficacy; distal outcomes were improved

(Continued)

TABLE 3.1   Key Considerations in Discovery Prephase *(Continued)*

Key Consideration	Explanation	Exemplar—ABLE Program
		quality of life and reduction of risk for mortality. Measures sensitive to change might include subjective appraisals of functional difficulty, self-efficacy, strategy use; objective measures of health care utilization, functional performance, depressive symptoms might also be relevant.
Quantify potential for improvement	Evaluate whether improvements will reflect small, medium, or large changes. Effect sizes will influence sample size considerations.	Reducing disability can minimize depression, morbidity, mortality, nursing home placement, hospitalization, risk of other types of relocations. Reductions in functional difficulties will be small but clinically significant.
Determine how problem is currently addressed	Through literature review, determine if there is an existing intervention and if it is effective for the targeted population. If not, then new intervention development will be warranted. Also, determine if there are proven protocols that may be useful.	There were no interventions developed or tested. Although there was previous evidence for role of home modifications, there were no proven protocols that could be combined into an intervention. Thus, ABLE had to be developed from the ground up.

of the problem and its personal and societal impact warrant moving forward with intervention development.

Specify the Populations Most at Risk for the Identified Problem

A third consideration that must occur in the discovery prephase is identifying the specific populations most at risk for the identified problem and for whom intervention development is most warranted. For example, depression in late life is common, and there are various effective depression treatments. However, older minority populations are differentially affected; depression tends to be underdetected and undertreated with most proven interventions not typically including these populations in their evaluations (Areán, & Unützer, 2003). Furthermore, there are numerous interventions for older Caucasians that have been tested in primary care settings. As depression in minority groups is underrecognized and undertreated in this setting, developing an intervention that specifically targets underserviced groups and is delivered in settings other than primary care to overcome persistent health disparities in access and treatment has become a recognized public health imperative (Gitlin, 2014).

For the ABLE Program, the groups identified as those most at risk for functional challenges at home were minority and low-income populations, representing the fastest growing segment of the aging population. Other subgroups affected included the oldest old, older adults living in poor housing stock, and those living alone and lacking resources to address their functional limitations. These groups all became targets for the ABLE Program (Gitlin, Winter, Dennis, & Hauck, 2008).

Determine the Pathways by Which the Identified Problem Occurs

A fourth consideration is to determine the primary pathway(s) by which a problem occurs. This necessitates identifying relevant and available theoretical or conceptual frameworks and examining if there is empirical evidence as to what contributes to the identified problem area. This in turn will help to explain how and why an intervention may have an impact on the outcomes being targeted, in subsequent evaluative phases.

Typically, multiple factors contribute to complex behavioral and health problems such as chronic disease, delirium, school-related problem behaviors, or social isolation. For example, falls are due to multiple causes including poor balance, environmental factors, sensory changes, certain medications and/or their combination, and a fear of falling. Hence, preventing or reducing falls requires a multifactorial approach to impact the different implicated pathways (Eldridge et al., 2005; Gillespie et al., 2012).

Similarly, complex health and social problems may require what is referred to as a "multimodal" approach. This would entail an intervention that combines different strategies that work through different modalities or pathways to achieve a desired outcome. For example, let's say of interest is improving lifestyle behaviors in middle-aged adults to reduce the risk of heart disease. A combination of approaches that impact different pathways contributing to risk of heart disease would be necessary; this might include physical exercise to improve physical strength and aerobic capacity; health eating habits to reduce fat and cholesterol levels; cognitive techniques to improve reframing daily habits and associated stressors; and stress reduction techniques to reduce situation stress.

Accordingly, it may be necessary to draw upon more than one theory base to understand complex problem areas that are being targeted for intervention (see Chapter 4 on theory). Furthermore, as problems occur within contexts, structures, and/or organizations, drawing upon organizational or systems theories or theories of implementation (see Chapter 19) may help to identify the contextual forces or factors that serve to perpetuate the problem area.

For the ABLE Program, several frameworks, the Disablement Model (Nagi, 1964; Verbrugge & Jette, 1994) and Motivational Theory of Life-Span Development (Heckhausen & Schulz, 1995; Heckhausen, Wrosch, & Schulz, 2010), were used to understand the primary pathways by which functional limitations have negative sequelae for older adults and impact daily quality of life. The Disablement Model suggests that intrinsic (e.g., cognitive and behavioral) and extrinsic (home environment) factors contribute to poor functional outcomes. Briefly, the Motivational Theory suggests the use of control-oriented strategies (e.g., compensatory techniques, seeking help, and using environmental adjustments) to accomplish meaningful activities and to exert control over behavior–event contingencies. Thus,

ABLE targeted both: extrinsic housing features that served as a barrier to daily performance through the provision of home modifications and assistive devices; and intrinsic coping strategies through the instruction in positive problem solving and cognitive reframing techniques as well as in the use of compensatory behavioral strategies (e.g., sit to perform meal preparation). A single bullet approach such as only improving home safety would not have resulted in the same desirable and expected outcomes.

Identifying the primary pathway(s) of the problem at the discovery phase will subsequently shape the level of complexity, content, and delivery characteristics of an intervention (see Chapter 5 on delivery characteristics).

Determine If Pathways Are Modifiable

A related consideration is to determine whether the identified pathway(s) of the selected problem area are amenable to change; and if so, what type and magnitude of change might be expected. Of importance is identifying triggers or contributors of the problem that are *modifiable* and thus can be addressed by an intervention. If a problem is due to factors that are intractable or not modifiable, and it is not possible to mitigate the problem, then an intervention is obviously not possible.

For example, certain personality types are a risk factor for negative or inappropriate behaviors; but personality is trait-based and not modifiable. However, the circumstances that elicit negative behavioral responses for specific personality types could be targeted through an intervention to mitigate inappropriate behaviors. More specifically, being male and having a history of aggressive behaviors are known risk factors for aggressive forms of behaviors in persons with dementia (Kunik et al., 2010). However, neither sex nor previous history or experiences are modifiable and thus cannot be targeted in an intervention. Yet an intervention could target other modifiable contributors such as reducing caregiver stress, increasing their understanding of dementia, and heightening awareness of the risk for aggressive behaviors.

The identification of modifiable factors in this stage of intervention development is critical. Through this identification process, it might be discovered that certain problems are due to multiple factors, some of which reflect "low-hanging fruit" or which could be addressed simply and if so, mitigate the problem. Alternately, an identified problem area may be rooted in individual behaviors, which in turn are supported by environmental forces. Take, for example, a weight loss intervention for low-income middle-aged adults that focuses on cooking and eating appropriate foods only. However, healthy foods may not be easily available in low-income neighborhoods of study participants. An intervention that focuses on individuals' behaviors exclusive to their living context may have an immediate benefit but not long-term impact on desired outcomes. Thus, a multimodal (e.g., targeting different pathways) and multicomponent (e.g., different strategies) intervention may be a preferred approach.

As to the ABLE Program (shown in Table 3.1), functional limitations may be due to an underlying pathology (e.g., irreversible arthritic processes) and impairments that are not necessarily modifiable. Although functional limitations may be partially addressed through exercise or reducing inflammation, the impact of functional limitations on quality of life is due primarily to the mismatch between persons' functional abilities and the physical and social environmental demands they confront. These latter factors can be modified. For example, persons with difficulty ambulating may not be able to ascend stairs easily to use a bathroom. They may compensate by restricting their living space to one floor, and/or they may choose to limit their fluid intake or discontinue a diuretic to reduce their need to use the bathroom. We may be able to enhance their balance and strength through exercise, but that may still not enable them to ascend stairs routinely to use a bathroom. However, installing a stair glide or creating a first floor powder room may address this mismatch. The ABLE Program was designed to optimize the fit between abilities, tasks, and environmental home features. The reduction of everyday difficulties in task performance was the primary outcome chosen to demonstrate intervention efficacy. Furthermore, it was hypothesized that reducing daily functional difficulties would result in enhanced engagement, quality of life, less health care costs, and a reduced risk for mortality. These are all outcomes that were demonstrated for the ABLE Program in a Phase III efficacy trial (Gitlin et al., 2006, 2009). Furthermore, examining the primary pathways will lead to identifying appropriate measures, which may serve as descriptors, modifiers, mediators, or primary or secondary outcomes of an intervention (see Chapters 14 and 15).

Specify Potential Outcomes

Yet another important consideration in this prephase of discovery is determining appropriate outcomes and their measurement for the targeted effect an intervention may induce. Initially, it is helpful to consider a wide range of potential outcomes and/or measures that may be possible from intervening to address an identified problem area. For example, if quality of life is the primary outcome, then it is helpful to consider a range of approaches for measuring this construct to determine which domains are most responsive to the intervention. Similarly, an intervention that is designed to reduce depressive symptoms will obviously include an outcome measure of depression. However, there are various aspects of depression that could be measured including symptom severity or diagnostic category, and there could be various intervention goals including symptom reduction, remission, or an a priori defined clinically significant change in depression score.

On the basis of theory, empirical evidence, and the scope and nature of the problem, outcomes can be categorized in different ways as either proximal, primary, secondary, distal, or mediators of an intervention. Proximal outcomes reflect the immediate effects of an intervention, and that may need to be impacted to achieve a primary outcome of greater interest. For example, if one is testing the role of exercise in reducing hypertension, the first outcome of interest is whether participants engage in the exercise as prescribed. Thus, exercise engagement (dose and intensity) reflects the proximal goal of such an intervention without which other outcomes of interest, such as lowered blood pressure, may not hypothetically be able to be achieved. In this regard, proximal outcomes represent the enactment of strategies provided in an intervention and serve as one indicator of fidelity (see

Chapter 12) and may also represent potential mediators to understand the pathways by which an intervention works. Whereas exercise participation represents the proximal outcomes, of primary interest and public health import is a clinically significant reduction in hypertension. Thus, the reduction of hypertension reflects the primary outcome of interest. There may also be outcomes of secondary interest that may occur as a consequence of an exercise intervention; for example, participants may experience better mood, less fatigue, reduced fall risk, and better sleep. These all represent potential secondary outcomes that could be measured.

The ABLE intervention involved different components, one of which was conducting a home safety assessment and providing recommendations for reducing home hazards. The implementation of these recommendations reflected a proximal, immediate outcome that was expected and measured. This in turn was hypothesized to lead to improved home safety, a primary outcome measure. Thus, home safety was one of several primary outcomes of interest. Additionally, in the ABLE Program, other strategies were introduced to support the safe performance of participants in daily activities of their choice. Thus, another primary outcome was a meaure of functional difficulty; a secondary outcome was self-efficacy managing daily self-care challenges.

Distal outcomes refer to those that the intervention may impact if proximal and primary goals are achieved. These outcomes may occur over time as a consequence of using the intervention strategies. In the ABLE Program, distal outcome measures included quality of life and mortality. It was hypothesized that reduced functional difficulty (primary outcome) and improved home safety (primary outcome) would lead to enhanced self-efficacy and quality of life (secondary outcomes) and reduced risk for mortality (distal outcome).

As one can see, the identification of proximal, distal, and primary and secondary outcomes also suggests potential causal mechanisms that can be tested formally using mediation analyses. So, for example, a mediator of the ABLE effect on mortality may have been a reduction in functional outcomes and the use of positive compensatory strategies (Gitlin et al., 2009).

Specifying outcomes, their respective measurement, and role (primary, secondary, mediator, etc.) for an identified problem is important at this prephase as subsequent evaluations can then evaluate which outcome is most appropriate to consider and which measures are most sensitive to the intervention. Chapters 14 and 15 explore in more depth measurement considerations and intervention outcomes.

Quantify the Potential for Improvement

The seventh consideration that needs to occur in the discovery phase is quantifying the potential for improvement in a problem area. Improvements from an intervention may be small, medium, or large and include both subjective and objective outcomes including cost (see Chapters 14 and 15 on measurement and Chapter 18 on cost). Projections of the effect size of an intervention can be derived from theory and existing evidence. Projections will inform sample size considerations in the evaluative phases that test for the outcomes of an intervention (see Chapter 9 on sampling considerations). An expected small impact on an intervention (referred to as "the effect size") will require the evaluation of the intervention with a large sample; alternately, an expected medium or large impact or effect size will not have the same requirements with respect to sample size. However, sample determination is not only a function of size but also includes other considerations such as sample composition and feasibility with respect to recruitment and attrition.

For the ABLE Program, at the time of its development, there was little empirical evidence as to what the effect for the main outcome, reduction in functional difficulties, might be possible to achieve. Pilot testing to advance the intervention was important in order to demonstrate proof of concept and if change in functioning could be achieved. This is an example of how these prephase considerations overlap with initial pilot testing, and this is referred to in Chapter 2 as "Phase I activity."

On the basis of pilot studies demonstrating proof of concept of the ABLE approach (Gitlin & Burgh, 1995; Gitlin, Schemm, Landsberg, & Burgh, 1996), it was subsequently hypothesized that a medium effect size could be achieved in reducing functional challenges and improving self-efficacy in managing daily challenges. Power calculations with this and other assumptions led to the conclusion that a Phase III efficacy trial would require a sample size of 319 study participants in order to demonstrate a medium effect of the intervention on functional difficulties when compared to a usual care control group.

Determine How the Problem Is Currently Being Addressed

The final consideration in the discovery phase involves determining how the problem is currently being addressed. This involves conducting systematic literature reviews to evaluate whether interventions for the problem area and targeted population exist. Here five scenarios may be possible, each of which may lead to a different subsequent developmental pathway. Figure 3.1 details these potential outcomes and their implications for how to proceed in developing an intervention along the pipelines discussed in Chapter 2.

One scenario and perhaps the most common that is discovered through a comprehensive literature review is that a theory-based intervention does not exist for the identified problem area. In this case, an intervention needs to be developed from "scratch" or from the ground up through Phase I testing, followed by the other phases along the pipeline.

A second scenario may be that there is not a proven intervention for the problem area of interest, but evidence-based protocols do exist for similar problems that could possibly be combined and applied to a new area. For example, behavioral activation is a powerful, evidence-based protocol that has been used to reduce depressive symptoms and improve self-care and medication management for distinct populations (Hopko, Lejuez, Ruggiero, & Eifert, 2003). This approach, however, might be useful in addressing the need to improve diabetes self-management. A behavioral activation protocol could be combined with perhaps another proven protocol for education or stress reduction. As each of these components has been previously shown to be feasible and acceptable for other problem areas, it might be possible to skip an initial pilot test of each of these components and move forward with either a strong pilot test of the new combination (Phase II) or efficacy testing (Phase III).

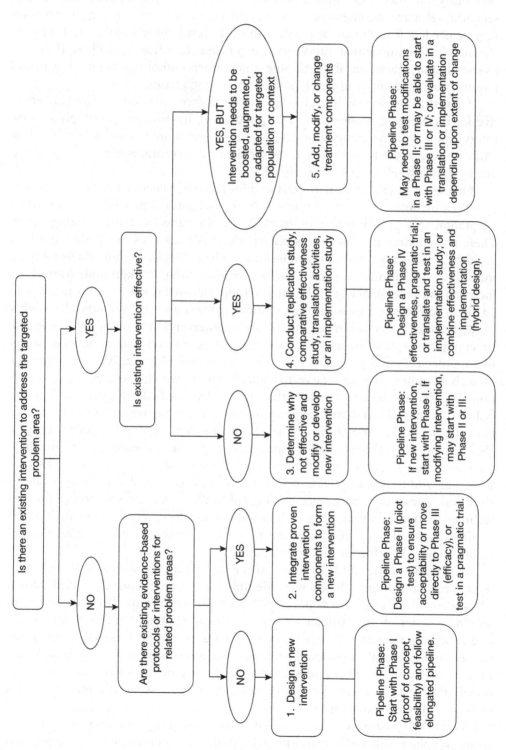

Figure 3.1 Five scenarios for intervention development.

Yet a third scenario is that one or more interventions may have been developed previously, but their evaluation resulted in poor or suboptimal outcomes. In this scenario, refinements, augmentations, and/or boosters to an existing intervention may be needed. If so, it may be possible to skip a few pilot test phases and evaluate the modified or augmented intervention in a Phase III (efficacy) or Phase IV (effectiveness) study. However, if developing a new intervention is warranted, it would require moving through all development and testing phases.

A fourth scenario may be that one or more interventions do exist and are effective for the targeted problem area and population. In this case, developing a new intervention is not necessary. However, it may be important to conduct a replication study or to compare two or more of these existing interventions to determine which one is more cost-efficient and beneficial.

Finally, an intervention may exist and found to be effective but not for the targeted population or context of interest. In this scenario, a new intervention or an adaptation to a proven intervention might be warranted and pilot testing occur. There is increasing interest in this scenario as it is unclear as to whether and how to adapt an existing proven intervention to enhance its fit to individuals who are from different cultural, linguistic, and/or socioeconomic backgrounds from those included in the original test of the intervention. Debated is whether it is possible to adapt an intervention to better fit a cultural context and still preserve the fidelity of the original intervention or whether a new intervention needs to be developed. Emerging conceptual models for adapting existing interventions support an adaptive approach (Bernal, Jiménez-Chafey, & Domenech Rodríguez, 2009). An example of such an approach is the Harvest Health Program, which was a cultural adaptation for older African Americans of the Chronic Disease Self-Management Program (CDSMP), an evidence-based program to improve self-management of chronic illness (Gitlin et al., 2008; Lorig, Sobel, Ritter, Laurent, & Hobbs, 2001). Harvest Health maintained the essential components of CDSMP, yet modifications included a name change to reflect a cultural meaningful symbol (e.g., one reaps what one sows); an additional introductory session to build trust and a working relationship; and course augmentations involving culturally relevant foods, stress reduction techniques, and communicating with racially/ethnically diverse physicians. Harvest Health was tested as a translational/implementation study (Chapter 2, Phase V) and shown to have benefits for this population.

In the case of the ABLE Program, at the time of its development, no other interventions or proven protocols were identified (see scenario one discussed above). Thus, the ABLE Program was developed from the ground up. This involved conducting a series of pilot studies to evaluate the acceptability and feasibility of its treatment components (e.g., whether energy conservation techniques, home modification and home safety protocol, and fall risk protocols were acceptable and used in a home environment) and identify potential outcome measures related to functional difficulties (main primary outcome), self-efficacy (secondary outcome), and quality of life (distal outcome).

As these five basic scenarios suggest, the considerations examined in this discovery prephase will yield critical knowledge that can inform how best to proceed with intervention development and the type of evaluation that will be needed.

SOURCES INFORMING DISCOVERY

Three important sources can inform the considerations described previously: systematic literature reviews, prospective studies, and simulation or modeling techniques. Similar to all phases and activities related to behavioral intervention research, it is always essential to begin the construction of an intervention by conducting systematic reviews of existing literature including gray matter, examining the epidemiological record, and identifying meta-analyses and/or systematic reviews. Epidemiological studies or research using large-scale population-based representative samples is particularly helpful for: identifying and quantifying the scope of a problem at both individual- and population-based levels; providing the evidence that the identified problem is a public health concern; and showing the magnitude of the problem. For example, epidemiological studies may be particularly helpful for identifying risk factors for a particular health problem. Either identifying findings from existing population-based studies or conducting secondary analyses with existing population-based data sets can inform how many people are affected, their characteristics, the impact of the problem area, and potential targets for intervention (Ebbeling et al., 2007).

For example, through an examination of the epidemiological literature, both the direct and indirect effects of alcohol misuse have been identified as major contributors to the risk for infection with HIV and transmission of HIV/AIDS. It may be that no level of alcohol consumption is appropriate for those infected by HIV. Thus, developing culturally suitable strategies that provide education to this effect may be a worthwhile intervention (Bernal et al., 2009).

Unfortunately, there continues to be large gaps between the epidemiological record and the targets selected in interventions in many fields (Gitlin, Marx, Stanley, & Hodgson, 2015; McBeth & Cordingley, 2009). An example of this gap can be found with caregiving interventions. Whereas population-based studies suggest that financial strain and physical burdens of care prompt nursing home placement (Spillman & Long, 2009), caregiver interventions to date have not attempted to intervene on these two contributing factors. Nevertheless, an important caveat is this. Although epidemiological research has much to offer, it is unclear whether interventions are indeed more effective if their targets are more aligned with those identified from such studies.

Discovery may involve small pilot testing or dynamically overlap with activities in Phase I (see Chapter 2, Figure 2.2). For example, conducting focus groups, surveys (online, face-to-face, mailings, Facebook), Delphi surveys, or needs assessments, or, as discussed earlier, engaging in secondary data analyses may help to more fully understand a problem area, identify what is meaningful to affected persons, and explore potential approaches to address the issue. Employing quantitative and qualitative methodologies (see Chapter 11 on mixed methods) including ethnographic, narrative approaches, or semistructured or open-ended in-depth interviews can capture the lived experience of individuals and inform the direction by which to develop an intervention (Zatzick et al., 2011).

Finally, applying simulation and modeling techniques to large data sets can be helpful for identifying potential targets for an intervention and examining under hypothetical scenarios associated costs and outcomes. Such approaches can assist in identifying whom or what to target prior to the prospective development of an intervention in order to maximize its impact (Anderson et al., 2014).

MAPPING AN INTERVENTION

On the basis of the information gleaned from the eight considerations outlined earlier, it should be possible to draft: the potential treatment goals of an intervention; its targeted population; its theory base; its specific objectives; primary (immediate, proximal), secondary, and distal measures; and the key potential components that will be delivered. In doing so, conducting a task analysis of a potential intervention can be helpful. A task analysis involves breaking down an intervention into its operational components to assure that there is complete alignment between the stated problem, targeted population, goals, objectives, and activities of an intervention and proposed outcomes.

Figure 3.2 provides an example of a task analysis of the Get Busy Get Better, Helping Older Adults Beat the Blues (GBGB) intervention. As illustrated, this approach is helpful for several reasons: it provides a visual for aligning the identified problem and treatment goals with specific treatment objectives, key activities and expected outcomes; it provides a roadmap for planning for fidelity or what will need to be monitored to assure that the intervention is delivered as intended (see Chapter 12); and it can serve as the basis for identifying other considerations such as staffing and budget needs, and feasibility and cost.

The GBGB intervention shown in Figure 3.2 was designed as a depression intervention for older African Americans and for screening by telephone and delivery in homes by senior center staff. Briefly, GBGB was based upon social, ecological, and behavioral frameworks for understanding depression among older African Americans with depressive symptoms. In keeping with these frameworks, the intervention goal was to reduce depressive symptoms and improve quality of life by mitigating negative environmental circumstances (e.g., difficulty traveling to physician's office, finance strain) infringing on mood and participation in positive activities. To meet this goal, the intervention had five objectives: to enhance participants' understanding of depression and ability to recognize their own symptoms; to identify unmet care needs; to link participants to needed services and resources; to enhance engagement in desired activities; and to reduce situational distress that may be preventing activity engagement. To meet each of these objectives, a series of activities was enacted as shown. The premise of the intervention is that each of these objectives works together to reach the treatment goal and is necessary in order to achieve the desired outcomes. By conducting this task analysis, it was determined that there are well-tested protocols for stress reduction and behavioral activation, which could be incorporated into the intervention. Furthermore, through pilot testing, it was discovered that pain from chronic diseases was not well addressed by any of the objectives, yet was interfering with the ability of participants to engage in meaningful activities. Also, motivational interviewing techniques were subsequently identified as important to use to boost the behavioral activation protocol. Thus, a new component on pain management was added to this intervention along

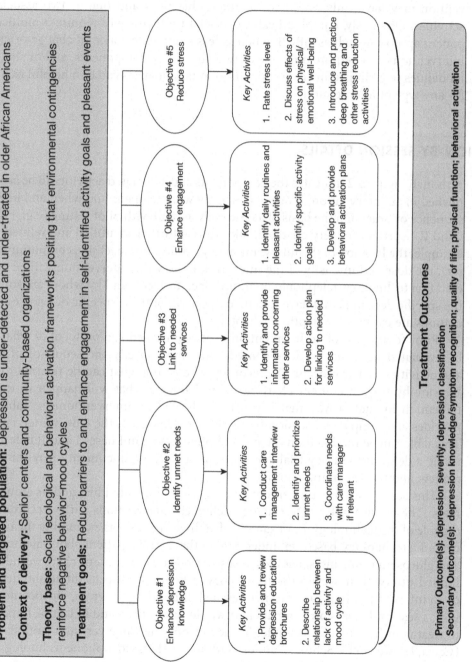

Figure 3.2 Tasks analysis of the Get Busy Get Better intervention.

with motivational interviewing techniques to better address the behavioral activation objective. This illustrates how a task analysis can serve as a working document to guide testing phases and intervention refinements.

Figure 3.2 reflects the anatomy of the GBGB intervention. However, an intervention may have only one, two, or three objectives and one or two associated activities. Obviously, complex health or social problems will require a multicomponent approach such as GBGB, whereas less complex behavioral change-oriented interventions may require only one or two objectives, components, and/or singular modalities (e.g., impacting cognition only). A task analysis can be a helpful exercise for any type of intervention.

SESSION-BY-SESSION DETAILS

Although Figure 3.2 indicates the components and associated activities to be accomplished in an intervention, it does not specify what happens and when and in what sequence or order. On the basis of a task analysis, and with pilot testing (e.g., Phases I and II), specific delivery characteristics can be further identified and refined. For example, the location of the intervention (e.g., office, home, clinic, community center), the dose and intensity of the intervention, how the intervention will be delivered (via technology, telephone, in groups, face-to-face), and by whom are some of the specific decisions that have to settled upon. All of these specific delivery considerations are explored in depth in Chapter 5.

Prior to any test of an intervention or its components, a protocol of what will be evaluated needs to be documented. One must specify the sequence of steps and activities that will occur. We recommend creating what can be referred to as a "session-by-session content chart" to help delineate what will happen in the intervention in such a way that it can be replicated by interventionists. Table 3.2 provides an example of a session-by-session description of the GBGB intervention. This table can be modified on the basis of pilot testing in Phases I and II before entering a definitive efficacy trial and serves as a working document for refining the content and flow of an intervention.

This session-by-session content chart is useful for individual and/or group formats. The applicability to technology-delivered interventions varies according to the role of the technology. For example, if an investigator was examining the usefulness of a technology-based reminder system that alerts a patient about medication- and glucose-monitoring schedules, a session-by-session content chart would have limited utility. If, however, the technology is being used to facilitate the delivery of an intervention (e.g., an Internet-based skill-building program, videoconferencing), a session-by-session content chart would have utility and in fact be important to treatment fidelity. For example, in the videophone caregiver intervention study (Czaja, Loewenstein, Schulz, Nair, & Perdomo, 2013), videophone technology was used to deliver an evidence-based intervention program that involved individual skill- building sessions led by a trained interventionist and facilitated caregiver support groups. To help ensure treatment fidelity and internal validity, detailed session-by-session protocols were developed for the individual skill-building sessions as illustrated in Table 3.3.

TABLE 3.2 Example of a Session-by-Session Content Chart of the Get Busy Get Better Intervention

Session	Location	Intervention Activities	Materials Needed
Screening	On-site senior center or via telephone	■ Assess for depression symptoms and eligibility for participation ■ Use Patient Health Questionnaire-9 (PHQ-9) ≥ 5 score as cutoff for participation	■ Referral form ■ Script explaining intervention
Session 1 (within 1 week of referral)	Home or senior center	■ Rapport building ■ Care management assessment ■ Review depressive symptoms ■ Introduce relationship between behavior and mood ■ Introduce and practice deep breathing ■ Referral and linkage to primary physician, if necessary	■ Clinical interview ■ Stress reduction handout
Sessions 2–3 (2nd and 3rd weeks from referral)	Home	■ On the basis of care management assessment, identify problem and potential resolution ■ Help make linkages with appropriate services, if necessary ■ Review ways to talk to one's doctor about symptoms ■ Review connection between behavior and mood ■ Complete forms together ■ Review deep-breathing technique	■ Documentation binder ■ Resource materials ■ Depression education materials
Sessions 4–5 (4th and 5th weeks from referral)	Home	■ Review care management plan ■ Review mood and activity forms and complete together daily activity recording and mood-rating forms ■ Identify list of pleasant events and meaningful activities of importance to person ■ Use problem solving to identify one activity that would make the person feel better ■ Break activity/task into small manageable steps ■ Rate likelihood of completing steps in week ■ Review deep breathing/ introduce stress reduction technique (counting; music)	■ Documentation binder ■ Behavioral activation rating forms

(Continued)

TABLE 3.2   Example of a Session-by-Session Content Chart of the Get Busy Get Better Intervention *(Continued)*

Session	Location	Intervention Activities	Materials Needed
Sessions 6–8 (every other week)	Home or telephone depending upon participant need and progress as measured by PHQ-9 and activation forms	■ Review depressive symptoms and condition ■ Review progress on all goals ■ Continue with second and third activity planning and tracking selecting new goals to attain ■ Validate accomplishments and support goal attainment	■ Documentation binder ■ PHQ-9
Sessions 9–10 (every other week	Home	■ Review depressive symptoms and conditions ■ Review all accomplishments ■ Encourage person to maintain gains and seek to attain new goals ■ Obtain closure	■ Documentation binder

TABLE 3.3   A Sample of a Session-by-Session Protocol Developed for the Videocare Project

VIDEOCARE
Phone Session # 2

Today's session will focus on common problem behaviors of dementia disorders. During the first part of our meeting, I will review common problem behaviors that have been identified by some caregivers in the past and practical suggestions for dealing with these problem behaviors. The second part of our meeting will be devoted to an open discussion to learn more about how some of these problem behaviors relate to your current situation. Please, feel free to take notes and share your own experience regarding today's topics.

Problem Behaviors of Dementia Disorders

Caring for someone with dementia is a difficult task, filled with everyday challenges. One of the biggest struggles caregivers face is dealing with problem behaviors. These can range from difficulties remembering recent and past events or persons to marked bizarre behaviors. Understanding the nature of these problem behaviors and using different strategies for dealing with difficult behaviors can help caregivers cope better with their loved one's changing levels of abilities and new conducts. The following are some practical suggestions for dealing with some of your loved one's behavior problems.

Tracking the problem: Many times caregivers are able to prevent the occurrence of a problem by becoming aware of the magnitude, frequency, and pattern behavior contributing to problem behavior. Before making any changes, it is always a good idea to track the severity of the problem by making notes of the frequency and possible triggers. That is, how serious is it, how many times does the problem occur, and what happened before the incident? The following are some suggestions to help you monitor the problem.

■ Keep a log of the seriousness, frequency, and possible trigger for your loved one's problem behavior. By keeping a log, not only will you be able to discover possible triggers associated with the behavior, but it will also give you an opportunity to determine if you are making progress in solving this problem.

(Continued)

TABLE 3.3   A Sample of a Session-by-Session Protocol Developed for the Videocare Project   (*Continued*)

Problem Behaviors of Dementia Disorders

- Make notes of any physical, emotional, and environmental conditions prior to the occurrence of the problem. You may find a pattern that can help you get a better understanding of the possible triggers.

Obtain medical advice regarding the problem behavior: A problem behavior may sometimes be the result of other medical problems, such as a negative reaction to a new medication or physical signs of pain or discomfort. Medical conditions can increase the frequency of a problem behavior aside from the cognitive limitation frequently associated with a diagnosis of dementia. A treating physician or a specialist, such as a psychologist or ear/nose specialist, can easily diagnose these problems. They will be able to point out the root of the problem and provide your loved one with adequate treatment. The following are some suggestions that can help you determine if your loved one's problem is due to another medical problem.

- Contact your loved one's treating physician and request an appointment to rule out possible medical causes for the problem behavior. You may need to request a referral to a specialist for further tests, if your treating physician is unable to address the problem.
- Make sure you are prepared when communicating with the doctors or related medical staff. That is, understand the nature of the problem (*refer to your log*), prioritize your concerns, bring a list of relevant medical information (*list of medications, etc.*), and something with which to take notes. We also suggest you arrive a few minutes before the appointment in case you need to fill out any paperwork or meet with another office staff member before meeting with the doctor.
- Listen to the communication menu, *Communication with Health Care Providers* on the E-Care Caregiver Network.

Common problem behaviors: Each person suffering from symptoms of dementia may exhibit different behavioral problems. We selected a few common problem behaviors that caregivers have identified for us as occurring at one point of their loved one's illness.

- **Wandering**

A person with symptoms of dementia may wander away from home or from their caregivers. There are some steps you can take to help reduce wandering and to protect the safety of your loved one if wandering does occur. It is helpful to engage the person in exercise such as walking and encourage movement to reduce restlessness and agitation. It also helps to involve your loved one in productive activities and to reassure them if they feel lost or disoriented. Always make sure that they have some kind of identification and that you have a recent photo of them readily available to help identify them should they become lost. Keep your doors locked and your home secure by installing deadbolt locks on the exterior doors. You should also inform your neighbors of the person's condition and keep a list of emergency phone numbers easily available. You may also want to enroll the person in the Alzheimer's Association Safe Return Program, a nationwide identification system designed to help with the safe return of people who wander and get lost. To find out more information on this program, use the resource guide to contact the Alzheimer's Association.

- **Perseveration (*repetitive speech/actions*)**

A condition of dementia can cause a person to exhibit unusual behaviors such as repetition of a word, a question, or an activity. This can be extremely frustrating to you as a caregiver. To help reduce problems with this type of behavior, you should try to stay calm and be patient and accept that the behavior is part of a disease. Try to identify if anything triggered the behavior and if there is something that the patient needs or wants. Also try to reassure the person and attempt to distract them. For example, you might have

(*Continued*)

TABLE 3.3 A Sample of a Session-by-Session Protocol Developed for the Videocare Project (*Continued*)

Problem Behaviors of Dementia Disorders

your loved one listen to music or take a short walk. Avoid reminding the person that he or she just asked the same question. In some cases, ignoring the behavior or question, though frustrating, may be effective. Also do not discuss plans until immediately prior to an event. You also might want to place signs or cue cards in easy-to-see places to remind the person of upcoming events such as dinner time. Finally, be sure to check with your physician to make sure the person is not in pain or suffering any side effects from prescription medications.

■ **Incontinence**

Many people with Alzheimer's disease or dementia develop problems with bladder control and begin to experience incontinence. This can be upsetting to the person and also be difficult for you as a caregiver. You can manage incontinence by changing the person's routine, clothing, or environment. However, at some point you need to accept that incontinence is a permanent condition of the disease. Initially, it is important to try to find the reason for the loss of control. It may be due to a medical condition, so make sure to discuss it with your physician. It may also be due to stress, problems in the environment, or clothing. To help manage problems with incontinence: develop a routine for taking the person to the bathroom and try to stick to it as much as possible; watch for signs that the person may need to use the bathroom and respond quickly; and try to identify when accidents occur so that you can plan ahead. Also make sure that there is a clear path to the bathroom and that it is easily identified and keep your loved one's clothing simple and practical so that it is easy to remove.Products such as pads or adult diapers may also be helpful. To help prevent problems with nighttime incontinence, limit the person's intake of fluids and drinks such as coffee, tea, or cola. You might also want to consider having a portable toilet near the bed. Finally, if an accident does occur, try to stay calm and be understanding and reassuring. Remember that accidents are embarrassing. Also, be willing to try different techniques and strategies, and remember what works for one person may not work for another.

■ **Communication**

A condition of dementia results in a number of changes that make it difficult for a person to understand and remember what others say. They may also have difficulty expressing their own thoughts and needs—this may be extremely frustrating for you as a caregiver and for the patient as it may contribute to their feelings of loneliness and fear. There are several things you can do to help improve communication and your relationship with your loved one. For example, it is important to reduce distractions and keep background noise to a minimum. You might want to set aside a "quiet place" where you can talk. Try to avoid mixed messages and saying things in front of the person that you do not want them to hear. Make your messages positive and easy to understand—use simple words and try to keep messages short. Also, ask questions and give instructions one step at a time and repeat things if needed. It might be helpful to use signs, labels, and written reminders. Also identify yourself if your loved one has trouble remembering who you are and address them by name. Speak calmly and try to maintain eye contact and stay near the person. It also may be helpful to act out activities you want the person to perform. Try to offer some type of affection such as a smile or a hug. Offer or supply a word if the person is having word-finding difficulties and repeat the last word if they forget what they are saying in midsentence. Remember that the words the person is saying may not reflect exactly what they want and they may repeat words or phrases. Repeat things back to make sure you understand. Finally, be patient and allow enough time for response and be careful not to interrupt or treat the person like a "baby" or as if they were not there.

(Continued)

TABLE 3.3 A Sample of a Session-by-Session Protocol Developed for the Videocare Project (Continued)

Problem Behaviors of Dementia Disorders

Personal hygiene

Personal appearance is important, and helping your loved one with grooming and dressing will allow him or her to maintain a sense of dignity and positive self-esteem. For a person with a condition of dementia, getting dressed can be frustrating and challenging. He or she may experience problems choosing what to wear, how to get clothing on and off, and managing buttons and zippers. To help your loved one with dressing, simplify the choices of clothing for the day and keep closets and drawers free of excess clothing. Help organize the process by establishing a routine and having the person get dressed at the same time each day. Lay out clothes in the order in which they should be put on or provide simple step-by-step instructions. Also, choose clothing that is simple and comfortable and easy to get on and off. For example, select clothing with elastic waists or Velcro instead of buttons, snaps, or hooks. Finally, plan a little extra time so that there is no time pressure.

Bathing can also be difficult and be frightening or unpleasant for a person suffering from dementia. If bathing is a problem, there are some things you can do to make it a more pleasant experience. Try to develop a routine time for the bath or shower, and plan the bath or shower for the day when the patient is most calm and agreeable. Prepare the bathroom in advance. For example, have the towels ready, draw the water in the bathtub and test the temperature, premeasure the shampoo, and keep the bathroom warm and comfortable. Tell the person what you are going to do, step-by-step, and allow him or her to do as much as possible. Respect the person's dignity and recognize that some people may be self-conscious; so have a robe or towel available. Make sure the bathroom is safe by checking the temperature of the water, avoid bubble baths or bath oils, and never leave the person alone in the bath or shower. You can also minimize safety risks by using a handheld shower, nonskid bath mats, a shower bench, and grab bars. Also make sure the floor is free from puddles. Finally, it may not be necessary to bathe everyday—sponge baths may be effective in between baths or showers.

Clinical Note: Review additional topics selected from the CHECK LIST.
Clinical Note: The therapist is encouraged to ask open-ended questions to help the caregiver relate his or her current situation to the information provided. The therapist should validate and track the information provided by the caregiver and link it to the session's educational material.
■ Of the behavior problems I reviewed today, which are you currently facing? ■ What strategies are you using to deal with your loved one's problem behavior? ■ Were there any strategies I covered that you would like to try? ■ What are other behavior problems about which you would like more information?
Clinical Note: Closure of session

1. Provide a brief summary of the material that was covered by *highlighting* and *punctuating* key points of the session through the experiences and comments given by the caregiver.
2. Encourage caregiver to *use the VIDEOCARE* to help him or her obtain more information on the session's topic (*Solutions to Common Problems Menu*).
3. Remind caregiver of the support group sessions.
4. Set the next phone session date.

(Continued)

CONCLUSION

There is no single or agreed upon approach for developing behavioral interventions. All interventions, however, must begin in a period of "discovery" referred to as a "prephase" in which we recommend eight key iterative considerations be accomplished. This discovery phase is critical and occurs regardless of the subsequent pathways that are followed for advancing interventions. The outcomes of this initial stage, directly and critically, inform the very next steps for advancing an intervention.

At the conclusion of a discovery period, one should have a clear understanding of the nature and scope of the identified problem, a specified population in need of an intervention, an understanding of what can be changed and how and why change may occur drawing upon theoretical and conceptual frameworks, identification of potential outcome measures, and knowledge of previous intervention attempts or applicable evidence-based strategies. Also, one should have an idea of how to proceed either with developing a new intervention, augmenting, or modifying an existing intervention, or with comparing interventions. The subsequent testing pathways that are followed are determined in large part by what is revealed in this period of discovery or by what the science requires in addition to the practical considerations including access to or availability of resources such as staff, space, populations, funding, and so forth. Noteworthy is that a discovery period may overlap dynamically with Phase I testing or may itself involve a series of small studies to advance the intervention idea.

In this chapter, we have also offered working tools (Tables 3.2 and 3.3 and Figure 3.1) to help map an intervention. These tools can help to break down the objectives and specific activities related to an intervention. An intervention itself is the heart of the matter and the basis from which all other design and testing decisions are made. Thus, carefully detailing the problem that is to be addressed and its essential features (e.g., contributing factors, at risk populations, pathways amenable to modification) warrants careful attention and continuous consultation with the research literature as well as key stakeholders and end users as suggested by both the elongated and iterative pipelines we have described in Chapter 2 (Figures 2.2 and 2.3).

REFERENCES

Anderson, S. J., Cherutich, P., Kilonzo, N., Cremin, I., Fecht, D., Kimanga, D., ... Hallett, T. B. (2014). Maximising the effect of combination HIV prevention through prioritisation of the people and places in greatest need: A modelling study. *Lancet, 384,* 249–256.

Areán, P. A., & Unützer, J. (2003). Inequities in depression management in low-income, minority, and old-old adults: A matter of access to preferred treatments? *Journal of the American Geriatrics Society, 51*(12), 1808–1809. doi:10.1046/j.1532-5415.2003.51569.x

Bartholomew, L. K., Parcel, G. S., & Kok, G. (1998). Intervention mapping: A process for developing theory and evidence-based health education programs. *Health Education & Behavior, 25*(5), 545–563.

Bernal, G., Jiménez-Chafey, M. I., & Domenech Rodríguez, M. M. (2009). Cultural adaptation of treatments: A resource for considering culture in evidence-based practice. *Professional Psychology: Research and Practice, 40*(4), 361–368.

Craig, P., Dieppe, P., Macintyre, S., Michie, S., Nazareth, I., & Petticrew, M. (2008). Developing and evaluating complex interventions: New guidance. *British Medical Journal, 337,* 979–983. doi:10.1136/bmj.a1655

Czaja, S. J., Loewenstein, D., Schulz, R., Nair, S. N., & Perdomo, D. (2013). A videophone psychosocial intervention for dementia caregivers. *The American Journal of Geriatric Psychiatry, 21,* 1071–1081.

Ebbeling, C. B., Pearson, M. N., Sorensen, G., Levine, R. A., Hebert, J. R., Salkeld, J. A., & Peterson, K. E. (2007). Conceptualization and development of a theory-based healthful eating and physical activity intervention for postpartum women who are low income. *Health Promotion Practice, 8*(1), 50–59.

Eldridge, S., Spencer, A., Cryer, C., Parsons, S., Underwood, M., & Feder, G. (2005). Why modelling a complex intervention is an important precursor to trial design: Lessons from studying an intervention to reduce falls-related injuries in older people. *Journal of Health Services Research & Policy, 10*(3), 133–142.

Fernández, M. E., Gonzales, A., Tortolero-Luna, G., Partida, S., & Bartholomew, L. K. (2005). Using intervention mapping to develop a breast and cervical cancer screening program for Hispanic farmworkers: Cultivando La Salud. *Health Promotion Practice, 6*(4), 394–404.

Gillespie, L. D., Robertson, M. C., Gillespie, W. J., Sherrington, C., Gates, S., Clemson, L. M., & Lamb, S. E. (2012). Interventions for preventing falls in older people living in the community. *Cochrane Database Systematic Review,* (9), CD007146.

Gitlin, L. N. (2014). The role of community and home-based interventions in late life depression. In C. S. Richards & M. W. O'Hara (Eds.), *The oxford handbook of depression and comorbidity* (pp. 511–527). New York, NY: Oxford University Press.

Gitlin, L. N., & Burgh, D. (1995). Issuing assistive devices to older patients in rehabilitation: An exploratory study. *American Journal of Occupational Therapy, 49*(10), 994–1000.

Gitlin, L. N., Chernett, N. L., Harris, L. F., Palmer, D., Hopkins, P., & Dennis, M. P. (2008). Harvest Health: Translation of the chronic disease self-management program for older African Americans in a senior setting. *The Gerontologist: Practice Concepts, 48*(5), 698–705.

Gitlin, L. N., Hauck, W. W., Dennis, M. P., Winter, L., Hodgson, N., & Schinfeld, S. (2009). Long-term effect on mortality of a home intervention that reduces functional difficulties in older adults: Results from a randomized trial. *Journal of the American Geriatrics Society, 57*(3), 476–481.

Gitlin, L. N., Marx, K., Stanley, I. H., & Hodgson, N. (2015). Translating evidence-based dementia caregiving interventions into practice: State-of-the-science and next steps. *The Gerontologist, 55*(2), 210–226. doi:10.1093/geront/gnu123

Gitlin, L. N., Schemm, R. L., Landsberg, L., & Burgh, D. (1996). Factors predicting assistive device use in the home by older persons following rehabilitation. *Journal of Aging and Health, 8*(4), 554–575.

Gitlin, L. N., Winter, L., Dennis, M. P., Corcoran, M., Schinfeld, S., & Hauck, W. W. (2006). A randomized trial of a multicomponent home intervention to reduce functional difficulties in older adults. *Journal of the American Geriatrics Society, 54*(5), 809–816.

Gitlin, L. N., Winter, L., Dennis, M. P., & Hauck, W. W. (2008). Variation in response to a home intervention to support daily function by age, race, sex, and education. *Journal of Gerontology: Medical Sciences, 63A*(7), 745–750.

Heckhausen, J., & Schulz, R. (1995). A life-span theory of control. *Psychological Review, 102*(2), 284–304.

Heckhausen, J., Wrosch, C., & Schulz, R. (2010). A motivational theory of life-span development. *Psychological Review, 117*(1), 32–60. doi:10.1037/a0017668

Hopko, D. R., Lejuez, C. W., Ruggiero, K. J., & Eifert, G. H. (2003). Contemporary behavioral activation treatments for depression: Procedures, principles, and progress. *Clinical Psychology Review, 23*(5), 699–717. doi:10.1016/S0272-7358(03)00070-9

Hou, S. I., Fernandez, M., & Chen, P. H. (2003). Correlates of cervical cancer screening among women in Taiwan. *Health Care for Women International, 24*(5), 384–398.

Koekkoek, B., van Meijel, B., Schene, A., & Hutschemaekers, G. (2010). Development of an intervention program to increase effective behaviours by patients and clinicians in psychiatric services: Intervention mapping study. *BMC Health Services Research, 10*(293), 1–11.

Kunik, M. E., Snow, A. L., Davila, J. A., Steele, A. B., Balasubramanyam, V., Doody, R. S., & Morgan, R. O. (2010). Causes of aggressive behavior in patients with dementia. *The Journal of Clinical Psychiatry, 71*(9), 1145–1152.

Lorig, K. R., Sobel, D. S., Ritter, P. L., Laurent, D., & Hobbs, M. (2001). Effect of a self-management program on patients with chronic disease. *Effective Clinical Practice, 4*(6), 256–262.

McBeth, J., & Cordingley, L. (2009). Current issues and new direction in psychology and health: Epidemiology and health psychology—Please bridge the gap. *Psychology and Health, 24*(8), 861–865.

McCannon, C. J., Berwick, D. M., & Massoud, M. R. (2007). The science of large-scale change in global health. *JAMA, 298*(16), 1937–1939.

McEachan, R. R., Lawton, R. J., Jackson, C., Conner, M., & Lunt, J. (2008). Evidence, theory and context: Using intervention mapping to develop a worksite physical activity intervention. *BMC Public Health, 8*(1), 326. doi:10.1186/1471-2458-8-326

Medical Research Council. (2000). *A framework for development and evaluation of RCTs for complex interventions to improve health.* Retrieved from www.mrc.ac.uk/documents/pdf/complex-interventions-guidance/

Nagi, S. Z. (1964). A study in the evaluation of disability and rehabilitation potential: Concepts, methods, and procedures. *American Journal of Public Health and the Nation's Health, 54*(9), 1568–1579.

Spillman, B. C., & Long, S. K. (2009). Does high caregiver stress predict nursing home entry? *Inquiry, 46*(2), 140–161.

Verbrugge, L. M., & Jette, A. M. (1994). The disablement process. *Social Sciences and Medicine, 38*, 1–14.

Zatzick, D., Rivara, F., Jurkovich, G., Russo, J., Trusz, S. G., Wang, J., … Katon, W. (2011). Enhancing the population impact of collaborative care interventions: Mixed method development and implementation of stepped care targeting posttraumatic stress disorder and related comorbidities after acute trauma. *General Hospital Psychiatry, 33*(2), 123–134.

FOUR

THEORY: A DRIVER OF BEHAVIORAL INTERVENTION RESEARCH

> *. . . there is nothing so practical as a good theory.*
> —Lewin (1951, p. 169)

Theory is one of the key drivers of behavioral intervention research. Nevertheless, its role in the development, evaluation, and implementation phases of a behavioral intervention is not clearly understood or fully recognized. Unfortunately, theory continues to be undervalued and underutilized and to receive little attention in the planning and publication of behavioral intervention research (Glanz & Bishop, 2010; The Improved Clinical Effectiveness through Behavioural Research Group [ICEBeRG], 2006).

The importance of theory in guiding intervention development, evaluation, and implementation should not be underestimated. The explicit use of theory can help to identify the treatment components and delivery characteristics of an intervention; to appraise the selection of outcome measures and an understanding of how and why desired outcomes are achieved; to inform as to the replication potential of a proven intervention; and to shed light as to why implementation is successful or not. Theories can also help to explain why some people actively engage in an intervention and others do not, thus informing intervention design and the selection of strategies for enhancing the delivery of an intervention to boost its effects for targeted individuals.

Interventions that are atheoretical or derived without a conceptual foundation do not advance an understanding of behavior change, how and why particular outcomes from an intervention are achieved, or how and why the implementation of the intervention is effective. Interventions that are grounded in a theory or conceptual framework tend to be more effective than those lacking one (Glanz & Bishop, 2010). Using theory also greatly enhances the potential for replication by helping to identify the essential components of an intervention that must be maintained and the most effective mechanisms for its implementation (Glanz & Bishop, 2010; ICEBeRG, 2006).

Our goal in this chapter is to examine the role of theory in behavioral intervention research. We first define theory and examine its specific and differential roles in each phase of the pipeline (Chapter 2). Through exemplars, we articulate the linkage of theoretical frameworks to treatment components and intervention delivery characteristics. Then we examine principles for selecting a theory/conceptual framework and the key challenges in using theories.

WHAT IS THEORY?

So, what is theory? Theory has been variably defined. For our purposes, we draw upon Kerlinger's definition of theory in his classic textbook, *Foundations of Behavioral Research* (1986), as it is comprehensive and useful. Kerlinger defines theory as

> a set of interrelated constructs, definitions, and propositions that present a systematic view of phenomena by specifying relations among variables, with the purpose of explaining or predicting phenomena. (p. 9).

In this definition, theory refers to a systematic way of understanding events, behaviors, and/or situations. It reflects a set of interrelated concepts, definitions, and propositions that explain or predict events and situations by specifying relationships among variables. Thus, the purpose of theory is to provide a roadmap or pathway among constructs, definitions, and propositions as well as their relationships to promote an understanding of the phenomenon of interest and to enable prediction of outcomes (DePoy & Gitlin, 2015). Simply put, the purpose of theory is to explain and predict events.

Theories differ with regard to scope and levels of abstraction and specificity and are often categorized into one of three levels, although there is not necessarily consensus on this nor which theories should be included in each of the levels. At the broadest level there are "grand theories," which function at a very high level of abstraction. This level of theory focuses mostly on social structure and social processes such as how financial strain affects psychosocial well-being.

Grand theories typically lack operational definitions or clarity as to the relationships among their propositions and constructs and are used to understand or encompass an entire field. Examples include critical theory or structuralism or Orem's self-care deficit theory (Bengtson, Burgess, & Parrott, 1997; Dowd, 1988; Taylor, Geden, Isaramalai, & Wongvatunyu, 2000).

In contrast, "midrange" theories can be derived from a grand theory and are less abstract. Midrange theories are composed of operationally defined propositions and constructs that are testable. This level of theory is the most useful for behavioral intervention research, and some of the most commonly used are described in Table 4.1.

Finally, "micro" level theories can be specific to particular populations, fields, or phenomena and have the narrowest scope and level of abstraction. Also referred to as "practice- or situation-specific" theories, they are useful in clinical situations or the study of small-scale structures. They typically focus on the individual level and/or social interactions, with symbolic interactionism, social phenomenology, and exchange theory as prime examples.

Regardless of level, a well-developed theory is one which yields testable hypotheses and has some empirical evidence to support its value. Although theories may be rooted in distinct philosophical traditions and categorized variably, that is not our concern here. Our approach is practical. For the purposes of this chapter, we use the terms "theory," "conceptual frameworks," and "models" interchangeably and view each as working tools for advancing behavioral interventions. We also do not differentiate between levels of theories (macro, mid, or micro). Our message

TABLE 4.1   Examples of Select Theories Commonly Used in Behavioral Intervention Research

Theory	Brief Explanation of Model
1. Health Belief Model (HBM) (Rosenstock, 1974)	People will be motivated to avoid a health threat if they believe they are at risk ("perceived susceptibility") for the disease/condition and if they deem it serious ("perceived severity"). These two necessary conditions—perceived susceptibility and perceived severity—converge to describe "perceived threat," the central construct of HBM. Perceived threat is also influenced by "cues to action," which are environmental stimuli such as advertisement campaigns and relatives who have the disease; cues to action extend this individual-level theory into an ecological perspective. An individual's decision to engage in health behaviors is further influenced by the counterbalance between "perceived barriers" and "perceived benefits." The HBM comprises all of these factors, moderated by demographic characteristics. In 1988, Rosenstock and colleagues added to the model an additional construct—"self-efficacy"—to capture individual perceptions of confidence to perform a behavior.
2. Health Action Process Approach (HAPA) (Schwarzer, 2008)	HAPA theorizes that *intention to change* is the most potent predictor of whether an individual will actually change his or her undesirable behavior to a more desirable one. Within this framework, HAPA proposes two stages of motivation: (1) "preintentional motivation" and (2) "postintentional volition." Preintentional processes (e.g., outcome expectancies, risk perception, action self-efficacy) result in the emergence of intention, whereas postintentional processes (e.g., maintenance self-efficacy, planning) result in the actual behavior being enacted.
3. Theory of Reasoned Action (TRA) (Ajzen & Fishbein, 1980)	An individual will engage in a health behavior if he or she has the *intention* to do so. Intention is composed of two main elements: "attitudes" and "subjective norms." Attitudes are operationalized as the belief that one's behavior will result in positive health outcomes ("behavioral beliefs") and is also dependent on the degree to which one values these positive health outcomes ("evaluation"). Subjective norms are operationalized as the appraisal of whether others will approve or disapprove of one's behavior ("normative beliefs") and whether or not the individual is affected by these normative beliefs ("motivation to comply").
4. Theory of Planned Behavior (TPB) (Ajzen & Madden, 1986)	TPB is incremental to TRA with the addition of the construct "perceived behavioral control." Perceived behavioral control is conceptualized as the degree to which an individual perceives a specific behavior as either *easy* or *difficult* to enact.
5. Life-Span Theory of Control (Heckhausen & Schulz, 1995) and Motivational Theory of Life-Span Development (Heckhausen et al., 2010)	Life-Span Theory of Control suggests that threats to, or actual losses in the ability to, control important outcomes may activate individuals to use strategies to buffer threats and losses. To the extent that control-oriented behavioral and cognitive strategies are used that are directed toward attaining valued goals, threats to, or actual losses of, control may be minimized and positive affect enhanced.

is simple: Interventions must be built upon theoretical and/or conceptual foundations. Theory/conceptual frameworks structure each phase of design, evaluation, and implementation of an intervention; as such, different theories/frameworks may be drawn upon and utilized depending upon phase, specific research questions being addressed, and the focus or objectives of a behavioral intervention.

DEDUCTIVE REASONING APPROACH

The use of theory in the context of behavioral intervention research reflects a deductive approach. That is, a theory is specified a priori to the formal evaluation of an intervention, and testable hypotheses are derived that articulate one or more pathways by which the intervention may have its desired effects. The hypotheses reflect the expected relationships between two or more concepts of the theory that can be evaluated and indicate what is expected to be observed on the basis of the principles of the theory (DePoy & Gitlin, 2015). It is important to point out that the outcomes of intervention research can also inform or refine theories or models of behavior. That is, the use of theory in intervention work reflects in part a test of the theory itself or its specific tenets, which in turn can prove, disprove, or advance the theoretical tenets.

The deductive use of theory in behavioral intervention research is in contrast to an inductive approach. A ground-up, generative, or inductive approach is used mostly for theory development or refinement and involves constructing or building theory using primarily qualitative methodologies.

An example of the utility of a conceptual framework in structuring an intervention and deriving specific hypotheses is illustrated by Rovner and colleagues' (2012) intervention to reduce cognitive decline in persons with a medical diagnosis of mild cognitive impairment (MCI-MD).

> We based this trial on the Disablement Process Model, which is a sociomedical model that describes how medical diseases affect functioning in specific body systems and lead to disability. The model posits that disability is part of a complex relationship between health conditions and contextual (i.e. environmental and personal) factors. In this model, a MCI-MD, as a possible preclinical AD state, reflects a physiologic dysfunction that results in diminished memory and initiative (disability), where environmental factors (i.e., activity participation) may "speed up" or "slow down" this core pathway. We propose to increase activity levels and thereby "slow down" progression to disability. (Rovner et al., 2012, p. 714)

As illustrated, this deductive, a priori use of a framework leads investigators to identify a target for the intervention (e.g., in the previous case, activity level) and the selection of expected outcomes (e.g., slower progression of memory loss).

ROLE OF THEORY ALONG THE PIPELINE

The specific role of theory in informing an intervention and its development depends upon the phase of the intervention along the pipeline. Figure 4.1 illustrates

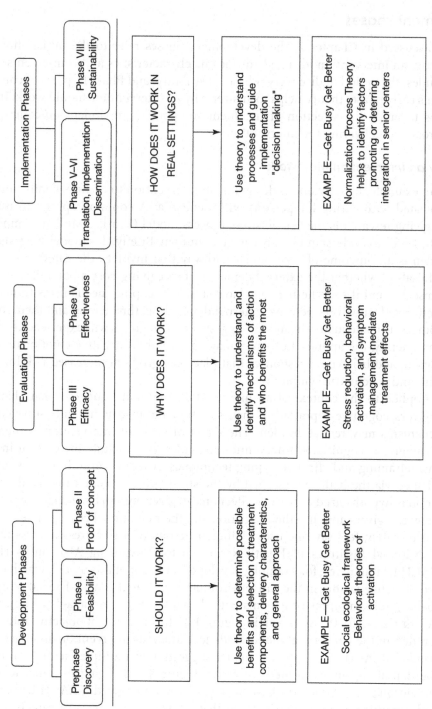

Figure 4.1 Role of theory in development, evaluation, and implementation phases.

the changing role of theory and the specific questions that a theory addresses at each phase of advancing an intervention.

Development Phases

As discussed in Chapter 2, the development phases refer to the initial efforts to identify an intervention idea and advance its characteristics and components. This includes: the period of discovery; Phase I, feasibility; and Phase II, proof of concept. In this early phase, theory helps to answer why an intervention should work. It also helps to guide the selection of treatment components, treatment outcomes, and approach to delivering the intervention.

Why an Intervention May Work

As an example, let's say one is designing an intervention to address family burdens associated with caring for persons with dementia. A common approach used in caregiving research is the classic stress process model (Pearlin, Mullan, Semple, & Skaff, 1990) to understand family caregiver burden. Briefly, this model suggests that burden is an outcome of a particular pathway that involves the caregivers' initial appraisals of whether the external demands of caregiving pose a potential threat to themselves and if so, whether they have sufficient coping mechanisms to manage effectively. If caregivers perceive external demands as threatening and their coping resources as inadequate, the model suggests that caregivers will experience burden. Consequently, the appraisal of stress may contribute to negative emotional, physiological, and behavioral responses that place caregivers at increased risk for poor health and psychiatric symptoms.

Applied to the context of an intervention, the model suggests that changing caregivers' cognitive appraisals of their situation and instructing in positive coping mechanisms may reduce burden. The target of such an intervention is therefore the caregivers' cognitions. Intervention activities may include instruction in cognitive reframing and effective coping techniques. A reduction in burden would be explained via the pathway outlined by the stress process model; that is, the intervention is hypothesized to have its effect on caregiver burden by changing cognition or how caregivers appraise their situation and their emotional coping style.

Alternately, let's say one uses a different iteration of the stress process model. The National Institutes of Health Resources for Enhancing Alzheimer's Health (REACH II) initiatives, for example, developed a variant of this model, which recognized objective factors in the care environment such as the lack of social resources or behavioral symptoms of persons with dementia (Schulz, Gallagher-Thompson, Haley, & Czaja, 2000). As shown in Figure 4.2, the inclusion of objective indicators of burden in the conceptual model leads to a different intervention approach. The expanded REACH stress process model suggests that multiple factors contribute to burden along the explicated pathways. Figure 4.2 thus suggests that to boost intervention impact, each of these factors should be targeted. REACH II therefore tested a multicomponent intervention that addressed five areas of caregiver risks for burden. These components and their associated activities included caregiver depression through the provision of education and mood management techniques including pleasant event activities; caregiver burden through the provision of

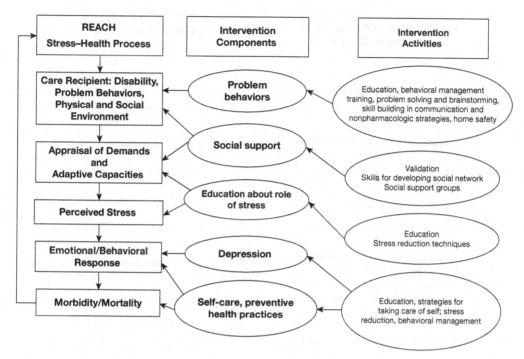

Figure 4.2 Role of theory in guiding treatment components and specific activities of the REACH II intervention.

education, instruction in stress reduction techniques, and specific skills to manage problem behaviors; self-care and healthy behaviors through the provision of education, helping caregivers track self-care practices; social support by providing opportunities to participate in tele-education and support sessions; and addressing problem behaviors through a structured problem-solving and brainstorming approach to identify specific strategies. As illustrated, even a seemingly small change to a conceptual model alters the intervention focus, its treatment components, and delivery characteristics.

Yet another example of the role of theory in intervention development is the Get Busy Get Better (GBGB) program designed to address depressive symptoms in older African Americans (Gitlin et al., 2012). This multicomponent intervention draws upon several complementary theoretical approaches. First, it uses a broad social ecological model of depression. This model suggests that situational factors (e.g., financial, housing, or health concerns) may provide low levels of positive reinforcement and minimal control, thus negatively impinging upon mood.

Second, GBGB draws upon behavioral theories of depression, which suggest that depressed affect is the consequence of environmental contingencies that decrease healthy responses within one's behavioral repertoire and increase avoidance of aversive stimuli (Hopko, Lejuez, Ruggiero, & Eifert, 2003). Behavioral theories further suggest that becoming activated can help individuals break the behavior–mood cycle by moving a person from avoidance to action (Hopko et al., 2003).

On the basis of these complementary frameworks, GBGB was designed to involve five conceptually linked components as shown in Figure 4.3: care management

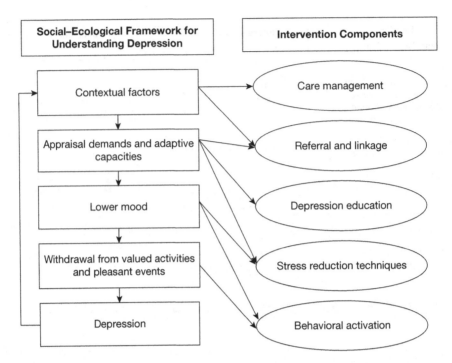

Figure 4.3 Theoretical frameworks informing the Get Busy Get Better intervention.

involving a comprehensive assessment to identify unmet needs; referrals and linkages to minimize situational or environmental stressors; education about depression symptoms and specific actions for self-management to enhance cognitive and behavioral self-awareness; instruction in stress reduction techniques to provide immediate relief from stressful situations; and behavioral activation by identifying a valued activity goal and specific steps to achieve it. The working hypothesis based on these conceptual frameworks is that treatment components operate in tandem such that each is necessary to bring about reductions in depression. This is a testable hypothesis that can be examined through mediation analyses in an evaluation phase, as discussed later.

Here is yet another example of how theory informs hypothesis generation, choice of treatment components, delivery characteristics and outcomes, and in turn the link to anticipated underlying mechanisms of an intervention designed to reduce maternal gestational diabetes mellitus (GDM) and delivery of a large for gestational age (LGA) infant.

The protocol presented here describes a complex behavioral intervention comprising dietary and physical activity changes which we have developed with the aim of improving glycemic control in obese pregnant women. The intervention is based on established control theory with elements of social cognitive theory. The primary hypothesis being tested is that an antenatal intervention package of low glycemic dietary advice combined with advice on increased physical activity will reduce the incidence of maternal GDM and LGA infants. A secondary hypothesis is that the intervention will reduce the risk of obesity in the child. (Briley et al., 2014, p. 3)

Selecting Delivery Characteristics

Thus far we have discussed how theory/conceptual frameworks frame an intervention, inform the targets of an intervention (e.g., cognition, behavior, social and/or physical environments) and provide an understanding as to why an intervention should work. However, theory can do even more at the development phases—it can help guide selection of delivery characteristics or the approach to delivering the intervention.

The specific approach to intervening or delivering an intervention may assume various forms depending upon the theoretical lens that is applied, practical considerations, and the empirical evidence as to what constitutes effective approaches. Chapter 5 examines delivery characteristics in depth. However, here our focus is on specifically the role of theory in informing the selection of delivery characteristics.

In our first example discussed earlier of a caregiver intervention to address burden through cognitive reframing, different delivery strategies could be employed on the basis of the theoretical lens that is adopted. For instance, adult learning theories emphasize situational-based and practice-oriented learning techniques. This could involve face-to-face sessions and learning through doing, which would be in contrast to a didactic and/or prescriptive approach. Alternatively, behavior change theories emphasize the role of peer-based and group-learning situations, suggesting the value of imparting new coping strategies through group meetings and exercises and peer-led programs.

The delivery characteristics of the REACH II intervention were shaped by several principles from adult-learning theories. These included: activities need to occur within the context in which the education and new skills would be applied or actually used; repeated exposure to new information and skills is needed for their integration into daily care routines; and education and skills are best offered and subsequently adopted when perceived as needed. Thus, the intervention was subsequently delivered in the home, activities were adjusted to areas of most concern to caregivers, and education was reinforced through the use of a telephone computer system (Belle et al., 2006). This illustrates the link of theory, models, and principles to the design of treatment components and delivery characteristics.

To illustrate these points further, we use, as an example, an intervention that is designed to reduce behavioral symptoms in persons with dementia through a nonpharmacologic approach. Behavioral symptoms, such as repetitive vocalizations, agitation, aggressiveness, wandering, rejection of care, and restlessness, are almost universal in dementia and can be troublesome to persons with dementia and their caregivers. Pharmacological approaches do not address the most troublesome behaviors, and their risks, including mortality, may cause more harm than the benefit derived (Gitlin, Kales, & Lyketsos, 2012).

Nonpharmacologic approaches conceptualize behavioral symptoms as, in large part, expressions of unmet needs (e.g., repetitive vocalizations for auditory stimulation); inadvertently reinforced behavior in the face of an environmental trigger (e.g., the patient learns that screaming attracts increased attention); and/or consequences of a mismatch between the environment and the patient's ability to process and act upon cues, expectations, and demands (Algase et al., 1996; Cohen-Mansfield, 2001). These approaches involve modifying cognitions, behaviors, environments, or precipitating events that may contribute to disturbances, or involve using compensatory strategies to reduce for persons with dementia their increased vulnerability to their environment (Kales, Gitlin, & Lyketsos, 2015). More specifically, one conceptual model, the Progressively Lowered Stress Threshold (PLST), proposes that, with disease progression, individuals with dementia experience increasing vulnerability and a lower threshold to stress and external stimuli (Hall & Buckwalter, 1987). One source of stress for persons with dementia is the complexity of routine activities of living and interactions with caregivers (formal and informal), which become increasingly challenging as the day progresses (Hall & Buckwalter, 1987). PLST suggests that, by minimizing environmental demands that exceed the functional capacity of an individual and by regulating activity and stimulation levels throughout the day, agitation can be reduced. Complementing this framework is the Competence–Environmental Press Model (CEPM; Lawton & Nahemow, 1973), which suggests that there are optimal combinations of environmental circumstances or conditions and personal competencies that result in the highest possible functioning for individuals. Obtaining the just-right-fit between an individual's capabilities and external demands of environments/activities results in adaptive, positive behaviors; alternately, environments/activities that are too demanding or understimulating may result in behavioral symptoms such as agitation or passivity in individuals with dementia. Similar to PLST, the CEPM suggests that environments/activities can be modified to fit any level of cognitive functioning and individual competencies in order to optimize quality of life. Both frameworks suggest that behaviors can be reduced or managed by modifying contributing factors that place too much demand or press on the individual with dementia. Such factors may include the physical environment (e.g., auditory and visual distractions), the social environment (e.g., communication style of informal/formal caregivers), or factors that are modifiable but which are internal to the individual themselves (e.g., discomfort, pain, fatigue).

Thus, to recapitulate, frameworks such as the Unmet Needs Model, the Progressively Lower Stress Threshold Process Model, or CEPM inform why nonpharmacologic approaches may effectively prevent, minimize, or manage troublesome behavioral symptoms. The stress process models described earlier in this chapter inform how minimizing an objective stressor such as behavioral symptoms may lower caregiver burden. So we now have a strong theoretical basis for a nonpharmacologic intervention and how it may impact both persons with dementia and family caregivers.

However, use of nonpharmacologic strategies for persons at the moderate to severe stage of dementia is totally dependent upon the willingness and ability of family caregivers to effectively implement them. Families may be so overwhelmed by the care situation that they are unable to use nonpharmacologic strategies although their use may be of potential help to them. Some caregivers may be more "ready" than others to learn about and enact strategies that require behavioral change on their part (e.g., employing different communication strategies or rearranging the physical environment), and their readiness may affect participation in and the benefits derived from the intervention for the person with dementia. Now we need a theory or conceptual framework to understand how to effectively engage families in the intervention process.

To this end, we can draw upon the Transtheoretical Model (TTM) (Prochaska, DiClemente, & Norcross, 1992). TTM has been widely used in behavior change interventions including smoking cessation, exercise, and other healthy lifestyle programs. The model suggests that to change and adopt new behaviors is complex and involves five incremental stages. These include precontemplation in which individuals do not consider changing their behavior, nor are they aware of the consequences of their behavior. Applied to caregivers, those at this stage may view behavioral symptoms of dementia as intentional and be unaware how their communications contribute to these symptoms. In contemplation, individuals are aware a problem exists and may begin to consider how to address the problem. At this stage, caregivers may understand behavioral symptoms as a disease consequence but not recognize the consequences of their own behaviors. The preparation stage is characterized by intention to take action and a positive orientation to behavior change; caregivers at this stage are ready to develop an action plan such as seeking information or learning about nonpharmacologic strategies. When behavior is consistently modified, individuals are considered to be in the action stage such as a caregiver who actively uses effective communication strategies. Maintenance occurs when the desired behavioral change is sustained for 6 months or more (Prochaska et al., 1992).

TTM can help inform effective approaches for intervening with families as illustrated in Figure 4.4. Families with an initially low level of readiness may require more education about dementia and behavioral symptoms than those at a high level of readiness. Similarly, those at a low level of readiness may need more time in the intervention. The interventionist may need to proceed slowly so as to not overwhelm the caregivers and to move them to a higher level of readiness in which they are willing and able to implement effective nonpharmacologic strategies. Thus, in this case example, the construct of readiness based in TTM can help inform how to tailor and deliver information and the pace of the intervention (Gitlin & Rose, 2014).

Evaluation Phases

Theory informs the evaluation phases (Phase III—efficacy; and Phase IV—effectiveness) of an intervention somewhat differently than we have discussed thus far (Figure 4.1). At this stage of an intervention's development, theory provides a basis for understanding the underlying mechanisms of action or how the intervention might result in positive outcomes. It also guides an understanding as to why and whether some groups or individuals may benefit from the intervention more than others (Gitlin et al., 2000).

More specifically, if an intervention is proven to be efficacious, then it is necessary to understand why and examine the pathways by which positive results have been achieved. Mediation and moderation analyses are typically the statistical approaches that are employed for these purposes. The specific hypotheses tested and variables selected for these analytic models must be informed by the theory or theories that underlie the intervention. As suggested earlier, the analyses in turn serve as a validation of the theory or theories and related hypotheses that frame the intervention. These analytic strategies help to examine the relationships among constructs and concepts of a theory and either verify, modify, refine, or refute them.

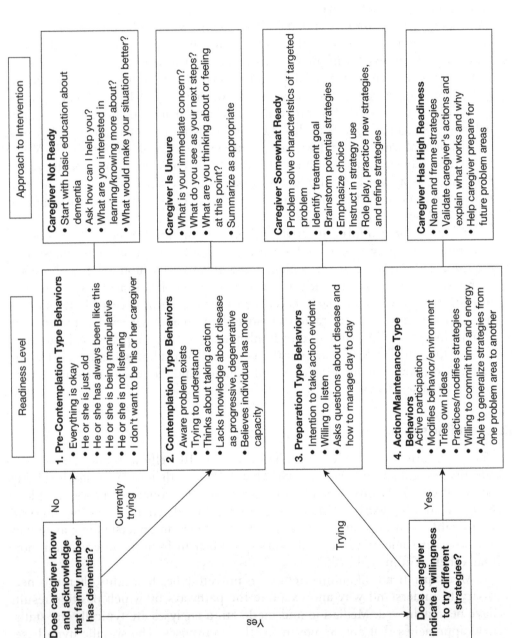

Figure 4.4 Use of behavioral change framework to guide delivery of an intervention.

In the earlier examples using the stress process models, one could evaluate whether an intervention reduces caregiver burden by mitigating an objective stressor such as the problem behaviors of persons with dementia. Similarly, one could test whether improving social support reduces burden. Mediation analyses could be used to test the independent and joint contributions of multiple mechanisms such as improving social support and reducing problem behaviors (Roth, Mittelman, Clay, Madan, & Haley, 2005).

The GBGB program was tested in an efficacy trial with 208 older African Americans. The Phase III trial demonstrated that the intervention group had reduced depressive symptoms and improved daily function and quality of life compared to a wait-list control group at 4 months. Furthermore, after receiving the intervention, the delayed treatment group similarly benefited (Gitlin et al., 2013). The social ecological model would suggest that multiple pathways were responsible for these outcomes. Behavioral activation theories would suggest that becoming behaviorally activated was the primary pathway in which depression reductions were achieved, although the other treatment components are necessary and support activation.

Mediation analyses confirmed that changes in depressive symptoms were achieved through multiple pathways and not exclusively through activation. The reduction of stress, the improvement of depression knowledge, use of self-management techniques, and activation, all variables linked to the applied broad theoretical framework of the intervention (Figure 4.3), were jointly responsible for the significant reductions in depressive symptomatology. That is, activation was not the only mechanism by which depression was reduced (Gitlin, Roth, & Huang, 2014). These findings support the theoretical models and suggest that a condition for engaging in behavioral activation is that immediate environmental stressors must be addressed in concert with helping people achieve behavioral change. The findings also have important implications for GBGB's translation and implementation into real-world settings. They suggest that all treatment components must be delivered in order to achieve positive benefits.

Furthermore, as the intervention was tailored to individual needs, differences in outcomes by demographic subgroups were not expected. This was shown to be the case through moderation analyses, which revealed that all participants benefited similarly as hypothesized; that is, men and women, those living alone or with others, and those with greater financial distress or without financial difficulties improved equally (Szanton, Thorpe, & Gitlin, 2014). This finding supports the notion that tailoring to the needs and personal behavioral goals of participants seems to be effective and an important delivery characteristic of this intervention.

To summarize, as the examples in this section demonstrate, theory at the evaluative phases can help guide selection of outcomes measures, explain mechanisms by which observed changes are achieved, and identify who may have benefited more or less and why.

Implementation Phases

Theory has still yet another role in the implementation phases of behavioral intervention research (Phase V—translation/implementation; Phase VI—diffusion/dissemination; Phase VII—sustainability). In these latter phases, theory informs an understanding of specific implementation processes such as the contextual barriers to, and supports of the adoption of, a proven intervention within settings and by interventionists and end users. Specifically, theory helps identify what components of the intervention could be modified or eliminated, the immutable elements or aspects that cannot be changed, organizational and contextual features impinging on implementation, and strategies for streamlining the intervention to enhance implementation potential. Using theory to identify and sort through contributory organizational or contextual characteristics is essential at this phase.

An exemplar is the use of Normalization Process Theory (NPT) to understand the potential of GBGB to be implemented in senior centers and other community-based agencies (May et al., 2009). This particular theory identifies four factors that can inform implementation potential. Briefly, these are "coherence" or whether an intervention is easy to describe and understand; "cognitive participation" or whether users consider it a good idea; "collective work" or how the program affects agency staff; and "reflexive monitoring" or how users of the program will perceive it.

As to the first factor, GBGB demonstrated high coherence: Staff and older African American participants alike understood and recognized the program and its benefits. As supporting positive mental health is the expressed mission of senior centers, GBGB fits within their organizational goals. With regard to cognitive participation, initially care managers responsible for screening for depressive symptoms did not value using a systematic screening tool and believed that their own appraisals were sufficient. However, through training, ongoing use, and supervisory support, care managers learned that their judgments were often incorrect and that screening afforded a more systematic and accurate approach to depression detection. Similarly, initially interventionists believed that they already practiced many of the elements of GBGB and therefore the intervention was not necessarily novel to them. This is a common reaction to behavioral interventions. However, with training and use, interventionists were able to differentiate GBGB from their own traditional mental health practices and became invested in the program. Older African American participants in the program found it highly valuable and perceived the program worthy of their investment of time and energy.

The third NPT factor, "collective work," presents as the most challenging for GBGB. As most senior centers or community-based agencies do not have the capacity to engage in depression care, GBGB would require a change in work practices and flow. Staff training and employment of skilled professionals would be critical to implement GBGB, and this may be difficult for agencies with limited budgets and staffing.

The fourth consideration, "reflexive monitoring," suggests that the value of GBGB was perceived positively by both interventionists and participants alike. Thus, NPT suggests two potential areas that present as critical challenges when implementing GBGB in real-world settings: accounting for and helping agencies adjust their work flow and payment mechanisms; and tweaking training efforts so that interventionists come to understand the benefits of the program sooner rather than later (Gitlin, Harris, McCoy, Hess, & Hauck, in press).

As specific theories have been developed to understand ways to embed evidence-based interventions in practice settings, Chapter 19 provides a more in-depth discussion of the role of theory in the implementation phase and specific theories that help to guide implementation processes.

SELECTING A THEORY OR CONCEPTUAL FRAMEWORK

There is not an agreed upon set of criteria, operational guidance, recipe, or step-by-step approach for selecting theories or conceptual frameworks to guide intervention development, evaluation, or their wide-scale implementation (French et al., 2012). However, we recommend several actions be taken. First, it is important to identify the specific phase along the pipeline that reflects the level of the intervention's development. Placement along the pipeline helps to anchor the specific research questions that will be asked and thus the role of the theory/conceptual framework (e.g., see Figure 4.1). Second, a literature review should be conducted to identify the ways in which the targeted problem area has been previously addressed, including the theories employed to understand it. Also, a literature review should be used to consider the empirical evidence as to how and why the problem area occurs, which may in turn help to suggest an appropriate theoretical framework for proceeding with an intervention. Third, selecting a theory/conceptual framework at any phase along the pipeline will depend upon one's intent, preferred approach to understanding and explaining phenomenon, and the target of change. As to the latter, different theories are needed depending upon whether the target of the intervention is at the individual (behavioral, cognitive, affective, knowledge), interpersonal, community, organization, or at the policy level (National Cancer Institute, 2005). Minimally, the theory or conceptual framework that is ultimately selected should be well developed and have some supportive empirical evidence for its basic tenets.

The Medical Research Council also recommends applying several self-reflective questions to guide theory selection (www.mrc.ac/uk/complexinterventionsguidance). These include what follows: Are you clear about what you are trying to do? What outcome are you aiming for? How will you bring about change? Does your intervention have a coherent theoretical basis? Have you used theory systematically to develop the intervention? These are essential questions that can guide theory selection.

The Improved Clinical Effectiveness through Behavioural Research Group (ICEBeRG) (2006) has identified six factors to consider when selecting a theory for implementation science. These include determining the origins of the theory (e.g., is there evidence to support its basic tenets?); examining the concepts of the theory and their interrelationships; evaluating the consistency of the theory (e.g., is there a logical structure?); considering the extent to which generalizations can be made on the basis of the theory and whether there is parsimony (e.g., can the theory be stated simply and clearly?); determining if the theory can generate testable hypotheses; and evaluating its utility (e.g., whether the theory is helpful in understanding or predicting outcomes).

COMMONLY USED THEORIES IN BEHAVIORAL INTERVENTION RESEARCH

As we have suggested, there is not a singular theory or conceptual framework that dominates behavioral intervention research or which is appropriate for use by all behavioral intervention studies. However, most effective public health and health promotion interventions tend to embrace or begin with an ecological perspective at the broadest level as shown with the earlier GBGB example (Glanz & Bishop, 2010;

Noar, 2005). Explanatory theories as to why behaviors occur and change theories to suggest best ways to influence behavior change are also very useful within the ecological perspective. Some of the most common theories framing behavioral intervention research include Social Learning Theory; Theory of Reasoned Action; Health Belief Model; Social Cognitive Theory, self-efficacy; Theory of Planned Behavior; and TTM of Stages of Behavior Change (Glanz & Bishop, 2010), and these are described in more detail in Table 4.1. Also, as shown by Table 4.1, theories are not static; they evolve and are refined over time as new data emerge that necessitate incremental changes to the tenets of the theory/model. For example, the Health Belief Model was originally proposed in 1974 (Rosenstock, 1974), but in 1988, it was expanded to include the construct of self-efficacy (Rosenstock, Strecher, & Becker, 1988). Further, Heckhausen and colleagues originally proposed the Life-Span Theory of Control in 1995, but in 2010, they presented an expanded version of the theory, the Motivational Theory of Life-Span Development on the basis of theoretical advancements and empirical research on goal engagement/disengagement (Heckhausen & Schulz, 1995; Heckhausen, Wrosch, & Schulz, 2010). The Life-Span Theory of Control sought to explain the processes by which individuals choose goals to optimize control. Their more recent theoretical work integrates this and other related models to provide a more comprehensive framework for understanding personal agency throughout the life span.

Similarly, the Theory of Planned Behavior extended the Theory of Reasoned Action by adding the construct of "perceived behavioral control," conceptualized as the degree to which an individual perceives a specific behavior as either easy or difficult to enact (Ajzen & Fishbein, 1980; Ajzen & Madden, 1986). Thus, theories are not static. Rather, they change and advance over time as hypotheses are tested and new data emerge that support or refute the propositions, relationships, constructs, and concepts suggested by a theory.

Table 4.1 is not an inclusive list nor should it be construed that these are the only theories to consider or use in behavioral intervention research. Rather, the table represents a starting point for considering ways to inform intervention development and evaluation.

USING MORE THAN ONE THEORY

As there are typically multiple determinants of health and behaviors, an intervention may need to be informed by more than one theory. This is particularly the case for complex health and psychosocial problems in which no single action alone may have a positive effect. Rather, a multicomponent approach informed by one or more theories may be more effective. As multiple pathways may need to be targeted to bring about the expected changes, one theoretical framework may complement another and together explain the different conduits by which the intervention has its impact. Similarly, if the intervention targets a dyad, let's say a caregiver and the person receiving care, different theories may be needed to articulate the specific pathways by which outcomes are achieved for each party, such as the example of an intervention targeting the behavioral symptoms of persons with dementia. These points are illustrated in the examples described earlier.

Furthermore, multiple theories may be necessary if an intervention is multi-modal. A multimodal intervention includes treatment components that intervene through different mechanisms of action. For example, an intervention designed to enhance cognitive abilities by impacting physiological reserve through a physical exercise program and cognitive reserve through a cognitive training program would require multiple theories to understand these distinct potential pathways.

The challenge in using more than one theory is to logically and systematically link them coherently (Michie & Prestwich, 2010). Here is an example of how investigators integrated different frameworks to form a strong rationale for an intervention designed to reduce risk for HIV and sexually transmitted diseases (STDs).

> The theoretical framework for the Eban HIV/STD Risk Reduction Intervention integrates components of social cognitive theory (SCT) and an Afrocentric paradigm into a relationship-oriented ecological framework that addresses multilevel risk and protective factors associated with HIV/STD risk reduction among African American HIV- serodiscordant couples. SCT informed the factors in the ecological model that are referred to as ontogenic- or personal-level and micro- or interpersonal-level factors. These SCT tenets are designed to build individual's and couples' self-efficacy, behavioral skills, and positive outcome expectancies with respect to HIV/STDs prevention. SCT behavior change strategies implemented in sessions include guided practice with rewards, modeling of behavioral skills (e.g., condom use) and communication and negotiation skills, and problem solving and decision-making. The intervention design incorporates an Afrocentric paradigm by organizing session content around discussions of one or more of the 7 principles of Nguzo Saba, which are aimed at addressing community-level or macro- structural-level factors. Through the use of these principles, African American couples learn to link the practice of safer sex to enhancement of cultural and gender pride and to an overall more positive way of living based on a healthy balance between self-protection and peer/community support. (NIMH Multisite HIV/STD Prevention Trial for African American Couples Group, 2008, pp. S16–S17)

Locher et al. (2011) also clearly explain how two theoretical approaches are used complementarily to inform the Behavioral Nutrition Intervention for Community Elders (B-NICE).

> The B-NICE study was guided by the theoretical approaches of the Ecological Model (EM) and Social Cognitive Theory (SCT). These theories are especially useful in combination with one another because they emphasize the reciprocal relationship that exists between individual behavior and the social environment; moreover, both have been recommended as particularly well-suited for addressing the problem of poor nutritional health in home-bound older adults. Specifically, we used an EM in designing particular components of the intervention and SCT in developing the manner in which the intervention was implemented. (Locher et al., 2011, p. 3)

Most behavioral interventions will require the use of more than one theoretical framework. To effectively use more than one theory, a clear explication of the link between theories and how each contributes to the intervention design is central.

CHALLENGES USING THEORY

Although using theory is essential to the development, testing, and implementation of an intervention, there are challenges. First, it may be difficult to find a theoretical base for a particular intervention approach. Some theories of interest may lack a strong empirical foundation. Applying theory to an identified problem area may not be straightforward. This is particularly the case for theories that are not well fleshed out or which do not have empirical support.

Second, a theory may suggest what needs to be changed, but not specifically how to induce change. As discussed earlier, the stress process model provides an understanding of what needs to be changed (e.g., cognition, external stressors) but not how to change it; augmenting it with the TTM can help inform the specific strategies to use when delivering an intervention to support desired changes.

A third challenge is that prevailing behavior change and health behavior theories tend to explain behavioral intentions or motivation, but they do not necessarily explain or predict actual behavior or behavior change. Other theories may need to be called upon to fill the gap between intention and actual behavior.

Yet another challenge is that many journals, particularly medical, do not encourage or support discussion of the theory base for an intervention. The theory base for an intervention is not even mentioned in the Consolidated Standards of Reporting Trials checklist that is used as a guide for reporting intervention work (see Chapter 24 for a discussion on publishing; see www.consort-statement.org/ for checklist of items). Most publications reporting the outcomes of a behavioral intervention study do not describe a theoretical foundation for the intervention. If a theoretical basis for the intervention is mentioned, it is done so briefly, often making it difficult to decipher connections between treatment components, measures, and outcomes. Thus, it is often difficult to understand how theory informs a published intervention as there is not an expectation that this needs to be articulated. As such, the role of theory and its importance tends to be minimized, and the replication potential of an intervention is potentially and inadvertently diminished.

Finally, a theory may not work. This may be due to various reasons: the choice of theory may not be appropriate or may not adequately explain the phenomenon of interest; the theory may lack clearly defined and testable relationships; the intervention informed by the theory may have been poorly developed and/or implemented (see Chapter 12 on fidelity); or the lack of significance may reflect a measurement error (see Chapter 14; ICEBeRG, 2006). If a theory does not work, it is important to determine the reasons why this might be the case. This can in turn lead to a refinement of the original theory, refutation of the theory, or modification of the intervention and measures to align better with theory.

CONCLUSION

In this chapter, we have shown that theory addresses three broad essential questions in behavioral intervention research: why the intervention should work (development phases), how the intervention does work (evaluation phases), and how the intervention works in real settings (implementation phases). Without a theory base, one cannot understand why an intervention should work, how it works and for whom, and how it is best implemented in real-world settings. Theories can help inform the selection of delivery characteristics and also guide decision making during the implementation phase concerning what elements of the intervention are immutable and what elements can be modified. As most, if not all, behavioral interventions need to be adapted for delivery in practice and service settings, this is a critical function during the translation/implementation/dissemination phases. Thus, theories/conceptual frameworks are highly practical tools that behavioral interventionists must use throughout the pipeline for advancing an intervention.

The choice of a theory is up to the investigator—there is no one magical theory or best conceptual framework. Furthermore, as most interventions are complex and designed to mitigate multifaceted problems, behaviors, or unaddressed needs, more than one theory most likely will need to be employed. Despite the challenges of using theory, without a theory, an intervention will have limited success.

REFERENCES

Ajzen, I., & Fishbein, M. (1980). *Understanding attitudes and predicting social behavior.* Englewood Cliffs, NJ: Prentice Hall.

Ajzen, I., & Madden, T. J. (1986). Prediction of goal-directed behavior: Attitudes, intentions, and perceived behavioral control. *Journal of Experimental Social Psychology, 22*(5), 453–474.

Algase, D. L., Beck, C., Kolanowski, A., Whall, A., Berent, S., Richards, K., & Beattie, E. (1996). Need-driven dementia-compromised behavior: An alternative view of disruptive behavior. *American Journal of Alzheimer's Disease and Other Dementias, 11*, 10–18. doi:10.1177/153331759601100603

Belle, S. H., Burgio, L., Burns, R., Coon, D., Czaja, S. J., Gallagher-Thompson, D., . . . Zhang, S. (2006). Enhancing the quality of life of dementia caregivers from different ethnic or racial groups: A randomized, controlled trial. *Annals of Internal Medicine, 145*(10), 727–738.

Bengtson, V. L., Burgess, E. O., & Parrott, T. M. (1997). Theory, explanation, and a third generation of theoretical development in social gerontology. *The Journals of Gerontology Series B: Psychological Sciences and Social Sciences, 52*(2), S72–S88.

Briley, A. L., Barr, S., Badger, S., Bell, R., Croker, H., Godfrey, K. M., . . . Oteng-Ntim, E. (2014). A complex intervention to improve pregnancy outcome in obese women; the UPBEAT randomised controlled trial. *BMC Pregnancy and Childbirth, 14*(1), 74.

Cohen-Mansfield, J. (2001). Nonpharmacologic interventions for inappropriate behaviors in dementia: A review, summary, and critique. *The American Journal of Geriatric Psychiatry, 9*(4), 361–381.

DePoy, E., & Gitlin, L. N. (2015). *Introduction to research: Understanding and applying multiple strategies* (5th ed.). St. Louis, Missouri: Elsevier/Mosby Year Book.

Dowd, J. J. (1988). The reification of age: Age stratification theory and the passing of the autonomous subject. *Journal of Aging Studies, 1*(4), 317–335.

French, S. D., Green, S. E., O'Connor, D. A., McKenzie, J. E., Francis, J. J., Michie, S, . . . Grimshaw, J. M. (2012). Developing theory-informed behaviour change interventions to implement evidence into practice: A systematic approach using the Theoretical Domains Framework. *Implementation Science, 7*, 38. doi:10.1186/1748-5908-7-38

Gitlin, L. N., Corcoran, M., Martindale-Adams, J., Malone, C., Stevens, A., & Winter, L. (2000). Identifying mechanisms of action: Why and how does intervention work? In

R. Schulz (Ed.), *Handbook on dementia caregiving: Evidence-based interventions for family caregivers* (pp. 225–248). New York, NY: Springer.

Gitlin, L. N., Fields-Harris, L., McCoy, M., Chernett, N., Jutkowitz, E., Pizzi, L. T., & Beat the Blues Team. (2012). A community-integrated home-based depression intervention for older African Americans: Description of the Beat the Blues randomized trial and intervention costs. *BMC Geriatrics, 12*, 4. doi:10.1186/1471-2318-12-4

Gitlin, L. N., Harris, L. F., McCoy, M. C., Chernett, N. L., Pizzi, L. T., Jutkowitz, E., . . . Hauck, W. W. (2013). A home-based intervention to reduce depressive symptoms and improve quality of life in older African Americans. *Annals of Internal Medicine, 159*(4), 243–252. doi:10.7326/0003-4819-159-4-201308200-00005

Gitlin, L. N., Harris, L. F., McCoy, M. C., Hess, E., & Hauck, E. E. (In press). *Delivery characteristics and acceptability of a home-based depression intervention for older African Americans: The Get Busy Get Better Program.* The Gerontologist, Practice Concepts.

Gitlin, L. N., Kales, H. C., & Lyketsos, C. G. (2012). Nonpharmacologic management of behavioral symptoms in dementia. *JAMA, 308*(19), 2020–2029. doi:10.1001/jama.2012.36918

Gitlin, L. N., & Rose, K. (2014). Factors associated with caregiver readiness to use nonpharmacologic strategies to manage dementia-related behavioral symptoms. *International Journal of Geriatric Psychiatry, 29*(1), 93–102. doi:10.1002/gps.3979

Gitlin, L. N., Roth, D. L., & Huang, J. (2014). Mediators of the impact of a home-based intervention (Beat the Blues) on depressive symptoms among older African Americans. *Psychology and Aging, 29*(3), 601–611. doi:10.1037/a0036784

Glanz, K., & Bishop, D. B. (2010). The role of behavioral science theory in development and implementation of public health interventions. *Annual Review of Public Health, 31*, 399–418.

Hall, G. R., & Buckwalter, K. C. (1987). Progressively lowered stress threshold: A conceptual model for care of adults with Alzheimer's disease. *Archives of Psychiatric Nursing, 1*(6), 399–406.

Heckhausen, J., & Schulz, R. (1995). A life-span theory of control. *Psychological Review, 102*(2), 284–304.

Heckhausen, J., Wrosch, C., & Schulz, R. (2010). A motivational theory of life-span development. *Psychological Review, 117*(1), 32–60.

Hopko, D. R., Lejuez, C. W., Ruggiero, K. J., & Eifert, G. H. (2003). Contemporary behavioral activation treatments for depression: Procedures, principles, and progress. *Clinical Psychology Review, 23*(5), 699–717. doi:10.1016/S0272-7358(03)00070-9

The Improved Clinical Effectiveness through Behavioural Research Group. (2006). Designing theoretically-informed implementation interventions. *Implementation Science, 1*, 4. doi:10.1186/1748-5908-1-4

Kales, H. C., Gitlin, L. N., & Lyketsos, C. G. (2015). Prevention, assessment and management of behavioral and psychological symptoms of dementia: The need for a tailored patient- and caregiver-centered approach. *BMJ, 350*. doi:10.1136/350:h369

Kerlinger, F. N. (1986). *Foundations of behavioral research* (3rd ed.). New York, NY: Holt, Rinehart & Winston.

Lawton, M. P., & Nahemow, L. E. (1973). Ecology and the aging process. In C. Eisdorfer & M. P. Lawton (Eds.), *The psychology of adult development and aging* (pp. 619–674). Washington, DC: American Psychological Association.

Lewin, K. (1951). *Field theory in social science: Selected theoretical papers* (D. Cartwright, Ed). New York, NY: Harper & Row.

Locher, J. L., Bales, C. W., Ellis, A. C., Lawrence, J. C., Newton, L., Ritchie, C. S., . . . Vickers, K. S. (2011). A theoretically based behavioral nutrition intervention for community elders at high risk: The B-NICE randomized controlled clinical trial. *Journal of Nutrition in Gerontology and Geriatrics, 30*(4), 384–402.

May, C. R., Mair, F., Finch, T., MacFarlane, A., Dowrick, C., Treweek, S., . . . Montori, V. M. (2009). Development of a theory of implementation and integration: Normalization Process Theory. *Implement Science, 4,* 29.

Michie, S., & Prestwich, A. (2010). Are interventions theory-based? Development of a theory coding scheme. *Health Psychology, 29*(1), 1–8.

National Cancer Institute. (2005). *Theory at a glance: A guide for health promotion practice* (2nd ed.). Washington, DC: U.S. Department of Health and Human Services, National Institutes of Health.

NIMH Multisite HIV/STD Prevention Trial for African American Couples Group. (2008). Eban HIV/STD risk reduction intervention: Conceptual basis and procedures. *JAIDS Journal of Acquired Immune Deficiency Syndromes, 49,* S15–S27.

Noar, S. M. (2005). A health educator's guide to theories of health behavior. *International Quarterly of Community Health Education, 24*(1), 75–92.

Pearlin, L. I., Mullan, J. T., Semple, S. J., & Skaff, M. M. (1990). Caregiving and the stress process: An overview of concepts and their measures. *The Gerontologist, 30,* 583–594.

Prochaska, J. O., DiClemente, C. C., & Norcross, J. C. (1992). In search of how people change. *American Psychologist, 47*(9), 1102–1114.

Rosenstock, I. M. (1974). The health belief model and preventive health behavior. *Health Education & Behavior, 2*(4), 354–386.

Rosenstock, I. M., Strecher, V. J., & Becker, M. H. (1988). Social learning theory and the health belief model. *Health Education & Behavior, 15*(2), 175–183.

Roth, D. L., Mittelman, M. S., Clay, O. J., Madan, A., & Haley, W. E. (2005). Changes in social support as mediators of the impact of a psychosocial intervention for spouse caregivers of persons with Alzheimer's disease. *Psychology and Aging, 20*(4), 634–644. doi:10.1037/0882-7974.20.4.634

Rovner, B. W., Casten, R. J., Hegel, M. T., & Leiby, B. E. (2012). Preventing cognitive decline in older African Americans with mild cognitive impairment: Design and methods of a randomized clinical trial. *Contemporary Clinical Trials, 33*(4), 712–720.

Schulz, R., Gallagher-Thompson, D., Haley, W. E., & Czaja, S. (2000). Understanding the intervention process: A theoretical/conceptual framework for intervention approaches to caregivers. In R. Schulz (Ed.), *Handbook on dementia caregiving: Evidence-based interventions for family caregivers* (pp. 33–60). New York, NY: Springer.

Schwarzer, R. (2008). Modeling health behavior change: How to predict and modify the adoption and maintenance of health behaviors. *Applied Psychology, 57*(1), 1–29.

Szanton, S. L., Thorpe, R. J., & Gitlin, L. N. (2014). Beat the Blues decreases depression in financially strained older African-American adults. *American Journal of Geriatric Psychiatry, 22,* 692–697. doi:10.1016/j.jagp.2013.05.008

Taylor, S. G., Geden, E., Isaramalai, S., & Wongvatunyu, S. (2000). Orem's self-care deficit nursing theory: Its philosophic foundation and the state of the science. *Nursing Science Quarterly, 13,* 104–110.

FIVE

DELIVERY CHARACTERISTICS OF BEHAVIORAL INTERVENTIONS

If we knew what it was we were doing, it would not be called research, would it?
—Albert Einstein

Behavioral intervention research is burgeoning and gaining recognition as playing a necessary and critical role in the development of strategies to address today's complex social and health care issues. Behavioral interventions address a wide range of issues and populations and can target individuals, communities, organizations, or the social, physical, or policy environments. Interventions can take many forms and may involve counseling, training, psychotherapy, education, skill building, stress management techniques, or some combination of activities. They may also target different aspects of behavior, such as coping skills, knowledge, self-management, or involve modifications to the physical and/or social environment. Many intervention programs are multifaceted and involve multiple components, objectives, and activities. Interventions also evolve and change throughout the phases of the pipeline over time, as new knowledge is gained from testing and from effective treatment approaches and methodological approaches. However, irrespective of the target population or the form of the intervention, behavioral intervention research is directed at gathering evidence regarding the impact of a program or protocol on an outcome(s) that is relevant to the problem of interest.

As discussed in Chapter 1, this type of research is complex, challenging, and costly. The researcher is faced with many decisions at all phases of the pipeline. As we discuss in this chapter, these decisions concern the content of the intervention, mode of treatment delivery, the duration of the intervention, and training and monitoring study interventionists. For example, if a researcher decides (after an extensive review of the literature) that he or she is interested in developing an intervention to alleviate the emotional distress of family caregivers, decisions will need to be made regarding the characteristics of the targeted sample (e.g., spouse vs. nonspouse, dementia caregiver vs. cancer caregiver); the aspect of caregiving or the care recipient that will be targeted (e.g., emotional well-being, problem behaviors, physical health, pain); sample size, the content, and duration of the intervention and how it will be delivered (e.g., face-to-face, computer, telephone); and how the impact of the intervention will be assessed. Clearly, this represents only a handful of issues that must be resolved.

Importantly, as discussed in Chapter 1, decisions regarding the characteristics of an intervention and an intervention trial cannot be made in a vacuum. Interventions occur within a context that includes multiple interacting levels such as the individual, the setting in which the intervention will be delivered, formal and informal networks and social support systems, the community, and the policy environment. All of these levels and the potential interactions among them need to be considered in the design of an intervention study. For example, if an intervention involves using a computer for treatment delivery, then issues such as the availability of the technology, the technology skills of the target population, and technology requirements (e.g., Internet/broadband access) will need to be addressed (see Chapter 7).

Our goal in this chapter is to provide an overview of the key factors that need to be considered in the design of the behavioral intervention itself. Our focus is specifically on the *delivery characteristics* of the intervention program (e.g., intervention content, dosage, delivery mode). Our objective is to highlight the multitude of factors that need to be considered when designing the delivery characteristics of a behavioral intervention study. Basically, this entails making decisions about what should be delivered, how it should be delivered and by whom, at what intensity, and for how long. Other decision points relate to materials, equipment, cost, and feasibility. Our intent is to provide a "roadmap" to guide the intervention protocol design process (Table 5.1). Other topics related to the design of an intervention study, such as sampling and ethical considerations and experimental methodologies, are covered in more depth in other chapters.

It is important to note that some of the topics related to designing delivery characteristics of an intervention (e.g., staff training) may have varying importance at various phases along the pipeline. However, even though some issues may not be relevant until the later phases, it is still important to understand what they are and consider them early on in the development of an intervention. Decisions that are made in the intervention development phases have a significant influence on the later phases of the pipeline. For example, the fidelity of an intervention program can be compromised if consideration is not given to staff training or protocols for monitoring treatment fidelity in the beginning of the intervention development process (see Chapter 12 for a discussion of fidelity).

Delivery characteristics are the backbone of an intervention and have a profound influence on the feasibility, timeline, and cost of a trial; the evidence regarding the impact of the intervention; and the likelihood that the intervention will be implemented on a broad scale. The challenge for the intervention researcher is to design intervention programs and research protocols that meet the standards for rigorous evaluation; address the needs and preferences of the targeted population; are effective with respect to outcomes; are feasible and can be replicated; and can ultimately be implemented in community and clinical settings. Purposely building in adaptability in the delivery characteristics is key to meeting these challenges as we have learned from moving interventions along the pipeline (e.g., flexible scheduling or dosing). Intervention research is an iterative process (see Chapter 2) where the outcomes and experiences of each phase inform the next phase of the pipeline; this is the case for every aspect of intervention work including the design of the delivery characteristics of an intervention, which is our focus here.

TABLE 5.1 Considerations in the Design of Delivery Characteristics

Delivery Characteristic	Factors
Treatment content	■ Theory/prior findings relevant to the content ■ Personnel involved in content decisions ■ Content to be delivered ■ Order or sequence of content ■ Number of components ■ Degree of flexibility/adaptability ■ Feasibility issues (e.g., cost) ■ Equipment requirements ■ Replicability ■ Participant burden ■ Safety ■ Protocols for informed consent and adverse event monitoring and reporting ■ Treatment manual of operation
Treatment dosage and duration	■ Duration of treatment ■ Amount of treatment ■ Strategy for measurement of dose ■ Feasibility ■ Participant burden ■ Criteria for intervention "completion" ■ Delivery schedule ■ Flexibility in schedule ■ Booster sessions ■ Protocol for tracking content
Delivery modality	■ Format of delivery (e.g., face-to-face, telephone, Internet) ■ Multimodal/single modality ■ Use of technology ■ Cost ■ Technical requirements ■ Skill and training requirements (participant and interventionist)
Delivery setting	■ Choice of setting (e.g., home vs. clinic) ■ Logistic requirements ■ Generalizability/external validity ■ Threats to internal validity ■ Single site versus multisite
Delivery approach	■ Prescriptive versus tailoring ■ Cultural adaptations ■ Aspects of the intervention that can be amenable to tailoring ■ Personnel involved in tailoring decisions ■ Criteria for tailoring ■ Protocols for documenting adaptations/tailoring
Staffing requirements	■ Size and nature of team (e.g., recruitment, coordinator, assessors, interventionists) ■ Skill level requirement for team ■ Characteristics (e.g., age, gender, language, culture/ethnicity) ■ Training protocols and criteria

(Continued)

TABLE 5.1 Considerations in the Design of Delivery Characteristics *(Continued)*	
Delivery Characteristic	**Factors**
	■ Strategies for team building ■ Protocols for communication ■ Protocols for meetings ■ Plan for monitoring and assessment ■ Safety protocols ■ Training for ethical conduct of research; resolution for adverse events

WHERE TO BEGIN: HELPING TO SHAPE THE TOPIC

Irrespective of the research experience of the investigator, conducting a literature review concerning the decisions that need to be made vis-à-vis delivery characteristics is an essential part of the research process and integral to the success of designing an effective intervention program. As discussed in Chapter 23, a succinct and current review of the literature is also critical for preparing a grant proposal for an intervention project that supports the design of the intervention. A current and thorough but succinct literature review demonstrates the relevance and uniqueness of the proposed study; introduces the theory guiding the intervention; and also informs the reviewers that the investigator is current and aware of recent theories, findings, and methodological approaches.

In general, a literature review, though sometimes tedious, serves many purposes. It provides insights into relevant theories and conceptual frameworks and also provides information on work that has been done to date, what needs to be done, and what works and what does not with regard to strategies for delivering a particular intervention. A literature review also provides valuable information on state-of-the-art methodologies for delivering interventions and roadblocks encountered by other researchers. This can help save time and effort. In other words, designing an intervention cannot be done in a vacuum; the selection of a delivery characteristic (e.g., use of face-to-face or group format) must be informed in part by prior research and hence the literature. Let's say an intervention is designed to help cancer patients modify their daily lifestyle to address pain. A literature review will reveal that providing education alone about cancer and pain management via a brochure will not be a sufficient form of delivery if the goal is behavioral change or modifying the way a person actively monitors pain.

An additional valuable aspect of a literature review that is often overlooked is that it helps to identify other researchers working in an area who can be called upon for expert consultation to further shape ideas about the intervention design or even to serve as collaborators. Today, conducting a literature search is relatively easy with the powerful search engines available on the Internet.

It is also always important to meet with other investigators and potential collaborators to learn from their experiences as to what works and what does not vis-à-vis the design of an intervention's delivery characteristics. The topics addressed in behavioral interventions and their design characteristics are complex and require a multidisciplinary team approach. Thus, obtaining input from other investigators is critical when deciding upon a particular delivery approach. For example, assume an investigator is interested in evaluating whether a cognitive training program has an impact on the cognitive abilities and brain functioning of older adults. In this case, the team might include a neuropsychologist who can provide advice on what domains of cognition should be targeted by the intervention and on measures that should be included in the study to assess change in cognitive abilities; an expert in neuroimaging; someone with expertise in cognitive aging; and a statistician. If the training involved computer-based games, the team would need to be expanded to include programmer/computer scientists. Each would bring a particular perspective and knowledge of his or her respective literature to help inform decision making as it concerns the delivery characteristics of the intervention. For example, decisions would need to be made as to the length of exposure a participant has to the computer-based game to evince a benefit; also, decisions would have to be made concerning the nature of the visuals used in the program and features that might motivate individual participation. All of these decisions need to be informed by theory, existing evidence, and direct experience that such experts can contribute. One challenge, of course, is fostering communication among team members (see Chapter 22) as they will represent different disciplines, speak a "different language," and may have a different perspective on the problem. However, in the long run, input from others reflecting various perspectives is often essential to designing the characteristics of a behavioral intervention. These types of meetings also foster "buy-in" to the project and foster teamwork.

FUNDAMENTAL INTERVENTION DELIVERY CHARACTERISTICS

Treatment Content

There are numerous issues that need to be resolved when designing the content of the intervention including the actual material/topics covered in the intervention, the number of components of the intervention (single vs. multicomponent), the structure of the intervention (e.g., order in which the topics are presented), the mechanisms of action (e.g., interactive skill building vs. instruction), and degree of flexibility/adaptability. Other issues relate to equipment and material requirements, feasibility, and participant burden (Table 5.1). Importantly, these issues need to be resolved for all of the conditions in a trial/intervention including control conditions.

The content of an intervention is the "active ingredient of an intervention" and should be shaped by consideration of a number of factors including the theory/conceptual framework guiding the intervention, prior research, the research questions, the target population of the intervention (e.g., individual, family) and associated characteristics, the stage of intervening (e.g., prevention, disease management), the area targeted (e.g., knowledge, skills, or the physical environment), and the intervention context. Other factors to consider are logistical problems as well as cost constraints and whether the treatment can be followed or replicated by others.

The theory guiding the intervention and prior research conducted in an area, as discussed earlier, helps to identify potentially malleable factors that may lead to changes in outcomes as well as mechanisms of action that are effective in realizing this change (Gitlin et al., 2000). The relationship between the means, ends, and intervening processes of a treatment in relation to the topic of interest or clinical problem needs to be clearly articulated (Kazdin, 1994). As discussed in previous chapters, the content and delivery characteristics of the Resources for Enhancing Alzheimer's Caregiver Health (REACH) II intervention (Belle et al., 2006) are shaped by a variant of the stress process model, the findings from REACH I, and principles of adult learning. The stress process model suggests that multiple factors contribute to caregiver burden and distress. Findings from the REACH I trial (Gitlin et al., 2003) indicated that active interventions were superior and that interventions should be tailored to the characteristics of the caregiver. The adult-learning literature also indicates that active learning approaches are superior, learning should take place in the context in which the new skills are applied, and education and skills are adopted when perceived as needed. Thus, the REACH II was multicomponent, delivered in the home, was tailored to the needs of the caregiver using a risk appraisal approach, involved a variety of mechanisms of action that actively engaged the caregiver (e.g., problem solving and skill building), and was matched to the treatment component and targeted trial outcomes. Other decisions regarding the intervention content in REACH II were related to the number and ordering of the intervention sessions, the nature of the handout materials, and the parameters around adaptability (e.g., what aspects of the intervention could be adapted such as delivery location, and who could make decisions about adaptability). Similar decisions had to be made for the content of the information-only control group condition.

In the Personal Reminder Information System Management (PRISM) trial (discussed previously) (Czaja et al., 2015), decisions concerning the delivery characteristics of the intervention concerned which features to include on the software system (e.g., e-mail, community resources) as well as the names, content, and structure of the features. For the Internet feature, a decision had to be made about whether access should be restricted to websites preselected by the research team or if the participants should have unrestricted access. In the end, the decision was made to support unrestricted access; however, a tab was included within this feature that included links to websites that the investigative team thought would be of particular relevance to the participants. The classroom feature was dynamic and contained scripted information, vetted videos, and links to other sites on a broad array of topics (e.g., cognitive health, traveling tips, nutrition). New material was placed in the classroom every month and remained in the "classroom library." In the design of this feature, specific decisions had to be made about the 12 monthly topics to be included, the order of the topics, the content for the topics, and the depth and literacy level of the information provided. The investigative team also had to select links to other sources of information and videos related to the featured monthly topic. In addition, similar materials had to be prepared for and delivered to those assigned to the attention control condition. Overall, the design and tailoring of the PRISM system and the material for the control condition were based on the available literature, the experience of the investigators, and knowledge about the characteristics of the target population and usability testing.

In all cases, it is important to pilot test the content of the intervention and the format in which it is delivered to receive input from other members of the research team as well as the targeted group. The content can also be shaped by input from members of a Community Advisory Board (CAB), Data Safety and Monitoring Board (DSMB), and a Scientific Advisory Board (SAB). The CAB can provide valuable advice about the relevance of the content for the target population and issues regarding feasibility. The DSMB is likely to provide input on issues related to participant burden, and an SAB might provide new ideas on topics, methods of treatment delivery, or challenges that might arise in the course of a trial based on the best evidence to date. As noted, the development of an intervention is an iterative process, and the content of an intervention should be refined through various feedback mechanisms and a purposeful, thoughtful approach.

Treatment Dosage and Duration

Two important delivery characteristics of an intervention are the *duration* or the time length of a treatment (e.g., 6 months, 12 months) and treatment *dose*, which refers to the amount of treatment. Dose is typically measured in terms of the number of sessions, contact time (e.g., minutes), number or frequency of contacts, or some combination (e.g., 12 weekly 60-minute sessions). Dose parameters may be applied to an interaction between a participant and a member of a research team (e.g., counseling session with a therapist), or some aspect of an individual's behavior (e.g., number of fruits or vegetables eaten, or minutes of exercise), or across several components of an intervention. In technology-based interventions, a dose parameter may reflect the number of uses of the system or an aspect of a particular software program. For example, in the PRISM trial, real-time data were collected on participants' use of the overall PRISM system as well as the use of each individual feature each day and over the 12-month duration of a trial.

A fundamental question in the design of the delivery characteristics of a behavioral intervention is: How much exposure, and to what, is enough? Clearly, this issue has a significant impact on treatment outcomes as well as the cost of a study, participant burden, and feasibility issues surrounding future implementation of an intervention at later stages of the pipeline. Insufficient doses of a treatment may contribute to Type II errors (the failure to reject a false null hypothesis; failing to detect the impact of a treatment that is present). On the other hand, large amounts of a treatment may negatively impact on the cost and feasibility of a trial and be burdensome to participants. This may in turn have a negative impact on participant retention, which can threaten the internal validity of a study. In addition, it may limit replication of the intervention and broad-scale implementation.

The goal, of course, is to find the optimal balance between demonstrating the effectiveness of a treatment (if there is one) and cost and feasibility issues. There is no one recommendation for the optimal dose. It depends on the nature of the intervention, the target population, and the context/setting. For example, the REACH II intervention trial involved 12 sessions (nine in-home face-to-face and three via technology) delivered over 6 months. A translation of the intervention was subsequently used in four Area Agencies on Aging (AAA). This version of the intervention was trimmed to enhance the feasibility of implementing the intervention in social service agencies and included seven sessions (four in-home face-to-face and three via telephone) delivered over 4 months. The results indicated that the translated version of the intervention appeared to be effective in terms of achieving a positive impact on caregiver outcomes such as burden, depression, and social support (Burgio et al., 2009).

Overall, determining the optimal dose of an intervention can be guided by a review of the relevant literature and through evaluation of the impact of the intervention in varying doses. For example, sequential, multiple assignment randomized trials (SMARTs) (Lei, Nahum-Shani, Lynch, Oslin, & Murphy, 2012) may be used to evaluate the impact of an intervention at varying doses. These types of designs allow for tailoring of the intervention components in the same trial.

Once the duration and dose of an intervention have been established, it is critically important to develop a system to track the planned and unplanned contact with study participants in all conditions during the course of a trial. This will allow the measurement of the dose delivered and the assessment of dose–response relationships. It is also important to determine how much dosage (e.g., number of sessions or time spent) of an intervention constitutes sufficient exposure and/or "completion" of the intervention protocol to evince a benefit. Additional factors to consider are issues related to the delivery schedule (e.g., once per week vs. once per month), flexibility in scheduling, and whether booster sessions are appropriate.

Delivery Modality and Setting

Delivery Modality

There are a variety of alternative ways to deliver an intervention such as face-to-face individual or group sessions, telephone or mail, or some technology-mediated format (e.g., the Internet, tablet computers). Each of these alternatives has associated strengths and weaknesses. Face-to-face individual sessions offer the potential benefits of greater therapeutic alliance and the ability to understand the context of an individual. However, this mode of treatment delivery can be costly and challenging with respect to scheduling. Alternatively, the increased use of the Internet has made Internet-based interventions more common. The advantages of using this delivery mode are that it can be more cost-effective (e.g., no travel on the part of the interventionists or the participants) and can offer enhanced flexibility with respect to scheduling and adaptability. Recent reviews (e.g., Tate, Finkelstein, Khavjou, & Gustafson, 2009) indicate that Internet-based behavioral interventions are efficacious. Potential challenges are associated with the technical development of the intervention, Internet access, and the technical skills of the study participants. Further, it can be more challenging to track treatment fidelity and to measure dosage (see Chapter 12).

Some interventions (e.g., REACH II) use a combination of modalities. In these cases, decisions have to be made regarding which components of the intervention will be delivered in a particular format. For example, in REACH II, decisions needed to be made regarding the number of face-to-face home visits versus the number delivered via the computer telephone system as well as which sessions were most amenable to each delivery format. Webb, Joseph, Yardley, and Michie (2010) conducted a review and meta-analysis of Internet-based interventions intended to promote health behavior changes. They found that more extensive use of theory in the development of the intervention was associated with a larger effect size as were interventions that incorporated more behavior change techniques. In addition, the effectiveness of Internet-based interventions was enhanced by the use of additional methods of communicating with patients such as text messages.

Delivery Setting

There are also various alternatives for the location in which an intervention is delivered. Location may include community-based settings, the home, a clinical setting, a residential facility, the workplace, or a research laboratory. Each of these settings has a unique set of characteristics that warrant consideration. In a research laboratory, the setting is much more controlled with respect to extraneous influences (e.g., pets, other family members), and thus one has more confidence about the internal validity of the study. However, it is artificial and there may be logistical problems for the participants in terms of travel, which may impact on recruitment and retention. Participants may also be uncomfortable in laboratory settings. Conducting interventions in home settings may be more comfortable, less stigmatizing if the intervention concerns a highly sensitive matter (e.g., depression, HIV prevention, sexual practices), and easier for study participants. However, this can also create logistical problems for the interventionist and add to trial costs (e.g., travel time of interventionists and travel costs). Home contexts also vary considerably in terms of factors such as clutter, cleanliness, pets, other family members, and safety that can impact on the delivery of the intervention. These factors can create unique challenges, especially if the intervention involves the use of some form of technology (Gitlin, 2003). In the PRISM trial, it was sometimes challenging to install computer systems in homes of participants owing to clutter and space constraints.

A general benefit of community settings is that they represent the context in which the intervention will be actualized and are familiar to participants. However, potential threats to both internal and external validity need to be carefully considered. In health care settings, the representativeness of patients and providers and settings is important (Glasgow, Bull, Gillette, Klesges, & Dzewaltonwski, 2002). Threats to internal validity include potential contamination (e.g., people in the same nursing home assigned to different treatments); confounding factors such as unanticipated changes in the community (e.g., weather events) or changes in organizational policy, missions, or practices; and issues with treatment fidelity. If a health care provider in a busy clinic is responsible for implementing the intervention or assessment protocols, he or she may take shortcuts or may not understand the importance of following standard procedures to assure the integrity of the delivery of an intervention. Thus strategies such as intervention manuals and booster-training sessions, to enhance treatment fidelity, need to be in place. CABs can also provide valuable input on how to best meet the challenges associated with implementing intervention programs in community settings. Community-based participatory research approaches are also helpful as they foster "buy-in" from the community and commitment to the project/intervention (see Melnyk & Morrison-Beedy, 2012 for more in-depth discussions of implementation in specific types of community settings).

The involvement of multiple sites at different institutions and locations poses a challenge to intervention delivery considerations. Expanding studies to more than one site is quite common in both efficacy and effectiveness trials (e.g., REACH I and II, Advanced Cognitive Training for Independent and Vital Elderly (ACTIVE). For the most part, multisite trials involve separate research teams but common research protocols and data collection strategies. Sometimes recruitment strategies and possibly the way in which an intervention is delivered may need to vary at the research sites to accommodate differences in the characteristics of target populations. Multisite studies often involve a separate data coordination site to provide oversight regarding data collection and also the delivery of the intervention. For example, in the REACH trials, the University of Pittsburgh served in this role. In the PRISM project, the University of Miami Miller School of Medicine assumed this role.

Decisions to engage in multisite trials require careful consideration as to how the delivery characteristics of an intervention will be implemented and monitored. These types of trials add considerably to cost and logistical considerations. Other important issues include establishing protocols for the research teams, treatment fidelity, data collection, storage, and transfer. In addition, the mechanisms for communication among team members within and across sites need to be clearly articulated, as do protocols for decision making, conflict resolution, and dissemination and publication activities.

Delivery Approach

There are also alternative approaches for delivery of an intervention. These include but are not limited to tailoring or adapting an intervention with respect to the characteristics of the participants (e.g., cultural tailoring) or the context in which it will be delivered; using a prescriptive one-size-fits-all approach; adapting a stepped care approach that adjusts the intensity or level of an intervention according to the stage of readiness/need of an individual; or a risk assessment approach that adjusts level of exposure by type and intensity of risk.

In general, the choice of delivery approach should be driven by the nature of the intervention, the relevant literature, and the phase of the pipeline. For example, within the caregiver intervention literature, it is generally found that multicomponent interventions that actively engage the caregiver yield better outcomes. Also, it may not be wise to use an adaptive approach at an early phase of the pipeline when an intervention is initially being developed or the feasibility of an approach is being evaluated.

If an adaptive delivery approach is chosen, decisions need to be made regarding which aspects of an intervention can be adapted, the extent or range of adaptability, who can make decisions regarding adaptability, and how an aspect of an intervention can be adapted. If an intervention involves two cognitive training sessions a week in a laboratory on separate days, a question may arise as to alternative scheduling for participants with transportation problems. Adaptations for these participants might involve scheduling two sessions on the same day (with a rest break) or allowing participants to complete one of the sessions at home. Irrespective of decisions concerning adaptability, protocols for adaptability must be in place and documented. Further, any adaptations made to a protocol must be tracked throughout a trial as they may interject biases into the outcomes that need to be evaluated in data analyses.

Staffing Issues

Who delivers an intervention is an important decision that must be made early on in the development of an intervention. The level of expertise needed for intervention delivery needs to be driven by the purpose of the intervention and the desired outcomes as well as other considerations. These include but may not be limited to the availability of the type of staff needed for the delivery of an intervention, whether staffing requirements will be able to be met if the intent is to disseminate and widely implement the intervention, and costs associated with training and supporting the level of expertise required. Balancing all of these factors and the implications for dissemination and wide-scale uptake of an intervention is further explored in Part IV. As noted, most behavioral interventions address complex issues that cannot be viewed from a single lens and may require multidisciplinary expertise in the delivery of different components of the intervention. For example, the Advancing Better Living for Elders (ABLE) program involved occupational therapists, physical therapists, and home modification specialists in the delivery of a six-visit intervention designed to improve daily function and enhance the ability of older frail adults to stay at home (Gitlin et al., 2009).

In terms of project staffing, important issues to consider include the number of needed staff and their roles and responsibilities; prior experience (e.g., experience with the target population or the intervention); and skill/certification/educational requirements (e.g., certified neuropsychologist, bilingual, at least a master's degree). It is a good idea to conduct a task analysis of the intervention and planned study design to identify staffing needs. This involves identifying the intervention objectives, specific activities, and how each will be delivered and by whom. Another important issue is ensuring that the roles and responsibilities of all of the team members are clearly specified and communicated within the team. A study manual (Manual of Operations [MOP], see Chapter 6) detailing all operations should be created that includes protocols for communication, lines of authority, and decision-making parameters. Protocols also need to be developed for staff training. Clearly, all members of the study team should understand the goals and aims of the study and be trained on all aspects of the protocol (including the protocols for both the intervention and comparison conditions). It is critically important that staff members understand the importance of adhering to the study protocol (e.g., delivery of the intervention) for all treatment conditions and also understand the importance of equipoise. Training should also be provided on the topical domain of the intervention (e.g., family caregiving) and on strategies for interacting with study participants so that staffs have the knowledge needed to adequately perform their role on the study. Other important training topics include staff safety protocols, resolution protocols for adverse events, ethical conduct of research and confidentiality, and data handling. To prevent drift among assessors and interventionists, the treatment fidelity plan should include protocols for monitoring and regularly scheduled booster training (see Chapter 12).

CHARACTERISTICS OF AN EFFECTIVE DELIVERY APPROACH

As discussed, there is not one specific mode, characteristic, or approach of delivery that will fit all behavioral interventions. Delivery characteristics need to be tailored to, and directed by, the specific goals and objectives of an intervention, the targeted population, and the context in which the intervention will be implemented among other factors. However, there are some general principles that can be applied when considering an intervention that focuses specifically on behavioral change. As changing behavior is complex, treatment delivery characteristics that are most effective have been found to include multiple components (e.g., education and skill building), tailoring messaging and content to participant characteristics and needs, integrating behavioral change strategies such as motivational interviewing, obtaining buy-in and using agreements/contracts, adjusting the pace of the intervention to meet abilities, needs, and readiness of participants, using problem solving and active approaches to involve persons, and activating persons through personal goal setting and/or peer support. Using education alone, a single-size-fits-all approach or didactic style has not been found to be effective when the desired outcome is behavioral change. Finally, it has also been found that typically more is better; that is, greater exposure or more treatment sessions tend to optimize outcomes for participants.

Nevertheless, it remains unclear whether there is a specific set of delivery characteristics that is most effective for other types of behavioral interventions. Intervention researchers must always comb the literature to understand emerging evidence as to what works best for which types of situations, populations, contexts, and intervention objectives, as we have discussed earlier.

CONCLUSION

Our goal in this chapter is to highlight issues related to decision making as it concerns the specific delivery characteristics of an intervention. The behavioral intervention researcher is faced with many decisions as to what the intervention will look like and how it will be delivered, and these decisions need to be made early on in the pipeline and then modified through various tests of the intervention. The process of developing the delivery characteristics of an intervention is iterative and generally includes numerous feedback loops between implementing a particular delivery strategy, evaluating its feasibility and outcomes, and modifying the strategy accordingly. Behavioral intervention studies also typically involve multidisciplinary teams that can provide different insights into delivering an intervention.

There is no one answer when determining treatment content, dosage, or delivery mode. Decisions regarding these issues should be driven by theory/conceptual framework guiding the intervention, prior research, the research questions, the target population, the stage of intervening (e.g., prevention, disease management), the area targeted (e.g., knowledge, skills, or the physical environment), the context of delivery, and the specific goals and objectives of the intervention.

The takeaway message is that delivery characteristics represent the backbone of an intervention and have a profound influence on: the feasibility, timeline, and cost of a trial; the evidence regarding the impact of the intervention; and the likelihood that the intervention will be implemented on a broad scale. Of course, there are other related issues that need to be considered in designing the delivery characteristics of an intervention such as the development of treatment manuals, protocols for monitoring, and resolution of adverse events and issues related to participant consent. These issues are discussed in later chapters.

REFERENCES

Belle, S. H., Burgio, L., Burns, R., Coon, D., Czaja, S. J., Gallagher-Thompson, D., . . . Zhang, S. (2006). Enhancing the quality of life of dementia caregivers from different ethnic or racial groups. *Annals of Internal Medicine, 145*(10), 727–738.

Burgio, L. D., Collins, I. B., Schmid, B., Wharton, T., McCallum, D., & DeCoster, J. (2009). Translating the REACH caregiver intervention for use by area agency on aging personnel: The REACH OUT program. *The Gerontologist, 49*(1), 103–116.

Czaja, S. J., Boot, W. R., Charness, N., Rogers, W. A., Sharit, J., Fisk, A. D., . . . Nair, S. N. (2015). The personalized reminder information and social management system (PRISM) trial: Rationale, methods, and baseline characteristics. *Contemporary Clinical Trials, 40,* 35–46.

Gitlin, L. N. (2003). Conducting research on home environments: Lessons learned and new directions. *The Gerontologist, 43*(5), 628–637.

Gitlin, L. N., Corcoran, M., Martindale-Adams, J., Malone, C., Stevens, A., & Winter, L. (2000). Identifying mechanisms of action: Why and how does intervention work? In R. Schulz (Ed.), *Handbook on dementia caregiving: Evidence-based interventions for family caregivers* (pp. 225–248). New York, NY: Springer.

Gitlin, L. N., Hauck, W. W., Dennis, M. P., Winter, L., Hodgson, N., & Schinfeld, S. (2009). Long-term effect on mortality of a home intervention that reduces functional difficulties in older adults: Results from a randomized trial. *Journal of the American Geriatrics Society, 57*(3), 476–481.

Gitlin, L. N., Winter, L., Corcoran, M., Dennis, M., Schinfeld, S., & Hauck, W. (2003). Effects of the home environmental skill-building program on the caregiver/care-recipient dyad: Six-month outcomes from the Philadelphia REACH initiative. *The Gerontologist, 43,* 532–546.

Glasgow, R. E., Bull, S. S., Gillette, C., Klesges, L. M., & Dzewaltonwski, D. A. (2002). Behavior change intervention research in healthcare settings: A review of recent reports with emphasis on external validity. *American Journal of Preventive Medicine, 23,* 62–69.

Kazdin, A. E. (1994). Methodology, design, and evaluation in psychotherapy research. In A. E. Bergen & S. L. Garfield (Eds.) *Handbook of psychotherapy and behavior change* (4th ed., pp.19–71). New York, NY: Wiley.

Lei, H., Nahum-Shani, I., Lynch, K., Oslin, D., & Murphy, S. A. (2012). A "SMART" design for building individualized treatment sequences. *Annual Review of Clinical Psychology, 8,* 21–48.

Melnyk, B., & Morrison-Beedy, D. (2012). *Intervention research: Designing, conducting, analyzing, and funding.* New York, NY: Springer.

Tate, D. F., Finkelstein, E. A., Khavjou, O., & Gustafson, A. (2009). Cost effectiveness of internet interventions: Review and recommendations. *Annals of Behavioral Medicine, 38,* 40–45.

Webb, T. L., Joseph, J., Yardley, L., & Michie, S. (2010). Using the internet to promote health behavior change: A systematic review and meta-analysis of the impact of theoretical basis, use of behavior change techniques, and mode of delivery on efficacy. *Journal of Medical Internet Research, 12*(1), e4. doi:10.2196/jmir.1376

SIX

STANDARDIZATION

Internal validity is the basic minimum without which any experiment is
un-interpretable: Did in fact the experimental treatments make a difference in
the experimental instance?
—Campbell and Stanley (1963)

As stressed throughout this book, a main goal of behavioral intervention research is to develop interventions that effectively address identifiable and documented public health issues, policy gaps, health disparities, or care approaches (Chapter 1). Behavioral intervention research is challenging, and the design, evaluation, and implementation of behavioral interventions require a systematic and well-documented approach. A systematic approach is required to establish confidence that an intervention has an impact on outcomes of interest. It also facilitates the ability of other researchers to replicate the intervention and, ultimately, the implementation of the intervention in community and clinical settings. Reports of intervention research trials should explain the methods used in the trial, including the design, delivery, recruitment processes, components of the invention, and the context (see Chapter 24). Unfortunately, in many instances, behavioral intervention researchers fall short in the reporting of study design and methods, which limits use of research findings, diminishes optimal implementation of intervention programs, wastes resources, and fails to meet ethical obligations to research participants and consumers (Mayo-Wilson et al., 2013). Often this is due to the lack of detailed protocols for, and documentation of, intervention activities.

Generally, as discussed in Chapter 14, internal validity refers to the reliability/accuracy of the results of a research trial—the extent to which the changes in outcome measures or differences between treatment groups can be confidently attributed to the intervention as opposed to extraneous variables (Kazdin, 1994). There are numerous factors that impact on internal validity, including historical events, maturation, repeated assessments, bias, and confounding factors. History or external events experienced differentially by groups can pose a threat to internal validity. For example, if an investigator is interested in evaluating a multisite workplace intervention to promote healthy eating and, during the course of the trial, some of the participating workplace sites change the food offerings at their cafeterias, it would be difficult at the end of the trial to attribute any changes in the eating habits of employees to the intervention. In this case, the event is out of the control of the investigator. However, the manner in which a trial is conducted is under the control of the investigator; as such, the investigator must track and document these types of events. Poorly conducted intervention trials increase the likelihood of confounding variables and biases, which in turn threaten the internal validity of the study.

In this chapter, we discuss issues related to the standardization of behavioral intervention research studies and address topics such as aspects of the trial that need to be standardized, tailoring, and strategies to enhance standardization such as manuals of operation (MOP) and training of research team members. Our intent is to highlight the importance of taking steps to ensure that research activities at all stages of the pipeline are of the highest quality, so that potential benefits of the intervention are maximized and potential threats to internal validity are minimized. Developing strategies for standardizing research protocols and methodologies is important at all stages of the pipeline. This is the case for the beginning stages of developing an intervention, which might involve observational studies, as well as for later stages, which generally involve experimental designs (Chapter 2). Standardization is essential to maintaining treatment integrity as discussed in Chapter 12. Finally, it is our experience that having detailed protocols and manuals for intervention activities (regardless of stage of its development) greatly facilitates the reporting of the results and the development of manuscripts. In fact, most refereed journals require that intervention trials adhere to the Consort Standards (Schulz, Altman, & Moher, 2010) for reporting randomized trials (see Chapter 24).

WHY IS STANDARDIZATION IMPORTANT?

Treatment fidelity refers to strategies used within an intervention study to monitor the implementation of the intervention to ensure that it is being delivered as intended. As discussed in Chapter 12, having a treatment fidelity plan enhances the reliability and validity of an intervention trial and is integral to the interpretation of study findings (Resnick et al., 2005). For example, if an investigator discovered after the completion of a trial that there was variation among the trial interventionists in the delivery of the intervention, it would be extremely difficult to interpret the findings of the study and understand if the outcomes were due to the treatment or to differences in interventionist behavior. Thus, in this case, we would learn very little about the impact of an intervention, which would be a waste of time, effort, and resources.

Standardization of the intervention protocol is a key element of treatment fidelity and has a significant impact on the internal validity of an intervention trial. It can also influence external validity. If, for example, differential inclusion/exclusion criteria were applied to study participants, it would be difficult to make statements about the generalizability of study outcomes. Standardization of the intervention protocol instills greater confidence that the intervention treatment was delivered consistently across participants as intended. This in turn reduces variability and potential biases, which results in greater confidence in the validity and reliability of the study outcomes. Standardization also enhances the ability of other investigators to replicate an intervention protocol, which is particularly important in multisite trials and in the implementation phase; the efficiency of a trial; and an investigator's ability to disseminate findings that emanate from a study.

For example, in the Personal Reminder Information System Management (PRISM) trial (Czaja, Loewenstein, Schulz, Nair, & Perdomo, 2014), which was a multisite trial that investigated the impact of a specially designed software program on the social connectivity and well-being of older adults at risk for social isolation, each site had multiple interventionists who implemented the intervention protocol (e.g., training the participants on the use of the software). The training program for the interventionists was standardized in that all interventionists were trained similarly and certified by the Miami site. This helped to ensure consistency among the interventionists and also reduced training costs, especially during the course of the project when new interventionists were brought on board.

WHAT NEEDS TO BE STANDARDIZED?

Now that we have established the importance of standardization, we will review aspects of an intervention protocol that need to be standardized—simply put, all of the elements of a protocol beginning with the study design through treatment delivery and assessment (Table 6.1). With respect to the study design, this must be established early on in a study as it sets the stage for other elements of the protocol. Unless adaptive and emerging trial design approaches are being used (see Chapter 2), the design of a study is rarely changed throughout the course of a trial. The participant inclusion/exclusion criteria must also be firmly established and well defined. For example, in the PRISM trial (Czaja et al., 2013), our target population was older adults "at risk for social isolation." We operationalized "at risk for social isolation" as living alone, not working or volunteering more than 5 hours a week and not spending time at a senior center or formal organization for more than 10 hours per week. Sometimes, in the beginning of a trial based on the recruitment data, the trial entry criteria may need to be adjusted. However, this should be done infrequently, be well justified, and be clearly specified. For example, early on in the PRISM trial, we learned that an inclusion criterion, "never having used a computer," was too stringent as some individuals reported that they had been exposed to a computer in their doctor's office or through a child or grandchild. Thus, this criterion was adjusted to "not having a computer at home, not having an e-mail address, and limited experience with a computer." The original and adjusted criterion were both documented and dated in a MOPs, which was continuously referred to in reporting results.

Another standardized approach is the consent. Clearly, as discussed in Chapter 13, the consent form must be consistent with the study protocol and as must be the process for obtaining consent. It is understood that in some cases there might be separate consent forms for subgroups of participants such as parents and children, but within subgroups the consent form and the process for consenting must be the same.

Participant screening protocols should also be standardized, as should the type of data collected during screening. Typically, a screening script and a screening

---

TABLE 6.1 Elements of an Intervention That Need to Be Standardized

Elements to Be Standardized

Inclusion/exclusion criteria

Consent protocols

Participant screening protocol
- Scripted
- Information collected

Data collection protocol
- Recruitment information—source—"How did the participant hear about the study?"
- Eligibility/noneligibility
- Categories of reasons for noneligibility
- Dropouts and reasons for dropouts
- Assessment protocol
  - Measures
  - Order of, and protocol for, administration
  - Who does the assessment
  - Blinding protocol
  - Data coding
  - Data storage and transfer

Treatment implementation
- Content
- Dosage
- Planned participant contacts
- Order/sequencing
- Nature of compensations
- Training of participants
- Protocol and documentation of unplanned contacts

Training of interventionist

Data-coding strategies

Protocols for reporting of adverse events/alerts and for event resolution

---

data form need to be developed. Screening data should include recruitment information (how did the individual hear about the study?), eligibility status, reasons for noneligibility (if appropriate), eligibility questions, and basic demographic information. Investigators also need to develop a system for tracking characteristics of participants who drop out of the study and the reasons for dropping out (Chapter 10).

There are numerous aspects of a data collection protocol that need to be standardized, including the measures and assessment instruments, protocol for the administration of measures/questionnaires, timing of assessments, team members responsible for the assessments, and blinding protocols. There should also be a specified procedure for data coding, data transfer, and data storage and for reporting and resolving adverse events and serious adverse events (Chapter 13). Table 6.2 presents a sample of the assessment battery used in the PRISM trial according to the order of administration of the measures and the format for administration. For this trial, measures were collected over the telephone at the follow-up assessments as it

TABLE 6.2   A Sample of PRISM Assessment Battery: Order and Format of Administration

Baseline—Mail	6 Months—Mail
Demographic information (Czaja et al., 2006a)	Demographic information
Technology, computer, Internet experience questionnaire (Czaja et al., 2006b)	Technology, computer, Internet experience questionnaire
Computer attitudes (Jay & Willis, 1982)	
Life Space Questionnaire (Stalvey, Owsley, Sloane, & Ball, 1999)	Computer attitudes
	Life Space Questionnaire
Formal care and services utilization (Wisniewski et al., 2003)	Formal care and services utilization
Technology Acceptance Questionnaire	
Computer proficiency (Boot et al., 2015)	Technology Acceptance Questionnaire
Ten-Item Personality Inventory (TIPI; Gosling, Rentfrow, & Swann, 2003)	Computer proficiency
	PRISM System/Control Group Evaluation
Baseline—In Person	**6 Months—In Person**
Mini-Mental State Exam (Folstein, Folstein, & McHugh, 1975)	STOFHLA
Fuld Object-Memory Evaluation (Fuld, 1978)	SF-36
Snellen Test of Visual Acuity	Perception of Memory Functioning
WRAT_T (Jastak & Wilkinson, 1984)	
Animal Fluency (Rosen, 1980)	**6 Months—Phone**
STOFHLA (Baker, Williams, Parker, Gazmararian, & Nurss, 1999)	Social Network Size
	Social Support
Reaction Time Task	Loneliness Scale
Stroop Color Name (McCabe, Robertson, & Smith, 2005)	Perceived Vulnerability Scale
Social Network Size (Berkman & Syme, 1979; Lubben, 1988)	
Shipley vocabulary (Shipley, 1986)	CESD
Trails A and B (Reitan, 1958)	Social Isolation
Social Support (Cohen, Mermelstein, Kamarack, & Hoberman, 1985)	Life Engagement Test
	Quality of Life
Loneliness Scale (Russell, 1996)	
SF-36 (Ware & Sherbourne, 1992)	
Digit Symbol Substitution (Wechsler, 1981)	
Letter Sets (Ekstrom, Frendch, Harman, & Dermen, 1976, pp. I-1, 80, 81, 84)	
Perception of Memory Functioning (Gilewski, Zelinski, & Schaie, 1990)	
Perceived Vulnerability Scale (Myall et al., 2009)	
CESD (Irwin, Artin, & Oxman, 1999; Radloff, 1977)	
Social Isolation (Hawthorne, 2006)	
Life Engagement Test (Scheier et al., 2006)	
Quality of Life (Logsdon, Gibbons, McCurry, & Teri, 2002)	

PRISM, Personalized Reminder Information and Social Management; STOFHLA, Short Test of Functional Health Literacy in Adults; SF-36, Short Form Health Survey; CESD, Center for Epidemiologic Studies Depression.

would have been difficult for assessors to remain blinded to treatment as the study involved technology that was placed in the homes of participants.

Finally, it is imperative to detail all of the elements of the treatment conditions including the control condition (if one is included in a trial). This includes the content; format of delivery (e.g., home vs. telephone); dosage and planned participant contacts; the ordering/sequencing of the content/components of the intervention; and protocols for participant compensation. It is also important to have plans for "unplanned contacts" and "what if scenarios." Of course, we realize that when dealing with human research participants it is difficult to predict unplanned events. We recommend developing a session-by-session plan if an intervention involves "sessions" (Chapter 3) and a protocol for tracking all participant contacts (planned and unplanned). The latter should include duration of contact, which will greatly facilitate dosage-outcome analyses. In addition, protocols for classifying, recording, reporting, and resolving adverse events and serious adverse events should be in place (see Chapter 13).

TAILORING OF INTERVENTIONS

A general principle guiding the development of interventions is that effective interventions are tailored/customized to the key risks, needs, and specific profiles of target populations and contexts (Chapter 1). A growing body of literature indicates that tailoring health information is more efficacious than a "one-size-fits-all approach" (e.g., Caiata Zufferey & Schulz, 2009; Noar, Benac, & Harris, 2007). A distinction can be made between *targeted* intervention strategies and *tailored* intervention strategies (Beck et al., 2010). Targeting intervention strategies refer to developing aspects of the intervention or intervention components to address certain characteristics of the population such as age, gender, or ethnicity. In intervention research, cultural adaptation, which refers to the *systematic* modifications of an intervention to consider language, culture, and context to be compatible with an individual's background and values (Barrera, Castro, Strycker, & Toobert, 2013), is common. This helps to reduce disparities in intervention access, facilitates recruitment of cultural minorities, and helps to ensure that interventions reach diverse subgroups and populations. An example is designing recruitment materials differently for different ethnic groups (Figure 6.1). This might include presenting the material in different languages and using different graphics and images. Other examples include using bicultural staff and incorporating familiar cultural traditions into intervention materials (Barrera et al., 2013).

Tailoring intervention strategies refers to modifying elements of an intervention so that they are uniquely individualized for an individual on the basis of some assessment. For example, in the REACH II trial, a questionnaire was used, referred to as the "risk appraisal," which identified areas that caregivers were at risk for, such as home hazards, lack of skills managing behaviors, or depressive symptoms. The risk appraisal was administered during the baseline assessment and then used to "tailor" the intervention to the specific needs of the caregiver.

Tailoring can also involve modifying the content according to the skill level or knowledge of the individual. The initial step in tailoring is selecting the

Caring for the Caregiver Network
A Research Study for Caregivers of Dementia and Alzheimer's Patients

The University of Miami Center on Aging is conducting a research study aimed to improve the lives of family caregivers.

Join us in our search to find ways to improve caregivers' ability to provide care to their loved ones and to reduce disparities in access to needed services and support among caregivers.

We are seeking English or Spanish speakers who are currently caring for a loved one diagnosed with Dementia or Alzheimer's disease.

Eligible participants may receive:
- A tablet computer during study participation
- Access to Web-based skill-building sessions
- Videos from experts, resources, information, and tips on caregiving or nutrition-related topics
- Compensation for time and participation

To learn more about this research study and how you may be eligible to participate, please contact the University of Miami Center on Aging.

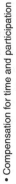

UNIVERSITY OF MIAMI
MILLER SCHOOL
of MEDICINE

 (XXX) XXX - XXXX   XXX.XXX@XXXXX.XXXX.edu

Red de Cuidado para Cuidadores
A Research Study for Caregivers of Dementia and Alzheimer's Patients

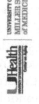

El Centro de Envejecimiento en la Universidad de Miami está realizando un estudio de investigación con el objetivo de mejorar la vida de los cuidadores.

Únete en nuestra búsqueda para encontrar formas de mejorar la capacidad de los cuidadores para atender a sus seres queridos y para reducir las disparidades en el acceso a los servicios y el apoyo entre los cuidadores.

Estamos buscando a personas que hablan inglesa o español que actualmente están cuidando a un ser querido diagnosticado con demencia o enfermedad de Alzheimer.

Los participantes elegibles pueden recibir:
- Una computadora de tableta para uso durante la participación en el estudio
- El acceso a sesiones de desarrollo de habilidades basadas en la Web
- Videos de expertos, recursos, información y consejos sobre temas relacionados con la nutrición y el cuidado
- Compensación por tiempo y participación

Para obtener más información sobre este estudio de investigación y cómo usted puede ser elegible para participar por favor póngase en contacto con El Centro de Envejecimiento en la Universidad de Miami.

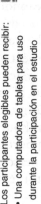

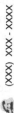 UNIVERSITY OF MIAMI
MILLER SCHOOL
of MEDICINE

(XXX) XXX - XXXX   XXX.XXX@XXXXX.XXXX.edu

Figure 6.1 Example of targeted recruitment material.

characteristics on which the intervention will be tailored. As noted by Beck et al. (2010), this should be driven by theories or prior research that demonstrates the association between these characteristics and study outcomes. Tailoring of an intervention might also involve modifying the intervention schedule or location of intervention delivery to correspond to an individual's needs. Adjusting the delivery of an intervention to accommodate an individual (within reason, of course) may help offset potential problems with attrition or delays in assessments.

So what are the implications of targeting and tailoring with respect to standardization? In short, the goals of standardization can still be achieved even if targeting or tailoring is part of the intervention protocol. The important consideration is planning and systematizing the strategies for targeting/tailoring the intervention materials or protocol. This cannot be done on an ad hoc basis. The plan for targeting/tailoring interventions needs to clearly articulate which aspects of the intervention can be modified, the boundaries of modifications, and who on the team can make decisions with respect to modifications. It must also include when modifications can occur and a systematic plan for making modifications. Of course, the essence or core elements of an intervention must be maintained. In addition, the cost and effort involved in targeting or tailoring an intervention must also be considered. For example, although it may be more convenient for a small group of participants to attend support group sessions on a Saturday evening, this might entail hiring an additional person on the research team who would be willing to adhere to this schedule. In this case, the benefits of maintaining a small number of participants would need to be carefully weighed against hiring an additional staff person.

STRATEGIES TO ENHANCE STANDARDIZATION

Manual of Operation

It is essential to develop a detailed MOP for a behavioral intervention study at any stage along the pipeline. We recognize that MOPs will be more detailed for larger scale efficacy and effectiveness trials; however, having a documented protocol is also important at the early stages (e.g., focus groups, usability studies). There are numerous advantages to developing and implementing MOPs in intervention research. One clear advantage is that they help to enhance the internal validity of a study by standardizing the treatment protocols. They also serve as a valuable tool for training interventionists and other team members and enhance the efficiency of training. We recommend having team members review the MOP before they begin any other formal training/certification process. The use of treatment manuals also facilitates the ability to have the interventions replicated across locations and at different points in time. In addition, having a detailed MOP greatly facilitates dissemination and the preparation of reports and articles related to the intervention. An example of the MOP developed for the PRISM project is presented in Figure 6.2. This shows the level of detail that is included in most MOPs for efficacy or effectiveness studies. In all cases, it is important to ensure that a MOP for a study is thorough so that no important details are missing and that the MOP is current. The MOP must also be understandable, usable, and available. In other words, a MOP that is written in highly technical language and hidden on the back of someone's bookshelf has limited utility. Finally, MOPs serve as a valuable training tool but do not suffice as a sole training mechanism.

Selection and Training of Team Members

As discussed in other chapters of this book (e.g., Chapters 5 and 22), the selection and training of team members is an important aspect of behavioral intervention research. Staffing considerations include the number of staff members, skill, educational and certification requirements, and allocation of functions and responsibilities. Staffing decisions clearly depend on the scope of the project and, of course, the budget. It is a good idea to conduct a task analysis of the intervention (Chapter 3) and planned study design to identify staffing needs (see also Chapter 5). Another important issue is ensuring that the roles and responsibilities of all of the team members are clearly specified and communicated within the team (discussed as well in Chapter 22). This information should be included in the MOP.

Protocols must also be developed for staff training and certification, and these protocols should all be included in the MOP (see Figure 6.2). All members of the study team should understand the goals of the study and be trained in all aspects of the protocol, including the protocols for both the intervention and comparison conditions. Staff members must also understand the importance of adhering to the study protocol (e.g., delivery of the intervention) for all treatment conditions. Training should also be provided on the topical domain of the intervention (e.g., family caregiving) and on strategies for interacting with study participants. Other important training topics include staff safety protocols, resolution protocols for adverse events, ethical conduct of research and confidentiality, and data handling. Finally, one-time training is rarely sufficient—we highly recommend booster training on a scheduled basis. All of these aspects are important aspects of standardizing study procedures.

Other Strategies to Enhance Standardization

Development of a plan to monitor the delivery of the intervention and of assessments is another important aspect of an intervention protocol (Chapter 12). This helps to prevent "burnout" and "drift" among interventionists and assessors, which can threaten internal validity. If an interventionist delivers an intervention for an extended period of time, it may become routine and thus he or she may take "shortcuts" or leave out important elements. Having a plan for monitoring the delivery of the intervention and a protocol for providing feedback can help to minimize this issue.

Finally, it is important to have regularly scheduled team meetings. This provides team members with an opportunity to discuss issues that may arise and to seek advice on situations that may be somewhat out of the ordinary. It also provides them with a chance to discuss aspects of the intervention/control group protocols or assessment protocols that are challenging or problematic. As noted in Chapter 22, having regularly scheduled team meetings also fosters team cohesiveness.

Table of Contents

	page
Section I. Background information	1
1. Description of the project/study design	1
2. Project timeline	4
3. Recruitment materials	4
Section II. Project flowchart, randomization procedures and scripts	1
1. Detailed project flowchart	1
2. Project scripts	2
A. Telephone screening	2
B. First home visit script	5
C. Condition assignment	7
D. PRISM-B training script	9
E. PRISM-C training script	14
F. Training follow-up telephone call	27
G. Telephone check-in calls	28
H. Monthly e-mail scripts	31
I. Script for Non-use of PRISM-C check-in call	32
J. Script for 6th/12th-month follow-up telephone assessment	33
K. Script for 6th/12th-month follow-up scheduler	34
L. Script for contacting disqualified participants due to FULD score	35
M. Script for re-administering FULD	36
Section III. Sample, recruitment, and retention	1
1. Inclusion/exclusion criteria	1
2. Recruitment guidelines	1
3. Screening protocol	1
4. Informed consent	2
5. Retention strategies	2
Section IV. Scheduling contacts	1
1. Protocol after screening interview	1
2. Protocol for lengthy lapse between screening, baseline, and installation	1
3. Protocol for rescheduling the home interview	1
4. Protocol for home interview	2
5. Protocol for non-use of PRISM-C	5
6. Protocol for making telephone assessment	5
7. Protocol for dealing with field challenges	6
8. Protocol for conducting 6th-month follow-up	7
9. Protocol for conducting 12th-month follow-up	7
10. Confidentiality	8
11. Managing interview challenges	9
Section V. Field trial overview	1
1. Flowchart	1
2. Description of PRISM	2
3. Contact description	3
4. Contact checklist	4
5. Description of control group (PRISM-B)	5
6. Enrolling/removing PRISM-C participants	5
7. Updating PRISM-C calendars	6
8. Adding/removing PRISM buddies	6
Section VI. Training protocols	1
1. PRISM-B condition	1
2. PRISM-C condition	6
Section VII. Adverse events	1
Section VIII. PRISM termination protocol	1
1. Script for PRISM-B 12th-month termination	1
2. Script for PRISM-C 12th-month termination	2
3. Instructions on how to apply the post-PRISM study default PC image	4
Section VIII. Certification protocol for assessors/interventionists	1

Appendix

- Flyer
- Brochure
- Delivery Assessment Form
- PRISM-B Buddy List Enrollment Form
- PRISM-C Buddy List Enrollment Form
- PRISM Adverse Events Form
- PRISM Classroom Topics and Subtopics List
- Letters:
  - PRISM-B classroom letters
  - Response card letter
  - Follow-up mail package questionnaire
  - Baseline mail package
  - Unable to reach over phone
  - Termination letter PRISM-B
  - Termination letter PRISM-C

Figure 6.2 Example of the manual of operations for the PRISM trial.

CONCLUSION

Behavioral intervention research is challenging and requires a systematic and well-documented approach. This is essential to having confidence that an intervention has an impact on outcomes of interest. It also facilitates the ability of other researchers to replicate the intervention and, ultimately, the implementation of the intervention in community and clinical settings. This does not imply that it is not possible to target intervention materials for subgroups within a sample or to tailor an intervention according to pre-established individual characteristics. Targeting intervention materials and tailoring also require a systematic and well-documented approach. In this chapter, we offer suggestions for enhancing the standardization of an intervention protocol. This includes developing a thorough and up-to-date MOP and a solid plan for training team members, which includes booster sessions. A plan for monitoring treatment integrity must also be in place, and there should be established mechanisms for communication within the research team. Adoption of these strategies for standardizing study protocols will greatly enhance the quality, accuracy, and reliability of the findings generated from an intervention research study.

REFERENCES

Baker, D. W., Williams, M. V., Parker, R. M., Gazmararian, J. A., & Nurss, J. (1999). Development of a brief test to measure functional health literacy. *Patient Education and Counseling, 38*, 33–42.

Barrera, M., Castro, F. G., Strycker, L. A., & Toobert, D. J. (2013). Cultural adaptations of behavioral health interventions: A progress report. *Journal of Consulting and Clinical Psychology, 81*, 196–205.

Beck, C., McSweeney, J. C., Richards, K. C., Roberson, P. K., Tsai, P., & Souder, E. (2010). Challenges in tailored intervention research. *Nursing Outlook, 58*, 104–110.

Berkman, L. F., & Syme, S. L. (1979). Social networks, host resistance, and mortality: A nine year follow-up study of Alameda county residents. *American Journal of Epidemiology, 109*, 186–204.

Boot, W. R., Charness, N., Czaja, S. J., Sharit, J., Rogers, W. A., Fisk, A. D., . . . Nair, S. (2015). Computer Proficiency Questionnaire (CPQ): Assessing low and high computer proficient seniors. *Gerontologist, 55*(3), 404–411. doi:10.1093/geront/gnt117

Caiata Zufferey, M., & Schulz, P. J. (2009). Self-management of chronic low back pain: An exploration of the impact of a patient-centered website. *Patient Education and Counseling, 77*(1), 27–32.

Campbell, D. T., & Stanley, J. (1963). *Experimental and quasi-experimental designs for research.* Chicago, IL: Rand McNally.

Cohen, S., Mermelstein, R., Kamarck, T., Hoberman, H. M. (1985). Measuring the functional components of social support. In I. G. Sarason & B. R. Sarason (Eds.), *Social support: Theory, research and applications* (pp. 73–94). Dordrecht, Netherlands: Martinus Nijhoff Publishers.

Czaja, S. J., Charness, N., Dijkstra, K., Fisk, A. D., Rogers, W. A., & Sharit, J. (2006a). *Demographic and Background Questionnaire* (CREATE-2006-02).

Czaja, S. J., Charness, N., Dijkstra, K., Fisk, A. D., Rogers, W. A., & Sharit, J. (2006b). *Computer and Technology Experience Questionnaire* (CREATE-2006-01).

Czaja, S. J., Loewenstein, D., Schulz, R., Nair, S. N., & Perdomo, D. (2013). A videophone psychosocial intervention for dementia caregivers. *American Journal of Geriatric Psychiatry, 21*(11), 1071–1081.

Ekstrom, R. B., French, J. W., Harman, H. H., & Dermen, D. (1976). *Manual for kit of factor-referenced cognitive tests—Letter sets.* Princeton, NJ: Educational Testing Service.

Folstein, M. F., Folstein, S. E., & McHugh, P. R. (1975). Mini-mental state: A practical method for grading the cognitive state of patients for the clinician. *Journal of Psychiatric Research, 12,*189–198.

Fuld, P. A. (1978). Psychological testing in the differential diagnosis of the dementias. In R. Katzman, R. D. Terry, & K. L. Biele (Eds.), *Alzheimer's disease: Senile dementia and related disorders* (pp. 185–193). New York, NY: Raven Press.

Gilewski, M. J., Zelinkski, E. M., & Schaie, K. W. (1990). The memory functioning questionnaire for assessment of memory complaints in adulthood and old age. *Psychology and Aging, 5,* 482–490.

Gosling, S. D., Rentfrow, P. J., & Swann, W. B., Jr. (2003). A very brief measure of the Big-Five personality domains. *Journal of Research in Personality, 37,* 504–528.

Hawthorne, G. (2006). Measuring social isolation in older adults: Development and initial validation of the friendship scale. *Social Indicators Research, 77,* 521–548.

Irwin, M., Artin, K. H., & Oxman, M. N. (1999). Screening for depression in the older adult: Criterion validity of the 10-item Center for Epidemiological Studies Depression Scale (CES-D). *Archives of Internal Medicine, 159,* 1701–1704.

Jastak, S., & Wilkinson, G. S. (1984). *The Wide Range Achievement Test-Revised: Administration manual.* Wilmington, DE: Jastak Associates.

Jay, G. M., & Willis, S. L. (1992). Influence of direct computer experience on older adults' attitude toward computers. *Journal of Gerontology: Psychological Sciences, 47,* P250–P257.

Kazdin, A. E. (1994). Methodology, design, and evaluation in psychotherapy research. In A. E. Bergen & S. L. Garfield (Eds.), *Handbook of psychotherapy and behavior change* (4th ed., pp. 19–71). New York, NY: Wiley.

Logsdon, R. G., Gibbons, L. E., McCurry, S. M., & Teri, L. (2002). Assessing quality of life in older adults with cognitive impairment. *Psychosomatics Medicine, 64,* 510–519.

Lubben, J. E. (1988). Assessing social networks among elderly populations. *Family & Community Health, 11,* 42–52.

Mayo-Wilson, E., Grant, S., Hopewell, S., Macdonald, G., Moher, D., & Montgomery, P. (2013). Developing a reporting guideline for social and psychological intervention trials. *Trials, 14,* 242.

McCabe, D. P., Robertson, C. L., & Smith, A. d. (2005). Age differences in stroop interference in working memory. *Journal of Clinical and Experimental Neuropsychology, 27,* 633–644.

Myall, B. R., Hine, D. W., Marks, A. D. G., Thorsteinsson, E. B., Brechman-Toussaint, M., & Samuels, C. A. (2009). Assessing individual differences in perceived vulnerability in older adults. *Personality and Individual Differences, 46,* 8–13.

Noar, S. M., Benac, C. N., & Harris, M. S. (2007). Does tailoring matter? Meta-analytic review of tailored print health behavior change interventions. *Psychological Bulletin, 133*(4), 673–693. doi:10.1037/0033-2909.133.4.673

Radloff, L. (1977). The CES-D scale: A self-report depression scale for research in the general population. *Applied Psychological Measures, 1,* 385–401.

Reitan, R. M. (1958). Validity of the trail making test as an indication of organic brain damage. *Perceptual and Motor Skills, 9,* 271–276.

Resnick, B., Inquito, P., Orwig, D., Yahiro, J. Y., Hawkes, W., Werner, M., . . . Magaziner, J. (2005). Treatment fidelity in behavior change research: A case example. *Nursing Research, 54,* 139–143.

Rosen, W. G. (1980). Verbal fluency in aging and dementia. *Journal of Clinical and Experimental Neuropsychology, 2*, 135–146.

Russell, D. W. (1996). UCLA Loneliness Scale (Version 3): Reliability, validity, and factor structure. *Journal of Personality Assessment, 66*, 20–40.

Scheier, M. F., Wrosch, C., Baum, A., Cohen, S., Martire, L. M., Matthews, K., . . . Zdaniuk, B. (2006). The Life Engagement Test: Assessing purpose in life. *Journal of Behavioral Medicine, 29*, 291–298.

Schulz, K. F., Altman, D. G., & Moher, D. (2010). CONSORT 2010 statement: Updated guidelines for reporting parallel group randomized trials. *Annals of Internal Medicine, 152*, 726–732.

Shipley, W. C. (1986). *Shipley Institute of Living Scale.* Los Angeles, CA: Western Psychological Services.

Stalvey, B. T., Owsley, C., Sloane, M. E., & Ball, K. (1999). The Life Space Questionnaire: A measure of the extent of mobility of older adults. *Journal of Applied Gerontology, 18*, 460–478.

Ware, J. E., & Sherbourne, C. D. (1992). The MOS 36-item short-form health survey (SF-36): Conceptual framework and item selection. *Medical Care, 30*, 473–483.

Wechsler, D. (1981). *Manual for Wechsler Memory Scaled Revised.* New York, NY: The Psychological Corporation.

Wisniewski, S. R., Belle, S. H., Marcus, S. M., Burgio, L. D., Coon, D. W., Ory, M. G., . . . Schulz, R. (2003). The Resources for Enhancing Alzheimer's Caregiver Health (REACH): Project design and baseline characteristics. *Psychology and Aging, 18*(3), 375–384.

SEVEN

THE USE OF TECHNOLOGY IN BEHAVIORAL INTERVENTION RESEARCH: ADVANTAGES AND CHALLENGES

RONALD W. BERKOWSKY AND SARA J. CZAJA

> *BITs not only provide new delivery media for mental health treatments,*
> *they also open the possibility for entirely new interventions.*
> —Mohr, Burns, Schueller, Clarker, and Klinkman (2013)

In a broad sense, technology refers to tools and machines that are used to perform real-world activities (e.g., communication technologies). Technology can be simple (e.g., hand tool), complex (e.g., computer), or "virtual" (e.g., software applications; Brian, 2009). Technology is ubiquitous within our society and has changed the way we learn, work, shop, interact, and communicate. The use of technology is also prevalent within the health care arena and increasingly being used for health care delivery and services. With this rapid growth in both the popularity and prevalence of technologies and the increased capabilities of technology, behavioral intervention researchers have also been incorporating various technology devices and applications into their research protocols. Technology is being used as a vehicle to deliver interventions, as a data collection tool, and to aid data analysis.

The use of technology in behavioral intervention research as a mechanism for treatment delivery holds promise. For example, technology-based interventions have proven to be both feasible and efficacious for a broad range of populations such as caregivers (e.g., Czaja, Loewenstein, Schulz, Nair, & Perdomo, 2013), older adults (e.g., Irvine, Gelatt, Seeley, Macfarlane, & Gau, 2013), and a variety of patient populations such as those with cancer (e.g., Børøsund, Cvancarova, Moore, Ekstedt, & Ruland, 2014; Freeman et al., 2014), diabetes (e.g., Piette et al., 2000), hypertension (e.g., Friedman et al., 1996), and depression (e.g., Mohr et al., 2005). The results of these studies also generally indicate that technology-based interventions are feasible and acceptable to target populations.

Technologies also afford behavioral intervention researchers unprecedented capabilities in data collection. For example, there is a plethora of monitoring technologies that can be used to monitor health indices and behavioral patterns and more are on the horizon. Technology applications are also impacting the way we store and analyze data. Overall, the intersection of technology developments and behavioral intervention research is exciting and holds great potential; however, it is not without challenges. The focus of this chapter is to explore the role of technology in behavioral intervention research. We discuss the application of technology to intervention delivery and the role of technology in data collection and provide examples of technology applications within each of these areas. We also discuss some of the advantages and challenges associated with technology-based approaches and highlight issues that warrant further investigation. As this field is broad and characterized by rapid change, and because there is a broad range of available technologies, we provide only a sample of examples of technology applications. Our intent is to illustrate how technology is emerging as an important component of behavioral intervention research.

TECHNOLOGY AND BEHAVIORAL INTERVENTIONS

Given the advantages associated with technology such as broader reach to target populations, flexibility in intervention delivery modes, and potential cost savings, technology is increasingly being used to deliver behavioral interventions to a wide variety of populations. By way of definition, behavioral intervention technologies (BITs) are generally referred to as ". . . the application of behavioral and psychological intervention strategies through the use of technology features to address behavioral, cognitive and affective targets that support physical, behavioral and mental health" (Mohr et al., 2013, p. 332). BITs can significantly contribute to behavioral intervention research by providing new and innovative means for delivering interventions, increasing access to these interventions, and providing the means for the development of novel interventions such as those that involve multimedia formats or robotic applications (e.g., cognitive coaching to support memory; see Czaja, 2015).

BITs include the use of a broad range of technologies such as telephone/ videoconferencing, mobile devices, Web-based interventions, wearable technologies (e.g., FitBit), and robotic devices to implement intervention strategies such as self-assessment and self-monitoring, psychoeducation, peer support goal setting, skill building and education, goal setting, and feedback (Mohr et al., 2013). Imbedded in our definition is an important distinction: technologies are typically used to deliver an intervention but are usually not the mechanism for behavior change. For example, Irvine and colleagues (2013) used the Internet to deliver an intervention, *Active After 55*, to enhance functional ability, mobility, and physical activity of sedentary older adults. The intervention was based on the theory of planned behavior, was designed to provide information and support, and included general assistance, tailored assistance and feedback, self-assessment, and general information, combined within a gain-framed messaging framework. The investigators found that those who received the intervention experienced gains in engagement in physical activities, self-efficacy, and quality of life as well as fewer perceived barriers to exercise. We (Czaja et al., 2013) used videophone technology to deliver a modified version of the REACH II multicomponent, psychosocial intervention (Belle et al., 2006) to minority family caregivers of patients with Alzheimer's disease. Caregivers who received the intervention reported less burden, higher social support, and more positive feelings about caregiving. They also found the technology to be acceptable and usable. In these examples, BITs provided a means to intervention delivery but were not the mechanism of the actual behavioral change.

The following sections of this chapter provide specific examples of the types of technologies frequently used in intervention delivery and the types of interventions being delivered via these technologies.

Telephone and Videoconferencing Technologies

Telephone and videoconferencing technologies are used frequently in behavioral intervention research to deliver interventions such as individual counseling, peer support/support groups, family support, education, and reminders. Use of these technologies as a mechanism for treatment delivery can offset some of the inconveniences and costs associated with traveling to an interventionist or vice versa. This may also help to reduce participant attrition (Mohr et al., 2012; Mohr, Vella, Hart, Heckman, & Simon, 2008). In fact, studies within the mental health arena have shown that behavioral interventions delivered via telephone or videoconferencing can be as effective as face-to-face therapy sessions for the treatment of depression (Khatri, Marziali, Tchernikov, & Shepherd, 2014), obsessive-compulsive disorder (Himle et al., 2006; Vogel et al., 2012), posttraumatic stress disorder (Germain, Marchand, Bouchard, Drouin, & Guay, 2009), and mood and anxiety disorders (Stubbings, Rees, Roberts, & Kane, 2013).

Telephone and videoconferencing technologies have also been found to be an effective format for intervention delivery for other targeted behaviors and populations. In our videophone study with minority family caregivers (Czaja et al., 2013), we conducted individual skill-building sessions and support group sessions via phone/video. We also included a library of short video clips by experts on topics related to caregiving, as well as a resource guide and an information and tips feature (see Figure 7.1). The interventionists also used the phone to send reminder messages to the caregivers. As noted, the intervention was efficacious with respect to caregiver outcomes and the caregivers found the support group sessions to be particularly valuable. A recent systematic review of telephone interventions for physical activity and dietary behavior change (Eakin, Lawler, Vandelanotte, & Owen, 2007) concluded that there is a solid evidence base supporting the efficacy of physical activity and dietary behavior change interventions in which the telephone is the primary method of intervention delivery. Videoconferencing-based interventions have also been shown to be effective within this domain. For example, the ("Virtual Small Groups for an Innovative and Technological Approach to Healthy Lifestyle"; Azar et al., 2015) demonstrated that a 12-week group weight-loss intervention program (based on the Diabetes Prevention Program) delivered via Web-based videoconferencing resulted in significant weight loss among overweight men.

Study participants also typically have positive perceptions of telephone- and videoconference-based interventions. In a study examining the effects of videoconferencing on the treatment of obsessive-compulsive disorder, Himle et al. (2006) found an overall clinical improvement in the participants' symptoms and high ratings of treatment satisfaction and therapeutic alliance. "The participants quickly accommodated to the videoconferencing environment and uniformly reported high levels of 'telepresence' resulting in a feeling that they were 'in the room' with the

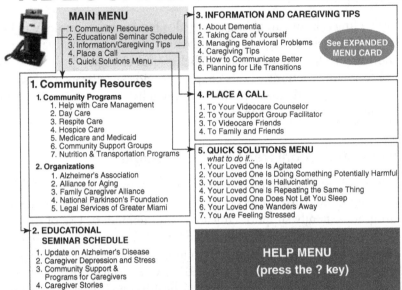

A VIDEOCARE PHONE MENUS

MAIN MENU
1. Community Resources
2. Educational Seminar Schedule
3. Information/Caregiving Tips
4. Place a Call
5. Quick Solutions Menu

3. INFORMATION AND CAREGIVING TIPS
1. About Dementia
2. Taking Care of Yourself
3. Managing Behavioral Problems
4. Caregiving Tips
5. How to Communicate Better
6. Planning for Life Transitions

See EXPANDED MENU CARD

1. Community Resources

1. Community Programs
1. Help with Care Management
2. Day Care
3. Respite Care
4. Hospice Care
5. Medicare and Medicaid
6. Community Support Groups
7. Nutrition & Transportation Programs

2. Organizations
1. Alzheimer's Association
2. Alliance for Aging
3. Family Caregiver Alliance
4. National Parkinson's Foundation
5. Legal Services of Greater Miami

4. PLACE A CALL
1. To Your Videocare Counselor
2. To Your Support Group Facilitator
3. To Videocare Friends
4. To Family and Friends

5. QUICK SOLUTIONS MENU
what to do if...
1. Your Loved One Is Agitated
2. Your Loved One Is Doing Something Potentially Harmful
3. Your Loved One Is Hallucinating
4. Your Loved One Is Repeating the Same Thing
5. Your Loved One Does Not Let You Sleep
6. Your Loved One Wanders Away
7. You Are Feeling Stressed

2. EDUCATIONAL SEMINAR SCHEDULE
1. Update on Alzheimer's Disease
2. Caregiver Depression and Stress
3. Community Support & Programs for Caregivers
4. Caregiver Stories

HELP MENU
(press the ? key)

B

AGITATION

- Try to assess what is causing your loved one to be agitated.
- Remain calm and redirect them by asking them what they need.
- Try and eliminate the source of the agitation.
- Avoid screaming or confrontation.
- Switch to a new activity.
- Offer something of comfort and speak in a calming voice.
- Walk away and give yourself some space.

VIDEOCARE

C

AGITACIÓN

- Trate de evaluar que es lo que esta potencialmente causando que su ser querido se ponga agitado.
- Manténgase calmado y redirija su atención por medio de preguntarle que es lo que quisiera hacer.
- Trate de eliminar la fuente de agitación.
- Evite gritar, confrontarle, o escalar en la agitación.
- Ofrézcale algo que le dé consuelo y hable con una voz calmada.
- Finalmente, aléjese, y dése su propio espacio.

VIDEOCARE

Figure 7.1 Videophone system. (A) Screen for main menu. (B) Screen for English version: sample of quick solutions for common problems. (C) Screen for Spanish version: sample of quick solutions for common problems.
Source: Czaja et al. (2013).

therapist" (p. 1827). Himle and colleagues (2006) had anticipated that the participants might be reluctant to express deep emotion owing to feeling self-conscious in an isolated environment (i.e., alone in a room with a technological device rather than a real live person), but their results found that this was generally not the case. Communicating via the telephone offers a certain degree of anonymity that is not possible in face-to-face interactions. In our work, we have also found high levels of willingness of our participants to engage in discussions with interventionists and with other caregivers in support groups. However, we have also found that it is important for the interventionists to display satisfaction with this format of intervention delivery, and the technology system must be easy to use.

Mobile Technologies

With the increased technical capabilities and adoption of mobile devices, mobile technologies, which typically refer to cell phones, smartphones, and tablet technologies, are increasingly being used as a format for intervention delivery. Mobile technologies can be used to send prompts and reminders to users via text, pop-up notifications, or audio/visual messages; to deliver educational programs and counseling; as a means for users to come in direct contact with medical personnel if needed; and as a way for interventionists/health care providers to provide suggestions for behavior modifications on the basis of real-time user-provided information.

In 2014, 64% of Americans owned a smartphone, 90% owned a cell phone, and 42% owned a tablet computer. Many people are dependent on smartphones for online access. This is especially true for those with lower education and ethnic minorities (Smith, 2015). Mobile phone penetration has also rapidly increased in less developed countries (Wilke & Oates, 2014) that often face considerable public health disparities and higher burdens of disease. Thus, mobile technologies present an opportunity for delivering health information and services to populations who frequently confront problems with access. Clearly, the use of "apps" as a means of delivering mobile health interventions is exciting as mobile technologies offer the potential for providing individualized support to large numbers of individuals.

Given the recent emphasis on health-related "apps" (applications), the term "mHealth" has emerged, which is an abbreviation for "mobile health," that is, the practice of medicine and public health supported by mobile devices (Adibi, 2015). The field has grown so tremendously that there is now an interactional conference that focuses on mHealth (mHealth Summit). mHealth represents a subsegment of eHealth that refers to the use of information and communication technologies, such as Internet-connected computers, for the delivery of health services and information.

Tran, Tran, and White (2012) conducted a review of apps targeted for the management of diabetes and found that individuals can successfully use "apps" such as *Diabetes Buddy*, *Diabetes Log*, and *Diabetes Pilot* (among others) to self-monitor blood glucose levels. Use of these "apps" can also facilitate a provider's access to a patient's data and his or her ability to provide feedback with regards to self-management practices. Mobile applications have also been shown to have a positive impact on individuals suffering from anxiety, bipolar disorders, and schizophrenia (Depp et al., 2010; Granholm, Ben-Zeev, Link, Bradshaw, & Holden, 2012; Heron & Smyth, 2010). With regards to diet and exercise, however (for which there are many applications currently on the market), the use of mobile apps has found mixed results. Studies have shown that, although individuals using mobile apps for weight loss can more successfully self-monitor and assess their diets and caloric intake, the weight-loss trajectories of app users tend not to be significantly different from those who do not use mobile technologies (e.g., Laing et al., 2014; Wharton, Johnston, Cunningham, & Sterner, 2014).

Social media–based interventions are also typically included in discussions of mobile technologies, as they are often accessed using mobile devices. Popular social media sites include Facebook and Twitter. Online support groups also represent a form of social media. Findings regarding the use of social media to deliver health interventions are mixed. For example, Bull and colleagues (Bull, Levine, Black, Schmiege, & Santelli, 2012) found that a social media–delivered sexual health intervention increased safe sex practices among young adults. In contrast, Cavallo and colleagues (2012) evaluated a social media–based physical activity intervention. They found that use of an online social networking group plus self-monitoring did not produce greater perceptions of social support or physical activity as compared to an education-only control intervention. Mohr et al. (2013) argue that many social media spaces remain unregulated by a moderator, such as a health care professional, and thus lack a driving force that is able to "steer" individuals in the right direction with regards to behavior change. Because social media has become pervasive and engrained in the fabric of popular culture, more research is needed to determine how to effectively use social media in behavioral intervention research.

In summary, mobile technologies are technologies that individuals can hypothetically have with them at all times (and always turned on), and these technologies have also become a primary means of communication in the United States and world population. Thus, mobile devices can provide access to therapies and interventions to a large number of people. However, behavioral intervention research in this area is still emerging. There is a need for more systematic evaluation of using mobile technologies to deliver interventions to establish stronger evidence of the efficacy and effectiveness of this approach and to establish guidelines for best practices with respect to implementation and evaluation.

Internet-Based Interventions

Use of the Internet as a format for intervention delivery is also becoming quite common. For a majority of the population, Internet use has become a primary means of communicating and information gathering and is often used on a daily basis. Recent data from the Pew Internet and American Life study indicate that most U.S. adults report access to and general use of the Internet (Pew Research Center, 2014). Thus, the Internet provides a natural, convenient, and cost-effective format for the delivery of an intervention. For example, similar to telephone- and videoconferencing-based interventions, interventions delivered online can reduce costs associated with a participant's need to travel to an intervention location or for an interventionist to travel to a participant's home (Griffiths, Lindenmeyer, Powell, Lowe, & Thorogood, 2006; Napolitano et al., 2003). Internet-based implementation of an intervention also allows participants to access intervention content at their convenience and in many cases anonymously.

An additional advantage of Internet-based interventions is the ability to offer a variety of features that can be customized for the target population or an individual. This includes: the use of multimedia formats such as text-based information supplemented by audio/video media, and animation; variations in font sizes and colors; and rich graphic displays. With the advent of applications such as Skype, these formats can also be complemented by the use of videoconferencing.

The Internet can be used for a wide variety of intervention activities such as the provision of information and interactive sessions/exercises, performance assessment, provision of automated feedback based on user-shared information, sending prompts and reminders (similar to mobile text messages, but through the use of pop-ups or through e-mails), and provision of social support. Intervention modules can also be organized in an adaptive manner where intervention components can be accessed only at certain times or after other components have been successfully completed, and can be updated in real time with new information (Mohr et al., 2013). The use of the Internet to deliver behavioral interventions is growing rapidly, and findings regarding the efficacy and effectiveness of these interventions across a broad array of populations and conditions are generally positive. For example, a meta-analysis examining Internet-based interventions designed to treat depression found that these interventions generally have a significant positive effect on reducing depressive symptoms (Andersson & Cuijpers, 2009). Positive outcomes for Internet-based interventions have also been shown for other target populations such as family caregivers (Marziali & Donahue, 2006), breast cancer patients (Owen et al., 2005), and behaviors such as diabetes self-management (McKay, King, Eakin, Seeley, & Glasgow, 2001) and medical decision making (Kobak, Engelhardt, & Lipsitz, 2006). Clearly, the Internet holds a great deal of promise with respect to the delivery of behavioral interventions. However, there are still issues that need to be addressed such as high rates of participant attrition, which are not uncommon (Bennett & Glasgow, 2009). Other issues include privacy, informed consent (see Chapter 13), and lack of access and technical skills for some segments of the population.

Other Emerging Technology Applications

In addition to the more prevalent technologies already discussed, intervention researchers have also begun to use other BITs to deliver interventions such as virtual reality applications and gaming. For example, research is emerging on the use of "virtual humans" (or "conversational agents") in changing patient behavior. Virtual humans are images of men and women programmed into a device or application that are made to interact with the user typically through the use of automated prompts or messages. How these images are employed and what dialogues they are given to exchange with the user are dictated by the researcher/therapist; the virtual human can act as an informational agent that instructs a user on how to perform an activity or when to take certain types of medication. The virtual human can also act as a coach or cheerleader providing motivation and words of encouragement to the user. Although the use of virtual humans in behavioral interventions is relatively new, there has been significant progress showing that use of these applications can be used to effectively change behaviors including physical activity, fruit and vegetable consumption, and breastfeeding (Bickmore, Schulman, & Sidner, 2013; Zhang et al., 2014).

Another growing body of research has focused on virtual environments or a "virtual world." A virtual world, as defined by Boulos, Hetherington, and Wheeler (2007), is a ". . . computer-based, simulated multi-media environment, usually running over the Web, and designed so that users can 'inhabit' and interact via their own graphical self representations known as avatars" (p. 233). One of the most popular virtual worlds currently available is Second Life, and research has shown that virtual worlds such as Second Life can provide innovative avenues through which health information can be presented and shared (by both individuals and organizations such as the U.S. Centers for Disease Control and Prevention) on such topics as HIV, sexually-transmitted diseases and sexual health, and perceptual abnormalities (e.g., hallucinations experienced by those suffering from a mental health disorder; Beard, Wilson, Morra, & Keelan, 2009). A recent study on the feasibility and efficacy of a behavioral treatment delivered through Second Life showed that virtual worlds can be used to help improve symptoms associated with social anxiety (Yuen et al., 2013).

A final application involves the use of gaming (the act of playing games) as a way to deliver a behavioral intervention. Mohr et al. (2013) argue that gaming can act as an avenue for researchers and therapists to deliver information to patients as well as to promote participation and adherence to intervention protocols. However, they also note that more work is needed to examine the efficacy of interventions that involve gaming, but the limited data that is available is promising. For example, a recent review conducted by Baranowski and Frankel (2012) demonstrated how gaming applications can be used to battle childhood obesity and help change dietary practices.

Potential Advantages and Challenges With Technology-Based Intervention Approaches

As noted early in this chapter, while the application of technologies for the delivery of interventions has vast potential, it is important to be aware of the potential advantages and disadvantages associated with these approaches. These advantages include potential cost savings because of reductions in costs (e.g., transportation costs) associated with office-based and in-home interventions; access to larger numbers of individuals who could potentially benefit from interventions; enhanced flexibility with respect to tailoring and presentation of information; and convenience. Many at-risk individuals in need of behavioral interventions may lack the means to access these interventions. For example, about 75% of primary care patients suffering from depression report at least one barrier that inhibits or prevents access to treatment, and the percentage of patients reporting such barriers are increased among rural populations (Mohr et al., 2010, 2013). BITs can help decrease such barriers. In addition to providing increased access of behavioral therapies to populations that experience barriers to receiving treatment, BITs also have the potential to contribute significantly to a research agenda through innovation. As outlined by Mohr et al. (2013),

> BITs not only provide new delivery media for mental health treatments, they also open the possibility for entirely new interventions. For example, mobile technologies can harness sensors and ubiquitous computing to provide continuous

monitoring and/or intervention in the patient's environment. Virtual reality creates simulated environments that afford a high degree of control in engineering the provision of therapeutic experiences. Gaming may provide teaching methods that are more engaging. These opportunities may also challenge and expand the limits of our knowledge regarding human behavior and behavior change processes. (p. 333)

However, use of technology-based approaches is not without challenges—although it is generally assumed that "everyone" has access and uses the latest technologies, there are still some segments of the population for whom access is challenging. This is especially true of populations with lower education/income and minority groups that may not be able to afford broadband access or rely on Internet connectivity outside the home—Pew finds that a much higher proportion of Black and Hispanic adults rely on Internet access outside the home compared to Whites (Zickuhr, 2013). Rural populations also utilize the Internet at a lower rate compared to suburban and urban groups (as much as 20% of rural populations are offline; Zickuhr, 2013); this can prove to be a significant hurdle for researchers testing an online intervention and who want to include participants living in a rural area. Other challenges include issues with adherence, the constant evolution of technology, and the constraints of skeuomorphisms.

Adherence

An intervention may potentially be incredibly beneficial and innovative, but it does little good if individuals do not adhere to the intervention protocol. The same is true for any behavioral intervention that involves technology: If a participant does not actually use the BIT, there will likely be no noticeable change in the outcome of interest. Murray (2012, p. e3) states, "Adherence to any specified intervention may be related to characteristics of the intervention, characteristics of the user, or characteristics of the condition addressed by the intervention." Predictors of adherence, as identified by Kelders, Kok, Ossebaard, and Van Gemert-Pijnen (2012) in systematic review of Internet-based health interventions, included: being involved in a randomized controlled trial intervention as opposed to an observational study; increased interaction with a counselor; *intended* use of BITs; increased updates (in the form of new information uploaded for participants or new "lessons" becoming available) in intervention content; and increased use of dialogue support (e.g., a BIT forwarding a message to a participant after successfully completing an intervention task). Adherence can be increased through a variety of mechanisms that depend heavily on the characteristics of the BIT, intervention, and study population—examples include rewards and incentives for participants for successfully adhering to the protocol (Thompson et al., 2008) or instituting periodic prompts to remind participants to use the BIT or increased interactivity (Fry & Neff, 2009).

Evolution of Technology

The evolution of technology can lead to *obsolescence*, or what Schueller, Muñoz, and Mohr (2013, p. 480) describe as, ". . . the rates at which technologies (and therefore the related interventions) become obsolete or updated." We see examples of this everyday where specific devices or applications are no longer popular, relevant, or compatible with other technologies. If a device or application is obsolete, it will be ineffective in a research environment. This is a big challenge for intervention researchers. The development of technology-based interventions can take considerable effort and time, and it is entirely possible that, when development is complete, a new technology or version of a technology will have emerged.

Examples of evolutions in technology abound (e.g., cell phones, software applications, and computer technology). For instance, currently behavioral interventions that use social media may be more successful if the intervention is based in such social media applications as Facebook or Twitter instead of a site such as MySpace, which, though popular a decade ago, is nowhere near as popular or prevalent as it once was. Operating systems fall in and out of favor, mobile technologies are constantly replaced or updated, and new technologies are constantly being developed. By remaining up-to-date, researchers can ensure that they are utilizing the technologies to their full potential. It is also important to recognize that many individuals in the user population may not see an advantage to constantly having to update and improve their technology systems, so they may not be willing to adopt newer versions of a technology.

Skeuomorphism

"In the physical world, a skeuomorph is an ornamental version of something that was, in an earlier product, a functional necessity. Fake shutter sounds in digital cameras. Fake candles in electric chandeliers. Fake grain in leatherette" (Pogue, 2013, p. 29). We see examples of skeuomorphs in technologies all the time, one of the most common being the use of a floppy disk icon to represent a "save" feature. Schueller et al. (2013) point out that psychological skeuomorphs are present in BITs, such as structuring the interventions into "sessions" or having BIT questionnaires administered on forms that resemble a paper-and-pencil document. The use of skeuomorphs may limit or constrain the potential of a BIT and may prevent the creative development of new interventions or the updating of old ones. This is not to say that skeuomorphs should be abandoned entirely, as they can be useful guides for researchers and participants alike; however, researchers must be cognizant of them so as to avoid the possible design constraints they unknowingly may impose.

Other Challenges

Additional concerns related to the use of BITs include (a) the potential of a BIT reinforcing an issue that it was initially designed to address and solve (e.g., social isolation) and (b) BITs not being a comparable substitute to the face-to-face interactions between patients and care providers (Griffiths et al., 2006). While BITs may allow for cost-effective methods for providing behavioral support to groups of individuals who normally would experience difficulty in accessing this support, the act of providing a low-cost intervention may in fact increase their feelings of isolation as the employment of a low-cost treatment option may reinforce the "low priority" of these individuals with regards to health and social services (Griffiths et al., 2006). As an example, those suffering from a stigmatizing mental health issue who are assigned to a Web-based intervention rather than a face-to-face intervention may psychologically feel as if they are "unworthy" of participating in a traditional intervention or that they are "not worth the time or effort" to medical personnel. This may force the group to feel even more marginalized and reinforce the stigmas they experience.

In addition, although BITs can increase access to behavioral therapies and treatments, such interventions may lack the personable attributes and the nuances of face-to-face interactions with physicians and study personnel. In effect, BITs may not provide the same personalized touch afforded by face-to-face interactions. This is not to imply that face-to-face interactions are always preferred, as there can be a great amount of discomfort experienced among patients in face-to-face situations, which can be potentially reduced through the use of a BIT (Bennett & Glasgow, 2009). However, there are cases wherein BITs have been shown to have less potent effects on patients compared to face-to-face interactions. An example is found in a study conducted by Mohr et al. (2012) comparing face-to-face cognitive behavioral therapy versus telephone-based therapy with individuals suffering from depression. The findings indicated that, while the telephone-based therapy was associated with lower attrition and patients saw comparable improvement in depression when compared to the face-to-face group, over time the group that received face-to-face therapy reported lower depression than the telephone group. It is important to recognize that Internet-based contact may be providing something different than face-to-face contact, and researchers should seek to assess these potentially different effects. However, some studies, such as those looking at online therapy effects on pain and headaches, find that online modalities are comparable to face-to-face interactions (Cuijpers, van Straten, & Andersson, 2008), highlighting the fact that continued research is needed in this area.

Some final considerations for researchers using BITs include access, usability, and privacy. Although BITs have the potential to deliver behavioral interventions to populations that may typically have difficulty accessing these interventions, as noted not all populations *have access to these technologies*. As pervasive as computer and smartphone technologies have become in daily life, there are pockets of people (such as those with lower socioeconomic status) who cannot afford these technologies; in addition, there are pockets of people (such as those in rural areas) who may not have Internet connectivity strong enough to support more complex multimedia interventions. Researchers and therapists must take this into account when potentially assigning clients/patients/study participants to a BIT treatment. Usability of the technology (and the need for training of targeted populations) must also be ascertained, as a lack of technical knowledge and experience can inhibit the effectiveness of the BIT (e.g., an older adult with very little Internet experience may become frustrated with navigating an online treatment for depression, which may lessen the treatment's efficacy). In addition, as with face-to-face interactions, steps must be taken to assure participant privacy and confidentiality when using BITs; an example may be to require a specific login so that only patients may access the BIT and to have any patient data that is collected through the BIT be stored on a secure server. Finally, the development of technology-based interventions necessitates the inclusion of technical personnel on the research team. These individuals may not be familiar with behavioral intervention research or the target populations; thus, it is extremely important that they receive training in the goals and objectives of the intervention, the study timeline and constraints, and the characteristics of the target population.

THE APPLICATION OF TECHNOLOGY IN DATA COLLECTION AND ANALYSIS

The use of technology in behavioral interventions is not limited to intervention delivery. Technologies can also provide advantages to the behavioral intervention researcher with respect to data collection and analysis. New technologies provide researchers with new tools to collect and analyze data and also afford researchers opportunities to collect *new types of data* that were previously thought to be unobtainable or difficult to obtain, for example, tracking the behavioral patterns of an individual or real-time continuous records of health indicators. The following section presents examples of possibilities of new technologies that are available with regards to data collection and assessment. The possibilities in this area are rapidly expanding as technology continues to evolve and improve. Our intent is to provide some insight into the possibilities offered by technology.

One of the more noticeable and positive developments in data collection afforded by technology is the move from using paper-and-pencil methods of collecting and recording data to performing these activities using a device such as a tablet. Use of devices such as tablet computers to record data (in comparison to a traditional paper-and-pencil method) can increase the efficiency and quality and decrease the costs associated with data collection and management. For example, collecting data via a tablet allows for the immediate transfer of data to the data management system for a study and eliminates the need for an additional data entry step in the process. These technologies (when designed properly) can be intuitive and easy-to-use for professionals of varying skill levels (Abernathy et al., 2008).

Another popular development with regard to technology and data collection is the proliferation of Web-based survey research. With traditional mail-in survey and telephone response rates decreasing dramatically over the past several decades (Dillman, Smyth, & Christian, 2009), Web-based surveys present researchers with a new method of engaging participants and distributing assessment instruments to a large number of people. Web-based surveys can be distributed through various avenues such as being e-mailed directly to potential research subjects, being shared on social media and in online forums, or being embedded into a website. Questionnaires can be built and programmed by the researcher to be tailored to the potential respondent and fit the needs of the study, and there are also a number of free online options (such as SurveyMonkey) that allow users to create surveys using premade templates. While survey response rates for Internet-only questionnaires may not be higher than those in traditional survey methods (Kaplowitz, Hadlock, & Levine, 2004), researchers may use a mixed-methods approach that incorporates Web-based instruments in the hopes of increasing overall response to a questionnaire. As noted in Chapter 13, issues related to informed consent can also be challenging.

In the case of Internet-based behavioral interventions, real-time data on the use of these interventions can be tracked remotely. As an example, if a researcher is evaluating an online intervention that is intended to relieve symptoms of depression, the researcher would be able to gather real-time information on the frequency with which the study participants accessed the intervention, when participants accessed the intervention, and the components of the intervention that they accessed on the site (such as opening a behavioral intervention module or posting a message on a support group message board). We tracked real-time participant usage data in the videophone study (Czaja et al., 2013). This type of data provides valuable information on how an intervention might need to be modified—for example, which components of the intervention engaged participants or were of low usage. In addition, it can help facilitate dosage–outcome analyses. There is software that exists (e.g., Morae) that allows researchers to record and visually track all activity completed on a device; a researcher conducting a study determining what a participant does on a behavioral intervention website can not only see what pages the participant visits or what links the participant clicks, but may also *see the cursor movements in real time* and gain additional insight as to the decision-making process used by participants when navigating the site. This opens up another exciting realm of analytics and level of understanding concerning how participants interact with treatment elements that has not hitherto been possible.

Mohr et al. (2013) outline another development in data collection that involves mobile technologies: passive data collection. In passive data collection, rather than having the technology user manually log in data regarding specific health practices or behaviors, the technology itself will log data using built-in or externally connected sensors. Examples of passive data collection can be GPS sensors that track the location of a user (which scientists can use to see where a user is and how much he or she is traveling, a potentially important piece of information in physical activity interventions) or sensors that record heart rate.

While mobile technologies can allow for passive data collection, other wearable technologies allow for similar data collection. A study done by Najafi, Armstrong, and Mohler (2013) tested accelerometers (in this case, sensors designed to monitor physical activity) to see whether sensors that could be worn as easily as inside a shirt could successfully track walking movements. They found that such technologies could actually help identify older adults who were at risk for falls. Many wearable technologies exist in the marketplace that can help track participant characteristics such as fitness level (e.g., Fitbit). Most of these devices also provide feedback to the user, which is in turn an intervention. New developments in sensing and wearable technologies are on the horizon. Examples include implantable devices such as implantable cardiac monitoring devices and stimulating devices and smart home applications that involve integrated networks of sensors—which may include a combination of safety, health and wellness, and social connectedness technologies—installed into homes or apartments to simultaneously and continuously monitor environmental conditions, daily activity patterns, vital signs, and sleep patterns.

Behavioral interventions conducted in an online environment also allow for the collection of qualitative data in addition to more quantitative survey responses and health measures. The most obvious example of online qualitative data is that found on social media sites or in online forums. In a study conducted by Frost and Massagli (2008), comments made by members of an online community called PatientsLikeMe were qualitatively analyzed to determine how members communicated their health status and opinions to other members and how members used the site to answer inquiries on their own health and behaviors. An advantage of using online discussions and forums is that online qualitative data produce "automatic transcripts"; there is no need for the researcher to use a recording device to capture an interview with a research subject nor is there a need for the researcher to be furiously scribbling down notes, because with analysis of online communication the "dialogues" between people are already written and ready for analysis (Im, 2006).

CONCLUSION

The technological evolution has granted behavioral intervention researchers new opportunities for delivering interventions that can enhance the cost-effectiveness and efficiency of intervention delivery. It also provides the opportunity to enhance access to these interventions for large numbers of people, especially those who have traditionally lacked access to these interventions because of financial constraints, geographic/travel concerns, fear of stigma, or other barriers. New technologies have also provided researchers and therapists tools that enhance data collection, management, and analysis. However, use of these technologies also gives rise to new challenges. Technology can have both beneficial and detrimental effects on behavioral interventions. Researchers need to be aware of the challenges and determine if and how technology is best used in a given intervention trial. In some cases, for example, it may not be optimal to use technology to deliver an intervention or some combination of technology and other more traditional formats for intervention. The answer to this issue depends on the stage of the pipeline, the objectives of the study, the target population, and feasibility constraints (e.g., budget, Internet access). In all cases when technology is employed in a trial, the issue of usability is paramount from the perspective of both the study participants and the research team.

A final thought on the use of BITs: Although it is common for behavioral scientists to employ the expertise of developers in the design and implementation of BITs, this relationship often fails to reach a true interdisciplinary or multidisciplinary level. Often a team of behavioral scientists will simply hire a developer to create a BIT to fit the needs of the behavioral scientists. In this instance, the developer has no say or influence over the research agenda and protocol itself and thus acts more as an employee instead of as a collaborator. The opposite can also be true, with computer engineers and scientists employing behavioral scientists in the development of interventions without a true collaborative atmosphere. Although the theoretical backgrounds and methodologies used by these groups may differ, they are able to work in tandem to develop a comprehensive research program that can potentially go beyond the individual limitations of each discipline (Schueller et al., 2013). For the behavioral sciences to fully enjoy the capabilities of technology in intervention research, these groups must learn to collaborate to develop methodologies that better cater to the needs of the research participants and study objectives.

REFERENCES

Abernathy, A. P., Herndon, J. E., Wheeler, J. L., Patwardhan, M., Shaw, H., Lyerly, H. K., & Weinfurt, K. (2008). Improving health care efficiency and quality using tablet personal computers to collect research-quality, patient-reported data. *Health Services Research, 43*, 1975–1991.

Adibi, S. (Ed.). (2015). *Mobile health: A Technology road map.* New York, NY: Springer.

Andersson, G., & Cuijpers, P. (2009). Internet-based and other computerized psychological treatments for adult depression: A meta-analysis. *Cognitive Behaviour Therapy, 38,* 196–205.

Azar, K. M., Aurora, M., Wang, E. J., Muzaffar, A., Pressman, A., & Palaniappan, L. P. (2015). Virtual small groups for weight management: An innovative delivery mechanism for evidence-based lifestyle interventions among obese men. *Translational Behavioral Medicine, 5*(1), 37–44.

Baranowski, T., & Frankel, L. (2012). Let's get technical! Gaming and technology for weight control and health promotion in children. *Childhood Obesity, 8,* 34–37.

Beard, L., Wilson, K., Morra, D., & Keelan, J. (2009). A survey of health-related activities on Second Life. *Journal of Medical Internet Research, 11,* e17.

Belle, S. H., Burgio, L., Burns, R., Coon, D., Czaja, S. J., Gallagher-Thompson, D., . . . Zhang, S. (2006). Enhancing the quality of life of dementia caregivers from different ethnic or racial groups: A randomized, controlled trial. *Annals of Internal Medicine, 145,* 727–738.

Bennett, G. G., & Glasgow, R. E. (2009). The delivery of public health interventions via the Internet: Actualizing their potential. *Annual Review of Public Health, 30,* 273–292.

Bickmore, T. W., Schulman, D., & Sidner, C. (2013). Automated interventions for multiple health behaviors using conversational agents. *Patient Education and Counseling, 92,* 142–148.

Børøsund, E., Cvancarova, M., Moore, S. M., Ekstedt, M., & Ruland, C. M. (2014). Comparing effects in regular practice of e-communication and web-based self-management support among breast cancer patients: Preliminary results from a randomized controlled trial. *Journal of Medical Internet Research, 16,* e295.

Boulos, M. N., Hetherington, L., & Wheeler, S. (2007). Second Life: An overview of the potential of 3-D virtual worlds in medical and health education. *Health Information & Libraries Journal, 24,* 233–245.

Brian, A. W. (2009). *The nature of technology.* New York, NY: Free Press.

Bull, S. S., Levine, D., Black, S. R., Schmiege, S., & Santelli, J. (2012). Social media-delivered sexual health intervention: A cluster randomized controlled trial. *American Journal of Preventative Medicine, 43,* 467–474.

Cavallo, D. N., Tate, D. F., Ries, A. V., Brown, J. D., DeVellis, R. F., & Ammerman, A. S. (2012). A social media-based physical activity intervention: A randomized controlled trial. *American Journal of Preventative Medicine, 43,* 527–532.

Cuijpers, P., van Straten, A., & Andersson, G. (2008). Internet-administered cognitive behavior therapy for health problems: A systematic review. *Journal of Behavioral Medicine, 31,* 169–177.

Czaja, S. J., (2015). Can technology empower older adults to manage their health? *Generations, 39,* 46–51.

Czaja, S. J., Loewenstein, D., Schulz, R., Nair, S. N., & Perdomo, D. (2013). A videophone psychosocial intervention for dementia caregivers. *The American Journal of Geriatric Psychiatry, 21,* 1071–1081.

Depp, C. A., Mausbach, B., Granholm, E., Cardenas, V., Ben-Zeev, D., Patterson, T. L., . . . Jeste, D. V. (2010). Mobile interventions for severe mental illness: Design and preliminary data from three approaches. *Journal of Nervous and Mental Disease, 198,* 715–721.

Dillman, D. A., Smyth, J. D., & Christian, L. M. (2009). *Internet, mail, and mixed-mode surveys: The tailored design method* (3rd ed.). Hoboken, NJ: Wiley.

Eakin, E., Lawler, S. P., Vandelanotte, C., & Owen, N. (2007). Telephone interventions for physical activity and dietary behavior change: A systematic review. *American Journal of Preventative Medicine, 32,* 419–434.

Freeman, L. W., White, R., Ratcliff, C. G., Sutton, S., Stewart, M., Palmer, J. L., . . . Cohen, L. (2015). A randomized trial comparing live and telemedicine deliveries of an imagery-based behavioral intervention for breast cancer survivors: Reducing symptoms and barriers to care. *Psychooncology, 24*(8), 910–918.

Friedman, R. H., Kazis, L. E., Jette, A., Smith, M. B., Stollerman, J., Torgerson, J., & Carey, K. (1996). A telecommunications system for monitoring and counseling patients with hypertension: Impact on medication adherence and blood pressure control. *American Journal of Hypertension, 9,* 285–292.

Frost, J. H., & Massagli, M. P. (2008). Social uses of personal health information within PatientsLikeMe, an online patient community: What can happen when patients have access to one another's data. *Journal of Medical Internet Research, 10,* e15.

Fry, J. P., & Neff, R. A. (2009). Periodic prompts and reminders in health promotion and health behavior interventions: Systematic review. *Journal of Medical Internet Research, 11,* e16.

Germain, V., Marchand, A., Bouchard. S., Drouin, M., & Guay, S. (2009). Effectiveness of cognitive behavioural therapy administered by videoconference for posttraumatic stress disorder. *Cognitive Behaviour Therapy, 38,* 42–53.

Granholm, E., Ben-Zeev, D., Link, P. C., Bradshaw, K. R., & Holden, J. L. (2012). Mobile assessment and treatment for schizophrenia (MATS): A pilot trial of an interactive text-messaging intervention for medication adherence, socialization, and auditory hallucinations. *Schizophrenia Bulletin, 38,* 414–425.

Griffiths, F., Lindenmeyer, A., Powell, J., Lowe, P., & Thorogood, M. (2006). Why are health care interventions delivered over the Internet? A systematic review of the published literature. *Journal of Medical Internet Research, 8,* e10.

Heron, K., & Smyth, J. M. (2010). Ecological momentary interventions: Incorporating mobile technology into psychosocial and health behaviour treatments. *British Journal of Health Psychology, 15,* 1–39.

Himle, J. A., Fischer, D. J., Muroff, J. R., Van Etten, M. L., Lokers, L. M., Abelson, J. L., & Hanna, G. L. (2006). Videoconferencing-based cognitive-behavioral therapy for obsessive-compulsive disorder. *Behavior Research and Therapy, 44,* 1821–1829.

Im, E. (2006). An online forum as a qualitative research method: Practical issues. *Nursing Research, 55,* 267–273.

Irvine, A. B., Gelatt, V. A., Seeley, J. R., Macfarlane, P., & Gau, J. M. (2013). Web-based intervention to promote physical activity by sedentary older adults: Randomized controlled trial. *Journal of Medical Internet Research, 15,* e19.

Kaplowitz, M. D., Hadlock, T. D., & Levine, R. (2004). A comparison of web and mail survey response rates. *The Public Opinion Quarterly, 68,* 94–101.

Kelders, S. M., Kok, R. N., Ossebaard, H. C., & Van Geemert-Pijnen, J. E. (2012). Persuasive system design does matter: A systematic review of adherence to web-based interventions. *Journal of Medical Internet Research, 14,* e152.

Khatri, N., Marziali, E., Tchernikov, I., & Shepherd, N. (2014). Comparing telehealth-based and clinic-based group cognitive behavioral therapy for adults with depression and anxiety: A pilot study. *Clinical Interventions in Aging, 9,* 765–770.

Kobak, K., Engelhardt, N., & Lipsitz, J. D. (2006). Enriched rater training using Internet based technologies: A comparison to traditional rater training in a multi-site depression trial. *Journal Psychiatric Research, 40,* 192–199.

Laing, B. Y., Mangione, C. M., Tseng, C., Leng, M., Vaisberg, E., Mahida, M., . . . Bell, D. S. (2014). Effectiveness of a smartphone application for weight loss compared with usual care in overweight primary care patients: A randomized, controlled trial. *Annals of Internal Medicine, 161,* S5–S12.

Marziali, E., & Donahue, P. (2006). Caring for others: Internet video-conferencing group intervention for family caregivers of older adults with neurodegenerative disease. *Gerontologist, 46,* 398–403.

McKay, M. R., King, D., Eakin, E. G., Seeley, J. R., & Glasgow, R. E. (2001). The diabetes network Internet-based physical activity intervention: A randomized pilot study. *Diabetes Care, 24,* 1624–1629.

Mohr, D. C., Burns, M. N., Schueller, S. M., Clarker, G., & Klinkman, M. (2013). Behavioral intervention technologies: Evidence review and recommendations for future research in mental health. *General Hospital Psychiatry, 35,* 332–338.

Mohr, D. C., Hart, S. L., Julian, L., Catledge, C., Honos-Webb, L., Vella, L., & Tasch, E. T. (2005). Telephone-administered psychotherapy for depression. *Archives of General Psychiatry, 62,* 1007–1014.

Mohr, D. C., Ho, J., Duffecy, J., Baron, K. G., Lehman, K. A., Jin, L., & Reifler, D. (2010). Perceived barriers to psychological treatments and their relationship to depression. *Journal of Clinical Psychology, 66,* 394–409.

Mohr, D. C., Ho., J., Duffecy, J., Reifler, D., Sokol, L., Burns, M. N., . . . Siddique, J. (2012). Effect of telephone-administered vs face-to-face cognitive behavioral therapy on adherence to therapy and depression outcome among primary care patients: A randomized trial. *JAMA, 307,* 2278–2285.

Mohr, D. C., Vella, L., Hart, S., Heckman, T., & Simon, G. (2008). The effect of telephone-administered psychotherapy on symptoms of depression and attrition: A meta-analysis. *Clinical Psychology: Science and Practice, 15,* 243–253.

Murray, E. (2012). Web-based interventions for behavior change and self-management: Potential, pitfalls, and progress. *Medicine 2.0, 1,* e3.

Najafi, B., Armstrong, D. G., & Mohler, J. (2013). Novel wearable technology for assessing spontaneous daily physical activity and risk of falling in older adults with diabetes. *Journal of Diabetes Science and Technology, 7,* 1147–1160.

Napolitano, M. A., Fotheringham, M., Tate, D., Sciamanna, C., Leslie, E., Owen, N., . . . Marcus, B. (2003). Evaluation of an Internet-based physical activity intervention: A preliminary investigation. *Annals of Behavioral Medicine, 25,* 92–99.

Owen, J. E., Klapow, J. C., Roth, D. L., Shuster, J. L., Jr., Bellis, J., Meredith, R., & Tucker, D. C. (2005). Randomized pilot of a self-guided Internet coping group for women with early stage breast cancer. *Annals of Behavior Medicine, 30,* 54–64.

Pew Research Center. (2014, January 9–12). *Internet users in 2014* (Pew Research Center Internet Project Survey). Retrieved from http://www.pewinternet.org/files/2014/02/12-internet-users-in-2014.jpg

Piette, J. D., Weinberger, M., McPhee, S. J., Mah, C. A., Kraemer, F. B., & Crapo, L. M. (2000). Do automated calls with nurse follow-up improve self-care and glycemic control among vulnerable patients with diabetes? *The American Journal of Medicine, 108,* 20–27.

Pogue, D. (2013). Out with the real. *Scientific American, 308,* 29.

Schueller, S. M., Muñoz, R. F., & Mohr, D. C. (2013). Realizing the potential of behavioral intervention technologies. *Current Directions in Psychological Science, 22,* 478–483.

Smith, A. (2015). *U.S. smartphone use in 2015.* Washington, DC: Pew Research Center. Retrieved from http://www.pewinternet.org/files/2015/03/PI_Smartphones_0401151.pdf

Stubbings, D. R., Rees, C. S., Roberts, L. D., & Kane, R. T. (2013). Comparing in-person to videoconference-based cognitive behavioral therapy for mood and anxiety disorders: A randomized controlled trial. *Journal of Medical Internet Research, 15,* e258.

Thompson, D., Baranowski, T., Cullen, K., Watson, K., Canada, A., Bhatt, R., . . . Zakeri, I. (2008). Food, fun, and fitness internet program for girls: Influencing log-on-rate. *Health Education Research, 23,* 228–237.

Tran, J., Tran, R., & White, J. R. (2012). Smartphone-based glucose monitors and applications in the management of diabetes: An overview of 10 salient 'apps' and a novel smartphone-connected blood glucose monitor. *Clinical Diabetes, 30,* 173–178.

Vogel, P. A., Launes, G., Moen, E. M., Solem, S., Hansen, B., Håland, T., & Himle, J. A. (2012). Videoconference- and cell phone-based cognitive-behavioral therapy of obsessive-compulsive disorder: A case series. *Journal of Anxiety Disorders, 26*, 158–164.

Wharton, C. M., Johnston, C. S., Cunningham, B. K., & Sterner, D. (2014). Dietary self-monitoring, but not dietary quality, improves with use of smartphone app technology in an 8-week weight loss trial. *Journal of Nutrition Education and Behavior, 46*, 440–444.

Wilke, R., & Oates, R. (2014). *Emerging nations embrace internet, mobile technology.* Washington, DC: Pew Research Center. Retrieved from http://www.pewglobal.org/files/2014/02/Pew-Research-Center-Global-Attitudes-Project-Technology-Report-FINAL-February-13-20146.pdf

Yuen, E. K., Herbert, J. D., Forman, E. M., Goetter, E. M., Comer, R., & Bradley, J. (2013). Treatment of social anxiety disorder using online virtual environments in Second Life. *Behavior Therapy, 44*, 51–61.

Zhang, Z., Bickmore, T., Mainello, K., Mueller, M., Foley, M., Jenkins, L., & Edwards, R. A. (2014). Maintaining continuity in longitudinal, multi-method health interventions using virtual agents: The case of breastfeeding promotion. *Intelligent Virtual Agents: Lecture Notes in Computer Science, 8637*, 504–513.

Zickuhr, K. (2013). *Who's not online and why.* Washington, DC: Pew Research Center. Retrieved from http://www.pewinternet.org/files/old-media//Files/Reports/2013/PIP_Offline%20adults_092513_PDF.pdf

EVALUATING INTERVENTIONS: ATTENTION TO DESIGN

In Part II, we move on to examine considerations related to evaluating interventions. We highlight those issues critical to behavioral interventions. First, as the value and benefit of an intervention are typically established through comparison to other treatments, services, programs, or usual care, we begin by examining various control group options and the criteria for selecting a control group for an intervention trial (Chapter 8).

Then we examine sampling considerations and methodologies for identifying participants for behavioral intervention studies across various stages of the pipeline, including the beginning development phases and efficacy or effectiveness evaluations (Chapter 9). We then discuss one of the most challenging activities in behavioral intervention research across the pipeline, the recruitment and retention of study participants (Chapter 10).

Next, we discuss an emergent approach in evaluating behavioral intervention research—the use of mixed methodologies (Chapter 11). These design approaches, which have the potential of maximizing our understanding of underlying mechanisms as to why and how an intervention may work and for whom, will greatly facilitate implementation processes.

We then discuss, in Chapter 12, a frequently neglected consideration at each phase of the pipeline—fidelity, or whether an intervention is implemented as it is intended. Without an understanding of fidelity, we can have little confidence that any observed treatment effects are (or not) "real."

Finally, as noted in Chapter 13, fundamental to the development and evaluation of behavioral interventions are ethical considerations.

The key "take home" points of Part II include the following:

- Selecting a control group is as important as designing the intervention as we learn about our interventions through a comparison to a control group or alternative treatment.
- Main considerations in selecting a study sample include the size of the sample and sample composition such that their characteristics should be copasetic with the goals of the intervention and representative of a larger target population.
- Recruiting and retaining study participants are important elements of study design, which demand deliberate consideration, effort, and time.

- A range of designs is available for mixing and integrating both quantitative and qualitative perspectives in an intervention study to maximize understandings of treatment effects and processes—what works for whom and why.
- Attending to treatment fidelity helps to establish confidence in findings regarding the impact of the intervention on targeted outcomes.
- Research ethics are a critical consideration and form the foundation of all evaluative actions in behavioral intervention research.

EIGHT

SELECTING CONTROL GROUPS: TO WHAT SHOULD WE COMPARE BEHAVIORAL INTERVENTIONS?

GEORGE W. REBOK

> *In the universe of effect sizes that make up our RCT evidence base for psychological interventions, control conditions remain dark matter, exerting effects that are unseen, ill-defined, and for the most part unquantified. While there have been disputes over which control conditions should be used, such debates have produced more heat than light.*
> —Mohr et al. (2009, pp. 282–283)

Selecting an appropriate control group is an essential component in the design of behavioral intervention studies. However, when designing protocols for these studies, often researchers do not pay sufficient attention to the control condition(s). Although the results of intervention studies typically are discussed in terms of the effects of a new treatment or therapy, any differences between the experimental and control conditions depend as much on the latter as they do on the former (Tansella, Thornicroft, Barbui, Cipriani, & Saraceno, 2006). Because control conditions can have variable effects, the choice of a control group can exert a substantial impact on research studies using the randomized controlled trial (RCT) design and other experimental and quasi-experimental designs. By definition, RCTs are comparative studies that evaluate differences in experience between two or more groups, and control conditions are the main method for removing unwanted sources of variation in accounting for those differences. Of the various control conditions, the condition where no alternative treatment is provided, also known as the "no-treatment control," often produces the largest effect size for behavioral interventions because it is least likely to positively affect the outcome (Mohr et al., 2009). However, even in this case, differences between the experimental and control conditions could be attenuated if nontreated control participants benefitted from repeated exposure to the outcome assessments, as in a longitudinal design.

Developing and testing behavioral interventions involve an iterative and incremental process of building an evidence base and then translating and implementing the intervention, disseminating it, and then scaling it up for sustainability within particular practice or community settings (Gitlin, 2013). During the different phases of the development, testing, and implementation of behavioral interventions, control groups may serve different purposes. They are most important during testing the efficacy (Phase III) and effectiveness (Phase IV) of an intervention through an RCT, but they also may play an important role in other phases such as testing for feasibility and preliminary effects (Phase II). The purpose of this chapter is to (a) describe the role of control conditions across different phases of intervention development; (b) identify key methodological and ethical challenges in the use of control groups; (c) provide empirical examples of control group selection and design in large-scale, community-based intervention trials; and (d) make recommendations about how to select and use the most appropriate control conditions for randomized behavioral intervention trials. Given the author's research interests and background, examples will focus on intervention trials to improve the cognitive health and well-being of older adults in order to illustrate the unique challenges that researchers face in control group selection in behavioral intervention studies. Many of the methodological and ethical issues discussed are relevant to different types of behavioral interventions with older adults as well as other age groups, such as those involving mental health, exercise, nutrition, and medication use.

WHEN AND WHY TO INCLUDE A CONTROL GROUP

Choosing an appropriate control group or condition(s) is always a critical decision in developing and evaluating a behavioral intervention and is most important when designing an RCT. Experimental research on psychological and behavioral interventions is usually implemented across a number of phases (Gitlin, 2013; Mohr et al., 2009; Schwartz, Chesney, Irvine, & Keefe, 1997). In thinking about control conditions, the investigator needs to consider the phase of intervention development: Phases I, II, III, IV, V, VI, and VII (see Table 8.1). Phase I trials are feasibility trials focused on developing and pretesting the acceptability, feasibility, and safety of the intervention components and development of the intervention manual. No control condition is needed. The second phase is exploratory and involves determining the frequency, duration, and intensity of a specific treatment intervention and defining the relevant outcomes. In this phase, the investigator would compare various doses of the intervention in order to determine the optimal frequency of contact or duration of treatment. The third phase would evaluate the efficacy of the intervention compared to the current standard treatment, or to usual care treatment if no standard of care or current best practice exists. A Phase III trial might also compare two common behavioral interventions that involve different assumptions about the mechanisms of action and likely outcomes (Schwartz et al., 1997). These trials typically include participants with comorbidities and multiple sites (Mohr et al., 2009). Phase IV studies are effectiveness trials that evaluate the transportability of the intervention to real-world settings. Phase IV trials may use a quasi-experimental design (e.g., case control) to evaluate the effect of a behavioral intervention in a health care setting where patients self-select to receive a particular intervention (Schwartz et al., 1997). In such cases, the investigator may need to statistically adjust for pretreatment differences between the cases and controls (e.g., socioeconomic status (SES) or preexisting medical conditions). In Phase V, most translational studies (see

TABLE 8.1 Suggested Control Conditions for Different RCT Phases

Phase	Objectives	Suggested Control Conditions
I	Develop and pretest intervention feasibility	None
II	Determine appropriate frequency, duration, and intensity; define relevant outcomes	Compare various doses of intervention
III	Evaluate efficacy of intervention as compared with standard treatment	Compare new treatment to standard
IV	Confirm effectiveness of intervention in "real-world" setting	Case control in clinical setting where participants self-select for intervention
V	Put intervention into practice, evaluate fidelity, test strategies for increasing reach, adoption	Compare effectiveness of different implementation strategies
VI	Distribute information about an intervention, scale up, translate for widespread diffusion	None
VII	Institutionalize an intervention program, policy, or practice	None

Note: Phases I–IV describe the traditional four-phase sequence for developing an intervention; phases V–VII have been added for translating, implementing, and institutionalizing the intervention (see Gitlin, 2013).
Source: Adapted from Schwartz et al. (1997).

Gitlin, Marx, Stanley, & Hodgson, 2015) use a pre–post design and do not include a control group. However, implementation studies can include a comparison group when the goal is to compare the effectiveness of different implementation strategies. The use of control groups in subsequent phases for the advancement of an intervention (Phase VI—diffusion/dissemination; and Phase VII—sustainability) is uncharted at this point, but it seems unlikely that control conditions are necessary.

Thus, control conditions are most important when evaluating the efficacy or effectiveness of behavioral interventions. The efficacy or the effectiveness of behavioral interventions is always determined relative to a control condition (Mohr et al., 2009). Efficacy, or "explanatory," trials usually precede effectiveness studies (also known as "pragmatic" studies) and refer to those trials conducted under optimal and controlled experimental conditions, whereas effectiveness trials are RCTs carried out in routine, "real-world" conditions. Because efficacy trials are aimed at determining the benefits of intervention for a specific group, they are necessary but not sufficient for establishing the effectiveness of interventions (Melnyk & Morrison-Beedy, 2012). However, the distinction between the two types of trials is a continuum rather than a dichotomy, and pure efficacy trials or pure effectiveness trials likely do not exist (Singal, Higgins, & Waljee, 2014).

WHY CONTROL GROUPS ARE IMPORTANT FOR THE RCT PHASES

The RCT is generally considered as the "gold standard" in evaluating the effects of psychological and behavioral interventions. The primary goal of an RCT is to determine whether an intervention works by comparing it to a control condition, usually either no intervention or an alternative intervention. Secondary goals may include identifying the factors (e.g., age, sex, health, cognitive status) that might moderate the effects of the intervention, and understanding the processes through which the intervention influences change (i.e., mediators or change mechanisms that bring about the intervention effect), according to the theory guiding the trial (Gitlin, 2013; West & Spring, 2007).

In an RCT, individuals or groups are assigned to treatment conditions at random (i.e., they have an equal probability of being assigned to the treatment or control). That helps ensure that the effects of the intervention can be causally attributed to the differences between the intervention and control, not to some extraneous factor(s). To the extent that the investigator can rule out alternative explanations and minimize systematic error (or bias), then the causal inference about the experimental effect is said to be "internally valid." If the results of the intervention can be generalized to a population of interest, that is, the population the intervention was designed to help, the intervention is said to be "externally valid." However, there are many factors that can threaten the internal and external validity of a study and lower confidence in the findings.

The original conceptualization of threats to validity was articulated by Campbell and Stanley (1966) and has changed very little over time. Common threats to internal validity that RCTs address include history, maturation, selection, temporal precedence, regression to the mean, attrition, and testing and implementation (Melnyk & Morrison-Beedy, 2012; West & Spring, 2007). There are also external threats to validity that can be addressed by RCTs, including sample characteristics, setting characteristics, and effects due to testing. However, RCTs have evolved and become increasingly more complex, creating new challenges for maximizing validity and minimizing bias (Mohr et al., 2009). For example, the use of a "usual care" group as a control may not be sufficient when the intervention requires an investment of time and energy that excludes all but the most highly motivated participants. In this case, any differences that emerge may be due to the composition of the samples participating in the intervention and control conditions (i.e., selection), and not to active ingredients of the intervention (Lindquist, Wyman, Talley, Findorff, & Gross, 2007).

Randomization of individuals or groups (e.g., schools, work sites, clinics, or communities) to an intervention or control condition represents the best strategy for ruling out alternative explanations, but it may not be possible to control for every conceivable threat to the internal validity of one's experiment (Melnyk & Morrison-Beedy, 2012). Today, behavioral interventions are conducted in the real-world of increasingly complex health care environments and diverse communities, which has increased their external or ecological validity, but which has also made it much more difficult to exert tight control over threats to internal validity. Thus, investigators are faced with inescapable trade-offs between internal and external validity, which makes it difficult or impossible to minimize threats to both at the same time (Freedland, Mohr, Davidson, & Schwartz, 2011).

Given the complexity of today's real-world environments, researchers have to weigh a variety of scientific, practical, and ethical issues and other considerations in choosing control groups for RCTs of behavioral interventions in health care and other settings (Westmaas, Gil-Rivas, & Silver, 2007). These considerations include the costs of the control conditions, feasibility, potential contamination, ethical issues, recruitment, retention, and sample size. As mentioned earlier, it may not be possible to control for every potential threat to internal validity. Rather, it may become necessary to control for whichever threats are deemed to be most important at the expense of remaining vulnerable to the less important ones (Freedland et al., 2011). In addition, it may be unethical to use a traditional control group if that deprives participants of treatments that have already been incorporated into routine health care practice (Freedland et al., 2011; Mohr et al., 2009).

TYPES OF CONTROL GROUPS FOR RCTs

Considerable heterogeneity exists in the forms of control conditions for RCTs of behavioral intervention research. Although there have been several attempts to address control group selection in the literature (Freedland et al., 2011; Mohr et al., 2009; Whitehead, 2004), there is currently little agreement or consistency among investigators about how to best design or select controls for behavioral intervention research. Different types of control conditions may have significantly different effects on the outcomes of RCTs (Cuijpers, van Straten, Warmerdam, & Andersson, 2008). Thus, ultimately the choice of controls may have a major impact on the evidence that underlies evidence-based research and practice (Mohr et al., 2009).

Control conditions vary in the magnitude of the impact that exposure to the condition is designed or expected to have on the trial's outcome variable(s) (Freedland et al., 2011). The no-treatment control, in which no alternative treatment is provided, is expected to have the least impact, as discussed previously, and the active alternative treatment control is considered the most impactful. In between are wait-list, attention/placebo comparison, and treatment component control groups.

Although there are many available choices for a control condition, none is perfect or suitable for all occasions. So, faced with many possibilities, which control(s) should the researcher choose? The choice depends on the specific research questions being asked, the existing state of knowledge about the intervention under study (Lindquist et al., 2007; West & Spring, 2007), and logistic issues/constraints (e.g., budgetary issues). Table 8.2 summarizes the different types of control/comparison conditions for RCTs of behavioral interventions and their relative advantages and disadvantages.

In the *no-treatment control*, outcomes for people randomly assigned to receive the treatment are compared to those people who receive no treatment at all. In clinical research, this group is often referred to as "treatment as usual." The main question is: "Does the treatment produce any benefit at all, over and beyond change due to passage of time or participating in a study?" One of the principal drawbacks of this type of control is that people randomized to no treatment may find their own treatment outside the bounds of the study. For example, in trials of cognitive interventions to improve memory performance in the elderly, researchers need to be concerned that participants who have concerns about their memory or who have been diagnosed with Alzheimer's disease or a related disorder may be less willing to accept an assignment to the no-treatment condition and to make a commitment

TABLE 8.2 Control/Comparison Group Selection for RCTs

Types of Groups	Definition	Pros	Cons
Control Groups			
No-treatment	Outcomes for people randomly assigned to those who receive treatment are compared to those who receive no treatment at all	Ability to assess test–retest or practice effects	People randomized to no treatment may find own treatment outside of the study Higher study dropout rates
Wait-list	People randomized to the treatment are compared to those on a wait-list to receive the treatment	Everyone in the study receives treatment sooner or later	People on the wait-list may still find treatment outside of the study People who are content to wait may be atypical or may have different expectancies for improvement Once wait-list participants receive the treatment, there is no long-term control for follow-up
Attention/placebo	New treatment is compared to a control intervention that delivers the same amount of support and attention, but does not include key components considered critical for the treatment	Tests whether the new treatment produces benefits beyond the effects due to nonspecific influences such as experimenter attention or positive expectations	People assigned to attention/placebo control may seek out treatment similar to the active intervention Attention/placebo controls may have differential expectations for improvement
Relative efficacy/comparative effectiveness	Head-to-head comparison between two or more treatments, each of which is a contender to be the best practice or standard of care	Assists consumers, clinicians, and policy makers to make informed decisions about what will assist health care at individual and population level	Requires large sample sizes in each treatment group to detect an effect Interventions may vary in so many ways that there is no common basis for comparison Subject to limitations such as missing data, incomplete follow-up, unmeasured biases, competing interests, and selective reporting of results

(Continued)

TABLE 8.2 Control/Comparison Group Selection for RCTs (Continued)

Types of Groups	Definition	Pros	Cons
Control Groups			
Parametric/dose finding[a]	Random assignment of people to different forms of interventions varying on factors such as number, length, duration of sessions, and so forth	Can be done early in treatment in order to determine the optimal dose or form of treatment Multiple levels of the variable under investigation can be examined	May be costly and time-consuming depending upon how many different factors one varies
Additive/ constructive comparison[a] (component control)	Those in the experimental group receive added treatment components that are hypothesized to add efficacy	Provides strong control by holding the two experimental comparisons equivalent except for the "add-on" Fewer ethical concerns because all components are considered efficacious	May be difficult to identify how to sequentially add or combine new treatment components Adding one or a few treatment components at a time may be a lengthy and costly process May have low statistical power because the treatment effect of the add-on component might be slight compared to the effect of the existing treatment
Treatment dismantling[a] (component control)	People randomized to receive the full efficacious intervention are compared to those randomized to receive a variant of that intervention minus one or more parts	Removing noneffective components may create a more cost-effective intervention Fewer ethical concerns because all components are considered efficacious	May be difficult to identify the active components of the treatment to drop May be costly to include the full efficacious intervention model from the beginning
Existing Practice Comparison Groups			
Treatment-as-usual (TAU); usual care (UC); routine care (RC)[b]	Control conditions are used to compare experimental interventions to existing treatments or clinical practices	Controls for many of the traditional threats to internal validity	Treatment provided by TAU, UC, or RC may vary considerably across patients and health care providers Outcomes may include variability from sources other than the treatment itself

[a]Adapted from West and Spring (2007).
[b]Adapted from Freedland et al. (2011).

not to seek other treatment during the intervention trial (Willis, 2001). They might decide to seek training on their own by buying a book or manual on cognitive improvement, by using an Internet-based memory training program, or through signing up for a training class outside of the study. They also may be more likely to drop out of the study, as new and more promising treatments become available, thus compromising the investigator's ability to do long-term assessments (Willis, 2001). They also may drop out if they feel that participation is too burdensome (e.g., an extensive assessment) relative to the benefits of participation. In such instances, it is important to actively monitor retention and what participants are doing with regard to engaging in other training-related activities outside the main intervention study.

To overcome some of the problems of the no-treatment control, many researchers employ some form of a *wait-list control design* in which the treatment is delayed rather than withheld, and the waiting period is equivalent to or longer than the length of the treatment. People randomized to the treatment are compared to people on a wait-list to receive the treatment. The advantage is that everyone in the study receives the treatment sooner or later. This may help reduce the likelihood that participants randomized initially to a no-treatment condition will be disappointed or resentful and seek out treatment on their own or drop out of the trial. However, depending on the length of the wait-period, this still may present a problem as some participants may not be content to remain on the wait-list, even for a relatively brief period of time, and may seek "off-study" treatments of their own. On the other hand, those who are content to remain on the list, especially for prolonged periods of time, may be atypical in some way (e.g., unusually cooperative or agreeable). Another potential problem in the use of wait-list controls is that expectations for improvement may differ between the treatment and the control groups (Whitehead, 2004). People on the wait-list may not expect that they will improve, even when they finally receive the treatment. Alternately, people on the wait-list may improve spontaneously on their own and then receive the treatment condition, although they no longer meet the initial study inclusion criteria. Finally, once the wait-list participants receive the treatment, there no longer exists a long-term control, limiting the possibility of testing the long-term effects of an intervention. Also, one needs to be careful as in some instances, for example, a couple of friends being randomized to different treatment conditions, there may be some "cross-condition" talk.

A usual design alternative to no-treatment controls is the *attention/placebo control*. Here, a new treatment is compared to a control intervention that delivers the same amount of contact and attention from the intervention agent, but none of the key active ingredients by which the new treatment is expected to cause change in the outcomes under study. This control tests whether the new treatment produces benefits beyond the effects owing to nonspecific influences such as experimenter attention, social support, or positive expectations. The optimal attention/placebo control should encompass none of the "active ingredients" of the treatment under evaluation (Gross, 2005). For example, attention controls may receive an intervention such as an educational seminar on health care that is not thought to include any of the critical intervention elements that may change participant behavior.

Masking (or blinding) is used in clinical trials to keep the group (e.g., the active placebo) to which the study participants are assigned not known or easily discerned by those who are "masked" (Schulz, Chalmers, & Altman, 2002; Stephenson &

Imrie, 1998; Viera & Bangdiwala, 2007). In "double-blind" trials, both study participants and the experimenter or health care provider are supposed to be unaware to which groups participants were allocated. In practice, this is often difficult to do, and it is not always clear which groups were actually masked. One of the main disadvantages of the placebo control is that participants who become unblinded and learn they are receiving placebo do more poorly than participants who do not know they are receiving placebo. Particularly in cases where neither the study participant nor the experimenter can be blinded, it is best that both the participants and research staff hold equal expectations about the merits of the intervention and control conditions (West & Spring, 2007). However, maintaining equivalent expectancies across groups, referred to as "equipoise," becomes more difficult when the treatment is lengthy, which is often the case when the intervention is dealing with serious, real-life issues (Willis, 2001). The ethical principle of clinical equipoise means that there must exist genuine uncertainty over whether or not the treatment will be superior to some alternative. If there is certainty about the superiority of the treatment relative to a placebo control, then the principle of equipoise is violated. These problematic issues have led investigators to question whether we should routinely use placebo controls in clinical research (Avins, Cherkin, Sherman, Goldberg, & Pressman, 2012). Other issues include the cost of including an attention control condition and ensuring the placebo group does not have active ingredients, which is often difficult to do in behavioral intervention trials. In addition, it is important to monitor issues surrounding treatment efficacy for the attention control condition to ensure that the intervention team is adhering to the protocol for the condition. They may not be as committed to this condition as they are to the treatment condition or understand the importance and purpose of including it in a trial.

A fourth type of control is known as the *relative efficacy/comparative effectiveness design*. This control condition addresses the question of whether a newly developed treatment works better than an existing best practice or standard of care. The treatments are thought to represent different conceptual approaches to the problem and have different hypothesized mechanisms of impact on outcomes. Use of this type of control requires large numbers of participants in each treatment group because all of the interventions being compared show promise or are known to work, so the expected differences between them are relatively small. The main questions in comparative effectiveness research are (a) which intervention works better and (b) at what relative costs (West & Spring, 2007). Although this might be thought to be a direct and useful way to compare interventions, several problems in using this design have been noted (Willis, 2001). First, when comparing two or more interventions, they often vary in so many ways (e.g., number of sessions, mode of delivery, degree of social contact) that there are few variables that can be held constant across treatment conditions. Differential expectations among the individuals who administer the interventions can also pose a major challenge to the internal validity of comparative effectiveness designs. Ideally, the interventions should be delivered at multiple sites by staff who have similar levels of training and expertise and hold similar expectancies about intervention effectiveness. Using a shared measurement framework across interventions also facilitates cross-study comparisons and helps reduce the problems associated with using different intervention protocols (Belle et al., 2003; Czaja, Schulz, Lee, Belle, & REACH Investigators, 2003).

OTHER TYPES OF CONTROL CONDITIONS

A fifth type of control condition is called *parametric/dose finding*. This type of control would typically be used early in the development of a new treatment. The goal here is to determine the optimal "dose" or format of treatment. Different forms of intervention that vary on factors such as number, length, or duration of sessions, the use of individual versus group sessions, or variations in the treatment setting comprise the conditions to which individuals are randomly assigned (West & Spring, 2007). Similar to a parametric/dose finding study, in the *additive/constructive comparison* condition, different randomized groups receive different versions of the treatment (West & Spring, 2007). This can be characterized as a "bottom-up" approach. Those in both the experimental and comparison conditions receive the same active intervention, but those in the experimental condition also receive an additional treatment component that is hypothesized to add efficacy. Investigators can use this type of control condition in the early phases of treatment development or after treatment is established as evidence-based to see if its efficacy can be improved even further. Alternatively, a "top-down" approach called *treatment dismantling*, also known as "component analysis," may be used. This approach uses a between-groups design where investigators compare individuals randomized to receive the full efficacious intervention to those randomized to receive a different form of that intervention, minus one or more parts (Lindquist et al., 2007; West & Spring, 2007). Usually, the treatment dismantling approach is used later in treatment development after the intervention's efficacy is well established. The goal is to develop more efficient and potentially more effective treatments by determining which components of the intervention are necessary and sufficient for maximum clinical change and which may be unnecessary. It essentially represents a "fine-tuning" of the intervention and is important with respect to treatment implementation. As West and Spring (2007, p. 17) state, "The aim from a public health perspective is often to find a low-cost, minimally intensive intervention that improves outcomes for a small percent of the population, which equates in absolute numbers to a large number of people being helped."

EXISTING PRACTICE COMPARISON CONDITIONS

As Freedland et al. (2011) have pointed out, there are several problems with the traditional control group hierarchy. First, it blurs the distinction between the control and comparison functions of control groups (e.g., controlling for threats to internal validity vs. actively comparing one treatment to another treatment to see which one is superior). Further, the traditional hierarchy is based on the questionable assumption that behavioral trials can be isolated from the health care settings in which they are conducted. Because participants in behavioral intervention trials frequently have access to nonstudy health care services, this rarely holds true in any RCT targeting physical or mental health problems. As discussed in Chapter 1 of this book, interventions are conducted within complex contexts that affect study designs and treatment outcomes and that need to be taken into account (see Chapter 1, Figure 1.2).

The increased usage of RCTs within complex, real-world environments has necessitated the development of other types of comparison conditions. One of these is known as an *existing practice comparison* condition. These are used to compare experimental interventions to existing treatments or clinical practices. Existing practice controls have played an important role in medical trials, but not in behavioral trials until recently. They are referred to by many different names, including *treatment-as-usual* (TAU), *usual care* (UC), *standard care* (SC), or *routine care* (RC) (Freedland et al., 2011; Thompson & Schoenfeld, 2007).

TAU controls use the treatments that are already in place by clinicians in the settings from which participants are recruited (Mohr et al., 2009). This implies that most people with the target problem in those settings ordinarily receive a particular treatment, which may not always be the case. The TAU approach to control is most often used to label control groups in psychotherapy studies, mental health services research, and behavioral intervention trials for substance abuse (Freedland et al., 2011). UC control groups are roughly equivalent to TAU controls. In this case, their use does not imply that participants receive a specific treatment of the target problem, although that may be true in some cases. For example, the UC for an RCT on a treatment for depression may encompass a wide variety of antidepressant medications, cognitive behavioral therapies, and clinical monitoring. Usually, the UC is determined by health care providers who are independent of the research team, but not always. A UC control may also be enhanced or modified by the researcher, that is, enhanced usual care (EUC) or constrained usual care (CUC) to overcome methodological or ethical problems that would be associated with ordinary UC (Freedland et al., 2011).

SELECTING CONTROL GROUPS: SAMPLE CASE OF COGNITIVE INTERVENTION TRIALS

Over the past two decades, there has been steadily growing interest in the development and testing of cognitive interventions for older adults to prevent cognitive decline and improve daily functioning and overall personal well-being (Gates, Sachdev, Fiatarone Singh, & Valenzuela, 2011; Gross, Parisi, et al., 2012; Stine-Morrow & Basak, 2011). For example, the Advanced Cognitive Training for Independent and Vital Elderly (ACTIVE) study was a large multi-site clinical trial of a cognitive intervention for community-dwelling older adults (Jobe et al., 2001; Rebok et al., 2014). ACTIVE was a randomized, controlled, single-masked trial using a four-group design consisting of three treatment arms and a no-contact control group (see Figure 8.1). Each treatment arm included ten 60- to 75-minute training sessions for one of three cognitive abilities (memory, reasoning, and attentional processing speed) thought to underlie everyday functional capacity. Assessors were masked to participant treatment assignment. Training exposure and social contact were standardized across the three interventions so that each intervention could serve as a social contact control for the other interventions. As described by Jobe et al. (2001, p. 456), the design allowed for testing of both social contact effects, as represented in the dashed lines in Figure 8.1 (via the contact control groups) and retest effects (via the no-contact control group) on outcomes. Being able to assess

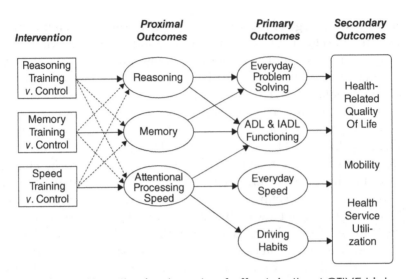

Figure 8.1 Hypothesized mode of effects in the ACTIVE trial.

Source: Jobe et al. (2001). ADL = activities of daily living; IADL = instrumental activities of daily living.

retest effects is an important advantage of a no-treatment or no-contact control in cognitive intervention research because the magnitude of practice effects may be substantial (Gross, Inouye, et al., 2012; Willis, 2001). Simply becoming familiar with the cognitive tests being administered and the testing routine can lead to significant improvement even without specific intervention.

The choice of an appropriate control group was a key issue in the development of the protocol for the ACTIVE trial (Jobe et al., 2001). There is no pharmacologic treatment or other usual care for normal older adults for cognitive performance. Therefore, usual care could be considered to be no care and thus no-contact was considered to be the equivalent control group to usual care. Moreover, previous investigations of cognitive training and occupational therapy interventions to improve functioning showed that a no-contact control group does not differ from a placebo social-contact group (Clark et al., 1997; Willis, Cornelius, Blow, & Baltes, 1983). One of the most elegant features of ACTIVE was that the design of the trial allowed multiple estimates of the nontreatment effects on the targeted abilities by estimating the influence of each training intervention (e.g., memory) on nontrained abilities relevant to the other two interventions (e.g., reasoning, attentional processing speed). The high degree of specificity of the effects reported given this design (e.g., see Ball et al., 2002; Willis et al., 2006) suggests that the generalized expectancy of doing well does not in itself play an important role in improving cognitive performance in the absence of target-specific training (Stine-Morrow & Basak, 2011).

In contrast to intervention trials such as ACTIVE that target specific cognitive skills or abilities, an alternative approach to intervention involves nonspecific stimulation of cognitive function via engagement in everyday stimulating cognitive, physical, and social activities (Fried et al., 2013; Park et al., 2013; Stine-Morrow et al., 2014). These stimulation/engagement approaches introduce special challenges when selecting appropriate controls. An example of an engagement model of cognitive intervention can be seen in the Baltimore Experience Corps trial (Fried et al., 2013). The Experience Corps® (EC) program is an innovative, community-based model for health promotion for older adults (Fried et al., 2004, 2013; Rebok et al., 2011) that involves volunteers aged 60 and older working with low-income, urban schools as mentors of children in grades K–3 for 15 hours a week throughout 2 academic school years. The program seeks to create meaningful, socially valued roles for older adults while simultaneously serving as a vehicle for health promotion by encouraging greater cognitive, physical, and social activity—all factors that have been shown to promote greater health and well-being and enhance cognitive fitness. The underlying two goals are to create a more active and healthier older population by engaging them in activities that can make a difference in society; and a student population having more educational needs met. A secondary benefit of Experience Corps design was the enhanced ability to create a positive learning environment in the classroom that results in schools having stronger academic performance.

An intention-to-treat, randomized, controlled effectiveness trial of the Experience Corps program recruited adults 60 and older who were eligible and randomized them to the intervention, Experience Corps participation, or to a usual volunteering opportunity, wait-list control (Fried et al., 2013). Those randomized to Experience Corps were assigned to serve for at least 1 year in a public elementary school, with grades Kindergarten through the third grade. Older adults randomized to the control arm were referred to the Baltimore City Commission on Aging and Retirement Education (CARE), where usual volunteer opportunities in Baltimore City, other than Experience Corps, were offered; these were selected to be of short duration and/or low time demand, such as volunteering at health fairs, city festivals, and senior center events. This was a usual care, low-activity control that was deemed more credible than a no-contact control because many older adults volunteer on their own, but usually for only a few hours a week and often for only limited periods of time. Those in the control arm were wait-listed for participation in Experience Corps after 2 years, should they remain interested. This proved to be a challenge as a few participants assigned to the control arm were not content to wait that long and tried to join the Experience Corps program without actually participating in the study. We also found that surprisingly few of the controls (about 20%) were actually still interested in joining the program after waiting 2 years, suggesting that their motivation or ability to participate may have decreased over time, or they may have found alternative volunteering opportunities.

As part of the Experience Corps trial, we also initially planned to randomize schools either to receive Experience Corps or to control status. Although randomization of schools was the gold standard to which we aspired, political realities made it impossible to randomize. For example, the city government wanted to select certain schools for participation on the basis of the level of educational need or political considerations. To maximize inference validity, we therefore identified control schools via a propensity score matching approach (Fried et al., 2013). Thus, it may not always be possible or feasible to carry out fully randomized trials in the complex environment of the real-world.

In a recent multimodal intervention study, Park and her colleagues used novel, real-world activities, which offer a degree of challenge and stimulation that can increase alongside increasing expertise (Park & Bischof, 2013). In their Synapse Project, a supported activity intervention, participants engaged in a new cognitively stimulating activity (i.e., quilting, digital photography, or both activities) for about 15 hours per week for 3 months (Park et al., 2013). The three intervention groups were compared to one of three control arms (social control, placebo, and no-treatment) over the 3 months. The social control group engaged in nonintellectual activities such as field trips and entertainment and socialized for 15 hours per week. In the placebo control condition, participants worked on cognitive tasks that relied on previous knowledge and did not require active learning. No-treatment controls were required to complete only a weekly checklist of their daily activities. The use of multiple controls in this study was important in helping the investigators isolate the effects of different types of activity. However, this advantage needs to be weighed against the increased costs of including multiple control groups and the need to recruit and assess more participants.

CONTAMINATION EFFECTS

In behavioral intervention trials, members of the control group may have access to the intervention, which can potentially affect the outcomes of interest. If the members of the comparison (control) group are actually affected by the intervention, then *contamination* or "spillover" is said to occur. Referred to as *contagion* in the case of experimental evaluation, contamination can pose a major threat to the investigator's ability to draw unambiguous conclusions about the effectiveness of the intervention under study. For example, suppose an investigator is trying to conduct a behavioral trial of an intervention to improve mood and reduce loneliness and isolation in a congregate living facility for older adults. He or she randomly assigns half of the residents in this community to the intervention group and half to the control condition. However, in this case, the potential of contamination effects from the intervention group to the control is very high because the residents of this community may talk to one another about the study and may even share intervention materials if they are available, given their close proximity and shared living space.

So, how should the investigator try to control for, or minimize, contamination? One possibility is to explicitly ask participants not to talk with one another about the study until the intervention trial is over. Although this may reduce the extent or severity of spillover, it will not entirely eliminate it, given that some residents may still share details of their experience with the interventions with those who are not in the treatment group. Also, this request may be perceived as burdensome to some study participants. These exchanges between participants can be difficult or impossible to document. Another related option is to try to limit access to the intervention materials, and ask intervention participants not to share materials with anyone. For example, in a memory-training study we conducted in a retirement community, all handouts were collected at the end of each training class, and participants were not allowed to take the intervention manuals home with them. However, there were still instances where participants asked to keep the handouts, or even tried to smuggle them out of the classroom; so the potential for sharing materials with others still may exist despite the investigator's best efforts.

A stronger approach to dealing with contamination involves the deliberate design of an intervention trial to minimize the possibility of spillover. For example, in the Baltimore Prevention trial with first and second graders, we used both *internal* and *external* control groups to derive a statistical estimate of how much spillover occurred from the intervention conditions to the control groups within 19 public elementary schools in Baltimore City (Dolan et al., 1993; Kellam, Rebok, Ialongo, & Mayer, 1994). Six of the 19 schools were randomly assigned to a classroom behavior intervention, 7 to a reading intervention, and the remaining 6 were assigned as no-treatment or external control schools. Because the latter schools had neither intervention, it was considered unlikely that contamination would have occurred through exposure to the intervention. However, we also employed internal controls within the 13 schools that had either the behavioral or reading interventions. By comparing the treatment effect size of the interventions under the two different types of control conditions, one can get an estimate of just how large the spillover effect might be. If no spillover effects had occurred, then one would expect there to be no difference in the treatment effect size under either comparison condition. However, if spillover occurred, then the treatment effects should be relatively larger in the external control schools, because the treatment effects may have been attenuated in the internal control schools owing to contamination of the control classrooms. However, in this digital age of electronic information sharing, even geographic distance of intervention sites does not guarantee control conditions, and contamination may still occur (Sanson-Fisher, Bonevski, Green, & D'Este, 2007). And these effects are exacerbated when the intervention is implemented at the community level such as in a school system or in community health care facilities.

ETHICAL ISSUES IN THE SELECTION AND USE OF CONTROL GROUPS

There are special ethical concerns in behavioral intervention trials related to the use of control groups because treatments are determined by chance (Street & Luoma, 2002). The arms of the intervention trial must be in *clinical equipoise*, which is central to the protection of human participants. The equipoise principle states that participants should be assured of receiving the best available standard therapy in any therapeutic study (Schwartz et al., 1997). Over the past several decades, clinical research has documented reduced morbidity and, in some cases, increased survival among medically ill populations receiving a psychosocial intervention (Schwartz et al., 1997). Given these effects, it is increasingly difficult to justify relying solely on a no-treatment control in many behavioral intervention studies. Although no-treatment controls have an appealing simplicity, as discussed earlier, they also raise ethical concerns. The use of these controls may be ethically defensible when the experimental treatment targets a problem without a treatment indication, or when the trial focuses on a population with no immediate risks (e.g., a trial for the prevention of depression; Mohr et al., 2009). However, the use of no-treatment controls may be less acceptable when the trial targets severe disorders, for which effective treatment is both indicated and available (e.g., a trial for patients with major depressive disorder).

Ethical issues are also raised when other control conditions are employed such as placebo controls (Emanuel & Miller, 2001; Schwartz et al., 1997). Where no effective treatment is available, the use of a placebo can be ethically justified. Placebos are also ethical when there exists no permanent harm in delaying active treatment for the duration of the trial. However, in the context of a treatment to prevent or delay death, it is difficult to defend the use of a placebo control. By denying treatment to controls, an investigator might run the risk of "resentful demoralization" on the part of the control group, which may lead them to seek out treatment similar to the active intervention. It may be inappropriate or unethical to ask control participants to avoid using a resource that has been demonstrated to be health enhancing (Schwartz et al., 1997). Even when there are debates about the efficacy of an intervention, and the scientific community remains neutral, ethical issues may still exist. Participants and their care providers may perceive benefit of the treatment when none exists.

There are also ethical issues involved in economic considerations in the design of behavioral intervention trials. Economic factors can influence trial design and the choice of treatment and control conditions. As Schwartz et al. (1997) point out, if resources are scarce, then the trial should be designed for clinically significant and economically feasible outcomes rather than focusing on statistical significance per se. In this case, the investigator might use less expensive, but perhaps less effective, commonly used treatments for a given control condition rather than a no-treatment control. The no-treatment control might be less costly because of lower sample size requirements, but the comparison conditions should be designed according to the treatment and effect sizes that are economically feasible in the real-world setting (Schwartz et al., 1997).

Finally, so-called "cluster RCTs" of behavioral interventions pose special ethical challenges because the intervention is delivered at the level of the group or community rather than at the individual level (Christie, O'Halloran, & Stevenson, 2009). In this case, it may be difficult to ensure individual choice when the intervention is delivered to the group. For example, if a health promotion intervention is delivered to an entire continuing care retirement community, individuals within that community may be exposed to the intervention whether they choose to be or not. Before starting a cluster RCT, investigators should determine if the intervention will actually be delivered to the community as a cluster without the possibility of individual choice. It is especially important for investigators to safeguard the rights and interests of the individual when designing and implementing cluster RCTs.

IMPACT ON RECRUITMENT AND ATTRITION

A great strength of RCTs is that each group is generally balanced on all characteristics, with any imbalance occurring by chance. However, during any trial, participants may be lost to follow-up, which reduces statistical power by decreasing sample size. In an RCT, there is an implicit trade-off between statistical power to detect an effect and the level of control over threats to validity (Mohr et al., 2009). Loss to follow-up can greatly influence the outcome of behavioral intervention trials (Dumville, Torgerson, & Hewitt, 2006). Bias may occur from attrition when there are different rates of attrition between the treatment group and the control group or the reasons for the attrition differ between the two groups (Tansella et al., 2006). This is an important source of bias, and that bias can remain large even when advanced statistical techniques, such as multiple imputation, are used to address the attrition. Thus, it is critical to minimize dropout from the control group. Suggestions for minimizing dropout include creating a research project identity; emphasizing the importance of the contribution of the control participants to the study results before randomization; developing a strong tracking system to be able to identify, locate, and determine the status of the control group members; and maintaining contact with them through telephone reminders, postcards, and newsletters (Miller & Hollist, 2007). Retention issues are discussed further in Chapter 10.

It is important when recruiting for behavioral intervention trials that the selection procedures do not yield a sample that is biased toward one or more treatment or control conditions. For example, participants might have a preference for a particular behavioral intervention, and this preference might lead to nonadherence and increased dropout rate, and even affect treatment response if a person gets randomized to his or her nonpreferred condition (Holroyd, Powers, & Andrasik, 2005). Potential participants who do not want a particular treatment condition or the control condition might be more likely to refuse randomization, or may not be as motivated to put forth their best effort. No ready solution to this problem is available at this time. The investigator should assess and report reasons for refusal of randomization and treatment preferences, and identify these as possible confounds, even if they cannot be completely controlled (Holroyd et al., 2005).

Additional information about how study participants' expectations and preferences impact treatment adherence, attrition, and outcomes should be collected routinely in RCTs, but seldom is. This failure to control for expectations is not a minor omission and may have serious consequences that may undermine any causal inference (Boot, Simons, Stothart, & Stutts, 2013). For example, Boot et al. (2013) examined the game-training literature and concluded that not controlling for expectations limits conclusions that can be drawn about the effectiveness of active videogame training in improving cognitive and perceptual abilities. Although they singled out videogame interventions for their review, they also pointed out that this is a broader problem affecting most behavioral interventions targeting mental health, education, and personal well-being. They recommend that researchers explicitly assess expectations, carefully choose outcome measures that are not influenced by differential expectations, and use alternative experimental designs that assess and manipulate expectation effects directly.

RECOMMENDATIONS AND CONCLUSIONS

Selecting appropriate control conditions in behavioral intervention research design and development is a critical decision. Choice of a control condition will depend upon several factors, including phase of intervention development, theory base, available resources, and ethical considerations. At the RCT phase, as should be apparent by this point, no RCT and no control condition are perfect. To help make more informed decisions about control group selection for RCTs, we recommend that the following points be taken into consideration. First, it is important to give as much attention to the selection of the control group as one does to the choice of the intervention. It has been our experience that researchers often think long and hard about which interventions to choose, but often approach control group selection as an afterthought. In this regard, avoid automatically selecting a no-treatment control as a default option, although there may be instances when no-treatment controls are called for, for example, to control for practice effects in cognitive intervention trials. Second, consider the use of multiple controls or comparisons, not always a single control condition. It may be the case that different types of controls are needed for a given study. For example, researchers may need to control for practice effects as well as the amount of social contact, as in the ACTIVE study (Jobe et al., 2001). Third, try to minimize differential dropout or attrition in the control condition by maintaining regular contact with control participants, by developing a strong tracking system, by creating a strong research project identity, and through emphasizing the importance of the control condition prior to randomization. More people may drop out of the control condition than the treatment condition, and often do so nonrandomly, creating problems interpreting the results of randomized clinical intervention trials. Fourth, it is important to pilot test control conditions if they involve some activity, and research staff should be trained in their delivery (Stephenson & Imrie, 1998). In addition, all unplanned contact in both treatment and control conditions should be logged. Finally, along with all of the previously mentioned considerations, researchers must become more aware of the broad array of theoretical, methodological, and ethical issues in control group selection (Gross, 2005). Such efforts should result in a better evidence base upon which to create standard best practice and policy. Having consistent evidence in a series of RCTs is generally considered to establish the intervention as "evidence-based" (i.e., it has sufficient data to support its use and broader scale adoption).

REFERENCES

Avins, A. L., Cherkin, D. C., Sherman, K. J., Goldberg, H., & Pressman, A. (2012). Should we reconsider the routine use of placebo controls in clinical research? *Trials, 13*(44), 1–7.

Ball, K., Berch, D. B., Helmers, K. F., Jobe, J. B., Leveck, M. D., Marsiske, M., . . . Willis, S. L. (2002). Effects of cognitive training interventions with older adults: A randomized controlled trial. *JAMA, 288*, 2271–2281.

Belle, S. H., Czaja, S. J., Schulz, R., Zhang, S., Burgio, L. D., Gitlin, L. N., . . . REACH Investigators. (2003). Using a new taxonomy to combine the uncombinable: Integrating results across diverse interventions. *Psychology and Aging, 18*, 396–405.

Boot, W. R., Simons, D. J., Stothart, C., & Stutts, C. (2013). The pervasive problem of placebos in psychology: Why active control groups are not sufficient to rule out placebo effects. *Perspectives on Psychological Science, 8*, 445–454.

Campbell, D. T., & Stanley, J. C. (1966). *Experimental and quasi-experimental designs for research*. Boston, MA: Houghton Mifflin Company.

Christie, J., O'Halloran, P., & Stevenson, M. (2009). Planning a cluster randomized controlled trial: Methodological issues. *Nursing Research, 58*, 128–134.

Clark, F., Azen, S. P., Zemke, R., Jackson, J., Carlson, M., Mandel, D., . . . Lipson, L. (1997). Occupational therapy for independent-living older adults. *JAMA, 278*, 1321–1326.

Cuijpers, P., van Straten, A., Warmerdam, L., & Andersson, G. (2008). Psychological treatment of depression: A meta-analytic database of randomized studies. *BMC Psychiatry, 8*(36), 1–6. doi:10.1186/1471-244X-8-36

Czaja, S. J., Schulz, R., Lee, C. C., Belle, S. H., & REACH Investigators. (2003). A methodology for describing and decomposing complex psychosocial and behavioral interventions. *Psychology and Aging, 18*, 385–395.

Dolan, L. J., Kellam, S. G., Brown, C. H., Werthamer-Larsson, L., Rebok, G. W., Mayer, L. S., . . . Wheeler, L. (1993). The short-term impact of two classroom-based preventive interventions on aggressive and shy behaviors and poor achievement. *Journal of Applied Developmental Psychology, 14*, 317–345.

Dumville, J. C., Torgerson, D. J., & Hewitt, C. E. (2006). Reporting attrition in randomised controlled trials. *BMJ, 332*, 969–971.

Emanuel, E. J., & Miller, F. G. (2001). The ethics of placebo-controlled trials—A middle ground. *The New England Journal of Medicine, 345*, 915–919.

Freedland, K. E., Mohr, D. C., Davidson, K. W., & Schwartz, J. E. (2011). Usual and unusual care: Existing practice control groups in randomized controlled trials of behavioral interventions. *Psychosomatic Medicine, 73*, 323–335.

Fried, L. P., Carlson, M. C., Freedman, M., Frick, K. D., Glass, T. A., Hill, J., . . . Zeger, S. (2004). A social model for health promotion for an aging population: Initial evidence on the Experience Corps® model. *Journal of Urban Health, 81*, 64–78.

Fried, L. P., Carlson, M. C., McGill, S., Seeman, T., Xue, Q.-L., Frick, K., . . . Rebok, G. W. (2013). Experience Corps: A dual trial to promote the health of older adults and children's academic success. *Contemporary Clinical Trials, 36*, 1–13.

Gates, N. J., Sachdev, P. S., Fiatarone Singh, M. A., & Valenzuela, M. (2011). Cognitive and memory training in adults at risk of dementia: A systematic review. *BMC Geriatrics, 11*(55), 1–14. doi:10.1186/1471-2318-11-55

Gitlin, L. N. (2013). Introducing a new intervention: An overview of research phases and common challenges. *American Journal of Occupational Therapy, 67*, 177–184.

Gitlin, L. N., Marx, K., Stanley, I., & Hodgson, N. (2015). Translating evidence-based dementia caregiving interventions into practice: State-of-the-science and next steps. *The Gerontologist, 55*(2), 210–216. doi:10.1093/geront/gnu123

Gross, A. L., Inouye, S. K., Rebok, G. W., Brandt, J., Crane, P. K., Parisi, J. M., . . . Jones, R. N. (2012). Parallel but not equivalent: Challenges and solutions for repeated assessment of cognition over time. *Journal of Clinical and Experimental Neuropsychology, 34*, 758–772.

Gross, A. L., Parisi, J. M., Spira, A. P., Kueider, A. M., Ko, J. Y., Saczynski, J. S., . . . Rebok, G. W. (2012). Memory training interventions for older adults: A meta-analysis. *Aging and Mental Health, 16*, 722–734.

Gross, D. (2005). On the merits of attention-control groups. *Research in Nursing & Health, 28*, 93–94.

Holroyd, K. A., Powers, S. W., & Andrasik, F. (2005). Methodological issues in clinical trials of drug and behavior therapies. *Headache, 45*, 487–492.

Jobe, J. B., Smith, D. M., Ball, K., Tennstedt, S. L., Marsiske, M., Willis, S. L., . . . Kleinman, K. (2001). ACTIVE: A cognitive intervention trial to promote independence in older adults. *Controlled Clinical Trials, 22*, 453–479.

Kellam, S. G., Rebok, G. W., Ialongo, N., & Mayer, L. S. (1994). The course and malleability of aggressive behavior from early first grade into middle school: Results of a developmental epidemiologically-based preventive trial. *Journal of Child Psychology & Psychiatry & Allied Disciplines, 35*, 259–281.

Lindquist, R., Wyman, J. F., Talley, K. M. C., Findorff, M. J., & Gross, C. R. (2007). Design of control-group conditions in clinical trials of behavioral interventions. *Journal of Nursing Scholarship, 39*, 214–221.

Melnyk, B. M., & Morrison-Beedy, D. (2012). *Intervention research: Designing, conducting, analyzing, funding.* New York, NY: Springer Publishing Company.

Miller, R. B., & Hollist, C. S. (2007). Attrition bias. *Faculty Publications, Department of Child, Youth, and Family Studies.* Paper 45. Retrieved from http://digitalcommons.unl.edu/famconfacpub/45

Mohr, D. C., Spring, B., Freedland, K. E., Beckner, V., Arean, P., Hollon, S. D., . . . Kaplan, R. (2009). The selection and design of control conditions for randomized controlled trials of psychological interventions. *Psychotherapy and Psychosomatics, 78,* 275–284.

Park, D. C., & Bischof, G. N. (2013). The aging mind: Neuroplasticity in response to cognitive training. *Dialogues in Clinical Neuroscience, 15,* 109–119.

Park, D. C., Lodi-Smith, J., Drew, L. M., Haber, S. H., Hebrank, A. C., Bischof, G. N., & Aamodt, W. (2013). The impact of sustained engagement on cognitive function in older adults: The Synapse Project. *Psychological Sciences, 25,* 103–112.

Rebok, G. W., Ball, K., Guey, L. T., Jones, R. N., Kim, H.-Y., King, J. W., . . . Willis, S. L. (2014). Ten-year effects of the ACTIVE cognitive training trial on cognition and everyday functioning in older adults. *Journal of the American Geriatrics Society, 62,* 16–24.

Rebok, G. W., Carlson, M. C., Barron, J. S., Frick, K. D., McGill, S., Parisi, J. M., . . . Fried, L. P. (2011). Experience Corps®: A civic engagement-based public health intervention in the public schools. In P. E. Hartman-Stein & A. La Rue (Eds.), *Enhancing cognitive fitness in adults: A guide to the use and development of community-based programs* (pp. 469–487). New York, NY: Springer.

Sanson-Fisher, R. W., Bonevski, B., Green, L. W., & D'Este, C. (2007). Limitations of the randomized controlled trial in evaluating population-based health interventions. *American Journal of Preventive Medicine, 33,* 155–161.

Schulz, K. F., Chalmers, I., & Altman, D. G. (2002). The landscape and lexicon of blinding in randomized trials. *Annals of Internal Medicine, 136,* 254–259.

Schwartz, C. E., Chesney, M. A., Irvine, M. J., & Keefe, F. J. (1997). The control group dilemma in clinical research: Applications for psychosocial and behavioral medicine trials. *Psychosomatic Medicine, 59,* 362–371.

Singal, A. G., Higgins, P. D. R., & Waljee, A. K. (2014). A primer on effectiveness and efficacy trials. *Clinical and Translational Gastroenterology, 5,* e45. doi:10.1038/ctg.2013.13

Stephenson, J., & Imrie, J. (1998). Why do we need randomised controlled trials to assess behavioural interventions? *BMJ, 316,* 611–613.

Stine-Morrow, E. A. L., & Basak, C. (2011). Cognitive interventions. In K. W. Schaie & S. L. Willis (Eds.), *Handbook of the psychology of aging* (7th ed., pp. 153–170). New York, NY: Elsevier.

Stine-Morrow, E. A. L. Payne, B. R., Roberts, B. W., Kramer, A. F., Morrow, D. G., Payne, L., . . . Parisi, J. M. (2014). Training versus engagement as paths to cognitive enrichment with aging. *Psychology and Aging, 29*(4), 891–906.

Street, L. L., & Luoma, J. B. (2002). Control groups in psychosocial intervention research: Ethical and methodological issues. *Ethics & Behavior, 12,* 1–30.

Tansella, M., Thornicroft, G., Barbui, C., Cipriani, A., & Saraceno, B. (2006). Seven criteria for improving effectiveness trials in psychiatry. *Psychological Medicine, 36,* 711–720.

Thompson, B. T., & Schoenfeld, D. (2007). Usual care in the control group in clinical trials of nonpharmacologic interventions. *Proceedings of the American Thoracic Society, 4,* 577–582.

Viera, A. J., & Bangdiwala, S. I. (2007). Eliminating bias in randomized controlled trials: Importance of allocation concealment and masking. *Family Medicine, 39,* 132–137.

West, A., & Spring, B. (2007). *Randomized controlled trials.* Retrieved November 15, 2014, from http://www.ebbp.org/course_outlines/randomized_controlled_trials/

Westmaas, J. L., Gil-Rivas, V., & Silver, R. C. (2007). Designing and implementing interventions to promote health and prevent illness. In H. S. Friedman & R. C. Silver (Eds.), *Foundations of health psychology* (pp. 52–70). New York, NY: Oxford University Press.

Whitehead, W. E. (2004). Control groups appropriate for behavioral interventions. *Gastroenterology, 126,* S159–S163.

Willis, S. L. (2001). Methodological issues in behavioral intervention research with the elderly. In K. W. Schaie & J. W. Birren (Eds.), *Handbook of the psychology of aging* (5th ed., pp. 78–108). San Diego, CA: Academic Press.

Willis, S. L., Cornelius, S. W., Blow, F. C., & Baltes, P. B. (1983). Training in research in aging: Attentional processes. *Journal of Educational Psychology, 75,* 257–270.

Willis, S. L., Tennstedt, S. L., Marsiske, M., Ball, K., Elias, J., Koepke, K. M., . . . Wright, E. (2006). Long-term effects of cognitive training on everyday functional outcomes in older adults. *JAMA, 296,* 2805–2814.

NINE

SAMPLING CONSIDERATIONS: IDENTIFYING APPROPRIATE PARTICIPANTS FOR BEHAVIORAL INTERVENTION RESEARCH

If you aren't taking a representative sample you won't get a representative snapshot.
—Nate Silver

An important aspect in the design of a behavioral intervention study at any stage along the pipeline is the selection of an appropriate sample. Clearly it would be ideal to include an entire population (e.g., all family caregivers of patients with Alzheimer's disease [AD] or all American adults with high blood pressure) in intervention research. This would enhance the external validity of the study or the extent to which results can be generalized to the population as a whole. However, in most cases, this is not feasible as populations are typically large and geographically diverse.

For example, estimates may vary slightly, but currently about 70 million American adults have high blood pressure (Centers for Disease Control and Prevention [CDC], 2015), and although rates of high blood pressure vary somewhat by geography (e.g., self-reported estimates tend to be higher in some areas of the southern United States as compared to areas in the northwest), there are adults with high blood pressure across the 50 states. Thus, it would not be possible for a researcher conducting a trial to evaluate a behavioral intervention for blood pressure control to include the entire target population, even if the study was multisite. Instead, investigators rely on samples (a subset of a population) to examine proof of concept and to test the feasibility, efficacy, and/or effectiveness of interventions as well as to attempt to generalize the findings and conclusions to an entire population.

Using a sample is advantageous for a number of reasons. Samples involve a smaller number of people and thus are less costly, more time efficient, and require less effort with respect to recruitment and data collection. In addition, it is easier to maintain treatment integrity with smaller numbers of people. Samples can also be selected to reduce heterogeneity. For example, AD is not a unitary disease, but has different symptom presentations at different stages of the disease progression. If an investigator was interested in testing the efficacy of a cognitive training intervention for people with AD, it would generally be more appropriate to evaluate the intervention with people at the mild stages of the disease as those in the later stages of the illness would be unlikely to benefit. Thus, in this case, a sample of the AD population with certain characteristics is more appropriate as opposed to the entire population of people with AD.

In selecting a sample for an intervention study, researchers must be aware of any potential bias in participant selection. Bias can lead to errors in the interpretation of results from an intervention study and limit the ability to generalize the findings to other groups of people. Referring to the blood pressure intervention example described earlier, assume the study involved a nutritional intervention and that the sample was restricted to White males. Obviously, the sample would be biased with respect to gender and ethnicity. The findings could not be generalized to other segments of the hypertensive population such as females and those from other ethnic groups, given differences in the characteristics of these segments of the population (e.g., body size, hormonal differences, cultural food preferences and patterns) that could have an impact on the effectiveness of the intervention.

It is clear that the selection of the sample is an essential consideration in behavioral intervention research. Who should be included in the evaluation of an intervention depends, of course, on the specific research question; the target population of the intervention; study design; and feasibility constraints with respect to budget, time, staff, and participant availability. Two important considerations are the composition of the sample and sample size. The sample should be representative of the target population on characteristics important to the research question and intervention and be of sufficient size to provide adequate power to test the study hypotheses. Unfortunately, oftentimes, researchers focus just on the size of the sample without giving adequate consideration to representativeness and feasibility issues. In this chapter, we discuss the topics of sample composition (who should be included in the evaluation of an intervention) and sample size as well as issues related to feasibility. We also discuss approaches to sampling and which sampling methods are most useful in behavioral intervention research. Our goal is to provide some guidelines to help optimize the selection of samples across the behavioral intervention pipeline.

SAMPLE CHARACTERISTICS

Sample Composition

A key consideration in the selection of a sample for an intervention study at any stage of the pipeline is the extent to which the sample is representative of the population for whom the intervention is intended on relevant characteristics. For example, within caregiver research, it is generally recognized that a "one-size-fits-all" approach is not efficacious with respect to the design of interventions, as caregivers vary along a number of dimensions: ethnicity/culture, gender, and age; caregiver experience, needs, and well-being; and caregiving demands, roles, and responsibilities. In the Resources for Enhancing Alzheimer's Caregiver Health II (REACH II) trial (Belle et al., 2006), the sample of caregivers included three different race/ethnic groups: White, African American, and Hispanic caregivers, who varied in age, relationship to the care recipient, and years in the caregiving role. This facilitated an analysis of whether the impact of the REACH II intervention varied by geographic, race/ethnic, and other characteristics of caregivers such as relationship to the person with dementia. Answers to these questions are important to help guide further refinements of an intervention and to determine if an intervention benefits some groups over others. Although participants in REACH II represented one of three race/ethnic groups, other subgroups were not represented such as Asian and Haitian caregivers. The exclusion of these groups limits the generalizability of findings from REACH II to these caregiver populations.

The composition of a sample is also important in another respect. The sample must possess the characteristics that the intervention intends to address or modify. Take, for example, a caregiver intervention that is designed to reduce depression and distress. As not all caregivers are depressed or find caregiving distressful, the sample for a study to test the effects of a depression intervention would need to include only a subset of caregivers—namely those who have depressive symptoms. Aligning the characteristics of the sample with the intent of an intervention through the specification of inclusion and exclusion study criteria is critical; otherwise, it would not be possible to adequately demonstrate whether the intervention has an impact or not and for whom.

In essence, a representative sample is one that accurately reflects the members of the population for whom the intervention is targeting; in other words, it is one that has strong external validity with respect to the target population of the intervention (Davern, 2008). Having a sample that is representative enhances the confidence with which the findings from a study can be generalized to the population that is the focus of the intervention. A sample that is not representative leads to bias or sampling error; certain groups may be overrepresented and others may be underrepresented, which impacts on the outcomes of the study. For example, in the Personalized Reminder Information and Social Management (PRISM) trial (Czaja et al., 2014), extensive pilot testing was used to evaluate the usability of the PRISM software before the implementation of an efficacy trial. The target population for the randomized controlled trial (RCT) was older adults (age 65+) who were at "risk for social isolation" and had minimal prior computer/Internet experience. If the sample for the pilot testing had included middle-aged adults with extensive computer or Internet experience, the findings regarding the software usability would have been biased and have limited generalizability to the target population. This illustrates the importance of carefully considering who the sample should be early on in the intervention development process and assuring representation of that sample through careful construction of study eligibility and ineligibility criteria and recruitment strategies.

Sample bias cannot be totally eliminated; however, it is important to attempt to minimize bias to the extent possible and also to understand the limitations imposed by the sample included in an evaluation of an intervention. Three factors influence the representativeness of a sample: sample size, sample attrition, and sampling method. With respect to sample size, the larger the sample the more likely it is to be representative of the target population and thus the less likely it is to be biased. Sample attrition can also lead to potential bias if those who drop out of a study have common characteristics (e.g., those who are older or who have less skill) as the remaining study participants will no longer be representative of the original sample.

This can lead to overestimation of the intervention effects or misestimating the effects. For example, assume an investigator is interested in evaluating the impact of a stress reduction intervention on the depression of family caregivers and the original sample includes caregivers with varying levels of depression. The results of the study indicate that the study is efficacious and results in a significant decrease in caregiver depression. However, during the course of the study, caregivers with high levels of depression have higher dropout rates. In this case, the impact of the treatment may be overestimated as the sample that received the intervention consists primarily of caregivers who have low levels of depression. Finally, sampling method can also influence bias as there are various ways to choose a sample, and as will be discussed later in this chapter, there are sampling methods that can be used to help ensure that the sample is representative of the target population.

In general, who should be included in a study depends on the objective(s) of the intervention and the research question(s), research design, available resources including budget, and sample availability. It is critical to characterize the target population of interest before a sample can be defined. For example, assume a researcher is interested in determining if an intervention that involves cognitive behavioral therapy delivered via videoconferencing is effective in alleviating symptoms among people with emotional disorders. It would be important to narrow and refine the research question to specify the type of emotional disorder (e.g., depression, bipolar disorder), age range (e.g., adolescents or adults), living arrangement of the participants (community-dwelling or hospitalized patients), and any restrictions with respect to medications or substance abuse. It would also be important to consider the availability and accessibility of a sample in terms of any potential geographic or time constraints in recruiting, enrolling, and retaining the targeted group. In the PRISM study, if the majority of the potential participants lived in an underserved area, Internet access may have been spotty, which would influence the size of the pool from which the sample can be drawn. This may also limit who may be able to enroll in the study and successfully engage in the intervention. The decisions made about sampling have implications for recruitment and retention strategies (Chapter 10).

Another important consideration in sampling is the inclusion of women and minorities. When designing interventions, it is important to consider culture/ ethnicity and gender as these factors can moderate or directly impact on the outcomes of an intervention. Many funding agencies, particularly in the United States, require applicants to clearly state if women and minorities are included in a study. In the United States, the National Institutes of Health (NIH) insists that women and members of minority groups must be included in all NIH-funded research, unless a clear and compelling rationale and justification are otherwise provided that their inclusion would be inappropriate with respect to the health of the subjects or the purpose of the research. This issue is considered in scientific peer review. As stated on the NIH website:

> Peer reviewers will also assess the adequacy of plans to include subjects from both genders, all racial and ethnic groups (and subgroups), and children, as appropriate, for the scientific goals of the research will be assessed. Plans for the recruitment and retention of subjects will also be evaluated. (NIH, 2015)

Of course, the nature and scope of diversity of the sample must be based on the research question posed; however, lack of diversity in a proposed sample must be clearly and adequately justified. For example, it would be reasonable to include only women in a study that is evaluating an intervention aimed at alleviating depression in women recently diagnosed with breast cancer, but it would not be reasonable to restrict the sample to White women. The NIH also requires consideration of the inclusion of children (<18 years of age), and a rationale must be provided in grant applications for their inclusion or exclusion. As noted by Kazdin (1999), there is a need to sample broadly, to evaluate the moderating role of sample differences, and to pursue mechanisms through which moderating factors may operate. Sampling broadly along a number of characteristics pertinent to the intervention also enables an intervention to have maximum "reach" to all those who are intended to benefit.

Sample Size

The size of a sample is also a critical consideration when developing and evaluating an intervention. Size will vary depending upon the phase along the pipeline. For example, the sample size needed for a small proof of concept study or for testing feasibility or usability of a component of an intervention will differ from a large efficacy trial. The size of a sample must be considered early on in the planning process of any evaluation, in particular, when the goal is to establish the efficacy/effectiveness of an intervention or to examine the comparative effectiveness between two interventions. This typically involves a comparison between two or more groups; that is, treatment versus control; or treatment A versus treatment B. In both cases, one can derive precise and accurate conclusions only with an appropriate sample size.

Whereas statistical power may not be a concern in the developmental phases of an intervention, it is extremely important in the evaluation phases when comparing two or more groups. The size of the sample influences the statistical power of the study—the extent to which the study can detect differences between groups. Power is a function of the criterion established for statistical significance (alpha level), the difference that exists between the groups (effect size) and the sample size (Kazdin, 1994). These four concepts are interrelated in the sense that, when three of them are known, the remaining one can be determined. To determine the sample size needed for a study, decisions can be made regarding the other three parameters: alpha, power, and effect size.

Building on an example from Kazdin (1994), assume you are interested in determining the needed sample size for a study evaluating the effectiveness of two different psychosocial interventions for family caregivers and your primary outcome is caregiver burden as measured by the Zarit Burden Interview (Zarit, Reever, & Bach-Peterson, 1980). The chosen alpha for the study is .05, the power is .80, and the estimated effect size is .40; based on available tables (Cohen, 1988), the needed sample size is 40 participants per group or a total of 80 caregivers. There are also computer programs available to conduct power analyses. If the required sample size is not feasible owing to availability of participants or budgetary/staffing issues, the alpha level can be varied or the power can be reduced slightly (e.g., .75). Estimates for an effect size can be obtained from prior research studies, the literature, or meta-analyses. It is generally recommended to select a conservative estimate of an effect size (Kazdin, 1994). Power estimates must also include any planned subgroup analyses in order to make sure that the comparisons of interest will be sufficiently sensitive to detect differences if, in fact, they exist. It is also important to plan for attrition—typically estimates of 15% to 20% are used, but rates can vary vastly depending upon the targeted population. For example, trials involving caregivers of individuals with dementia can have attrition rates as high as 50% over a short time frame (e.g., 6 months) because of the vulnerabilities of this population and high risk for hospitalizations and death. However, in the previous example, to achieve sufficient power after accounting for an estimated attrition of 20%, a sample of 96 participants would be needed.

It is important to derive sample size estimates prior to the beginning of a study to ensure that the study is sufficiently powered. For most funding agencies, power calculations are an important element of the proposed methodology for which an investigator will be evaluated. Power calculations are also now required by many refereed journals when reporting a randomized intervention trial. Understanding the required number of participants is also important with respect to planning the study recruitment strategy, budget, staffing requirements, and timeline. It may also allow an investigator to make any necessary adjustments to the study design, although this is not particularly desirable. For example, if, upon entry into the field, the required sample size is not obtainable, a decision might be made to reduce the number of experimental groups, or assume effect sizes will be challenging to detect.

For example, assume that an investigator is interested in examining the impact of computer gaming on the cognitive functioning of older adults by comparing computer gaming with crossword puzzles. The initial plan may be to examine this across three age groups: younger, middle-aged, and older. Thus, the study design would be a 2 (gaming vs. crossword puzzles) × 3 (age group) design. However, a power analysis indicates that the required sample size to achieve an effect size of .75 at an alpha level of .05 is 35; thus, a total sample size of 210 participants (35 per 6 cells) would be needed to achieve the desired power. After accounting for attrition (20%), the actual number would be 252 participants or 42 per cell. The investigator might determine that it would not be feasible to recruit this number of participants and thus could decide to eliminate the younger age group as inclusion of this group was not critical to the goals of the research.

Obtaining the appropriate number of participants in a study is a critical aspect of behavioral intervention research. At the efficacy/effectiveness phase, a small sample size may lead to a falsely negative Type II error (accepting the null hypotheses that there is no difference between study groups), and there is a risk that an effective intervention may not be recognized. Of course, a very large sample size is also not recommended as it is costly and can result in a waste of resources and unnecessarily increase the duration of a study. Sometimes, a sampling procedure involves *oversampling* where a large portion of individuals with a particular characteristic are sampled. This strategy is used to help ensure that the study will have sufficient data for a particular group or subgroups. For example, it may be the case that an investigator is recruiting from a geographic region where the prevalence of a particular ethnic/racial group represents a small portion of the population. In this case, an investigator might *oversample* individuals from this ethnic/racial group to ensure that this group is sufficiently represented in the sample.

Suffice it to say that, at the study design phase, there is often a tension between feasibility issues, cost constraints, sample size, and composition considerations. All of these issues need careful consideration before trial implementation as sampling decisions have significant implications for recruitment efforts (Chapter 10) and the internal and external validity of the study. In the following section, we discuss various sampling methods.

SAMPLING METHODS

The process of selecting a representative sample for a study is called "sampling." There are two main categories of sampling approaches: *probability sampling* and *nonprobability sampling*. Within these categories, there are various methods or procedures that are used to select samples for intervention studies, particularly at the trial phase. These approaches are summarized in Table 9.1. The choice of sampling approach and procedure should be based on the intent of the intervention, specific research goals and questions, the study design, information available about the target population, resources available, and the stage along the pipeline. For example, one typically does not use a probability sampling approach when conducting focus groups early on in the pipeline to gather initial information about perceptions of the need for an intervention. As discussed later in this chapter, this type of approach is more likely to be used when engaged at different stages in the pipeline or in survey research. Before we discuss these strategies, we define the concept of "sampling frame"—a key concept in sampling.

A *sampling frame* is the "list" or source material that is used to select a sample from a population. For example, if you were conducting a study that was evaluating an intervention to foster safe sex practices among high school students in a particular school region, the sampling frame would be a list of all registered high school students in that region. Examples of sampling frames include an electoral register, telephone directories, employment records, school class lists, patient files in a clinic or hospital, organizational lists, and so on. A sampling frame must be representative of the target population. Oftentimes, a complete sampling frame does not exist. For example, assume that one is relying on use of a telephone directory to conduct a survey about the prevalence of family caregiving within a particular geographic region. This sampling frame would be incomplete, as it would not include people with unlisted numbers or those who have temporary cell phones.

A sampling frame may also be unavailable. A work organization, for example, may not be willing to provide a list of employees; a clinic may not be willing to share the names of patients. In other cases, a sampling frame may not exist because the target population is challenging to identify or reach or may remain hidden—for example, those whose behaviors are illegal (e.g., drug abusers) or individuals who are reluctant to be identified as having a particular characteristic (e.g., persons affected with a specific illness or condition) (Magnani, Sabin, Saidel, & Heckathorn, 2005). As described later, in these cases, other methods such as "snowball sampling techniques" (an initial number of the sample is identified and recruited and helps to identify other individuals to be included in the sample) are used to identify and recruit research samples. In these cases, it is difficult to recruit a representative sample.

TABLE 9.1   Summary of Sampling Methods

Sampling Method	Summary Description
Probability sampling	All elements (e.g., individuals, skilled living facilities) in the target population have some opportunity of being included in a sample, and the probability of being included in the sample is known for each element in the population.
Simple random sampling	Each member of the population has an equal probability of being included in the sample.
Systematic sampling	Selecting every *n*th unit of the target population from a list that is randomly ordered.
Stratified sampling	Dividing a population into groups or strata (e.g., age group, race/ethnicity) and then randomly selecting from that group.
Cluster sampling	Generally a two-staged process. Initially, the total population is divided into clusters or groups, and then a random sample of clusters is selected. In the second stage, a random sample is selected from within each of these clusters.
Nonprobability sampling	Sample members are selected on the basis of availability. In others words, everyone in the target population does not have a chance of being included in the sample; the selection of members is nonrandom.
Convenience sampling	Sample members are selected on the basis of convenience—they are available and convenient (e.g., caregivers who attend community support groups).
Quota sampling	Similar to convenience sampling, but the goal is to select a certain quota or number of members of a sample that have a certain characteristic (e.g., socioeconomic status).
Purposive sampling	Sampling a specific group of individuals to address a very specific need or purpose (e.g., those who did not do well in a particular training program).
Snowball sampling	Gathering data from a few members of the target population and then asking those members for information regarding the location of other potential members of the population.
Adaptive allocation sampling	Adaptive allocation sampling, similar to cluster sampling, is a staged sampling approach. The initial sample is obtained using a conventional approach such as random sampling and then that sample is examined to determine if there are some geographic areas that exhibit more of the behavior/phenomena of interest on the basis of observations from a few select variables.

Probability Sampling

Probability sampling techniques allow an investigator to specify the probability that a participant will be selected from a population. With probability sampling, all elements (e.g., individuals, skilled living facilities) in the target population have some opportunity of being included in a sample, and the probability of being included in the sample is known for each element in the population. Use of probability sampling techniques increases the likelihood that the sample included in a study is representative of the target population. There are four basic types of probability sampling techniques: random sampling, systematic sampling, stratified sampling, and cluster sampling. We briefly review each of these techniques in the following sections.

Random Sampling

Random sampling refers to a procedure whereby each member of the population has an equal probability of being included in the sample. Thus, the probability of someone will be included in the sample in $1/N$ (N = size of the population) (e.g., if the population has 100 people, the probability of someone being included in the sample is .01 or 1%). The procedures for selecting a random sample can be as simple as selecting names from a hat if the population is small or using a table of random numbers if the population is larger. The advantage of using this approach is that the findings of a study can be generalized to a population with computable estimates of error. However, a disadvantage of using this approach is that the population might be spread out geographically (e.g., across different cities), which creates problems with feasibility. For example, assume the target population for an intervention study was spousal caregivers of patients with breast cancer in the United States. Clearly, this population would be spread across the 50 states, which would make it difficult to contact, recruit, and enroll a random sample of caregivers. Also, as noted, the sampling frame for a population may be incomplete or difficult to obtain. For this reason, behavioral intervention researchers rarely engage in pure random sampling.

An issue that is often discussed in the context of random sampling is *sampling with replacement* and *sampling without replacement,* which refers to methods used to select a random sample. Though not immediately relevant to behavioral intervention research, it is good to have basic familiarity with the concepts. Sampling with replacement means that, once a person is selected for a sample, he or she is put back into the population and could be sampled again; in other words, the person could be sampled again. Sampling without replacement means that, once a person is selected, he or she is not put back into the population for resampling (Frerichs, 2008). In general, sampling with replacement is a "more random" sample because in each case individuals have the same probability of being selected for inclusion in the sample. Referring back to our earlier example, with a sample size of 100, in this case the first person who is selected has a 1% probability of being selected. If that person is returned to the sample, the second person also has a 1% chance of being selected; however, that is not the case if the first person is not put back into the sample, thus they do not have the same probability of being selected. This distinction has relevance to statistical theories of sampling. However, in behavioral intervention research, the most common method of sampling is without replacement. We typically do not want to resample the same individuals. As noted, however, it is important to be aware of the distinction.

A cautionary note is that random sampling is not to be confused with random assignment of participants to a treatment condition. In this latter case, individuals are first selected on the basis of the study inclusion/exclusion criteria and then assigned using random methods to the different treatment conditions. This helps to ensure that the participants within the groups are as similar as possible and thus, if group differences on an outcome of interest are found, the differences are more likely due to treatment as opposed to differences within the composition of the groups.

Systematic Sampling

Systematic random sampling involves selecting every nth unit of the target population from a list that is randomly ordered—for example, every 10th spousal caregiver of breast cancer patients. It is important that the population listed is not ordered in some way to create a bias, for example, in this case, if every 10th caregiver was Caucasian or lived in the southern part of the United States.

Stratified Sampling

Stratified random sampling involves dividing a population into groups or strata and then randomly selecting from that group. The strata might be age, gender, cultural/ethnic group, level of experience, or level or duration of a disease. Researchers use this technique to ensure that subgroups of a population have an equally likely chance of being included in a sample. For example, in our caregiver example, assume that the population of caregivers is 50% White Caucasian, 30% Black/African American, 10% Hispanic, and 10% Asian, and the goal is to examine if responses to the intervention vary by race/ethnicity. Using stratified random sampling, the population could be divided into racial/ethnic groups, and then individuals would be randomly selected from each of these groups. Using this strategy would guarantee that the sample would include members from all of the race/ethnic groups. A *proportional stratified sample* is one in which the size of each strata in the sample is proportional to the size of the strata in the population; whereas in a *disproportional stratified sample*, the size of the strata is not proportional to the actual size in the population.

Again, stratified random sampling should not be confused with stratified random assignment of participants into treatment groups. For example, in the REACH II trial, convenience sampling procedures were used to recruit study participants. However, the randomization scheme was stratified by race/ethnicity to ensure that equal numbers of Black/African Americans, Latino/Hispanics, and Caucasian/Whites were included in the intervention and enhanced (information only) control conditions.

Cluster Sampling

Cluster sampling techniques are used when a complete sampling frame for a population is unavailable. It is typically a two-staged process. Initially, the total population is divided into clusters or groups, and then a random sample of clusters is selected. In the second stage, a random sample is selected from within each of these clusters. A common example of this approach is geographical sampling where clusters are based on geographical areas (e.g., neighborhoods). For example, assume that the development of an intervention that is targeting teenagers with substance abuse problems involves conducting interviews with social workers in New York City, the targeted area. The interviews are designed to collect initial input as to the need for, and format/content of, the intervention. However, a complete list of social workers in the targeted area may not be available. Thus, one strategy would be to select agencies in the area that are likely to employ social workers. In addition, the city is large and the agencies are dispersed across neighborhoods (e.g., SoHo, Upper East Side, Upper West Side). Using two-stage clustering techniques would entail initially selecting a random sample of neighborhoods (large clusters) and then a smaller random sample of agencies (small clusters) within these select neighborhoods to include in the sample. One would then recruit social workers from these clusters. An advantage of cluster sampling is that it can be more economical and reduce costs such as, in this case, travel.

Nonprobability Sampling Techniques

Probability sampling methods are not always practical and are not typically used in intervention research. Rather, nonprobability sampling techniques are commonly used. Using these sampling methods, it is not possible to specify the probability or likelihood of specifying and then selecting one individual over another. In other words, in behavioral intervention research, not everyone in the target population has an equal chance of being included in the sample. Thus, the sample may not be representative of the population, which threatens the external validity of the study or the extent to which one can generalize intervention outcomes from the sample to the population. For this reason, it is important to clearly specify the key characteristics of the population being targeted by the intervention and then to select a sample as representative of that population as possible. For example, assume a researcher is interested in evaluating the efficacy of a computer-training program for seniors with low computer literacy; it would be important to select older adults of both genders, mixed ethnic/racial backgrounds, of a fairly broad age range (e.g., 65+ years), with limited computer skills. Individuals with strong computer skills in the training program should be excluded from the study. If they were to be included, it would limit the extent to which one could generalize findings to the main population of interest. Furthermore, those with high skill levels may rate the class as too simplistic or slow in pace. As noted in Chapter 10, it is important to clearly specify criteria for including and excluding individuals early on in the development of the intervention. Identifying who will most likely benefit from an intervention and who will not is part of the initial work of an interventionist in the discovery phase of the pipeline (Chapter 3).

The most common methods of nonprobability sampling are convenience sampling, quota sampling, purposive sampling, snowballing techniques, and adaptive allocation. Each of these techniques will be described in the following sections. However, before beginning a review of these techniques, we will begin this section with a brief discussion of *adaptive sampling* since adaptive sampling techniques (e.g., snowball sampling and adaptive allocation sampling, which are described later) are often used when conducting research with populations such as people at high risk for infection, substance abusers, or people who are homeless or severely mentally ill. Adaptive sampling approaches involve using information gained during initial sampling of participants to redirect sampling strategies (Thompson & Collins, 2002). In the substance abuse example provided earlier, an initial sample of drug users might be asked for names of other users with whom they interact. These individuals are then approached to determine if they would be willing to participate in the study (of course, they would not be enrolled without consent). In this case, additional study participants are added on the basis of social network information obtained through contact with initial members of the sample as opposed to the information established prior to the beginning of recruitment. In other words, information gathered during initial sampling is used to inform future sample efforts. Adaptive sampling designs generally involve those that are based on social networks (e.g., snowballing) and those that are based on geographic location (adaptive allocation design). We provide a brief overview of these techniques later. However, as noted by Thompson and Collins (2002), statistical theory and procedures for estimating population quantities for these designs are still evolving (see Thompson & Collins, 2002 for a more complete discussion of these issues). It is also important to give careful consideration to ethics and human subject issues (see Chapter 13). For example, someone may be uncomfortable providing the name of someone else who is also involved in illicit behaviors. Overall, adaptive designs offer many advantages when dealing with challenging health and human service issues in which common approaches to reaching out to the targeted population do not suffice. However, it is important to be aware of the limitations of these approaches, especially with respect to their implications for external validity.

Convenience Sampling

Convenience sampling is one of the most commonly used sampling methods in behavioral intervention research. Convenience samples are based on individuals who are available, are interested in participating in a study, and, of course, who meet study inclusion/exclusion criteria. These samples are often obtained through access to a particular group (e.g., students in a class), advertisement, community outreach activities (e.g., speaking at a support group), clinical lists, or participant registries. As is common in behavioral intervention research, in the PRISM study (Czaja et al., 2014) it was not possible to randomly select 300 persons aged 65+ who lived alone and who were "at risk" for social isolation from a list of the total population of individuals meeting this criteria. Instead, a variety of recruitment activities (e.g., radio and newspaper advertisements, outreach to community agencies serving these populations) were employed at each of three participating sites to identify, recruit, and enroll study participants who were representative of the population the intervention was intended for on relevant characteristics.

Clearly, convenience samples have limitations, particularly with concerns about generalizing to the population level. Thus, they limit the ability of intervention studies to fully examine the external validity of the findings of the study since every member of the population does not have a chance of being included in the sample and thus the sample does not truly represent the population at large. However, the external validity of convenience samples can be increased by ensuring that the sample is as representative of the target population as possible and by minimizing sample bias as much as possible.

Quota Sampling

Quota sampling is similar to convenience sampling, but in this case the goal to select a certain quota or number of individuals with a particular characteristic (age group, race/ethnicity, gender, socioeconomic status). It is the nonprobability version of stratified random sampling. As described earlier in the REACH II study, the goal was to enroll equal numbers of Black/African American, Caucasian/White, and Latino/Hispanic caregivers. This approach has some utility in intervention research and can be applied when the research question seeks to examine treatment effects on different discrete populations.

Purposive Sampling

Purposive sampling is a type of nonprobability sampling that serves a specific need or purpose and involves sampling a specific group of individuals such as those who did not do well in a particular training program or caregivers who have participated in select community support groups. It may not be possible to specify the entire population and access to the entire population may be difficult; thus the investigator attempts to include whoever is available from the target group. This type of sampling is referred to as "purposive sampling" because individuals included in the sample fit a specific purpose or description. Purposive strategies are used to enhance understanding of the opinions/experiences of selected individuals or groups participating in an intervention study. It is frequently used when applying a mixed methods approach to understand the processes of adopting an intervention, using imparted strategies, or examining underlying mechanisms (see Chapter 11 on mixed methods).

Generally, three types of cases are optimal in purposive sampling: typical cases, those who are "average"; deviant or extreme cases, those who are at the high or low end of some phenomenon of interest; and negative or disconfirming cases, those who represent exceptions to the rule (e.g., experience an opposite reaction to an intervention) (Devers & Frankel, 2000). For example, in an evaluation of a basic computer skills–training program designed for older adults (Czaja, Lee, Branham, & Remis, 2012) and implemented at several sites, some class participants performed less well than others. In this case, purposive sampling can be used to interview this group of poor performers to gain an understanding of the challenges and difficulties they experienced and how the training program might be redesigned to better serve their needs. As with any sampling strategies, the research questions and goals must be clearly understood prior to the selection of a purposive sample.

Snowball Sampling

As discussed earlier in this chapter, snowball sampling is used when the members of a target population are difficult to locate. This sampling technique involves gathering data from a few members of the target population and then asking those individuals for information regarding the location of other potential members of the population. The example provided earlier in this chapter involved drug abusers. Snowball sampling is unlikely to yield a representative sample and is sometimes used at an exploratory stage of intervention development to gain initial insight into a problem area from which to design an intervention. It can also be combined with other sampling techniques. For example, in an evaluation of an intervention for family caregivers, one source of potential participants may be caregivers who attend community support groups or receive services from community agencies. After enrollment, these caregivers might be asked to recommend the program to someone else they may know in similar circumstances. This type of sampling could also be considered a form of snowballing. As mentioned previously, careful consideration must be given to human subject issues when using this type of sampling approach.

Adaptive Allocation Sampling

Adaptive allocation sampling, similar to cluster sampling, is a staged sampling approach. The initial sample is obtained using a conventional approach such as random sampling and then that sample is examined to determine if there are some geographic areas that exhibit more of the behavior/phenomena of interest on the basis of observations from a few select variables (Thompson & Collins, 2002). For example, assume a researcher is interested in evaluating an educational intervention to help remediate problems with childhood asthma. An initial random sample of households within a city is taken and prevalence of children with asthma is evaluated. In certain areas of the city, there appears to be a higher concentration of children with asthma; thus, a larger sample of households is chosen from these neighborhoods for potential inclusion in the study (for more detailed information on adaptive designs, see Thompson, 1990).

CONCLUSIONS AND GENERAL RECOMMENDATIONS

Regardless of the phase along the pipeline for the development of an intervention, behavioral intervention research involves dealing with samples. It is too costly, not feasible, and unnecessary to include entire populations to develop and evaluate an intervention. Thus, the selection of a sample is critical at each juncture along the pipeline and needs careful consideration and planning as it can impact the conduct of the research as well as the external validity of the study outcomes. Unfortunately, consideration of the pros and cons of the various methods for selecting a sample is often a neglected part of designing and evaluating an intervention.

The primary issues in sample selection as it concerns behavioral intervention research include the composition of the sample and assuring it conforms to the purpose of the intervention; the size of the sample and assuring it enables an appropriate test of the intervention particularly in comparative studies; and the method of obtaining the sample. Of course, the decisions concerning these three areas should be informed by existing theory, the research goals and questions, the availability of the target population, and feasibility constraints including resources, budget, staffing, and know-how. In this chapter, we summarized various methods for obtaining a sample and highlighted some of the advantages and disadvantages associated with key approaches.

At any stage of the pipeline, it is important to define the target population; review the relevant literature to identify population characteristics that are aligned with the purpose of the intervention (e.g., in a caregiver study, the living arrangement of the caregiver and care recipient may be important; thus, an investigator might want to include only those who live together); determine the necessary sample size; specify the sampling frame (where participants are likely to located); determine the sampling method; review available resources and constraints; and implement the recruitment plan (see Chapter 10). Finally, it is important to be aware of the limitations inherent in a chosen sampling approach and ultimately the sample included in a study, as these will impact the extent to which the findings from a study can be generalized to the target population.

REFERENCES

Belle, S. H., Burgio, L., Burns, R., Coon, D., Czaja, S. J., Gallagher-Thompson, D., . . . Zhang, S. (2006). Enhancing the quality of life of dementia caregivers from different ethnic or racial groups. *Annals of Internal Medicine, 145*(10), 727–738.

Centers for Disease Control and Prevention. (2015). *High blood pressure.* Retrieved from http://www.cdc.gov/bloodpressure/

Cohen, J. (1988). *Statistical power analysis for the behavioral science* (2nd ed.). Hillsdale, NJ: Erlbaum.

Czaja, S. J., Boot, W. R., Charness, N., Rogers, W. A., Sharit, J., Fisk, A. D., . . . Nair, S. N. (2014). The personalized reminder information and social management system (PRISM) trial: Rationale, methods, and baseline characteristics. *Contemporary Clinical Trials, 40*, 35–46.

Czaja, S. J., Lee, C. C., Branham, J., & Remis, P. (2012). OASIS connections: Results from an evaluation study. *The Gerontologist, 52*, 712–721.

Davern, M. (2008). Representative sample. In P. Lavrakas (Ed.), *Encyclopedia of survey research methods* (pp. 721–723). Thousand Oaks, CA: Sage.

Devers, K. J., & Frankel, R. M. (2000). Study design in quality research—2: Sampling and data collection strategies. *Education for Health, 13*, 263–271.

Frerichs, R. R. (2008). *Rapid surveys.* Retrieved from http://www.ph.ucla.edu/epi/rapid surveys/RScourse/RSbook_ch3.pdf

Kazdin, A. E. (1994). Methodology, design, and evaluation in psychotherapy research. In A. E. Bergen & S. L. Garfield (Eds.), *Handbook of psychotherapy and behavior change* (4th ed., pp. 19–71). New York, NY: Wiley.

Kazdin, A. E. (1999). The meanings and measurement of clinical significance. *Journal of Consulting and Clinical Psychology, 67*, 332–339.

Magnani, R., Sabin, K., Saidel, T., & Heckathorn, D. (2005). Review of sampling hard-to-reach and hidden populations for HIV surveillance. *AIDS, 19*, S67–S72.

National Institutes of Health (2015). Writing your application. Accessed on July 20, 2015, from http://grants.nih.gov/grants/writing_application.htm

Thompson, S. K. (1990). Adaptive cluster sampling. *Journal of America Statistical Association, 85*, 1050–1059.

Thompson, S. K., & Collins, L. M. (2002). Adaptive sampling in research on risk-related behaviors. *Drug and Alcohol Dependence, 68*, 57–67.

Zarit, S. H., Reever, K. E., & Bach-Peterson, J. (1980). Relatives of the impaired elderly: Correlates of feelings of burden. *The Gerontologist, 20*(6), 649–655.

TEN

RECRUITMENT AND RETENTION: TWO OF THE MOST IMPORTANT, YET CHALLENGING, TASKS IN BEHAVIORAL INTERVENTION RESEARCH

DANIEL E. JIMENEZ AND SARA J. CZAJA

The research participants who volunteer or give permission for themselves, their clinical and health data, and their tissues to be used in clinical research are the heart of the clinical research enterprise.
—Sung et al. (2003, p. 1279).

Over the past 50 years, as a result of breakthroughs in basic biomedical and behavioral intervention research, many strategies for improving health and quality of life have been discovered, and there has been an unprecedented supply of information related to them. Development of these discoveries and translation to individuals, communities, and clinical settings are predicated upon the participation of diverse study participants in intervention trials (George, Duran, & Norris, 2014; Sung et al., 2003). A carefully developed, implemented, and evaluated recruitment and retention plan ensures adequate representation in intervention studies from diverse groups of individuals (e.g., age, gender, ethnicity), which in turn is essential to support the generalizability of interventions that will ultimately positively impact the health and well-being of populations (Hendricks-Ferguson et al., 2012; Sung et al., 2003). Given the pace of discovery in biomedical science and the increased complexity of health and social issues, there will be an increased need for behavioral intervention research. Accordingly, the number of behavioral intervention research studies will continue to increase (Sung et al., 2003) and in turn, there will be an increased demand for research participants from diverse populations.

It is well established that the effective recruitment and retention of individuals in behavioral intervention research trials are critical to the development of a successful intervention at all stages of the pipeline. Yet, despite the long history of intervention research, recruitment and retention of study participants remain a central challenge to most investigators (Sung et al., 2003). There are two main goals of recruitment: to enroll participants into a study who are representative of the target population and to enroll sufficient numbers of participants to meet the sample size and power requirements for the study. Many studies fall short on recruitment and fail to achieve these goals or to do so within a reasonable time frame. Practical considerations include one's budget and access to resources such as staff to help with recruitment and retention. Allocation of funds to this effort is critical as it takes resources to assure adequacy in recruitment methodology and also to employ effective retention strategies. Time taken to recruit research participants is important for both logistical and scientific reasons. From a logistics standpoint, lagging recruitment results in higher costs, frustration, and issues related to treatment fidelity and staff effort. From a scientific standpoint, lagging recruitment may make the trial outdated (e.g., a new intervention may be introduced), or supplanted by other researchers who address the research questions sooner. This could delay the time that an effective intervention could be actually implemented in community settings. Recruitment lags can also adversely impact those already enrolled in a trial (Friedman, Furberg, & DeMets, 2010). For example, participants enrolled in a group therapy study would have to wait an indefinite amount of time to receive a much needed treatment owing to a delay in recruiting the required number of participants for the group. Moreover, recruitment lags generate concern from the funding agency about the ability of the research team to successfully conduct the trial.

Retention, the process of keeping participants in a study, also poses many challenges, especially in longitudinal studies or studies that involve vulnerable populations such as those who are ill or older (e.g., the "older old"). High rates of participant dropout are costly and have a significant impact on the external validity of the research findings. For example, high rates of attrition can lead to sampling biases if participants with certain characteristics (e.g., educational level or age) are more likely to drop out of a study and can also cause unevenness among study groups (e.g., those in the control group have higher rates of attrition than those in the intervention group or vice versa). Obviously, attrition has important implications for sample size and the statistical power of a study.

Overall, problems with recruitment and retention: disrupt study timelines; create additional workload for study staff and problems with frustration, low morale, and additional costs; pose threats to the internal and external validity of a study; and can ultimately lead to the abandonment of a trial. A common reason for problems with recruitment and retention is a lack of knowledge of recruitment issues and planning on the part of the investigator or study team. Often, investigators have an unrealistic view of the availability of participants and the effort required to enroll and maintain participants in a study. As noted by Friedman and colleagues (2010), "successful recruitment depends on developing a careful plan with multiple strategies, maintaining flexibility, establishing interim goals, preparing to devote the necessary effort and obtaining the sample size in a timely fashion" (p. 103).

Unfortunately, in the intervention literature, reports of the baseline characteristics or the results of an intervention trial typically provide limited detail describing recruitment procedures or the "success rates" of the various methods used to enroll participants. In fact, a review of 172 randomized controlled trials (RCTs) published in high-impact medical journals over a year's period (April 1, 1999 to April 1, 2000) (Gross, Mallory, Heiat, & Krumholz, 2002) indicated that only a small percentage provide detailed information about patient recruitment processes. Thus, researchers generally have little guidance when developing recruitment plans.

The goals of this chapter are twofold: (a) to describe the most common barriers to successful recruitment and retention and (b) to provide strategies that can be used to enhance the enrollment and retention of participants in behavioral intervention research. Our emphasis is on ways to enhance recruitment and retention efforts and avoid common pitfalls and problems. Recruitment and retention will always be a challenge, and there is no magic formula to ensure complete success. However, having an awareness of the challenges and strategies to meet them can help to improve the efficiency and effectiveness of the recruitment process. We begin with a discussion of common challenges concerning recruitment and retention that confront investigators in behavioral intervention trials. We then describe general strategies to enhance recruitment and retention followed by specific recommendations for recruiting and retaining the desired, representative sample.

COMMON ISSUES WITH RECRUITING STUDY PARTICIPANTS

As noted, recruitment of study participants is often a challenge for investigators at all stages of the pipeline, but this is especially the case in the efficacy and effectiveness phases when an intervention is being evaluated. Common problems include difficulty identifying targeted participants, the need to change participant inclusion/exclusion criteria, slow rates of recruitment, and failure to meet recruitment goals. For example, a review of 114 multicenter randomized controlled trials (RCTs) conducted in the United Kingdom between 1994 and 2002 (McDonald et al., 2006) indicated that less than 31% of the trials achieved their original recruitment goals; about half (53%) needed to extend their recruitment timeline; and the majority (63%) reported problems early in the trial with recruitment.

There are numerous challenges to recruitment, especially for certain study populations such as older adults, minorities, or those with a chronic or debilitating illness. Recognizing that each intervention study, target population, and context is unique, in this section we discuss common issues and challenges in recruitment and factors that deter or enhance participation in behavioral intervention research. Having an understanding of these issues early on in the intervention pipeline will facilitate enrollment of study participants and ultimately enhance the efficiency and cost-effectiveness of a study and the strength of the evidence regarding the impact of the intervention. Recruitment strategies can be developed on a broad platform and then adapted to meet the particular specificities of targeted groups and contexts. When recruitment materials and methods resonate within the target community, members of that community are more likely to participate in the research trial (George et al., 2014).

Challenges to Recruitment

Challenges to recruitment are multifaceted and include a lack of planning or knowledge on the part of the research team; factors related to the study design and resources allocated to recruitment; and characteristics of the target population and contextual/environmental factors. In this section, we provide a summary review of these challenges.

Lack of Planning

A common problem with recruitment is investigators' overestimation of the pool of individuals who conform to the study inclusion criteria and be willing to enroll in a trial. This is commonly known as the recruitment "funnel effect" (Spilker & Cramer, 1992). It generally results from a lack of knowledge of the characteristics of a community or recruitment site, relevant data on prevalence of a population characteristic (e.g., Internet access), or a chronic condition in the catchment area. Relaxing the inclusion criteria (assuming that it does not negatively impact on the study or outcomes), enhancing the catchment area, and increasing canvassing efforts are potentially effective ways to rectify this problem. For example, in a recent trial examining the efficacy of a software application to enhance the well-being and quality of life of older adults at risk for social isolation (Czaja et al., 2015), the original study inclusion criteria stipulated that participants could not have prior exposure to computers or the Internet. However, this criterion had to be modified as it quickly became obvious that it was not reasonable given the ubiquitous dispersion of computer technology. Participants may have had exposure by completing an online form at a doctor's office or through a relative. Therefore, the criterion was changed to the inclusion of persons who did not have a computer at home and only minimal computer and Internet use in the past 3 months.

Investigators may also place too much reliance on surrogate sources of recruitment such as referrals from a health care provider or contacts within an agency or organization. It is important to recognize that, although people within these organizations have the best intentions, they are typically busy with their own workplace demands. A research project that they are not actively involved in may not be a priority or be forgotten with increased work demands.

Study-Related Factors

The study design may also pose barriers. Participation in research, specifically behavioral interventions, often requires a time commitment that many participants are unwilling or unable to give. Participants often face time and financial constraints owing to competing demands of needing to work (even sometimes multiple jobs), or being the primary caretaker of children and/or relatives, or being the single head of a household (Adeyemi, Evans, & Bahk, 2009; Herring, Montgomery, Yancey, Williams, & Fraser, 2004; Wyatt et al., 2003). Logistical issues such as the need to travel to the research site, lack of transportation, or reservations about the neighborhood of the site may also prevent interest in participation. Randomization presents a particular challenge to recruitment because participants may prefer to make a choice rather than to be assigned to the available group options, fearing they may end up in a group contrary to their preference such as a control group (Broome & Richards, 2003; also see Chapter 8 on control group selection). In addition, excessive restrictions on eligibility may limit the ability to generate an adequate sample size needed for statistical power and representation of the target population (Yancey, Ortega, & Kumanyika, 2006).

Participant Factors

There are numerous participant-related factors that may prevent a person from enrolling in a research project. Having an awareness of these issues can help with the development of strategies to minimize them. In general, demographic characteristics such as a person's age, health status, socioeconomic status (SES), and cultural/ethnic identity influence recruitment. Higher rates of refusal are often found among persons with less education or less income or lower health knowledge (Gul & Parveen, 2010). It is also typically more difficult to recruit minorities and older adults or dyads (e.g., patient and caregiver).

A historic problem and well-documented barrier to recruitment that continues to pose a formidable barrier to research participation, especially among minority populations, is mistrust of research and the research process (Crawford Shearer, Fleury, & Belyea, 2010; George et al., 2014). The Tuskegee Study is just one example of the history of systematic abuse and mistreatment in both health care and medical research for African Americans (Scharff et al., 2010). As a consequence of that incident, for many African Americans, their mistrust in research participation is associated with the perception that research will benefit Whites or the research institution and not people of color (Katz et al., 2008; Scharff et al., 2010). Similarly, Native Hawaiians have reported mistrust related to the fear of purposeful mistreatment and that the researcher's agenda is not to serve their community (Gollin, Harrigan, Calderón, Perez, & Easa, 2005). Among Latinos, there is the fear that participating in research may lead to deportation (Calderón et al., 2006). Such mistrust in itself is likely to lead to stigmatizing attitudes toward participation in clinical research (Jang, Chiriboga, Herrera, Tyson, & Schonfeld, 2011; Link & Phelan, 2014). In fact, recruitment of minority populations continues to be a challenge for many intervention trials and has become a priority of funding agencies such as the National Institutes of Health. The need for increased ethnic minority recruitment reflects the changing demographic composition of the United States, which is increasingly multiethnic and pluralistic. Increased proportions of minorities in intervention studies will also allow for subgroup analyses to examine if race/ethnicity moderates the outcomes and will enhance the generalizability of the findings to diverse groups (Yancey et al., 2006).

In the context of behavioral intervention research, stigma may be related to the study topic of interest (Conner et al., 2010; Jimenez, Bartels, Cardenas, & Alegría, 2013; Zúñiga, Blanco, Martínez, Strathdee, & Gifford, 2007). This in turn may negatively impact recruitment. For example, participants may be reluctant to participate in research for fear of the social repercussions of disclosing sexual preference, HIV status, or substance abuse (Brooks, Newman, Duan, & Ortiz, 2007). For those struggling with mental illness, the lack of acceptance and support from family members may manifest itself in deciding whether to participate or not in a study (Jimenez et al., 2013).

Recruitment of older adults may also pose challenges. This group may be fearful about the research process or simply lack the stamina to participate if a study is effortful in terms of time or energy demands. Their family members may also advise them against participating because of concerns that they are being exploited. Special challenges arise when recruiting individuals with cognitive impairments or life-threatening illnesses. Often, recruitment in these cases involves a surrogate or caregiver, and there are ethical issues to consider concerning the consent process and data collection protocols (see Chapter 13).

Lack of effective strategies for communicating effectively to potential participants, such as tailoring recruitment materials to the characteristics of the target population, also represents a barrier to recruitment. For example, among non– or limited–English-speaking racial/ethnic minority participants, the lack of bilingual research staff and informational material in languages other than English is a barrier (Calderón et al., 2006; Giarelli et al., 2011). Similarly, advertisements in magazines, newsletters, newspapers, and on radio have proven to be ineffective ways of communicating with participants who are very familiar with digital media and technologies (Griffin, O'Connor, Rooney, & Steinbeck, 2013). The literature also suggests that effective means of advertising vary as a function of ethnicity/culture. For example, in the Personal Reminder Information and Social Management System (PRISM) for Seniors trial, it was found that the Hispanic participants responded more favorably to community outreach activities, whereas the primary sources of recruitment for African American participants were more varied and included community outreach, flyers/brochures, and word of mouth (Czaja et al., 2015).

Other participant-related factors that may influence enrollment decisions include safety concerns related to perceived risks associated with the intervention and privacy concerns related to the use or potential exposure of personal data.

Contextual Factors

Contextual and sociocultural variables also influence enrollment of participants. The characteristics of the research site may deter potential participants from enrolling in a trial. For example, the perceived safety of the neighborhood, parking facilities, travel distance, and other factors such as cleanliness and access to snacks are important variables. Sociocultural factors such as values and belief systems of the participants or the perceptions of the research institute by the community also need to be considered.

COMMON ISSUES IN RETENTION

Unfortunately, enrolling participants into a study is not the end of the story; once participants are enrolled, strategies are needed to ensure that they will remain in the study. As noted, retention of participants is often challenging, especially in longitudinal studies. Common issues with retention include participant death, changes in location or residence, illness or other changes in status such as increased job or caregiving responsibilities. Participants may also lose interest in a project or become dissatisfied if the study does not meet their expectations. They may also decide not to participate if they are unhappy with their group assignment following randomization. Study design factors such as time demands, requirements of the intervention, or burdensome assessment protocols can also contribute to high rates of attrition. Overcoming these challenges takes careful planning and concerted effort on the part of the investigative team. In the following section, we discuss some strategies for alleviating problems with recruitment and participant retention.

STRATEGIES TO ENHANCE RECRUITMENT AND RETENTION

General Strategies

Although the barriers described previously can seem daunting, there are strategies that can be used to enhance the efficiency and effectiveness of the recruitment process and participant retention. Of course, every study is different, so these strategies need to be adapted to the characteristics of the target population, context, and the intervention.

First and foremost, it is essential to have a recruitment plan and this plan must be developed early on in the pipeline. A key part of this plan must be obtaining information on the recruitment "environment" in order to obtain accurate estimates of the number of potential individuals who meet study entry criteria. If it appears that the numbers are low relative to recruitment goals, it might be necessary to expand the catchment area, and/or reexamine inclusion and exclusion criteria. It is also important to analyze the requirements and demands of participation to identify potential barriers to study enrollment and retention such as excessive time demands or transportation costs. In addition, it is important to understand the characteristics of the target population within the recruitment catchment area. The plan should also include sources for recruitment, a recruitment timeline, and contingencies in case there are recruitment lags (e.g., additional recruitment sources that might be tapped). There should also be a plan for maintaining enrolled participants (e.g., birthday greetings, check-in calls).

Sufficient resources must be allocated to both recruitment and retention. All too often investigators underestimate the cost and personnel effort associated with enrolling and maintaining participants in a study. Systems and personnel must be in place to identify and engage potential participants and to determine eligibility. Sufficient staff must be allocated to recruitment, and monies must be set aside in study budgets for recruitment efforts (e.g., costs for advertisements or travel costs of staff to attend community meetings). Staff must also be educated about the importance of participant recruitment, the recruitment timeline, and participant retention. They should also have training in working with the target population. For example, in the PRISM trial, the staff received basic training on aging and effective strategies for interacting with older adults. Culturally congruent research staff, who share similar personal characteristics (e.g., age, race/ethnicity, diagnosis) as the individuals being recruited, has been identified as an important facilitator to participant enrollment (George et al., 2014). This seems to increase trust in the research process and also allows participants to relate to and communicate with research staff in their own language and rhythm of expression (Calderón et al., 2006). Sometimes, it is helpful to have a community representative, such as an outreach worker from the target population, serve as a recruitment agent. For example, in African American communities, having a deacon or church member work with the ministers of churches may prove helpful.

Another critical aspect of recruitment is the need to establish collaborations with key members of the community and recruitment sites. These collaborations can take time and effort to foster and should be in place early in the pipeline as one is developing an intervention. Community leaders and agency representatives need to be clear about the goals and scope of the research, participant inclusion and exclusion criteria, the requirements of participation, and potential costs/benefits to the participants. It is also important to maintain frequent contact with these individuals, to not make excessive time or effort demands on them, and to maintain contact with them throughout the study.

A plan should also be in place for monitoring recruitment and retention. This is important not only for the effective implementation of the study, but also for the subsequent publication of the study results. A database for monitoring recruitment and retention should be established for the study that should include information regarding recruitment status relative to the study timeline, source of recruitment (e.g., "How did you hear about the study?"), reasons for refusal or ineligibility, actual enrollment, as well as data related to attrition (e.g., date of dropout, reasons for leaving the study). This type of data provides valuable information about adherence to the study recruitment timeline and overall effectiveness of recruitment strategies. The Consolidated Standards of Reporting Trials (CONSORT) requirements (see Chapter 24) for RCTs provide clear guidance on these issues. Data of this type can help identify fruitful sources of recruitment, problems with current strategies, and the study requirements; and it can allow corrective action to be taken early on. For example, in the PRISM trial, it was discovered that one of the factors influencing enrollment was randomization—potential participants wanted to receive computer training. Thus, the design was modified such that for those randomized to the control group (noncomputer group), the opportunity to receive computer training upon completion of the trial was provided. Although this reflected an increased cost to the trial, it effectively addressed the enrollment issue. Figure 10.1 presents an example of a graphic display depicting the number of persons inquiring about a study, the target enrollment number, and the actual enrollment number. This type of graphic provides a quick visual of month-by-month recruitment progress to help guide recruitment planning.

The nature and method of communicating with potential participants and community representatives are also critical to recruitment and retention outcomes.

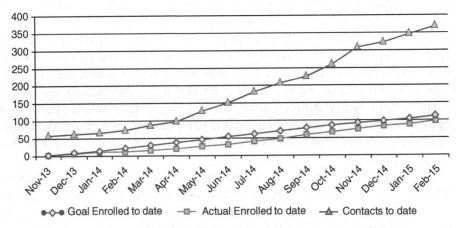

Figure 10.1   Example of a study enrollment graph (cumulative to date).

Understanding the benefits of participating in the study may positively influence participant enrollment as may compensation for participation. Highlighting "the good" that can come out of their participation—not only for themselves but to their community—can be a powerful facilitator. When participants view their participation in research as altruistic—helping family members and the community in the present and future, advancing medical knowledge—then they may be much more likely to volunteer for a study (George et al., 2014). Participants must also clearly understand the goals and objectives of the study, requirements of their participation, and risks/benefits. Issues related to safety and privacy must also be addressed. For example, if individuals perceive that participation will help them achieve personal goals (e.g., weight loss studies, access to health care), they may be more likely to participate in a study (Brooks et al., 2007; Calderón et al., 2006; Farmer, Jackson, Camacho, & Hall, 2007; Zúñiga et al., 2007). Communication can take many forms such as flyers, advertisement in newspapers/radio, outreach talks, announcements in libraries and other public spaces, mailings, and so forth. Irrespective of the format of the communication, it must be done in a way that is understandable by participants and that is also approved by an institutional review board.

Depending upon the monetary resources available for a study, compensation might include monetary incentives for participation, free lunch, or free health screens (Chao et al., 2011; DeFreitas, 2010). The compensation must be meaningful to individuals relative to their time and effort commitments; however, it cannot be too great as to be or appear to be coercive. Attention also needs to be paid to participants' perceptions concerning the risk of exploitation (Brugge, Kole, Lu, & Must, 2005). If participants feel that the risk of exploitation is minimal or nonexistent, they will be much more motivated to enroll in a study.

Addressing the potential logistical barriers of a study may also help enrollment. Every effort should be made to make participation as convenient as possible. This may include soliciting employer support to allow participants to take time off to attend appointments (Wyatt et al., 2003), helping with child or eldercare (Calderón et al., 2006), arranging for transportation (Crawford Shearer et al., 2010), or compensating for transportation costs. Other strategies such as having flexible hours for participants and scheduling assessment or intervention sessions on weekends or in the evening or at a convenient place may also facilitate recruitment. Involving community consultants to understand the needs and values of the targeted population and guide recruitment and retention decisions can be instrumental in deriving an effective plan of action.

Another major concern of researchers conducting behavioral intervention trials is to decrease attrition and achieve the required follow-up contacts to meet study goals. This is a particular challenge for longitudinal studies or those involving older participants or those who are ill or frail. Participant attrition is also influenced by study characteristics such as the number and timing of follow-up contacts, the complexity of the treatment protocol, incentives for continued participation logistical issues, and skills of the research staff. Thus, some of the same strategies to enhance recruitment, such as minimizing the logistical inconveniences of study participation, establishing mutual investment in the research process, tailoring the intervention materials, and providing some form of compensation, are helpful with respect to minimizing participant attrition. It is also critical to train staff so that they have a comfortable and respectful relationship with the participants, conduct follow-up assessments in a timely manner, and understand the importance of retention. In addition, where appropriate, it is important to maintain contact with participants, especially those in control conditions, with check-in calls, messages, and thank-you notes for participation.

Methods of Recruitment

Recruitment methods impact the enrollment of a representative sample as well as the types of participants entered into a trial, which in turn impacts study outcomes and the generalizability of the findings and the translation of the intervention into practice. However, investigators often place a low priority on comparing different recruitment methods (Huynh et al., 2014). As a result, there is little understanding of the key barriers and facilitators for specific populations or what the driving issues are regarding recruitment and retention as they relate to intervention research. Investment of time and resources to learn what methods may work in distinct communities to improve community acceptance of clinical research and thus improve participation is important (George et al., 2014; Morrison, Winter, & Gitlin, 2014).

Recruitment strategies can be broadly classified into the following categories: medical referral, community outreach, mass media, direct contact, personal referral, incentives, and registries (Huynh et al., 2014). Medical referral is health professionals inviting participants to the study. Community outreach involves mobilizing the community to promote the study at local fairs, churches, or community-organized events. Mass media refers to using public service announcements and advertisements to inform potential participants about the study. Direct contact involves mailing, telephoning, or e-mailing potential participants. Personal referral includes word-of-mouth referral by friends and family to the study. Incentives include cash or prizes to compensate for the participants' time in the study. Finally, registries refer to the use of clinical databases (e.g., electronic medical records) to identify potential participants for the study. Given that the recruitment process is expensive, and time and labor intensive, it is essential that researchers know how to effectively and efficiently use each of these strategies and identify what works best for the targeted community/population. For example, for studies involving family caregivers, speaking at support groups can be effective as well as working with organizations that serve older adults such as the Alzheimer's Association or Easter Seals. African Americans tend to respond to outreach activities through churches, whereas Hispanics tend to respond more to radio advertisements or community outreach. Recently, technology has also opened up new venues for participant recruitment. Given that individuals are increasingly using the Internet for health information and forms of social support, researchers are in turn using Internet communities as recruitment sites for research participants. There are both free and paid (e.g., browsers search ads) online recruitment methods. Clearly, one of the advantages of this approach is the potential to reach larger numbers of participants. However, a challenge is that certain segments of the target population may not have access to the Internet such as those in the older cohorts or of low SES.

Generally, recruitment approaches that involve a variety of methods and active approaches (e.g., outreach talks) tend to be more beneficial than passive approaches (e.g., flyers). Given the expense and effort associated with recruitment, it is important to track which methods provide the most yield with respect to participant enrollment.

Planning for Recruitment and Retention

The following are eight recommendations for developing an effective recruitment and retention plan. These recommendations are summarized in Table 10.1.

TABLE 10.1   Summary of Recommendations for Developing an Effective Recruitment and Retention Plan

Recommendation	Summary
1. Conduct an analysis of the environment, target population, and the intervention	■ Identify the prevalence rates of the target population in the catchment area ■ Identify the characteristics of the target population (e.g., living arrangements, literacy, distance from intervention site) ■ Conduct an analysis of the intervention (e.g., inclusion/exclusion criteria; study participation requirements—number of sessions, location)
2. Establish a recruitment timeline and identify recruitment staff	■ Develop a timeline for target enrollment (Figure 10.1) ■ Identify recruitment personnel ■ Clearly identify the roles and responsibilities with respect to recruitment/retention among project team members

3. Develop a recruitment and retention database	■ Database should include information regarding
	  ■ Source of recruitment (e.g., newspaper ad)
	  ■ Reasons for ineligibility
	  ■ Reasons for lack of interest
	  ■ Dropout date
	  ■ Reason for dropout

4. Adopt a community-based participatory approach for recruitment and retention	■ Identify community members and key stakeholders in organizations to help with the recruitment process ■ Obtain advice from community members on sources of recruitment and strategies for recruitment ■ Actively involve community members in recruitment efforts
5. Establish a Community Advisory Board (CAB)	■ The CAB should involve a variety of community stakeholders ■ Establish project "buy-in" from the CAB ■ Outline clear objectives for the CAB and mechanisms for involvement ■ Establish a timeline for meetings and a convenient meeting venue

(Continued)

TABLE 10.1 Summary of Recommendations for Developing an Effective Recruitment and Retention Plan (Continued)

Recommendation	Summary
6. Build trust with the community/target population	■ Identify a variety of methods for communicating with the community ■ Clearly express the goals, importance, and any benefits associated with the study ■ Clearly express the importance of community participation ■ Train study team members in communication skills and recruitment strategies ■ Schedule regular meetings on topics related to recruitment/retention
7. Minimize potential inconveniences associated with study participation	■ Be flexible with respect to study scheduling and location of participation ■ Provide compensation for transportation ■ Provide tokens of appreciation ■ Be understanding of participant constraints and attempt to accommodate
8. Pilot test recruitment materials	■ Review materials with CAB and other members of the study team ■ Review materials with representative members of the target population ■ Obtain Institutional Review Board approval prior to pilot testing

Recommendation 1: Conduct an Analysis of the Environment, the Target Population, and the Intervention

To avoid the recruitment "funnel effect" and obtain an accurate estimation of the pool of potential participants, it is important to conduct an analysis of the community/catchment area with respect to prevalence rates of the target population. This should be done in early phases of intervention development and might involve examining registries, census data, or data from previous trials. An analysis of the characteristics of the population should also be conducted. For example, questions related to the location of participants (e.g., "Do most of the participants live in locations remote to the study site?"), health literacy, and SES are important with respect to the design of recruitment efforts and materials. Finally, it is important to do an analysis of the intervention to have a clear understanding of essential inclusion/exclusion criteria, requirements associated with participation, and potential barriers to participation.

Recommendation 2: Establish a Recruitment Timeline and Identify Recruitment Staff

A second important step is the establishment of a realistic recruitment timeline and a plan for allocating staff to recruitment activities. The timing for beginning the recruitment process is important—it should begin prior to the actual date when data collection will commence; however, the window between the startup of recruitment efforts and the actual beginning of data collection should not be too long or participants may lose interest in the study. It is also helpful, if resources permit, to hire research team members including a recruitment coordinator with personal characteristics (e.g., age, race/ethnicity) similar to the target population. This has been shown to be an effective facilitator of the recruitment process because potential participants from the target community may feel more comfortable divulging personal information to someone from their own community (Areán, Alvidrez, Nery, Estes, & Linkins, 2003; Mendez-Luck et al., 2011). Allowing participants to communicate with study personnel in their preferred language and in a manner in which they feel comfortable fosters trust and enthusiasm and ultimately facilitates study enrollment (Calderón et al., 2006; Hendricks-Ferguson et al., 2012). In addition, research staff from the representative communities may also be more sensitive to participants' reactions to research and can provide feedback to the investigators about how to improve the recruitment and retention methodologies. In all cases, staff must be well trained and knowledgeable about the study, participants, community, and the importance of recruitment.

Recommendation 3: Develop a Recruitment and Retention Database

It is important to establish a database to record data related to recruitment and retention. This should include information on recruitment sites, their activities and yield of enrollees, issues such as source of participants, reasons for ineligibility, reasons for lack of interest (if a participant declines), and timing of, and reasons for, attrition.

Recommendation 4: Adopt a Community-Based Participatory Research Approach for Recruitment and Retention

Community-based participatory research (CBPR) is an approach to research that engages the community in every stage of the research process. In a CBPR approach, community members are equal partners with researchers in shaping the study questions, developing the intervention and a recruitment and retention plan, collecting data, and interpreting and disseminating results (Israel et al., 2005).

On the basis of CBPR principles, community members actively participate in the development of a plan for recruitment and retention and facilitate the recruitment process. This can be extremely helpful to enrollment and retention for several reasons. First, a CBPR approach elevates the value of the research for the community and researchers. Collaborating with community members to identify salient issues important to a particular population (bottom-up approach) rather than identifying an issue that may not be reflective of a community's needs (traditional top-down approach) may improve a population's enthusiasm and participation in clinical research (De las Nueces, Hacker, DiGirolamo, & Hicks, 2012). Second, a CBPR approach creates a bridge between researchers and the community. Community members are viewed as partners, not subjects. Therefore, the community is likely to become more invested in the research and study outcomes. Lastly, a CBPR helps to establish a mutual trust.

Methods for community engagement vary according to the values, needs, and previous research experience of the community and the needs and characteristics of the study. Community Advisory Boards (CABs) have emerged as one strategy for establishing partnerships that promote community consultation in socially sensitive research (Morin et al., 2008).

Recommendation 5: Establish a Community Advisory Board

CABs involve stakeholders from various arenas including education, health care, childcare, public health, local churches, community service agencies, and the general community. These community members often serve as validation and advocacy for the research team. They lend instant credibility to the researchers, which is essential in gaining access to communities that have been underrepresented in research and perhaps not familiar with or trusting of academia or the research process (McHenry et al., 2015; Mendez-Luck et al., 2011). In addition to serving as advocates for both the community and researchers, CABs also advise study investigators on recruitment and retention strategies and other study procedures. This includes suggestions for recruitment sites and strategies for how best to tailor recruitment and retention efforts in order to increase the chances of finding and keeping potentially eligible participants. This targeted approach helps to eliminate additional time and expense involved in screening large numbers of noneligible community residents. In addition, CABs can also advise on how to communicate effectively and how to build trust within the population of interest.

Recommendation 6: Build Trust With the Community/Target Population

Advertisement of a study is an essential aspect of the recruitment process. Techniques such as posters, flyers, brochures, public service announcements, and radio scripts are the most common methods used. As noted, online advertisement is also becoming popular. An important task of the CABs is to review these materials and make sure that message is culturally appropriate and congruent with how the target population identifies and perceives the nature and goals of the study. For example, "depression" is a stigmatizing term among many Hispanics (Jimenez et al., 2013); "feeling blue," a common description of depression relevant to African Americans (Gitlin et al., 2013), bears no meaning when translated into Spanish. In this instance, a CAB could help researchers to avoid stigmatizing terms and provide a description of the study purpose and protocol in a manner that is understandable and nonthreatening.

Prior studies have reported that face-to-face contact is the most effective way to build trust and recruit the targeted populations (Areán et al., 2003; Gonzalez, Gardner, & Murasko, 2007; Greaney, Lees, Nigg, Saunders, & Clark, 2006). Community events (e.g., health fairs, county festivals) are appropriate settings for effectively introducing information about the study. This allows researchers to interact with attendees in a face-to-face situation and shed the "ivory tower" reputation of academia. In addition, this is an opportunity for researchers to overcome the stigma associated with potentially sensitive topics. For example, researchers involved in an intervention trial that is evaluating a cognitive-training study for persons with mild cognitive impairment (MCI) could offer memory screens alongside blood pressure checks and diabetes screens at a health fair. Paired alongside these less stigmatizing health screens, the memory screens can be used as a trust-building launch for education about dementia as well as an opportunity to introduce more specific information about study participation.

Communication among study personnel is also an essential component of any recruitment and retention plan that will help to sustain successful recruitment in clinical research studies. Regularly scheduled meetings or conference calls for project staff provide an opportunity to discuss and monitor recruitment rates. This will also help foster camaraderie within the team and motivate team members to meet projected recruitment goals and gain from the experiences of other project staff (Hendricks-Ferguson et al., 2012).

Recommendation 7: Minimize Potential Inconveniences Associated With Study Participation

For many participants, the largest obstacles are time and transportation related. To help overcome the competing demands barrier, research staff should be creative in the scheduling and the location of the research interviews. If participants are available only on evenings and weekends, then study staff's schedules could be altered to be available during these times. Also, in-home assessments (if possible) can be offered to participants who are unable to leave the home because of either childcare or health reasons. If in-home assessments are not possible, then transportation to and from the research offices or parking should be provided. Participants should feel that they are valued. Details such as providing them with a cold bottle of water, a light snack (if the interview is long), and financial compensation are ways that researchers can convey their appreciation for the inconvenience that study participation may entail.

Recommendation 8: Pilot Test Recruitment Materials and Methods

Pilot testing of recruitment materials and strategies with representatives of the target population or the CAB can also be quite helpful. It can provide information on the appropriateness and potential effectiveness of the recruitment methods and estimates of the response rates. The Institutional Review Board must approve all recruitment materials (flyers, brochures, etc.) and strategies (changes to study protocol, public service announcements, etc.) prior to pilot testing.

CONCLUSION

As discussed throughout this chapter, enrolling and maintaining participants in behavioral intervention trials are a challenging, yet critical, aspect of the research process. There is not one single recommended approach for successfully recruiting participants. Successful recruitment and retention of participants depend upon careful planning and overcoming barriers related to fear and mistrust of science, stigma, communication, aspects of the study design, and available resources (e.g., staff and budget). Each culture and community has its own unique barriers and concerns. The challenge for investigators is to develop recruitment methods that address the issues specific to a target population and community, rather than to try to develop a one-size-fits-all approach. However, CBPR models suggest that a framework can be a helpful approach as it helps foster partnerships with the community, trust in the research process, and an understanding of the needs and characteristics of the target population. In order for recruitment and retention to be successful, the research team must work in concert with the community to fit recruitment and retention strategies to the needs and characteristics of the community. Each project requires thoughtful consideration of the study environment, research tasks, community resources, budgetary constraints, and any special needs or obstacles within the target population.

As the public's investment in behavioral intervention research continues to increase, it is imperative that clinical research be conducted with participant samples that are large enough to reliably test the research hypotheses and diverse enough to reflect a representative sample and thus ensure the validity and generalizability of the findings.

REFERENCES

Adeyemi, O. F., Evans, A. T., & Bahk, M. (2009). HIV-infected adults from minority ethnic groups are willing to participate in research if asked. *AIDS Patient Care and STDS, 23*(10), 859–865.

Areán, P. A., Alvidrez, J., Nery, R., Estes, C., & Linkins, K. (2003). Recruitment and retention of older minorities in mental health services research. *The Gerontologist, 43*(1), 36–44.

Brooks, R. A., Newman, P. A., Duan, N., & Ortiz, D. J. (2007). HIV vaccine trial preparedness among Spanish-speaking Latinos in the US. *AIDS Care, 19*(1), 52–58.

Broome, M. E., & Richards, D. J. (2003). The influence of relationships on children's and adolescents' participation in research. *Nursing Research, 52*(3), 191–197.

Brugge, D., Kole, A., Lu, W., & Must, A. (2005). Susceptibility of elderly Asian immigrants to persuasion with respect to participation in research. *Journal of Immigrant and Minority Health, 7*(2), 93–101.

Calderón, J. L., Baker, R. S., Fabrega, H., Conde, J. G., Hays, R. D., Fleming, E., & Norris, K. (2006). An ethno-medical perspective on research participation: A qualitative pilot study. *Medscape General Medicine, 8*(2), 23–30.

Chao, S. Z., Lai, N. B., Tse, M. M., Ho, R. J., Kong, J. P., Matthews, B. R., . . . Rosen, H. J. (2011). Recruitment of Chinese American elders into dementia research: The UCSF ADRC experience. *The Gerontologist, 51*(Suppl. 1), S125–S133.

Conner, K. O., Copeland, V. C., Grote, N. K., Rosen, D., Albert, S., McMurray, M. L., . . . Koeske, G. (2010). Barriers to treatment and culturally endorsed coping strategies among depressed African-American older adults. *Aging and Mental Health, 14*(8), 971–983.

Crawford Shearer, N. B., Fleury, J. D., & Belyea, M. (2010). An innovative approach to recruiting homebound older adults. *Research in Gerontological Nursing, 3*(1), 11–18.

Czaja, S. J., Boot, W. R., Charness, N., Rogers, A. W., Sharit, J., Fisk, A. D., . . . Nair, S. N. (2015). The personalized reminder information and social management system (PRISM) trial: Rationale, methods and baseline characteristics. *Contemporary Clinical Trials, 40,* 35–46.

DeFreitas, D. (2010). Race and HIV clinical trial participation. *Journal of the National Medical Association, 102*(6), 493–499.

De las Nueces, D., Hacker, K., DiGirolamo, A., & Hicks, L. S. (2012). A systematic review of community-based participatory research to enhance clinical trials in racial and ethnic minority groups. *Health Services Research, 47,* 1363–1386.

Farmer, D. F., Jackson, S. A., Camacho, F., & Hall, M. A. (2007). Attitudes of African American and low socioeconomic status white women toward medical research. *Journal of Health Care for the Poor and Underserved, 18*(1), 85–99.

Friedman, L. M., Furberg, C. D., & DeMets, D. L. (2010). Recruitment of study participants. In L. M., Friedman, C. D. Furberg, & D. L. DeMets (Eds.), *Fundamentals of clinical trials* (pp. 183–197). New York, NY: Springer.

George, S., Duran, N., & Norris, K. (2014). A systematic review of barriers and facilitators to minority research participation among African Americans, Latinos, Asian Americans, and Pacific Islanders. *American Journal of Public Health, 104*(2), e16–e31.

Giarelli, E., Bruner, D. W., Nguyen, E., Basham, S., Marathe, P., Dao, D., . . . Nguyen, G. (2011). Research participation among Asian American women at risk for cervical cancer: Exploratory pilot of barriers and enhancers. *Journal of Immigrant and Minority Health, 13*(6), 1055–1068.

Gitlin, L. N., Harris, L. F., McCoy, M. C., Chernett, N. L., Pizzi, L. T., Jutkowitz, E., . . . Hauck, W. W. (2013). A home-based intervention to reduce depressive symptoms and improve quality of life in older African Americans: A randomized trial. *Annals of Internal Medicine, 159*(4), 243–252.

Gollin, L. X., Harrigan, R. C., Calderón, J. L., Perez, J., & Easa, D. (2005). Improving Hawaiian and Filipino involvement in clinical research opportunities: Qualitative findings from Hawaii. *Ethnicity and Disease, 15*(4, Suppl. 5), 111–119.

Gonzalez, E. W., Gardner, E. M., & Murasko, D. (2007). Recruitment and retention of older adults in influenza immunization study. *Journal of Cultural Diversity, 14,* 81–87.

Greaney, M. L., Lees, F. D., Nigg, C. R., Saunders, S. D., & Clark, P. G. (2006). Recruiting and retaining older adults for health promotion research: The experience of the SENIOR project. *Journal of Nutrition for the Elderly, 25,* 3–22.

Griffin, H. J., O'Connor, H. T., Rooney, K. B., & Steinbeck, K. S. (2013). Effectiveness of strategies for recruiting overweight and obese generation y women to a clinical weight management trial. *Asia Pacific Journal of Clinical Nutrition, 22*(2), 235–240.

Gross, C. P., Mallory, R., Heiat, A., & Krumholz, H. M. (2002). Reporting the recruitment process in clinical trials: Who are these patients and how did they get there? *Annals of Internal Medicine, 137*(1), 10–16.

Gul, R. B., & Parveen, A. A. (2010). Clinical trials: The challenge of recruitment and retention of participants. *Journal of Clinical Nursing, 19,* 227–233.

Hendricks-Ferguson, V. L., Cherven, B. O., Burns, D. S., Docherty, S. L., Phillips-Salimi, C. R, Roll, L., . . . Haase, J. E. (2012). Recruitment strategies and rates of a multi-site behavioral intervention for adolescents and young adults with cancer. *Journal of Pediatric Health Care, 27*(6), 434–442.

Herring, P., Montgomery, S., Yancey, A. K., Williams, D., & Fraser, G. (2004). Understanding the challenges in recruiting Blacks to a longitudinal cohort study: The Adventist health study. *Ethnicity and Disease, 14*(3), 423–430.

Huynh, L., Johns, B., Liu, S. H., Vedula, S. S., Li, T., & Puhan, M. A. (2014). Cost-effectiveness of health research study participant recruitment strategies: A systematic review. *Clinical Trials, 11*(5), 576–583.

Israel, B. A., Parker, E. A., Rowe, Z., Salvatore, A., Minkler, M., López, J., . . . Halstead, S. (2005). Community-based participatory research: Lessons learned from the centers for children's environmental health and disease prevention research. *Environmental Health Perspectives, 113*(10), 1463–1471.

Jang, Y., Chiriboga, D. A., Herrera, J. R., Tyson, D. M., & Schonfeld, L. (2011). Attitudes toward mental health services in Hispanic older adults: The role of misconceptions and personal beliefs. *Community Mental Health Journal, 47*(2), 164–170.

Jimenez, D. E., Bartels, S. J., Cardenas, V., & Alegría, M. (2013). Stigmatizing attitudes toward mental illness among racial/ethnic older adults in primary care. *International Journal of Geriatric Psychiatry, 28*(10), 1061–1068.

Katz, R. V., Green, B. L., Kressin, N. R., Kegeles, S. S., Wang, M. Q., James, S. A., . . . McCallum, J. M. (2008). The legacy of the Tuskegee syphilis study: Assessing its impact on willingness to participate in biomedical studies. *Journal of Health Care for the Poor and Underserved, 19*(4), 1168–1180.

Link, B. G., & Phelan, J. (2014). Stigma power. *Social Science and Medicine, 103*, 24–32.

McDonald, A. M., Knight, R. C., Campbell, M. K., Entwistle, V. A., Grant, A. M., Cook, J. A., . . . Snowdon, C. (2006). What influences recruitment to randomised controlled trials? A review of trials funded by two UK funding agencies. *Trials, 7*(9), 1–8. doi:10.1186/1745-6215-7-9

McHenry, J. C., Insel, K. C., Einstein, G. O., Vidrine, A. N., Koerner, K. M., & Morrow, D. G. (2015). Recruitment of older adults: Success may be in the details. *The Gerontologist, 55*(5), 845–853.

Mendez-Luck, C. A., Trejo, L., Miranda, J., Jimenez, E., Quiter, E. S., & Mangione, C. M. (2011). Recruitment strategies and costs associated with community-based research in a Mexican-origin population. *The Gerontologist, 51*(Suppl. 1), S94–S105.

Morin, S. F., Morfit, S., Maiorana, A., Aramrattana, A., Goicochea, P., Mutsambi, J. M., . . . Mutsambi, J. M. (2008). Building community partnerships: Case studies of community advisory boards at research sites in Peru, Zimbabwe, and Thailand. *Clinical Trials, 5*(2), 147–156.

Morrison, K., Winter, L., & Gitlin, L. N. (2014). Recruiting community-based dementia patients and caregivers in a nonpharmacologic randomized trial: What works and how much does it cost? *Journal of Applied Gerontology.* Advance online publication. doi:10.1177/0733464814532012

Scharff, D. P., Matthews, K. J., Jackson, P., Hoffsuemmer, J., Martin, E., & Edwards, D. (2010). More than Tuskegee: Understanding mistrust about research participation. *Journal of Health Care for the Poor and Underserved, 21*(3), 879–897.

Spilker, B., & Cramer, J. A. (1992). *Patient recruitment in clinical trials.* New York, NY: Raven Press.

Sung, N. S., Crowley, W. F., Genel, M., Salber, P., Sandy, L., Sherwood, L. M., . . . Rimoin, D. (2003). Central challenges facing the national clinical research enterprise. *JAMA, 289*(10), 1278–1287.

Wyatt, S. B., Diekelmann, N., Henderson, F., Andrew, M. E., Billingsley, G., Felder, S. H., . . . Fuqua, S. (2003). A community-driven model of research participation: The Jackson heart study participant recruitment and retention study. *Ethnicity and Disease, 13*(4), 438–455.

Yancey, A. K., Ortega, A. N., & Kumanyika, S. K. (2006). Effective recruitment and retention of minority research participants. *Annual Review of Public Health, 27*, 1–28.

Zúñiga, M. L., Blanco, E., Martínez, P., Strathdee, S. A., & Gifford, A. L. (2007). Perceptions of barriers and facilitators to participation in clinical trials in HIV-positive Latinas: A pilot study. *Journal of Women's Health, 16*(9), 1322–1330.

ELEVEN

MIXED METHODS IN BEHAVIORAL INTERVENTION RESEARCH

JOSEPH J. GALLO AND SU YEON LEE

Imagination is the highest form of research.
—Albert Einstein

Mixed methods used in behavioral interventions have the advantage of drawing strengths from both quantitative and qualitative approaches rather than using one approach alone. Beyond the strict use of quantitative methods, qualitative methods can provide rich, detailed, and comprehensive knowledge on various processes of intervention development and testing: building theory relevant to behavioral health, developing and validating instruments, assessing context and processes involved in behavioral health interventions, and pointing toward acceptable and sustainable ways to implement and disseminate the intervention.

The goals of this chapter are to define mixed methods approaches to provide a rationale for using mixed methods in behavioral intervention research; to introduce basic concepts and types of mixed methods designs; to highlight approaches for incorporating mixed methods in developing, testing, and implementing behavioral interventions; to understand mixed methods study outcomes in the context of scaling up intervention; and to consider challenges of using mixed methods in interventions. Investigators with well-considered research questions and aims can be creative and imaginative in how to deploy mixed methods to make their intervention relevant and effective for diverse community and service settings. From designing interventions that take into account cultural factors to the study of implementation processes for established interventions, mixed methods can play an important role across the entire spectrum of the intervention development pipeline.

WHAT ARE MIXED METHODS?

Mixed methods research is characterized by the combination of quantitative and qualitative methods to address the depth (e.g., individual perspective on why an intervention does or does not work) and breadth (e.g., mediation analysis) of research questions (Johnson, Onwuegbuzie, & Turner, 2007). Mixed methods research involves the integration of quantitative and qualitative approaches to study designs, data collections, and data analyses. Some "qualitative" approaches involve numeric methods (e.g., cultural consensus analysis; Romney, Batchelder, & Weller, 1987), while some "quantitative" approaches based on statistics involve qualitative judgments (e.g., the number of classes in a latent class model; van Smeden, Naaktgeboren, Reitsma, Moons, & de Groot, 2014). We should state at the outset that the terms "quantitative" and "qualitative" are shorthand for broad approaches often characterized as "numeric" (statistical, objective) or "text" (interpretive, subjective). Depending on the type of mixed methods study, quantitative or qualitative methods may have a more primary role, with an emphasis on the respective theoretical assumptions, study designs, and analytical approaches.

Quantitative and qualitative frameworks have developed from distinct disciplinary worldviews (DePoy & Gitlin, 2015). Quantitative methods are derived from positivist assumptions that are ideal for establishing cause-and-effect relationships (determinism), identifying key variables to describe a phenomenon (reductionism), measuring a construct (measurement), or testing a hypothesis (deductive logic)—an *etic* or "culturally neutral" perspective. Qualitative approaches are framed from constructivist or realistic worldviews that seek insight and interpretation of the context in which interventions take place at individual, social, and organizational levels—an *emic* or "culturally unique" perspective (Robins et al., 2008). Often quantitative approaches (exemplified by the fields of biostatistics and epidemiology) seek to generalize replicable results from the sample to the population (e.g., using a standardized depression questionnaire to estimate the prevalence of depression in the population from results in a sample). In contrast, qualitative approaches (exemplified by the fields of anthropology and sociology) seek to understand the scope of a domain (e.g., understanding the experience and concept of depression from the point of view of an individual from a certain culture).

Mixed methods maximize the strengths and counterbalance the weaknesses of quantitative and qualitative approaches in a single study or program of research. Purposeful and planned integration of quantitative and qualitative approaches is a key feature of mixed methods. Thinking carefully about the purposes and stages of intervention design allows investigators to build strong ties between the research question, methods, and theory. Driven by the needs and goals of the research, investigators should make specific and planned efforts to integrate quantitative and qualitative methods at all stages of the pipeline—study design, data collection, analysis, and interpretation. In the rest of this chapter, we describe how mixed methods can be used across the intervention pipeline to the design and development and evaluation of interventions to implementation in community and clinical settings.

WHY USE MIXED METHODS TO DEVELOP AND EVALUATE BEHAVIORAL INTERVENTIONS?

Mixed methods can bridge the gap between evidence generated from "ideal" intervention conditions (e.g., careful selection of participants after excluding "complex" cases with multiple comorbidities, high level of training and experience among interventionists) and the adoption of evidence-based practices for diverse populations in real-life settings. Although numerous novel behavioral interventions are funded and tested every year, knowledge gained from research is often slow or ineffective in resolving real-life problems, involving poor access to health services, engagement, and outcomes of health services. Quantitative approaches alone cannot fully describe the attitudes toward, and dissatisfaction with, aspects of current models of health care services by patients, families, clinicians, and administrators or areas of needed improvement (Becker & Newsom, 2003; Rössler, 2012). An in-depth qualitative analysis that assessed dissatisfaction in health care among African American patients with chronic illness found that low-income patients compared to middle-income patients were particularly dissatisfied with health care associated with lower resources available at care sites serving low-income patients, dealing with more bureaucracy in health care, and lack of health insurance (Becker & Newsom, 2003). Such depth of knowledge on dissatisfaction with health care among low-income African Americans with chronic illness would not have been available with a standard quantitative study that adjusts for socioeconomic status. In addition to quantitatively assessing the clinical, functional, and behavioral outcomes of interventions, qualitative methods take into account the contexts in which interventions are deployed at individual, social, and organizational levels.

Epidemiologic investigations involve statistical approaches to identify causes of diseases and environmental or social conditions/trends, to measure exposure, to count cases, and to guide treatment or prevention (Goodman, Buehler, & Koplan, 1990). Quantitative methods provide ways to reliably assess intervention outcomes, but not necessarily how or why an intervention worked or failed, or why uptake of an intervention was poor. Qualitative methods can fill in such important information by obtaining the participant's perspective. As the leading causes of mortality have shifted from communicable diseases to noncommunicable diseases, multiple methods are required to understand complex relationships, often tied to a specific context or culture, that influence the onset and persistence of behavioral health problems (Murray, Vos, & Lozano, 2012). While investigators have used some form of "mixed" methods (e.g., combining epidemiologic and anthropologic approaches; Trostle, 1986, 2005) for some time, the use of "mixed methods" has recently emerged as a cohesive set of strategies to address individual motivational factors as well as contextual and environmental factors that contribute to disease burden (Creswell & Plano Clark, 2011; Tashakkori & Teddlie, 2003).

In order to flexibly respond to a changing landscape of behavioral health, we need effective interventions that are successfully implemented in community and clinical settings (Midgley, 2006). Without consideration of the contextual factors that influence uptake by patients, practitioners, and organizations, even effective interventions are unlikely to lead to substantial change in public health (The National Academy of Medicine, formerly known as the Institute of Medicine [IOM], 2006; National Institute of Mental Health, 2008; U.S. Department of Health and Human Services, 2001). The IOM *Quality Chasm* report called attention to the need for "outside the box" thinking related to the redesign of health care, including a strong focus on preferences and patient (person)-centered care, and evidence-based clinical decision making (IOM, 2006). Obtaining the "insider" perspective seeks to understand the patient's point of view, employing methods that are designed to elicit the patient's cultural model of illness and health. Understanding how providers view and adapt an intervention also is critical to translate interventions along the "pipeline" from research into practice.

The value of mixed methods has also been recognized by the National Institutes of Health (NIH). In 2011, the NIH Office of Behavioral and Social Science Research (OBSSR) convened a work group to develop guidelines for mixed methods proposals in the health sciences (Creswell & Plano Clark, 2011). NIH OBSSR published and widely disseminated the "Best Practices for Mixed Methods Research in Health Sciences" to aid investigators using mixed methods to prepare for competitive funding applications and to assist reviewers and staff to properly evaluate mixed methods applications and papers (Creswell, Klassen, Plano Clark, Clegg Smith, & Meisser, 2011). In 2014, several NIH Institutes funded a Mixed Methods Research Training Program for the Health Sciences (R25MH104660; Joseph J. Gallo, Principal Investigator). The need for training in mixed methods was clear because many investigators are seeking to gain insight on how context and culture influence the adoption and adaptation of behavioral interventions (Creswell et al., 2011). An increase in proposals submitted to NIH using mixed methods reflects the growing awareness of the importance of this approach in addressing population and behavioral health (Plano Clark, 2010) in fields such as nursing (Morse & Niehaus, 2009), medicine (Albright, Gechter, & Kempe, 2013; Creswell, Fetters, & Ivankova, 2004), mental health (Wittink, Barg, & Gallo, 2006), cardiovascular health (Curry, Nembhard, & Bradley, 2009), palliative care (Farquhar, Ewing, & Booth, 2011), public health (Curry, Shield, & Wetle, 2006), global health (Bass et al., 2013; Betancourt et al., 2011; Nastasi et al., 2007), implementation science (Bradley et al., 2009; Greenhalgh et al., 2010), health policy (Brannen & Moss, 2012), and health disparities (Apesoa-Varano & Hinton, 2013; Stewart, Makwarimba, Barnfather, Letourneau, & Neufeld, 2008).

WHAT ARE KEY MIXED METHODS DESIGNS?

There are many possible typologies for constructing a mixed methods design (Nastasi, Hitchcock, & Brown, 2010). We use the terminology of Creswell and Plano Clark because of its simplicity to delineate mixed methods study types (Creswell & Plano Clark, 2011). In this chapter, we only scratch the surface.

The diagrams in Figure 11.1 are a simplification of countless possibilities in which quantitative and qualitative approaches (often called "strands" in a research design) are mixed, at the data collection step, in data analysis, in data interpretation, or at multiple levels of the study design. What we discuss in this section are the basic structures of mixed methods study designs. How the "mix" of quantitative and qualitative "strands" is configured in a particular study must be justified by the goals of the study and the questions to be answered by the research as well as the stage of pipeline in intervention development. Sequential designs (exploratory and explanatory sequential designs) have data collection performed in sequence so that the results of one strand influence the data collection for the next strand. In concurrent designs, the data collection for the strands is embedded in one another, often with one method being primary. In this section, we outline key mixed methods designs and end with a note on sampling for mixed methods designs.

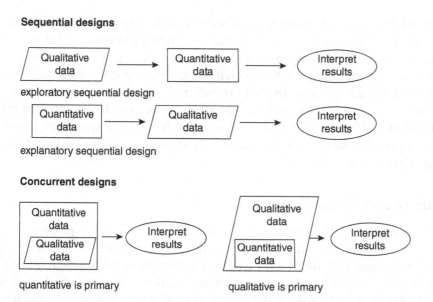

Figure 11.1 Basic mixed methods designs that deploy qualitative and quantitative methods sequentially or concurrently.
Source: Adapted from Creswell and Plano Clark (2011).

Exploratory Sequential Design

In an exploratory sequential design, qualitative data are collected prior to the collection of quantitative data (Figure 11.1). This type of design is likely to be familiar to many investigators as it is commonly used as a strategy to design an instrument or questionnaire or to gather information to guide the content of an intervention (e.g., focus group: a guided discussion that systematically investigates what a diverse group of people thinks of a set of research questions). The qualitative component helps "discover" or "uncover" the range of domains and the words people use to express constructs; the goal is not to generalize the study results to the larger population. In other words, the salience of ideas (or themes) comes from the meaning participants ascribe to constructs, not from counting the number of persons or calculating proportions of persons who express a particular idea. Although qualitative methods do not use a standardized set of questions for every respondent, participants are able to express attitudes, beliefs, feeling, and constructs that are most important to them. For instance, in the northern region of Australia, Nagel and others initially qualitatively interviewed local aborigines to understand their perspective of mental health, then incorporated an aboriginal concept of mental health in a randomized controlled study of a brief motivational intervention (Nagel, Robinson, Condon, & Trauer, 2009).

In the context of behavioral intervention development, an exploratory sequential design with an initial qualitative exploration of patients' perceptions of an intervention can guide the adaptation and administration of a larger scale intervention that is then based on quantitative methods of assessment (i.e., outcomes assessed with standardized questionnaires). Pilot studies of a new intervention need to incorporate ways for participants to provide feedback about how to make recruitment and informed consent procedures effective as well as to gauge feasibility and acceptability of the intervention, and for making modifications to the intervention to be more palatable to participants (Audrey, 2011). The active incorporation of patient feedback resembles a patient-centered design process commonly used in research and systems designs, and the NIH recognizes the needs for research development centered around the patients' perspectives (Office of Disease Prevention, 2015). Mixed methods provide a tool to systematically integrate quantitative and qualitative approaches so that interventions and care systems are consistent with patients' experiences and concepts.

Explanatory Sequential Designs

An alternative to the exploratory sequential design is the explanatory sequential design in which the quantitative data collection comes first, followed by qualitative data collection (Figure 11.1). Investigators who select this design often do so because there is some need for an explanation of the quantitative findings from study participants. An example of the use of an explanatory sequential design would be interviewing persons who did not seem to benefit from the intervention (based on the quantitative assessments typically used in a trial) to find out how the intervention could be modified. Participants may have useful feedback about aspects of the intervention that were helpful, or aspects that they found unhelpful or would not use. This information can be used to refine an intervention for the next phase of intervention testing or implementation (e.g., to understand the concepts of depression that are important to older adults) (Barg et al., 2010).

In an explanatory sequential design, it is important to carefully select participants to maximize the information specific to the research question. For example, participants who were enthusiastic users of an intervention or, on the other hand, who engaged only minimally with the intervention may provide more critical information on their responses to the intervention than a random sample of participants. Perhaps the purposive sampling might include both participants who did and who did not engage in the intervention to understand the reasons behind their decisions. In the explanatory sequential design, emphasis is placed on understanding not only whether an intervention works, but for whom, under what circumstances, and why an intervention did (or did not) have the desired effects—all questions for which mixed methods approaches are well suited.

Concurrent Designs

In some cases, the research questions or circumstances of the research settings require that the data collection be essentially concurrent, often referred to as "embedding" one strand in another, typically with one strand dominating (Figure 11.1). For concurrent designs, less emphasis is placed on how one strand informs the next, and more on making inferences or drawing conclusions from the concurrent strands. In a design in which the quantitative methods are primary, participants might undergo extensive structured assessments using standard assessment instruments (e.g., behavioral change measures), but some participants might be selected for more detailed evaluation (e.g., what a participant who received an intervention experienced), to understand processes in intervention implementation (e.g., what practitioners really do) or to study mediation (e.g., through the use of selected case studies to understand causal pathways; Weller & Barnes, 2014). Iloabachie and colleagues (2011) examined the effectiveness of an Internet-based intervention for depression among adolescents and concurrently collected quantitative survey and qualitative interview data. Over time, the authors were able to assess quantitative outcomes (helpfulness and attitude change) along with qualitative themes reflecting adolescent experience. Embedded designs in which the qualitative methods are the primary method of data collection can also be envisioned. An example would be assessing personal characteristics (e.g., age) or outcomes (e.g., response to an intervention) in a study employing primarily qualitative interview methods. Doing so might be important for investigators who want to compare themes or ideas across groups defined by the quantitative characteristics (i.e., comparing men and women, or persons at different levels of functional impairment).

Sampling

For different quantitative and qualitative strands of mixed methods study designs mentioned earlier, a mix of quantitative and qualitative sampling methods can be used in a single research inquiry. When using mixed methods, investigators need to be aware of different expectations for the rigor of methods used for sampling across quantitative and qualitative approaches. Assumptions about the nature of reality (ontology) and how we know what we know (epistemology), assumptions not typically examined critically by investigators, determine sampling, data collection, and data analysis methods that need to be made explicit for the effective combination of quantitative and qualitative approaches (Creswell & Clark, 2010; Creswell & Miller, 2000; Dellinger & Leech, 2007).

As with any sampling method, sampling in mixed methods must consider not only *how* sampling was carried out, but *why* a particular sampling strategy was used, how the sampling strategy was supported by theory, and how the sampling strategy was consistent with the aims of the study (Glaser & Strauss, 1967). As a general rule, sampling strategies for quantitative studies aim to recruit a number of participants to provide sufficient statistical power for the primary outcomes. In addition, quantitative studies seek to sample randomly and systematically with a view to generalize the findings to the population of interest (see Chapter 10 for discussion on sampling). In contrast, the goal of sampling for qualitative strands will not be generalizable to the population; instead there is purposive recruitment of participants who will likely bring valuable insights and perspectives that maximally inform the research question. When considering sample size in qualitative work, keep in mind that often the goal is to obtain a breadth of views (e.g., the scope of a domain), not generalization. Sampling strategies with both goals (representativeness, informativeness) may be deployed in mixed methods in the designs discussed earlier. For example, random sampling may be the foundation for selecting participants for a large-scale survey or intervention study, whereas purposive sampling may be based on participants with specific characteristics (e.g., minority groups, or persons who did or who did not respond to a treatment).

MIXED METHODS IN THE INTERVENTION PIPELINE

Mixed methods may be valuable throughout the pipeline—in the development of the intervention, during the evaluation of the intervention, and after the completion of the follow-up and assessment of outcomes. Typically, quantitative methods are used to assess intervention outcomes (shown in the upper right of Figure 11.2, adapted from Sandelowski, 1996), but qualitative methods may be introduced before, during, and after a trial (lower half of Figure 11.2). Qualitative approaches are most frequently used to develop an instrument, to understand strategies for successful recruitment, to find areas for intervention adaptation, to understand the processes of an intervention, to evaluate fidelity and other implementation factors, to explain outcomes, to provide feedback to improve intervention, and to understand mediators and moderators. As discussed in Chapter 16, qualitative methods are also sometimes used to gather information on the clinical significance of an intervention.

Traditional efficacy and effectiveness clinical trials focus on improving individual-level clinical and functional outcomes. For example, the National Institute of Mental Health (NIMH) is leading efforts to move toward an "experimental medicine approach" that generates knowledge about "mechanisms" underlying a disorder or a service use pattern (see Dr. Insel's overview at http://www.nimh.nih .gov/about/director/2014/a-new-approach-to-clinical-trials.shtml). An emphasis is on understanding mechanisms and designing studies in such a way that even if an intervention has minimal effects, it will be possible to inform future improvements or modifications to the intervention (O'Cathain, Murphy, & Nicholl, 2007). Mixed methods are essential to achieving these objectives as it is no longer tenable for an investigator to answer only the question: Does this work? The investigator must also be prepared to address the questions: Why didn't this work? Why didn't this

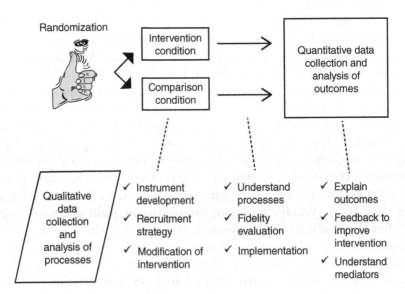

Figure 11.2 The role and timing of using quantitative and qualitative approaches in randomized clinical trials.

Source: Adapted from Sandelowski (1996).

work for this group? Why didn't this intervention reach the people for whom it was intended?

Mixed methods have the potential to discover, explain, or (dis)confirm mediators or moderators not traditionally identified through quantitative methods. Though quantitative methods in randomized controlled trials (RCTs) have been regarded as the gold standard for efficacy and effectiveness research, active integration of qualitative methods in behavioral intervention research facilitates the identification of complex procedural, contextual, and interpersonal factors underlying efficacy or effectiveness of interventions (Neuman, 2006). The *emic*, or insider's perspective of cultural, interpersonal, and environmental contexts, provides a more complete understanding of the processes that determine success or failure of an intervention. Evidence-based practices that are appropriate for diverse groups and contexts in which the intervention will be deployed are more likely to be integrated into complex and evolving health systems.

EXAMPLES OF MIXED METHODS APPROACHES IN THE INTERVENTION DEVELOPMENT PIPELINE

In this section, we describe examples of studies employing mixed methods along the intervention development pipeline—intervention development, intervention evaluation in efficacy and effectiveness trials, implementation in diverse community and service settings, and understanding results. Mixed methods can augment an RCT or intervention design by gathering exploratory data before, during, or after a trial (Creswell & Plano Clark, 2011). Mixed methods studies provide insight by giving study participants a chance to describe how an intervention might be modified before full deployment, or to explain outcomes observed of a trial (Farquhar et al., 2011).

Intervention Development

Barg and colleagues (2006) examined how patient notions of depression differed from or were similar to standard definitions. Older adults were administered a structured interview assessing symptoms of depression ("quantitative methods"), but also were asked to provide the investigators with ideas about depression and its treatment in their own words in semistructured interviews (a form of a qualitative method that uses a set of open-ended questions to gather ideas from the interviewee; Barg et al., 2006). What emerged was a concept of depression that included loneliness as a prominent component, with evidence drawn from both semistructured interviews and quantitative assessment. These findings have led to strategies that employ community members to deliver interventions to isolated older adults, to be more in line with conceptions of depression held by older adults.

Nastasi and colleagues (2007) used a multiphased mixed methods design for the Sri Lanka Mental Health Promotion Project, conducted in the Central Province of Sri Lanka. The group used formative research to identify and refine individual and cultural constructs and variables that explain or predict mental health, violent behavior, and academic achievement among Sri Lankan youths and teachers. Researchers conducted focus group interviews with students and teachers, individual interviews with school administrators, and observed participants in schools to identify culture-specific definitions of mental health constructs, such as "stress." On the basis of the theories generated with a combination of interviews and school-based observations, the researchers developed scales—using factor analysis—that assessed culturally specific values of adolescents' competency and prominent stressors. Those highly targeted psychological measures for the Sri Lankan context were administered to students across six schools and were quantitatively analyzed. This formative research phase led to the design of a mental health promotion program that used a RCT to test the effectiveness of an intervention that used culturally appropriate coping strategies and peer support activities. During the program implementation, researchers collected information on program acceptability, cultural relevance and social validity, integrity, and immediate impact of the intervention. The quantitative and qualitative results consistently found that girls, but not boys, became more aware of feelings of distress and limited helpfulness of social support for situations over which they had little control. Girls also had a heightened sense of responsibility in problem solving of complex family problems. Teachers found new roles in contributing to students' social and emotional development, and students sought emotional support from them outside of the immediate intervention settings.

Within a Randomized Trial

Intervention studies may carry out quantitative and qualitative interviews in parallel throughout the follow-up interval for intervention and control groups. Cramer and colleagues (2011) tested the feasibility and acceptability of group cognitive behavioral therapy (CBT) for women with depression, using both quantitative and qualitative methods over time. The Patient Health Questionaire-9 measured depressive symptoms, while qualitative interviews with all participants, clinicians, and community staff sought to understand the acceptability and feasibility of the intervention. The authors provided both quantitative and qualitative interpretation of their findings. Quantitative findings demonstrated the effectiveness of group-based CBT for women with depression. Qualitative findings described that the intervention was well-received by participants and the intervention acted as a catalyst for changing negative thoughts and bringing positive change in taking up new jobs, volunteer work, and other activities salient to the participants. High engagement in treatment was largely due, according to the participants, to support and encouragement provided by facilitators. Qualitative approaches provided insight into the experiences of participants in the intervention trial, expanding on factors that were most salient to participants beyond what quantitative data collection methods revealed.

Implementation Studies

An important distinction needs to be made between intervention components and implementation components. Intervention components (usually studied in efficacy or effectiveness studies under controlled conditions) are aspects of the intervention designed to create change (e.g., to improve patient-level symptoms and functioning). Implementation components refer to the elements needed to implement the core intervention components and to enhance acceptability and feasibility of a new evidence-based practice in a real setting (Fixsen, Naoom, Blase, Friedman, & Wallace, 2005). Implementation is defined as "a set of activities designed to put into practice" an intervention program (Fixsen et al., 2005). For example, the core intervention components of the chronic care model include a patient registry and self-management strategies (Wagner, Austin, & Von Korff, 1996); the implementation components concern how those components are carried out in clinical or community settings. Important aspects of implementation may include practitioners' attitudes toward changing their care practices and the willingness of organizational leadership to adopt an intervention.

In implementation, quantitative methods are commonly used to study outcomes while qualitative methods are used to understand process (Palinkas et al., 2011). Process involves understanding what actually happens in practice settings when an intervention is implemented, for which qualitative methods are well suited because of the focus on gaining the perspective of people in the practice setting. Failure to adapt treatments in ways that increase organizational and community "fit" may explain why research-proven interventions are often not disseminated or maintained (Hoagwood, Burns, & Weiss, 2002). When developing behavioral strategies and putting interventions into practice, mixed methods provide a framework to ensure that the interventions incorporate real-world concerns. Mixed methods inform several implementation issues: how to adapt an intervention to a specific context, what strategies are used to implement interventions in practice settings, and how elements of the implementation strategy influence patient-centered outcomes.

An example of using mixed methods through implementation of an intervention comes from a study of the development, testing, and scale-up of an integrated care management of type 2 diabetes and depression program aimed at improving medical adherence (Bogner, Morales, de Vries, & Cappola, 2012). Initial qualitative interviews with patients and families indicated how to adapt Wagner Chronic Care Model to incorporate core intervention components needed for patients with diabetes and depression comorbidity. A RCT was then used to test the efficacy of the integrated care intervention in improving adherence to medication treatment. Furthermore, focus groups and semistructured interviews were employed to assess interventionists' views on the successes and challenges of the intervention as well as organizational factors (e.g., cost-effectiveness and hospital administrators' attitudes concerning the intervention) that served as important implementation factors for the scalability of the intervention. Mixed methods were also used to identify policy- and environmental-level factors that influence maintenance and sustainability of an integrated care intervention in a health care setting. All of these efforts toward careful development of intervention and implementation components using mixed methods led to improved patient outcomes not only in the research trials but also in practice settings.

Understanding Outcomes

Mixed methods can provide a more complete understanding of the results or outcomes of an intervention study. Midgley, Ansaldo, and Target (2014) used a qualitative approach nested in a randomized control study called Improving Mood With

Psychoanalytic and Cognitive Behavioral Therapy (IMPACT). The intervention was designed to treat adolescent depression in the United Kingdom and to prevent relapse. Before the intervention, all adolescents and parents underwent qualitative interviews to assess the issues that brought them to treatment, as well as their hopes and expectations about the therapy. At the posttreatment follow-up, families were interviewed regarding their experiences of therapy over time with the focus on treatment outcomes and cultural and contextual factors that affected the outcomes. In addition, participants identified outcomes that were important to them that the investigators did not expect.

For community-based participatory research, mixed methods are important to gain both *emic* and *etic* perspectives (Ahmed, Beck, Maurana, & Newton, 2004). Because mixed methods research designs place high value on the stories behind the numbers—both in exploratory designs where the experiences and insights of the community under study inform the quantitative investigation, and in explanatory designs where they illuminate the quantitative data—mixed methods are especially attractive to community partners whose interest is in improving practice and outcomes suitable to a context. As such, mixed methods provide a valuable bridge between researchers and community partners, which is essential to the successful implementation of an intervention.

Mixed methods strategies are essential to understanding what must be adapted in evidence-based models to ensure successful outcomes for different patients and in different communities. The Federal Coordinating Council for Comparative Effectiveness Research (CER) defined CER broadly, asserting that it is patient-centered, "real-world" research that can help patients, clinicians, and other decision makers assess "the relative benefits and harms of strategies to prevent, diagnose, treat, manage, or monitor health conditions and the systems in which they are made" (Congressional Budget Office of the Congress of the United States, 2007; National Institutes of Health, n.d.). A misleading assumption is that all participants respond to an intervention in the same way, no matter the context. In the real-world, people come to the treatment with different preconceived notions about what is wrong and what to do about it. Tension between "patient-centeredness" and application of an "evidence base"—between incorporating context and general applicability of evidence ("generalizability")—keeps treatments that might be beneficial (e.g., depression treatment) from getting to people who could benefit from the treatments (e.g., persons with medical comorbidity such as diabetes who are sometimes poorly adherent to lifestyle changes and medical regimens; Ciechanowski, Katon, & Russo, 2000; Gonzalez et al., 2008). Mixed methods can offer insight into how an intervention works or does not work, and for whom and in what context.

CHALLENGES IN MIXED METHODS RESEARCH

Despite the many benefits of mixed methods, challenges arise in using and integrating multiple analytic approaches. One of the challenges in using both quantitative and qualitative approaches in designing and testing interventions is to have sufficient time and resources allocated to ensure sufficient rigor for both approaches. Though a qualitative approach using participant interviews and observations may yield detailed information, sampling for qualitative approaches typically involves a small number of people (often <50). Such sample sizes typically preclude the use of statistical testing (e.g., of differences in participant characteristics according to themes that emerged in qualitative interviews; Wittink et al., 2006). The key criterion is to ensure representativeness of the main themes, perceptions, and insights (as we continue to talk to people, do new themes emerge or have we reached "saturation" in that no new themes emerge?), as opposed to estimating a population parameter (which may depend on random selection of a sample large enough to provide statistical power). Another challenge is the initiation of collaboration with investigators who are used to restricting their data collection strategies to quantitative methods to adequately allocate resources to collect and analyze qualitative data from observations, narratives, and visual data (George, 2011). In analysis of mixed data, findings from one strand may be contradictory or discordant with the other strand. Although this may be a challenge or viewed as a weakness, such discrepancies can lead to new insights about the processes or measurements we might otherwise not question.

Fostering transdisciplinary research teams for mixed methods behavioral health research poses a pressing challenge (Kessel, Rosenfeld, & Anderson, 2008). In order to maximize the use of mixed methods in RCTs, principal investigators of clinical trials may benefit from including researchers and staff who are trained in qualitative and mixed method approaches, beginning at the study design stage (Robins et al., 2008). Robins and colleagues (2008) have emphasized that "mixed" teams benefit from time set aside for problem solving and discussions about study design, underlying epistemological assumptions, and interpretations.

CONCLUSION

In this chapter, we provided an overview to the use of mixed methods approaches in intervention development, evaluation, and implementation. The basic mixed methods designs discussed in this chapter provide a starting point for using mixed methods in developing, evaluating, and implementing behavioral interventions in real-world settings. Readers wishing for more details may refer to several excellent resources on mixed methods (Creswell et al., 2011; Creswell & Plano Clark, 2011; Curry & Nunez-Smith, 2014; Tashakkori & Teddlie, 2010). Readers wishing to have more in-depth information on writing mixed methods for publication or proposals may find the article of Dahlberg and colleagues helpful (Dahlberg, Wittink, & Gallo, 2010). For rapid immersion in the concepts of mixed methods, Creswell has written a short introduction (Creswell, 2014).

In January 2015, President Obama shared a major policy initiative in precision medicine, with the goal of "delivering the right treatments, at the right time, every time to the right person" (Office of the Press Secretary, 2015). Use of mixed methods approaches can enrich the development, evaluation, and scale-up of behavioral health interventions in a patient-centered manner. Having rich contextual information along with quantitative intervention outcomes data may lead to the reduction of the 17 plus years time lag between evidence generation to clinical practice (Westfall, Mold, & Fagnan, 2007). We urge investigators to incorporate mixed methods in intervention development, testing, and implementation in practice settings to ensure that the interventions developed will reach the diverse persons who are meant to benefit.

REFERENCES

Ahmed, S. M., Beck, B., Maurana, C. A., & Newton, G. (2004). Overcoming barriers to effective community-based participatory research in US medical schools. *Education for Health, 17,* 141–151.

Albright, K., Gechter, K., & Kempe, A. (2013). Importance of mixed methods study in pragmatic trials and dissemination and implementation research. *Academic Pediatrics, 13*(5), 400–407.

Apesoa-Varano, E. C., & Hinton, L. (2013). The promise of mixed-methods for advancing Latino health research. *Journal of Cross-Cultural Gerontology, 28*(3), 267–282. doi:10.1007/s10823-013-9209-2

Audrey, S. (2011). Qualitative research in evidence-based medicine: Improving decision-making and participation in randomized controlled trials of cancer treatments. *Palliative Medicine, 25,* 758–765.

Barg, F. K., Huss-Ashmore, R., Wittink, M. N., Murray, G. F., Bogner, H. R., & Gallo, J. J. (2006). A mixed methods approach to understand loneliness and depression in older adults. *Journal of Gerontology: Social Sciences, 61*(6), S329–S339.

Barg, F. K., Mavandadi, S., Givens, J. L., Knott, K., Zubritsky, C., & Oslin, D. W. (2010). When late-life depression improves: What do older patients say about their treatment? *The American Journal of Geriatric Psychiatry, 18*(7), 596–605.

Bass, J. K., Annan, J., McIvor Murray, S., Kaysen, D., Griffiths, S., Cetinoglu, T., . . . Bolton, P. A. (2013). Controlled trial of psychotherapy for Congolese survivors of sexual violence. *The New England Journal of Medicine, 368*(23), 2182–2191. doi:10.1056/NEJMoa1211853

Becker, G., & Newsom, E. (2003). Socioeconomic status and dissatisfaction with health care among chronically ill African Americans. *American Journal of Public Health, 93*(5), 742–748. doi:10.2105/Ajph.93.5.742

Betancourt, T., Myers-Ohki, S. E., Stevenson, A., Ingabire, C., Kanyanganzi, F., Munyana, M., . . . Beardslee, W. R. (2011). Using mixed-methods research to adapt and evaluate a family strengthening intervention in Rwanda. *African Journal of Traumatic Stress, 2,* 32–45.

Bogner, H. R., Morales, K. H., de Vries, H. F., & Cappola, A. R. (2012). Integrated management of type 2 diabetes mellitus and depression treatment to improve medication adherence: A randomized controlled trial. *The Annals of Family Medicine, 10*(1), 15–22. doi:10.1370/afm.1344

Bradley, E. H., Curry, L. A., Ramanadhan, S., Rowe, L., Nembhard, I. M., & Krumholz, H. M. (2009). Research in action: Using positive deviance to improve quality of health care. *Implementation Science, 4,* 25. doi:10.1186/1748-5908-4-25

Brannen, J., & Moss, G. (2012). Critical issues in designing mixed methods policy research. *American Behavioral Scientist, 56*(6), 789–801.

Ciechanowski, P. S., Katon, W. J., & Russo, J. E. (2000). Depression and diabetes: Impact of depressive symptoms on adherence, function, and costs. *Archives of Internal Medicine, 160*(21), 3278–3285.

Congressional Budget Office of the Congress of the United States. (2007). *Research on the comparative effectiveness of medical treatments.* Washington, DC: Author.

Cramer, H., Salisbury, C., Conrad, J., Eldred, J., & Araya, R. (2011). Group cognitive behavioural therapy for women with depression: Pilot and feasibility study for a randomised controlled trial using mixed methods. *BMC Psychiatry, 11*, 82. doi:10.1186/1471-244X-11-82

Creswell, J. W. (2014). *A concise introduction to mixed methods research.* Thousand Oaks, CA: Sage.

Creswell, J. W., & Clark, V. P. (2010). *Designing and conducting mixed methods research* (2nd ed.). Los Angeles, CA: Sage.

Creswell, J. W., Fetters, M. D., & Ivankova, N. V. (2004). Designing a mixed methods study in primary care. *The Annals of Family Medicine, 2*, 7–12. doi:10.1370/afm.104

Creswell, J. W., Klassen, A. C., Plano Clark, V. L., Clegg Smith, K., & Meisser, H. F. (2011). *Best practices for mixed methods research in the health sciences.* Washington, DC: Commissioned by the Office of Behavioral and Social Sciences Research (OBSSR).

Creswell, J. W., & Miller, D. L. (2000). Determining validity in qualitative inquiry. *Theory into Practice, 39*(3), 124–130. doi:10.1207/s15430421tip3903_2

Creswell, J. W., & Plano Clark, V. L. (2011). *Designing and conducting mixed methods research* (2nd ed.). Washington, DC: Sage.

Curry, L., & Nunez-Smith, M. (2014). *Mixed methods in health sciences research: A practical primer.* Thousand Oaks, CA: Sage.

Curry, L., Shield, R., & Wetle, T. (Eds.). (2006). *Improving aging and public health research: Qualitative and mixed methods.* Washington, DC: American Public Health Association.

Curry, L. A., Nembhard, I. M., & Bradley, E. H. (2009). Qualitative and mixed methods provide unique contributions to outcomes research. *Circulation, 119*, 1442–1452. doi:10.1161/CIRCULATIONAHA.107.742775

Dahlberg, B., Wittink, M., & Gallo, J. J. (2010). Funding and publishing integrated studies: Writing effective mixed methods manuscripts and grant proposals. In A. Tashakkori & C. Teddlie (Eds.), *Handbook of mixed methods in social & behavioral research* (2nd ed., pp. 775–802). London, England: Sage.

Dellinger, A. B., & Leech, N. L. (2007). Toward a unified validation framework in mixed methods research. *Journal of Mixed Methods Research, 1*(4), 309–332. doi:10.1177/1558689807306147

DePoy, E., & Gitlin, L. N. (2015). *Introduction to research: Understanding and applying multiple strategies* (5th ed.). St. Louis, MO: Elsevier.

Farquhar, M. C., Ewing, G., & Booth, S. (2011). Using mixed methods to develop and evaluate complex interventions in palliative care research. *Palliative Medicine, 25*(8), 748–757. doi:10.1177/0269216311417919

Fixsen, D. L., Naoom, S. F., Blase, K. A., Friedman, R. M., & Wallace, F. (2005). *Implementation research: A synthesis of the literature.* Tampa, FL: University of South Florida.

George, D. R. (2011). Intergenerational volunteering and quality of life: Mixed methods evaluation of a randomized control trial involving persons with mild to moderate dementia. *Quality of Life Research, 20*(7), 987–995. doi:10.1007/s11136-010-9837-8

Glaser, B. G., & Strauss, A. L. (1967). *The discovery of grounded theory: Strategies for qualitative research.* New York, NY: Aldine Publishing.

Gonzalez, J. S., Peyrot, M., McCarl, L. A., Collins, E. M., Serpa, L., Mimiaga, M. J., & Safren, S. A. (2008). Depression and diabetes treatment nonadherence: A meta-analysis. *Diabetes Care, 31*(12), 2398–2403.

Goodman, R. A., Buehler, J. W., & Koplan, J. P. (1990). The epidemiologic field investigation: Science and judgment in public health practice. *American Journal of Epidemiology, 132*(1), 9–16.

Greenhalgh, T., Stramer, K., Bratan, T., Byrne, E., Russell, J., & Potts, H. W. (2010). Adoption and non-adoption of a shared electronic summary record in England: A mixed-method case study. *BMJ, 340*, c3111. doi:10.1136/bmj.c3111

Hoagwood, K., Burns, B. J., & Weiss, J. R. (2002). A profitable conjunction: From science to service in children's mental health. In B. J. Burns & K. Hoagwood (Eds.), *Community treatment for youth: Evidence-based interventions for severe emotional and behavioral disorders* (pp. 327–338). New York, NY: Oxford University Press.

Iloabachie, C., Wells, C., Goodwin, B., Baldwin, M., Vanderplough-Booth, K., Gladstone, T., . . . Van Voorhees, B. W. (2011). Adolescent and parent experiences with a primary care/Internet-based depression prevention intervention (CATCH-IT). *General Hospital Psychiatry, 33*, 543–555.

Institute of Medicine (US) Committee on Crossing the Quality Chasm: Adaptation to Mental Health and Addictive Disorders. (2006). *Improving the quality of care for mental and substance-use conditions: Quality chasm series.* Washington, DC: National Academies Press.

Johnson, R. B., Onwuegbuzie, A. J., & Turner, L. A. (2007). Toward a definition of mixed methods research. *Journal of Mixed Methods Research, 1*(2), 112–133. doi:10.1177/1558689806298224

Kessel, F., Rosenfeld, P. L., & Anderson, N. B. (2008). *Interdisciplinary research: Case studies from health and social science* (2nd ed.). New York, NY: Oxford University Press.

Midgley, G. (2006). Systemic intervention for public health. *American Journal of Public Health, 96*(3), 466–472.

Midgley, N., Ansaldo, F., & Target, M. (2014). The meaningful assessment of therapy outcomes: Incorporating a qualitative study into a randomized controlled trial evaluating the treatment of adolescent depression. *Psychotherapy, 51*(1), 128–137. doi:10.1037/a0034179

Morse, J. M., & Niehaus, L. (2009). *Mixed method design: Principles and procedures.* Walnut Creek, CA: Left Coast Press.

Murray, C. J. L., Vos, T., & Lozano, R. (2012). Disability-adjusted life years (DALYs) for 291 diseases and injuries in 21 regions, 1990–2010: A systematic analysis for the Global Burden of Disease Study 2010 (Erratum in: *Lancet* 2013, *381*(9867), 628. AlMazroa, M. A., Memish, Z. A. [added]). *Lancet, 380*(9859), 2197–2223. doi:10.1016/S0140-6736(12)61689-4.

Nagel, T., Robinson, G., Condon, J., & Trauer, T. (2009). Approach to treatment of mental illness and substance dependence in remote indigenous communities: Results of a mixed methods study. *Australian Journal of Rural Health, 17*, 174–182.

Nastasi, B. K., Hitchcock, J. H., & Brown, L. M. (2010). An inclusive framework for conceptualizing mixed methods design typologies: Moving toward fully integrated synergistic research models. In A. Tashakkori & C. Teddlie (Eds.), *Sage handbook of mixed methods in social and behavioral research* (pp. 305–338). Thousand Oaks, CA: Sage.

Nastasi, B. K., Hitchcock, J., Sarkar, S., Burkholder, G., Varjas, K., & Jayasena, A. (2007). Mixed methods in intervention research: Theory to adaptation. *Journal of Mixed Methods Research, 1*(2), 164–182.

National Institute of Mental Health. (2008). *National Institute of Mental Health strategic plan.* Washington, DC: National Institutes of Health.

National Institutes of Health. (n.d.). *NIH Research portfolio online reporting tools (RePORT): NIH RePORTER.* Retrieved from http://projectreporter.nih.gov/reporter.cfm

Neuman, W. L. (2006). *Social research methods: Qualitative and quantitative approaches* (6th ed.). Boston, MA: Pearson Education.

O'Cathain, A., Murphy, E., & Nicholl, J. (2007). Why, and how, mixed methods research is undertaken in health services research in England: A mixed methods study. *BMC Health Services Research, 7*, 85. doi:10.1186/1472-6963-7-85

Office of Disease Prevention. (2015). *Panel cites need for individualized, patient-centered approach to treat and monitor chronic pain.* Retrieved from http://www.nih.gov/news/health/jan2015/odp-12.htm

Office of the Press Secretary. (2015, January 30). *Remarks by the president on precision medicine.* Retrieved from http://www.whitehouse.gov/the-press-office/2015/01/30/remarks-president-precision-medicine

Palinkas, L., Aarons, G., Horwitz, S., Chamberlain, P., Hurlburt, M., & Landsverk, J. (2011). Mixed methods designs in implementation research. *Administration and Policy in Mental Health and Mental Health Services Research, 38,* 44–53.

Plano Clark, V. L. (2010). The adoption and practice of mixed methods: U.S. trends in federally funded health-related research. *Qualitative Inquiry, 16*(6), 428–440.

Robins, C. S., Ware, N. C., dosReis, S., Willging, C. E., Chung, J. Y., & Lewis-Fernandez, R. (2008). Dialogues on mixed-methods and mental health services research: Anticipating challenges, building solutions. *Psychiatric Services, 59*(7), 727–731. doi:10.1176/appi. ps.59.7.727

Romney, A. K., Batchelder, W. H., & Weller, S. C. (1987). Recent applications of cultural consensus theory. *American Behavioral Scientist, 31,* 163–177.

Rössler, W. (2012). Stress, burnout, and job dissatisfaction in mental health workers. *European Archives of Psychiatry and Clinical Neuroscience, 262*(2), 65–69. doi:10.1007/s00406-012-0353-4

Sandelowski, M. (1996). Focus on qualitative methods: Using qualitative methods in intervention studies. *Research in Nursing and Health, 19,* 359–364.

Stewart, M., Makwarimba, E., Barnfather, A., Letourneau, N., & Neufeld, A. (2008). Researching reducing health disparities: Mixed-methods approaches. *Social Science & Medicine, 66*(6), 1406–1417.

Tashakkori, A., & Teddlie, C. (Eds.). (2003). *Handbook of mixed methods in social and behavioral research.* Thousand Oaks, CA: Sage.

Tashakkori, A., & Teddlie, C. (Eds.). (2010). *Handbook of mixed methods in social & behavioral research* (2nd ed.). Thousand Oaks, CA: Sage.

Trostle, J. (1986). Early work in anthropology and epidemiology: From social medicine to the germ theory, 1840 to 1920. In C. R. Janes, R. Stall, & S. M. Gifford (Eds.), *Anthropology and epidemiology: Interdisciplinary approaches to the study of health and disease* (pp. 35–57). Dordrecht, Netherlands: D. Reidel Publishing Company.

Trostle, J. A. (2005). *Epidemiology and culture.* New York, NY: Cambridge University Press.

U.S. Department of Health and Human Services. (2001). *Mental health: Culture, race and ethnicity. A supplement to mental health: A report of the surgeon general.* Rockville, MD: U.S. Department of Health and Human Services, Substance Abuse and Mental Health Services Administration, Center for Mental Health Services.

van Smeden, M., Naaktgeboren, C. A., Reitsma, J. B., Moons, K. G., & de Groot, J. A. (2014). Latent class models in diagnostic studies when there is no reference standard—A systematic review. *American Journal of Epidemiology, 179,* 423–431.

Wagner, E. H., Austin, B. T., & Von Korff, M. (1996). Organizing care for patients with chronic illness. The *Milbank Quarterly, 74*(4), 511–544.

Weller, N., & Barnes, J. (2014). *Finding pathways: Mixed-method research for studying causal mechanisms.* New York, NY: Cambridge University Press.

Westfall, J. M., Mold, J., & Fagnan, L. (2007). Practice-based research—"Blue highways" on the NIH roadmap. *JAMA, 297*(4), 403–406. doi:10.1001/jama.297.4.403

Wittink, M. N., Barg, F. K., & Gallo, J. J. (2006). Unwritten rules of talking to doctors about depression: Integrating qualitative and quantitative methods. *Annals of Family Medicine, 4*(4), 302–309.

TWELVE

ARE TREATMENT EFFECTS REAL? THE ROLE OF FIDELITY

LAURA N. GITLIN AND JEANINE M. PARISI

> *I have not failed. I have just found 10,000 things that do not work.*
> —Thomas Edison

A multisite intervention study to improve exercise adherence among cardiac patients reports large and statistically significant benefits overall for the treatment groups; yet, outcomes vary by site with some demonstrating null findings.

A home-based intervention that provides stress reduction techniques to parents caring for children with chronic illness demonstrates positive results with parents also reporting a strong bond with interventionists with whom they felt comfortable in confiding.

A proven intervention for self-management of chronic illness is replicated in multiple senior centers, but demonstrates varying levels of effectiveness by site.

These are common scenarios in behavioral intervention research. Each of these scenarios raises questions as to whether treatment effects reported from the evaluations of the interventions are attributable to the intervention itself, are consequences of other unmeasured factors, or reflect inadequate or inconsistent implementation of the intervention protocols. In the multisite study, exercise adherence scenario, unaccounted for variations in dose, intensity, or different motivational styles of interventionists may be at play; in the study on parental outcomes, formation of a strong therapeutic alliance versus the specific stress reduction techniques of the intervention may account for reported benefits; and for the multisite self-management study, poor adherence to the delivery of the intervention at some sites may explain variations in outcomes and differences in effectiveness levels reflecting threats to internal and external validity.

These examples showcase the critical need to attend to what is known as "fidelity." Fidelity, also referred to as "implementation fidelity," "fidelity of implementation," "intervention or treatment fidelity," or "treatment integrity," is a multidimensional construct that, at its most basic or fundamental level, refers to

213

whether an intervention is implemented as designed or intended (Bond, Evans, Salyers, Williams, & Kim, 2000; Gearing et al., 2011; Mowbray, Holter, Teague, & Bybee, 2003; Perepletchikova & Kazdin, 2005).

The consideration of fidelity is critical in every phase of advancing an intervention (developing the intervention, evaluating the intervention's efficacy and effectiveness, and implementing the intervention in a practice setting). Without an understanding of the level of fidelity achieved, it is impossible to determine whether an outcome from an evaluative study was due to the intervention itself or other potential competing factors, especially if the intervention was not delivered as intended. Similarly, without fidelity, it would be impossible to evaluate whether an intervention could be replicated effectively in the future (Gearing et al., 2011).

Although essential to behavioral intervention research, fidelity is an often overlooked study design element (Hardeman et al., 2008). Most intervention reports fail to include an adequate description of a fidelity plan, how fidelity was measured, or the level of protocol adherence achieved through fidelity monitoring (Dane & Schneider, 1998; Gearing et al., 2011). Moreover, reviews of published interventions have found that fidelity is rarely reported. For example, only 3.5% of psychosocial interventions published between 2000 and 2004 sufficiently addressed fidelity (Perepletchikova, Treat, & Kazdin, 2007). Similarly, a review of 63 social work intervention studies revealed that the majority lacked critical information concerning intervention delivery (e.g., mention of training, treatment manuals, and supervision) to adequately assess study outcomes (Naleppa & Cagle, 2010). Likewise, in a review of high-impact journals publishing education intervention research between 2005 and 2009, Swanson and colleagues (2011) found considerable inconsistencies in fidelity reporting. Even in articles that did provide fidelity information, the authors found fewer than 10% included data about the quality of implementation. Thus, across many disciplines, fidelity tends to be underemphasized or hidden, and outcomes of fidelity monitoring are rarely reported in behavioral intervention research.

The purpose of this chapter is to provide a comprehensive overview of the meaning and importance of fidelity and to describe specific strategies for addressing fidelity. We begin by briefly reviewing the historical use of the term to highlight the evolution of this construct and its varied definitions over time. Next, we examine the multiple roles and purposes it serves at different junctures along the intervention pipeline. Finally, we consider strategies for addressing fidelity and discuss the key challenges in advancing fidelity plans in the design and testing of behavioral interventions.

EVOLUTION AND HISTORICAL USES OF THE CONSTRUCT OF FIDELITY

The construct of "fidelity" has been a concern of, and an emphasis in, many fields of study over the past several decades. The construct has been advanced in separate, yet parallel, fashions within respective disciplines. It has long been a topic of discussion in educational research, where efforts have been directed toward translating and assuring scalability and quality of the replication of evidence-based programs in educational settings. Similarly, in program evaluation and implementation sciences, fidelity has been, and continues to be, a primary driver and main focus of research attention. Hence, different models for ensuring replication with fidelity have emerged from each of these respective fields of inquiry (Tomioka & Braun, 2013).

In behavioral intervention research, interest in fidelity has been highly influenced by developments in psychological research. Table 12.1 outlines the ways in which fidelity has been defined and differentially operationalized.

As shown, in the 1970s, researchers began to raise the critical issue of causality as it pertained to the outcomes reported for psychotherapeutic interventions. Variations and anomalies in the implementation of treatments brought to the forefront nagging concerns as to whether positive outcomes could be solely ascribed to the tested therapeutic intervention or to other observed and unobserved factors. Suspected confounding factors included, for example, the skill level of the therapist, dosage, participant readiness, and strength of the therapeutic alliance (Cook, Campbell, & Day, 1979; Sechrest & Yeaton, 1981; Yeaton & Sechrest, 1981). Unfortunately, early trials of psychotherapeutic interventions were not designed to disentangle these and other potential confounders from treatment effects to address these concerns.

Moncher and Prinz (1991) were among the first researchers to formally use the term "fidelity" in reference to treatment integrity or whether a given treatment was delivered as intended. They extended the scope of the construct to include the notion of treatment differentiation, arguing that it was not only important to ensure treatment integrity but also to clearly and demonstrably differentiate multiple treatments from one another. The goal of fidelity was to achieve transparency and to demystify what often was reported as the "black box" of an intervention.

Lichstein, Riedel, and Grieve (1994) followed with further refinements of this construct. They suggested that treatment integrity involved three critical components: delivery (whether the intervention is delivered as intended by interventionists), receipt (whether the study participant receives the intended intervention), and enactment (whether the participant uses or enacts the cognitive or behavioral skills imparted in the intervention). They illustrated these three components with the following scenario: On the basis of clinical guidelines, a nurse practitioner provides a patient with a prescription for hypertension medication; this is the delivery aspect of fidelity. Next, the patient must fill the prescription, which reflects evidence of receipt of treatment. Finally, after receiving the prescription, the patient must self-administer the prescribed medication, reflecting evidence of enactment of the intended intervention. In this scenario, to conclude with confidence that an observed positive change in the patient's blood pressure is due to the prescribed medication, all three components need to be evaluated affirmatively. A deviation in delivery, receipt, and/or enactment from the protocol could impede benefits (Lichstein et al., 1994).

Alternately, deviations from the protocol may inadvertently contribute to a positive outcome. Consider this scenario. Perhaps the patient takes the prescription from the nurse but forgets or chooses not to have the prescription filled by a pharmacist; or conversely, perhaps the patient has the prescription filled but then decides not to take the medication. Instead, the patient chooses to use alternative strategies such as changing diet, initiating an exercise program, and/or practicing stress reduction techniques. These alternative practices, and not the medication,

TABLE 12.1 Key Definitions and Components of Fidelity Over Time

Authors/Citations	Definitions	Design	Training	Implementation	Delivery	Dose	Adherence	Receipt	Enactment	Responsiveness	Differentiation	Competence
Moncher & Prinz (1991)	Fidelity of treatment in outcome research refers to confirmation that the manipulation of the independent variable occurred as planned. Verification of fidelity is needed to ensure that fair, powerful, and valid comparisons of replicable treatments can be made.	✓	✓	✓	✓	✓	✓				✓	
Lichstein et al. (1994)	Adequate levels of independent treatment components (delivery, receipt, and enactment) are prerequisite to asserting whether a valid clinical trial has been conducted.			✓			✓	✓				
Dane & Schneider (1998)	Defined as the degree to which specified procedures are implemented as planned				✓		✓			✓	✓	

Components Considered

(Continued)

TABLE 12.1 Key Definitions and Components of Fidelity Over Time (Continued)

Authors/ Citations	Definitions	Components Considered										
		Design	Training	Implementation	Delivery	Dose	Adherence	Receipt	Enactment	Responsiveness	Differentiation	Competence
Dusenbury, Brannigan, Falco, & Hansen (2003)	Fidelity of implementation refers to the degree to which teachers and other program providers implement programs as intended by the program developers. While there is agreement generally about what is intended when research refers to fidelity, in fact, fidelity has come to refer to a broad and loosely collected set of specific definitions.	✓				✓	✓			✓	✓	
Bellg et al. (2004)	Treatment fidelity refers to the methodological strategies used to monitor and enhance the reliability and validity of behavioral interventions. It also refers to the methodological practices used to ensure that a research study reliably and validly tests a clinical intervention.	✓	✓		✓			✓	✓			

(Continued)

TABLE 12.1 Key Definitions and Components of Fidelity Over Time (Continued)

Authors/ Citations	Definitions	Design	Training	Implementation	Delivery	Dose	Adherence	Receipt	Enactment	Responsiveness	Differentiation	Competence
Santacroce et al. (2004)	Intervention fidelity, defined as the adherent and competent delivery of an intervention by the interventionist as set forth in the research plan, is fundamental to the inference of validity in nursing intervention research.						✓					✓
Gresham (2005)	Refers to the degree to which treatments are implemented as intended. Treatment integrity is concerned with accuracy and consistency with which therapeutic procedures (independent variables) are implemented and how these procedures affect treatment outcome (dependent variables).	✓	✓				✓				✓	
Prohaska & Peters (2007)	Methodologic strategies used to monitor and enhance reliability and validity of behavioral interventions. Method to ensure that essential elements of the intervention, and only the intervention, account for the outcomes	✓	✓		✓			✓	✓			

(Continued)

TABLE 12.1 Key Definitions and Components of Fidelity Over Time (Continued)

Authors/ Citations	Definitions	Components Considered										
		Design	Training	Implementation	Delivery	Dose	Adherence	Receipt	Enactment	Responsiveness	Differentiation	Competence
Wilson et al. (2010)	Degree to which the protocol was implemented as planned					✓		✓				
Strijk et al. (2011)	The extent to which the intervention was implemented as planned		✓		✓	✓		✓		✓		
Gearing et al. (2011)	Intervention fidelity refers to the extent to which core components of interventions are delivered as intended by the protocols.	✓						✓				
Zauszniewski (2012)	Defined as competent delivery of the intervention that adheres to a prescribed protocol	✓	✓				✓	✓				
Tomioka & Braun (2013)	Degree of adherence to delivering the program, as well as the adapter's competence in delivering the program						✓					✓

may produce lower blood pressure. Without evaluating all three treatment components of fidelity, the nurse might conclude inaccurately that it was the hypertension medication treatment alone that positively lowered the patient's hypertension level.

For each component of fidelity, Lichstein and colleagues (1994) emphasized several considerations. First, strategies need to be introduced that "induct," or enhance, the probability of effective delivery, receipt, and enactment. For example, the use of detailed treatment manuals, checklists, and a standardized protocol for training and certifying interventionists can enhance the consistency and integrity of delivering an intervention. Second, both qualitative and quantitative measures can be used to document the extent to which each of the three components of fidelity is achieved.

One of the first large-scale, multisite behavioral trials to formally employ the Lichstein et al. (1994) model was the National Institutes of Health Resources for Enhancing Alzheimer's Caregiver Health initiatives (REACH I, 1995–2001; and REACH II, 2001–2006). In REACH I, six sites tested a different novel caregiver intervention and developed specific strategies for enhancing and tracking the delivery, receipt, and enactment (Burgio et al., 2001). In REACH II, one complex, multilevel intervention was tested across five sites utilizing a shared fidelity plan. For both REACH I and REACH II, strategies to induct fidelity included, but were not limited to, the development and use of well-constructed manuals of procedures and detailed treatment manuals, training and certification of interventionists using active learning techniques (including role-play, demonstrations, monitoring delivery through direct observation and audiotaping, and coding of treatment sessions for level of protocol adherence), and supervisory sessions for course corrections and prevention of drift. The concentrated level of attention to fidelity efforts in the REACH initiatives set a high scientific bar for the conduct of caregiver intervention studies in particular that had not previously been achieved in this area (Burgio et al., 2001; Chee, Gitlin, Dennis, & Hauck, 2007; Gitlin et al., 2003). The level of fidelity rigor achieved in the REACH initiatives also brought into question whether the inconsistent findings reported previously for the initial wave of caregiver intervention research were due, in part, to inconsistencies in treatment implementation across sites and a consequence, at least in part, to the lack of attention to treatment fidelity (Callahan, Kales, Gitlin, & Lyketsos, 2013).

Building on these previous efforts, the Health Psychology Workgroup for the National Institutes of Health (NIH)-sponsored Behavior Change Consortium (Ory, Jordan, & Bazzarre, 2002) developed what is now considered the classic explication of fidelity (Bellg et al., 2004). This workgroup defined fidelity as reflecting two interrelated components: "methodological strategies used to monitor and enhance the reliability and validity of behavioral interventions" and "methodological practices used to ensure that a research study reliably and validly tests a clinical intervention" (Bellg et al., 2004, p. 443). The NIH workgroup definition integrated the approach defined by Lichstein and colleagues (1994) with trial design considerations. Thus, four integral aspects of fidelity are emphasized: (a) adherence to trial design protocols, (b) treatment delivery, (c) treatment receipt, and (d) treatment enactment. Attention to all four components has become the recommended approach in behavioral intervention research.

Since the NIH guidelines were proposed, additional fidelity definitions have been suggested, often reflecting specific research contexts (e.g., public health, nursing, worksite evaluation) (Prohaska & Peters, 2007; Santacroce, Maccarelli, & Grey, 2004; Strijk, Proper, van der Beek, & van Mechelen, 2011). For instance, Carroll and colleagues (2007) conducted a critical review of existing fidelity models and proposed a new conceptual framework. Their model suggested that intervention outcomes are dependent primarily upon adherence, and its subcomponents including intervention content, coverage, frequency, and duration can be moderated by such factors as intervention complexity, facilitation strategies, and quality of delivery. However, adherence alone may not capture the complexity of the intervention and interactions among core components of fidelity. This model was formally tested by Hasson (2010) using a multiple case study method. In an investigation of the implementation processes of three intervention studies conducted in complex health or social care environments, the framework was modified to include two additional moderating factors: context and recruitment (Hasson, 2010).

Gearing and colleagues (2011) evaluated 24 meta-analyses and review articles on fidelity published over the past 30 years and concluded that attention should be given to the four aspects suggested by the NIH workgroup: design, training, monitoring of intervention delivery, and intervention receipt. More recently, Tomioka and Braun (2013), in conjunction with Hawaii's Healthy Aging Partnership, developed a four-step protocol for assuring replication with fidelity as follows: (a) deconstruct the program into its components and prepare a step-by-step plan for program replication; (b) identify agencies ready to replicate the program and sponsor excellent training to local staff who will deliver and coordinate it; (c) monitor the fidelity of program delivery using standardized checklists; and (d) track participant outcomes to assure achievement of expected outcomes. As the need for implementing evidence-based practices for health promotion continues, guidelines and protocols will become even more critical for the successful adaptation and replication of evidence-based approaches in diverse communities.

Although there is general agreement concerning the importance of fidelity in behavioral intervention research, there remains a lack of consensus concerning its definition, essential elements, assessment, and scope. Nevertheless, an important take-home point is that, as one develops an intervention, it is critical to consider fidelity. Behavioral intervention researchers have numerous emerging conceptual models and approaches to consider, with the models of Bellg and colleagues (2004) and Lichstein and colleagues (1999) now considered the classic approaches.

FIDELITY CONSIDERATIONS ALONG THE INTERVENTION PIPELINE

The specific aspects of fidelity that should be considered may vary depending upon the particular phase of an intervention along the pipeline (see Chapter 2). Nevertheless, there are neither documented best practices nor evidence concerning the preferred approach to fidelity at each development, evaluation, or implementation phases. Regardless, it seems reasonable to suggest that some attention be conferred to fidelity when developing and evaluating an intervention, possibly as early as in Discovery and Phase I (selection of a theory base, treatment elements, and delivery characteristics, determining feasibility) and Phase II (pilot testing, evaluation of outcomes and effect sizes). Developing a plan for enhancing and monitoring fidelity and evaluating the feasibility of this plan, as well as the validity of fidelity measures, would best occur in tandem with identifying the essential ingredients of an intervention protocol. Furthermore, attending to fidelity early on would provide some measure of confidence that the intervention is worthy of advancing. For example, examining whether interventionists are able to learn a complex intervention and adhere to its delivery, or that participants adequately receive intervention components, would provide important preliminary evidence for validating the value of the approach and also allow for "real-time" changes to be made early on in the intervention development process. Nevertheless, although there may be much value in attending to fidelity during the initial stages of intervention development, practical limitations such as inadequate funding, minimal staffing, and limited resources may make this the ideal rather than a reality.

In the evaluation phases, particularly in an efficacy trial (Phase III), the role of fidelity is clear. It is to assure that an intervention is implemented per protocol and that adherence to the established study design features and procedures is achieved. The goal of a fidelity plan in this phase is to maximize internal validity by minimizing "noise" from external sources such as differences in interventionists' backgrounds and approaches to delivering an intervention.

The importance of measuring and monitoring fidelity in an efficacy trial cannot be overstated. Poor fidelity can have a critical impact on the interpretation of results at any developmental phase of an intervention, but particularly in a definitive efficacy study. Without proper documentation and/or measurement of fidelity, it is not possible to evaluate whether inconsistent, ambiguous, or unsuccessful outcomes from a trial reflect a failure of the intervention or failure to implement it as intended (Chen, 1990; Hohmann & Shear, 2002). Failed implementation is the most common reason for the lack of positive outcomes (Mills & Ragan, 2000). This is aptly illustrated by early psychotherapy research in which therapists did not always adhere to treatment techniques yielding studies with inconsistent outcomes (Bond et al., 2000).

Another way to understand the impact of failed implementation in an efficacy trial is through the lens of Type I and Type II errors. The lack of adequate fidelity monitoring and evaluation may lead to the risk of a Type I error or accepting positive outcomes as a signal that the intervention works when unknown contaminants may actually be responsible for the desired effects (Hohmann & Shear, 2002; Spillane et al., 2007). As such, undetected errors in delivery can result in positive results for ineffective treatments, yet such treatments may not be replicable. Alternately, if results are not significant, researchers run the risk of a Type II error by erroneously rejecting a treatment that may have been poorly or inconsistently implemented.

Fidelity is also important in effectiveness studies (Phase IV). In Phase IV evaluations, the focus is on testing an intervention in different settings and with diverse populations that may differ from those included in the original efficacy trial. The concern at this evaluative phase is with external validity or being able to generalize the intervention to a broader arena including other settings and populations. With regard to fidelity, the focus is with obtaining a balance between streamlining or modifying the intervention to better fit the practice context and maintaining the integrity of the intervention for which it was originally designed and tested. Maintaining fidelity to the identified core immutable principles and features of an intervention is essential; however, the demands of a delivery context may require that adaptations to the intervention be made. A balance between being flexible and maintaining treatment integrity can be difficult to achieve and, to date, there is no consensus as to how much flexibility or deviation from a protocol can be allowed or for what aspects of the protocol. As to the latter, it may be that changing dose, visit schedule, or level of expertise of an interventionist is required to enable the intervention to be embedded into a practice setting. Yet, the effect of such changes may not be well understood or previously evaluated in earlier phases of the intervention's development. It may be that adapting interventions leads to better and more appropriate adoption and reach; yet, an adapted intervention may then need to be submitted to further rigorous testing if it is transformed too much from its original form (Washington et al., 2014). Figure 12.1 summarizes the role of fidelity in the different evaluative phases of a behavioral intervention and the tension between the demands for internal and external validity.

In implementation and sustainability phases, the emphasis of fidelity is on the accurate replication of an intervention and identifying the barriers to, and facilitators of, implementation integrity within a delivery context. Without attention to fidelity in previous evaluative phases and the in-depth knowledge of how an intervention has been delivered, received, and enacted, it is not possible to replicate or generalize to other settings (Bass & Judge, 2010). Further, the effectiveness of scaling up and rolling out an intervention will depend upon the ability of other practice sites to replicate the original intervention or make adaptations to fit their context. In this respect, standardization of the intervention is critical (see Chapter 6 on standardization).

Although assuring fidelity and accurate replication of an intervention is essential in the translation and implementation phases, efforts to do so are challenging. The fidelity approach used in the evaluation phases may need to be streamlined to reflect the realities and resources of the practice setting. For example, whereas monitoring and rating treatment sessions via audio or video for adherence are a

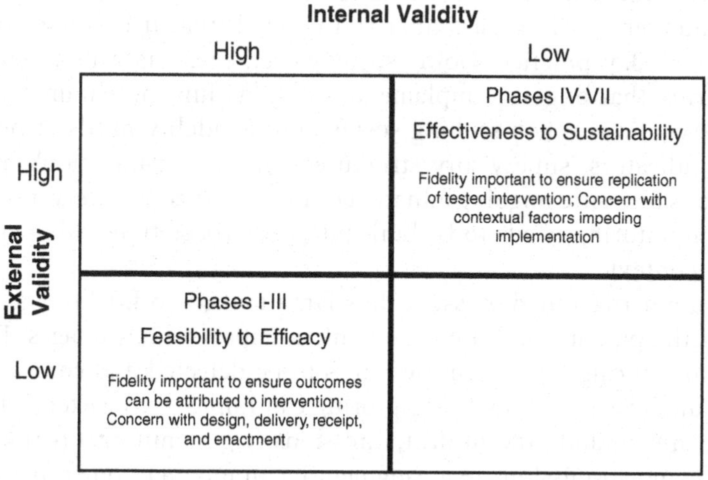

Figure 12.1 Role of fidelity in development, testing, and implementation phases.

common fidelity practice in an efficacy trial, these are impractical in a translation phase. Clinical sessions are not typically audiotaped, and in the few cases where this is possible, neither agencies nor clinical personnel typically have the time to review and code recordings to assess fidelity.

Consider the case of the Skills$_2$Care^R program. This intervention was initially tested as part of the NIH REACH I initiative. In this efficacy trial, audiotapes of 10% of intervention sessions were listened to and rated by two research staff along various dimensions (Gitlin et al., 2003) using a monitoring form similar to the one shown in Table 12.2. A score was derived reflecting the level of adherence achieved for that session; also, strengths and concerns were documented, and then shared with interventionists in one-on-one supervisory sessions in order to provide course corrections early in the trial. Subsequently, common errors detected across interventionists were discussed at group supervisory sessions. Reasons for their occurrences were explored, and solutions were derived and documented.

However, when the Skills$_2$Care^R program was translated and implemented in busy home care practices (Gitlin, Jacobs, & Earland, 2010), this approach was not feasible. Other approaches had to be adopted, such as having supervisors review session-by-session checklists that documented the elements delivered in sessions. Indicators of fidelity were subsequently built into the documentation of each contact with clients, and checklists were developed for ease of use by clinical supervisors. Understanding the challenges that present at the implementation phases can inform the development of fidelity strategies and measures early on in the process of building an intervention. Integrating fidelity processes into the intervention protocol may help researchers avoid the need to reconfigure fidelity approaches in the latter phases of rolling out an intervention.

The role of fidelity in dissemination and then in the maintenance or the sustainability phase of an intervention is unknown. In disseminating a proven program, of importance is to specify what can and what cannot be modified in terms of treatment delivery characteristics. As to sustainability, it is unclear as to what constitutes an effective fidelity plan when an intervention is fully integrated and being maintained in a delivery setting. The goal of sustainability is to normalize an intervention in a particular setting such that it becomes habituated and part of everyday practice. Doing so, however, presents a new set of challenges for assuring that ongoing implementation is within the parameters of the original intervention. When seeking sustainability, fidelity needs to be aligned with quality indicators, supervisory structures, and an organization's quality control procedures to assure ongoing adherence. To normalize an intervention in practice, fidelity monitoring needs to be built into the expectation and operations of that delivery context.

To summarize our discussion thus far, attention to fidelity is critical at every phase of the pipeline and doing so confers important advantages. First, monitoring and measuring fidelity enable errors to be detected and course corrections to be instituted. Second, fidelity monitoring can improve consistency in the delivery of the treatment and prevent drift, omissions (e.g., omitting a particular treatment element), and co-missions (e.g., augmenting an intervention with a new treatment element) or their co-occurrence. Third, attending to fidelity helps to further define and refine an intervention.

TABLE 12.2   Example of a Monitoring Checklist for a Dementia Caregiver Intervention Session

Interventionist: _____
Reviewer: _____

Date of Session: _____
Date Reviewed: _____

	Effectively Met (2)	Partially Met (1)	Not Met (0)	N/A	Comments
Preparedness					
1. Did interventionist appropriately greet the caregiver and the person with dementia?					
2. Did interventionist accurately describe the Tailored Activity Program and the specific purpose of Session 1?					
3. Did interventionist have all necessary materials available?					
a. Documentation binder					
b. Education materials					
c. Assessment tools					
4a. Was interventionist able to answer questions asked by caregiver concerning the session and/or research study?					
4b. If not, did he or she indicate that he or she would check with supervisor and get back to respondent within a day or two?					
Professionalism					
1. Did interventionist speak in a clear audible voice?					
2. Was the volume of interventionist's voice appropriate?					
3. Did interventionist use a calm voice?					

(Continued)

TABLE 12.2   Example of a Monitoring Checklist for a Dementia Caregiver Intervention Session   (Continued)

Interventionist: _____

Date of Session: _____

Reviewer: _____

Date Reviewed: _____

	Effectively Met (2)	Partially Met (1)	Not Met (0)	N/A	Comments
4. Was interventionist polite?					
5. Did it appear that sufficient rapport was established between interventionist and caregiver/person with dementia?					
6. Were interruptions and/or other unexpected occurrences handled professionally?					
7. Was the caregiver/person with dementia treated with respect and his or her wishes adhered to?					
8. Did interventionist use nonmedical and nontechnical language?					
9. Did interventionist express confidence and enthusiasm in the intervention?					
Flow and Compliance: **Did the interventionist . . .**					
1. Demonstrate knowledge of intervention goals and objectives?					
2. Clearly introduce session goals?					
3. Stay focused on session goals?					
4. Indicate the intervention includes eight sessions over 3 months, discussing flexibility of meeting schedule?					

(Continued)

TABLE 12.2 Example of a Monitoring Checklist for a Dementia Caregiver Intervention Session (*Continued*)

Interventionist: _____   Date of Session: _____
Reviewer: _____   Date Reviewed: _____

	Effectively Met (2)	Partially Met (1)	Not Met (0)	N/A	Comments
5. Actively engage caregiver in telling his or her story (e.g., asking what a typical day is like)?					
6. Confirm and discuss behaviors identified in interview and/or new or upsetting behaviors?					
7. Periodically ask caregiver if he or she had any questions or understood the purpose of the session and/or points being made?					
8. Refer to information caregiver provided during interview?					
9. Provide and review educational materials and discuss in context of each target behavior?					
10. Obtain closure for the session (e.g., reviews what was accomplished, sets up next session, provides homework, reviews strategies to try)?					

Score:
Summary of strengths, concerns:
Action plan:

DEVELOPING A FIDELITY PLAN

Consistent with previous definitions (Bellg et al., 2004; Gearing et al., 2011; Lichstein et al., 1994) and our own experiences, we recommend that a fidelity plan attend to four aspects: the study design, and the delivery, receipt, and enactment of an intervention. We also recommend that strategies be introduced to *enhance*, *monitor*, and *measure* each of these four aspects. An example of a fidelity plan is shown in Table 12.3.

Strategies for Assuring Study Design Integrity

With regard to study design and to ensure trial integrity, a fidelity plan might include, but does not have to be limited to, the development of a Manual of Procedures for implementing the overall trial design, as well as specific interview protocols, codebooks, and certification procedures for training interviewers and other research staff. External collaborators, advisory boards, or Data and Safety Monitoring Boards (DSMBs) can also help monitor fidelity or suggest strategies for fidelity assessment. Randomization efforts should be conducted by an independent investigator who is not part of the project team. In addition, periodic reports should be submitted to a DSMB (see Chapter 13), or another external advisory or oversight board for their fair and impartial review of data collection and fidelity-monitoring procedures.

Strategies for Delivery

To enhance the consistent and accurate delivery of an intervention, strategies to enhance, monitor, and measure this aspect may include the purposeful and careful selection, training, and certification of interventionists. Further, ongoing and regular meetings with interventionists in which feedback as well as direct observations, review of audiotaped sessions, or the use of monitoring checklists to quantify adherence to session protocols is provided, can be used to both monitor and measure fidelity among interventionists. Furthermore, the use of study folders, checklists, and forms to track dose and intensity can also be helpful strategies (Spillane et al., 2007).

Strategies for Receipt

To enhance, monitor, and measure receipt of an intervention, participants can be asked to demonstrate a particular skill or knowledge of material or to complete worksheets that reinforce the information provided as part of the intervention. Ongoing assessment and monitoring of knowledge or skill attainment can provide an understanding of what is (or is not) working, to address participants' questions and to identify barriers to participation. To this end, checklists or measures of the level of receptivity or understanding of the participant and pre- and posttest readiness and knowledge and skills assessments may be useful.

Strategies for Enactment

Lastly, fidelity should include enhancements for enactment and ways to monitor and measure this aspect. Enhancement for enactment may include providing ongoing

TABLE 12.3 Example of a Fidelity Plan

Domain	Enhancements	Monitoring Procedures	Measurement

Trial design	■ Based on theory
	■ Manual of Procedures
	■ External oversight by DSMB and IRB
	
	Interviewing
	■ Interviewer manuals with question-by-question codebook
	■ Interviewer training and certification procedures
	■ Weekly/biweekly interviewer meetings in which interviews are presented and discussed
	■ Weekly tracking reports for follow-up interview scheduling
	■ Double-check coding of all interviews by others than interviewer
	■ Maintain blinding to study allocation
	■ Maintain detailed list of coding decisions, which are routinely referred to
	
	Randomization
	■ Randomization forms developed by statistician who does not reveal allocation and blocking scheme
	■ Randomization occurs by a researcher who is not part of the project team
	
	Alerts and Adverse Event Tracking
	■ Training in event-tracking form
	■ Weekly review of events with principal investigator (PI)
		■ Periodic reports to and review by DSMB or other oversight board
		■ Regular investigator meetings
		
		■ Audiotape of interview sessions and random review of more than 10% using a monitoring form from which to derive quantification of adherence to protocol
		■ Direct observation of select interviews and ratings concerning
		  ■ Adherence to protocol
		  ■ Omissions
		  ■ Commissions
		  ■ Drift
		  ■ Competence
		
		■ Periodic checks of randomization forms and allocations by statistician
		■ Monitoring of randomization infractions using protocol-tracking forms
		
		■ Weekly reviews by project manager and PI to assure all alerts/adverse events have been documented and addressed adequately
		■ Completion of tracking forms
		■ DSMB and IRB oversight of adverse event tracking
			■ Off protocol-tracking forms
			
			■ Completed certification forms
			■ Quality control questions at end of interview
			■ Interviewer best guess as to group assignment
			■ Study follow-up satisfaction interview of participants to assure quality of delivery
			■ Ratings from monitoring forms used to review audiotape and/or videotape sessions
			
			■ Number of protocol violations
			
			■ Number of alerts and timely resolution
			■ Number of adverse events and resolution

(Continued)

TABLE 12.3   Example of a Fidelity Plan *(Continued)*

Domain	Enhancements	Monitoring Procedures	Measurement
Delivery Is the intervention delivered as intended?	**Interventionist** ■ Use of a treatment manual ■ Systematic training program ■ Certification process in which interventionist demonstrates knowledge and competencies ■ Use of interactive training including role-play to enhance learning ■ Ongoing regular meetings to review case presentations ■ Audiotaped sessions ■ Direct observation of sessions	■ Ongoing regular meetings to monitor cases and documentation ■ Completion of session-by-session tracking forms of activities per intervention session ■ Observation of select intervention sessions ■ Review of audiotapes for ■ Adherence to protocol ■ Omissions ■ Commissions ■ Drift ■ Competence	■ Knowledge test (pre–post) ■ Post evaluation of training by interventionists ■ Monitoring checklists that provide quantification of adherence to session protocols
	Delivery to End User (Participant) ■ Use of a range of techniques to enhance knowledge and skill acquisition ■ Calendar to track use of strategies ■ Study folder with study materials	■ Completion of a "delivery assessment form" at completion of each session. Form documents treatment elements including dose and time spent	■ Quantification of dose and intensity ■ Checklist of activities completed at each session
Receipt Did participant receive intervention as intended?	■ Participant provides return demonstration of a particular skill ■ Use of worksheets for reinforcement of information provided ■ Approach tailored to readiness of participant	■ Checking in at each session to evaluate what works and what is not working and address questions ■ Identification of barriers to participation	■ Checklist of level of receptivity, understanding of participant ■ Readiness ratings pre and post
Enactment Did caregiver use knowledge and/or skills as prescribed during, between, and after sessions?	■ Validation of knowledge and skills	■ Review of strategies provided ■ Videotaping of select sessions	■ Measure of use or proximal outcome expected from intervention ■ Checklist of observed engagement ■ Follow-up survey of continued use of strategies ■ Observation checklist used by interventionist to rate participant use of strategies

DSMB, Data and Safety Monitoring Board; IRB, Institutional Review Board; PI, Principal Investigator.

validation of a participant's knowledge and skills and progress in an intervention, as well as having procedures in place for continued monitoring and measurement of skills and adherence to the intervention protocol. Such strategies may include review or booster sessions, as well as use of follow-up surveys or observations to assess current level of engagement and use of previously taught skills and strategies (see Table 12.3).

CONSIDERATIONS IN DEVELOPING A FIDELITY PLAN

Considerations when developing a fidelity plan include tailoring to the particular characteristics of an intervention study and the level of complexity needed to achieve an adequate approach.

With regard to tailoring, there is no single plan, form, questionnaire, or approach that can be used across all intervention studies to address fidelity. Strategies need to be customized to the nuances of the study. To illustrate the tailoring of strategies to a study and the range of approaches available to investigators, we highlight the fidelity plan by Washington and colleagues (2014) for their educational intervention (Families Matter in Long-Term Care) to improve family involvement and promote better resident, family, and staff outcomes in 6 nursing homes and 18 residential care/assisted living settings. The authors describe their plan as follows:

> Several fidelity strategies were conceived at the design phase. First, a participant would receive a full dose of the intervention by attending the entire workshop and implementing a service plan. To encourage workshop attendance, letters were mailed to families and an announcement about the upcoming workshop was posted in the community newsletter. To track attendance, participants were asked to sign in. Also, all participants received a certificate of completion, and staff members who attended the workshop received continuing education credits. During the workshop, participants practiced creating meaningful service plans. A supply list was provided to families to aid in the development of the service plans. These supplies were made available to families to ensure that they possessed the materials required to successfully perform the activities (for example, watering pots, pedometers, art supplies). To track adherence to the service plans, families were to have ongoing contact with the interventionist by way of follow-up telephone calls at one month, three months, and five months after service plan development and postcard reminders at months two and four. During the calls, participants would be asked whether a service plan was created; if not, why not; and if so, to what extent it was being followed as planned. (Washington et al., 2014, pp. 2–3)

Another important consideration in developing a fidelity plan is the level of its complexity. The complexity of a fidelity plan may range from high to low depending upon several factors including the characteristics of the intervention, study design, and resources available to the investigative team. Multicomponent interventions and complex study designs will necessitate complex, multifaceted fidelity plans. Alternately, a simple intervention and design require less fidelity monitoring and measurement. This simple linear relationship between complexity of the study design and intervention and the subsequent fidelity plans is expressed in Figure 12.2.

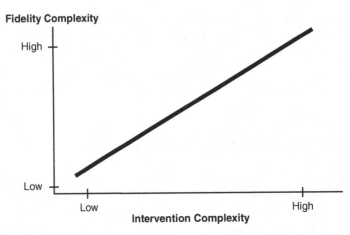

Figure 12.2   Relationship between intervention and fidelity with respect to their complexities.

Consider a single focused intervention such as one offering education on a particular topic (e.g., pain management in cancer care). When compared to a no-treatment control group, the fidelity plan would be rather straightforward and focus on the delivery of education, that is, whether the information provided was adequately received and understood by participants. In comparison, a fidelity plan for a multicomponent intervention that has several objectives (e.g., pain reduction, functional improvement, and improved activity engagement during cancer care) and multiple activities (e.g., education, behavioral activation, compensatory strategies) would be more complex. Enhancements, monitoring, and measuring of each treatment component and key activities would need to occur.

Take, for example, the multicomponent home-based intervention Get Busy Get Better: Helping Older Adults Beat the Blues (GBGB). GBGB, an intervention for African Americans 55 years of age or older with depressive symptoms (Gitlin et al., 2012, 2013), is designed to reduce depressive symptoms and improve overall well-being. Delivered by a social worker at home over eight 1-hour sessions, the intervention involves five treatment components: care management, referral and linkage, depression education and symptom detection, stress reduction, and behavioral activation. A fidelity plan for this type of intervention is necessarily multifaceted and complex. It involves enhancements to delivery, receipt, and enactment of each of its five treatment components, as well as monitoring and measuring them throughout the trial. For this trial, enhancements included creating treatment manuals, a standard training and certification approach for interventionists, structured clinical supervision, and use of motivational interviewing techniques to increase likelihood of enacting behavioral activation plans. To measure fidelity, randomly selected audiotapes were reviewed and rated for interventionist adherence, along with case presentations with feedback and the introduction of course corrections. This monitoring revealed that, at the start of the trial, a few of the interventionists were deviating from the protocol, which necessitated retraining, closer supervision, and, in one case, dismissal of the interventionist from the trial. As highly complex treatments increase the risk of lapses in treatment integrity, a carefully crafted fidelity plan is important.

The complexity of a trial design will also impact the intricacy of the fidelity plan. Trial designs that involve two or more treatment conditions or a comparative effectiveness study in which two active treatments are compared will require more complex fidelity plans. A fidelity plan would have to ensure integrity of the delivery, receipt, and enactment of each treatment condition and also how differentiation between the two treatment groups will be determined.

Illustrating this point is a study by Carpenter and colleagues (2013), which used a three-group randomized controlled trial comparing slow deep breathing (intervention), fast shallow breathing (attention control), and treatment as usual for management of menopausal hot flashes. They describe their fidelity plan as follows:

> The three-group design enabled blinding of participants and staff who were told the study compared two breathing programs to usual care. The breathing programs differed on the active ingredient (e.g., breath rate) but were otherwise similar in terms of appearance and content. Materials were delivered via an express mailing courier with delivery confirmation. Participants interacted with non-blinded staff to ensure that they understood and could use the materials (treatment receipt), but were otherwise using the materials at home on their own to self-manage their hot flashes. . . . Staff developed and closely followed a detailed set of standard operating procedures to ensure that study blinding, random assignment, and participant contacts occurred as planned. Any deviations to standard operating procedures were recorded carefully into a protocol deviations log, including any instances where staff or participants were unblinded to study condition. The log included the participant number, date of the event, study visit number, description of the event, reasons for the event, and any corrections or response to the event that were necessary. (Carpenter et al., 2013, p. 61)

As shown, various strategies were employed to assure adherence to each of the three conditions.

Staffing and budgetary resources also influence the level of complexity of a fidelity plan. Complex study designs and interventions require greater resources to enhance, monitor, and measure fidelity than simpler designs and interventions. When resources are limited, then identifying the most important elements that need to be enhanced, monitored, and measured is critical.

In the initial development and also evaluation phases, a minimal fidelity plan might include basic enhancements to delivery such as use of a manual and training protocol as well as monitoring delivery through direct observation of select intervention sessions or review of select audiotaped sessions. In the translation and implementation phases, attention to the adequate training of interventionists and assuring that the essential components of an intervention are delivered as intended are basic considerations. For dissemination, specification of what can be modified and what is immutable could minimally be provided.

Comprehensive and more elaborate fidelity plans, if resources permit, may include extensive measurement strategies that combine qualitative and quantitative approaches, or mixed methods. A mixed-methods approach may provide a fuller and more nuanced evaluation of fidelity (see Chapter 11; see also Albright, Gechter, & Kempe, 2013) and may afford multiple ways of seeing, hearing, and making sense of the implementation of a behavioral intervention (Greene, 2007). For example, an education intervention, administering a standardized scale to quantify knowledge attainment, could be combined with focus group methodology to obtain an in-depth understanding of how participants received and engaged with the intervention (e.g., treatment receipt and enactment). A mixed-methods approach complements the strengths and offsets the relative disadvantages of any one particular methodological approach and, therefore, provides important understandings of implementation processes (Albright et al., 2013).

CHALLENGES IN ENHANCING, MONITORING, AND MEASURING FIDELITY

We have identified six challenges concerning fidelity for which further attention is needed in order to advance this aspect of behavioral intervention research. These include the lack of guidelines, adequate funding, measures, reporting requirements, understanding of its analytic role, and understanding of its role in comparative effectiveness studies.

Foremost is the lack of firm guidance as to how to best enhance, monitor, and measure the core components of fidelity, especially given the wide variations in fidelity definitions, frameworks, and models employed in intervention studies. It is unclear as to whether certain enhancement strategies are more effective than others and which enhancements work best for which types of interventions, populations, and settings. Also unclear are best practices concerning supervisory approaches, the impact of course corrections on trial outcomes, which training techniques of interventionists are most effective, and what are the most optimal strategies for delivering effective interventions and enhancing their receipt and enactment. As enhancement, monitoring, and measurement approaches remain idiosyncratic and tailored to specific interventions, comparing fidelity strategies across intervention studies to derive best practices has not been feasible.

Gearing and colleagues (2011) provide the most comprehensive guidelines and practices to date on the basis of their systematic review of 24 meta-analyses and review articles reporting on fidelity. Nevertheless, the lack of written documentation concerning best fidelity practices leaves investigators dependent upon a limited set of publications on this topic and their own experiences. Fortunately, new studies are emerging to examine this issue. For example, Stirman and colleagues (2013) are investigating whether clinicians receiving post-workshop support subsequently deliver a cognitive processing therapy with better consistency (fidelity) and whether this in turn improves patient outcomes. Their study is in progress and as such, results are not available. However, findings from their study will be useful in helping to establish coaching and supervisory approaches when testing behavioral interventions.

A second challenge is funding for developing and implementing fidelity plans as it requires resources including staffing, time, and sufficient funding (Spillane et al., 2007). In the early phases of intervention development in which resources are focused on the end goal of feasibility and safety, fidelity considerations can easily be viewed as less important and relegated to a back seat, if addressed at all. In evaluation phases (efficacy and effectiveness), some minimal fidelity plan is required, but again the extent to which fidelity is enhanced, monitored, and measured can vary widely across trials depending upon available resources and their allocation.

The importance of attending to fidelity must be matched by resources that can be allocated to this endeavor.

The third challenge is measurement. Currently, there are no standardized assessments or measures for different aspects of fidelity. Investigators typically create their own monitoring forms and measurement approaches. Given the significant limitations in time and funding, most investigator-developed fidelity measures are not submitted to a validation process. Additionally, fidelity measures tend to be study specific; hence, comparison of fidelity outcomes across intervention studies on similar dimensions is not always possible. In order to derive an understanding of acceptable levels of adherence and impact on outcomes for different interventions, objective, well-validated measures are needed along with the development of measurement strategies that integrate both objective and subjective appraisals of fidelity. A related point is that it is unclear as to the causal pathways between fidelity and trial outcomes. Different levels of adherence among interventionists or different adherence levels to intervention strategies by study participants may impact trial results; yet, these relationships have not been systematically considered (Hardeman et al., 2008).

The fourth challenge concerns the need for better reporting guidelines and requirements for grant applications and publications. Grant reviewers are not necessarily instructed in nor may they understand the need to evaluate the quality and effectiveness of a fidelity plan for a proposed intervention study in a grant application. In a grant application, a fidelity plan should be presented near the end of the design section and after the description of the intervention. Page limitations, however, can constrain the level of detail provided for a fidelity plan (up to 12 pages for most NIH applications). Including a detailed description of a fidelity approach can be challenging. Providing a table describing enhancements, monitoring approaches, and measures of each fidelity component (study design, delivery, receipt, and enactment) may be one strategy for overcoming space limitations.

Similarly, journal reviewers of a manuscript reporting treatment outcomes may not critically appraise whether an acceptable level of adherence was obtained (Naleppa & Cagle, 2010). Most checklists for reporting trials, such as the 2010 Consolidated Standards of Reporting Trials (CONSORT) (see www.consort-statement.org/), do not explicitly include the need to report fidelity methods, measures, or outcomes.

Additionally, there are limited opportunities to include fidelity plans and outcomes in a comprehensive report. In main trial outcome papers, fidelity considerations are typically consigned to a few sentences as part of the description of the intervention that confirm treatment integrity was monitored and achieved. An exemplar is the publication by Barsky and Ahern (2004), which reports the results of a randomized trial designed to test a cognitive behavior therapy program for hypochondriasis. The authors appropriately address fidelity in a brief description as follows:

> Treatment fidelity was assessed by auditing audiotapes of randomly selected therapy sessions from all 3 therapists; adherence to the CBT manual was excellent. Receipt of the consultation letter was acknowledged by 96.8% of the primary care physicians. (pp. 1465–1466)

As most journals have word limitations, this is a typical minimalist statement that authors have begun to appropriately include and which is expected.

Although fidelity considerations are not yet part of main stream clinical trial literature, there is increasing awareness of the importance to do so. Consequently, more attention will be afforded to this aspect of intervention development, and we suspect and hope that more careful disclosure of fidelity plans and outcomes will be required. At a minimum, in a trial outcome paper, a brief overview of a fidelity plan and adherence results should be presented after a description of an intervention and before the discussion section (Davidson et al., 2003). Also, researchers are now reporting fidelity outcomes in publications separate from the main trial outcome publication so that more careful delineation of the fidelity plan and results can be presented. Examples of this approach include the publication of Long and colleagues (2010) on therapist fidelity with a multicomponent cognitive behavioral intervention for posttraumatic stress disorder; or the publication of Hardeman and colleagues (2008) on adherence to behavior change techniques used in a physical activity intervention.

Yet another issue is the role of fidelity in analyses. It is unclear whether an indicator of adherence level should serve as an outcome, a covariate, a moderator, or a mediator. It may be that for some interventions, a certain level of exposure or enactment is required for a benefit to be achieved. In Lichstein and colleagues' (1994) example of a hypertension medication intervention, benefits may occur only if a patient strictly conforms to the medication dosing; for the GBGB, enactment of only one of three behavioral activation prescriptions may be needed to realize a benefit (Gitlin et al., 2013). A fidelity plan that included appropriate design and measurement features could help to address these key questions.

Finally, a sixth challenge is the role of fidelity in comparative effectiveness research. As the focus in this type of trial is the comparison of two distinct interventions, assuring fidelity to each treatment arm and assuring that each is differentiated from the other are critical.

CONCLUSION

Although there is an increasing recognition of, and attention to, the importance of fidelity, there is still a lack of clarity in the definition and operationalization of this construct. Moreover, there is inconsistency in the methods employed for measuring fidelity, and fidelity results are rarely reported in publications of behavioral intervention research. Nevertheless, it is clear that the cost of low fidelity is substantial and may include the rejection of an effective program, the acceptance of an ineffective program, or the inability to replicate a program.

As discussed, fidelity has a different role depending upon the phase of development of a particular intervention. In development phases, attention to fidelity enables an evaluation of the feasibility of implementation; whereas, in the evaluation phases, attention to fidelity helps to optimize an understanding of treatment outcomes and whether a desired outcome is due to the intervention itself or the way it was implemented, or if other potential factors are responsible for outcomes. Its role further changes in the implementation phases; here, fidelity becomes an important outcome in its own right (Proctor et al., 2011) and serves as a key indicator of the replication potential of the intervention. However, the role of fidelity and how fidelity plans are implemented when seeking to sustain an intervention are not clear and remain uncharted.

As an intervention is being developed, evaluated, and implemented, careful attention needs to be given to fidelity. Specifically, attention should be given to three activities: enhancing, monitoring, and measuring four components that are study design, and the delivery, receipt, and enactment of the intervention itself. The level of complexity of a fidelity plan that is executed will reflect several factors: the phase of intervention development, purpose of fidelity, the characteristics of the intervention itself (e.g., its treatment components, dosage, and activities), financial and staffing resources, and intricacy of the study design (e.g., type of control group employed). As addressing fidelity requires resources, fidelity plans can be challenging to implement. At a minimum, some form of tracking of study design and intervention processes is critical to provide a level of assurance that an intervention is being delivered as intended.

REFERENCES

Albright, K., Gechter, K., & Kempe, A. (2013). Importance of mixed methods in pragmatic trials and dissemination and implementation research. *Academic Pediatrics, 13*(5), 400–407. doi:10.1016/j.acap.2013.06.010

Barsky, A. J., & Ahern, D. K. (2004). Cognitive behavior therapy for hypochondriasis: A randomized controlled trial. *JAMA, 291*(12), 1464–1470.

Bass, D. M., & Judge, K. S. (2010). Challenges implementing evidence-based programs. *Generations, 34*(1), 51–58.

Bellg, A. J., Borrelli, B., Resnick, B., Hecht, J., Minicucci, D. S., Ory, M., . . . Czajkowski, S. (2004). Enhancing treatment fidelity in health behavior change studies: Best practices and recommendations from the NIH behavior change consortium. *Health Psychology, 23*(5), 443–451.

Bond, G. R., Evans, L., Salyers, M. P., Williams, J., & Kim, H. (2000). Measurement of fidelity in psychiatric rehabilitation. *Mental Health Services Research, 2*(2), 75–87.

Burgio, L., Lichstein, K. L., Nichols, L., Czaja, S., Gallagher-Thompson, D., Bourgeois, M., . . . REACH Investigators. (2001). Judging outcomes in psychosocial interventions for dementia caregivers: The problem of treatment implementation. *The Gerontologist, 41*(4), 481–489.

Callahan, C. M., Kales, H. C., Gitlin, L. N., & Lyketsos, C. G. (2013). The historical development and state of the art approach to design and delivery of dementia care services. In H. de Waal, C. G. Lyketsos, D. Ames, & J. O'Brien (Eds.), *Designing and delivering dementia services* (pp.17–30). Hoboken, NJ: Wiley-Blackwell.

Carpenter, J. S., Burns, D. S., Wu, J., Yu, M., Ryker, K., Tallman, E., & Von Ah, D. (2013). Strategies used and data obtained during treatment fidelity monitoring. *Nursing Research, 62*(1), 59–65. doi:10.1097/NNR.0b013e31827614fd

Carroll, C., Patterson, M., Wood, S., Booth, A., Rick, J., & Balain, S. (2007). A conceptual framework for implementation fidelity. *Implementation Science, 2*(40), 1–9.

Chee, Y. K., Gitlin, L. N., Dennis, M. P., & Hauck, W. W. (2007). Predictors of adherence to a skill-building intervention in dementia caregivers. *The Journals of Gerontology. Series A, Biological Sciences and Medical Sciences, 62*(6), 673–678.

Chen, H. (1990). *Theory-driven evaluations.* Newbury Park, CA: Sage.

Cook, T. D., Campbell, D. T., & Day, A. (1979). *Quasi-experimentation: Design & analysis issues for field settings.* Boston, MA: Houghton Mifflin.

Dane, A. V., & Schneider, B. H. (1998). Program integrity in primary and early secondary prevention: Are implementation effects out of control? *Clinical Psychology Review, 18*(1), 23–45.

Davidson, K. W., Goldstein, M., Kaplan, R. M., Kaufmann, P. G., Knatterud, G. L., Orleans, C. T., . . . Whitlock, E. P. (2003). Evidence-based behavioral medicine: What is it and how do we achieve it? *Annals of Behavioral Medicine, 26*(3), 161–171.

Dusenbury, L., Brannigan, R., Falco, M., & Hansen, W. B. (2003). A review of research on fidelity of implementation: Implications for drug abuse prevention in school settings. *Health Education Research, 18*(2), 237–256.

Gearing, R. E., El-Bassel, N., Ghesquiere, A., Baldwin, S., Gillies, J., & Ngeow, E. (2011). Major ingredients of fidelity: A review and scientific guide to improving quality of intervention research implementation. *Clinical Psychology Review, 31*(1), 79–88.

Gitlin, L. N., Belle, S. H., Burgio, L. D., Czaja, S. J., Mahoney, D., Gallagher-Thompson, D., . . . Schulz, R. (2003). Effect of multicomponent interventions on caregiver burden and depression: The REACH multisite initiative at 6-month follow-up. *Psychology and Aging, 18*(3), 361–374. doi:10.1037/0882-7974.18.3.361

Gitlin, L. N., Harris, L. F., McCoy, M., Chernett, N. L., Jutkowitz, E., Pizzi, L. T., & Beat the Blues Team. (2012). A community-integrated home-based depression intervention for older African Americans: Description of the Beat the Blues randomized trial and intervention costs. *BMC Geriatrics, 12*(4), 1–11. doi:10.1186/1471-2318-12-4

Gitlin, L. N., Harris, L. F., McCoy, M. C., Chernett, N. L., Pizzi, L. T., Jutkowitz, E., . . . Hauck, W. W. (2013). A home-based intervention to reduce depressive symptoms and improve quality of life in older African Americans: A randomized trial. *Annals of Internal Medicine, 159*(4), 243–252. doi:10.7326/0003-4819-159-4-201308200-00005

Gitlin, L. N., Jacobs, M., & Earland, T. V. (2010). Translation of a dementia caregiver intervention for delivery in homecare as a reimbursable Medicare service: Outcomes and lessons learned. *The Gerontologist, 50*(6), 847–854. doi:10.1093/geront/gnq057

Greene, J. C. (2007). *Mixed methods in social inquiry.* San Francisco, CA: Jossey-Bass.

Gresham, F. M. (2005). Treatment integrity and therapeutic change: Commentary on Perepletchikova and Kazdin. *Clinical Psychology: Science and Practice, 12*(4), 391–394.

Hardeman, W., Michie, S., Fanshawe, T., Prevost, A. T., Mcloughlin, K., & Kinmonth, A. L. (2008). Fidelity of delivery of a physical activity intervention: Predictors and consequences. *Psychology and Health, 23*(1), 11–24.

Hasson, H. (2010). Systematic evaluation of implementation fidelity of complex interventions in health and social care. *Implementation Science, 5*(67), 1–9. doi:10.1186/1748-5908-5-67

Hohmann, A. A., & Shear, M. K. (2002). Community-based intervention research: Coping with the "noise" of real life in study design. *American Journal of Psychiatry, 159*(2), 201–207.

Lichstein, K. L., Riedel, B. W., & Grieve, R. (1994). Fair tests of clinical trials: A treatment implementation model. *Advances in Behaviour Research and Therapy, 16*(1), 1–29.

Long, M. E., Grubaugh, A. L., Elhai, J. D., Cusack, K. J., Knapp, R., & Frueh, B. C. (2010). Therapist fidelity with an exposure-based treatment of PTSD in adults with schizophrenia or schizoaffective disorder. *Journal of Clinical Psychology, 66*(4), 383–393.

Mills, S. C., & Ragan, T. J. (2000). A tool for analyzing implementation fidelity of an integrated learning system. *Educational Technology Research and Development, 48*(4), 21–41.

Moncher, F. J., & Prinz, R. J. (1991). Treatment fidelity in outcome studies. *Clinical Psychology Review, 11*(3), 247–266.

Mowbray, C. T., Holter, M. C., Teague, G. B., & Bybee, D. (2003). Fidelity criteria: Development, measurement, and validation. *American Journal of Evaluation, 24*(3), 315–340.

Naleppa, M. J., & Cagle, J. G. (2010). Treatment fidelity in social work intervention research: A review of published studies. *Research on Social Work Practice, 20*(6), 674–681. doi:10.1177/1049731509352088

Ory, M., Jordan, P. J., & Bazzarre, T. (2002). The Behavior Change Consortium: Setting the stage for a new century of health behavior change research. *Health Education Research, 17,* 500–511.

Perepletchikova, F., & Kazdin, A. E. (2005). Treatment integrity and therapeutic change: Issues and research recommendations. *Clinical Psychology: Science and Practice, 12*(4), 365–383.

Perepletchikova, F., Treat, T. A., & Kazdin, A. E. (2007). Treatment integrity in psychotherapy research: Analysis of the studies and examination of the associated factors. *Journal of Consulting and Clinical Psychology, 75*(6), 829–841.

Proctor, E., Silmere, H., Raghavan, R., Hovmand, P., Aarons, G., Bunger, A., . . . & Hensley, M. (2011). Outcomes for implementation research: Conceptual distinctions, measurement challenges, and research agenda. *Administration and Policy in Mental Health and Mental Health Services Research, 38*(2), 65–76.

Prohaska, T. R., & Peters, K. E. (2007). Physical activity and cognitive functioning: Translating research to practice with a public health approach. *Alzheimer's & Dementia, 3*(2), S58–S64.

Santacroce, S. J., Maccarelli, L. M., & Grey, M. (2004). Intervention fidelity. *Nursing Research, 53*(1), 63–66.

Sechrest, L., & Yeaton, W. E. (1981). Assessing the effectiveness of social programs: Methodological and conceptual issues. *New Directions for Program Evaluation, 1981*(9), 41–56.

Spillane, V., Byrne, M. C., Byrne, M., Leathem, C. S., O'Malley, M., & Cupples, M. E. (2007). Monitoring treatment fidelity in a randomized controlled trial of a complex intervention. *Journal of Advanced Nursing, 60*(3), 343–352. doi:10.1111/j.1365-2648.2007.04386.x

Stirman, S. W., Miller, C. J., Toder, K., & Calloway, A. (2013). Development of a framework and coding system for modifications and adaptations of evidence-based interventions. *Implementation Science, 8*(65), 1–12.

Strijk, J. E., Proper, K. I., van der Beek, A. J., & van Mechelen, W. (2011). A process evaluation of a worksite vitality intervention among ageing hospital workers. *International Journal of Behavioral Nutrition Physical Activity, 8*(58), 1–9.

Swanson, E., Wanzek, J., Haring, C., Ciullo, S., & McCulley, L. (2011). Intervention fidelity in special and general education research journals. *The Journal of Special Education, 47*(1), 3–13. doi:10.1177/0022466911419516

Tomioka, M., & Braun, K. L. (2013). Implementing evidence-based programs: A four-step protocol for assuring replication with fidelity. *Health Promotion Practice, 14*(6), 850–858. doi:10.1177/1524839912469205

Washington, T., Zimmerman, S., Cagle, J., Reed, D., Cohen, L., Beeber, A. S., & Gwyther, L. P. (2014). Fidelity decision making in social and behavioral research: Alternative measures of dose and other considerations. *Social Work Research, 38*(3), 154–162. doi:10.1093/swr/svu021

Wilson, M. G., Basta, T. B., Bynum, B. H., DeJoy, D. M., Vandenberg, R. J., & Dishman, R. K. (2010). Do intervention fidelity and dose influence outcomes? Results from the move to improve worksite physical activity program. *Health Education Research, 25*(2), 294–305. doi:10.1093/her/cyn065

Yeaton, W. H., & Sechrest, L. (1981). Critical dimensions in the choice and maintenance of successful treatments: Strength, integrity, and effectiveness. *Journal of Consulting and Clinical Psychology, 49*(2), 156–167.

Zauszniewski, J. A. (2012). Intervention development: Assessing critical parameters from the intervention recipient's perspective. *Applied Nursing Research, 25*(1), 31–39.

THIRTEEN

ETHICAL CONSIDERATIONS IN BEHAVIORAL INTERVENTION RESEARCH

Research is a public trust that must be ethically conducted, trustworthy, and socially responsible if the results are to be valuable.
—University of Minnesota (2003)

Behavioral intervention research by its nature involves human participants; thus, ethical considerations with respect to the involvement and treatment of research participants is a critical issue at all phases of the pipeline and throughout the research process. Because of its importance and owing to many horrific incidents that have occurred with research participants (e.g., The Tuskegee Syphilis Trial), ethical considerations are critical and reflect fundamental principles as to how to conduct behavioral intervention research. Also, ethical conduct in research is increasingly being scrutinized by funding agencies and research institutions, and there is greater oversight.

Many countries have specific ethical standards for the conduct of research. In the United States, there are many guidelines and requirements at the federal, local, and institutional levels, with which investigators must comply when conducting research with human participants. Professional organizations such as the American Psychological Association also have research ethics policies. In fact, most universities/research institutions have offices/programs dedicated to research ethics that go beyond Institutional Review Boards (IRBs) to include ongoing seminars, training courses, and consultant services to help ensure that the research conducted by investigators within the institution adheres to the highest ethical standards. At all institutions throughout the United States, and consistent with the policy of the National Institutes of Health (NIH), investigators and in fact all members of a research team, including community partners, must complete training and become certified in the ethical conduct of research before they can engage in any type of research with human participants and receive research grant awards. Although these requirements may sometimes seem to be a nuisance or hinder the progress of behavioral intervention research, they are designed to ensure adherence to fundamental ethical behavior. These requirements underscore the importance of carefully considering ethical issues. Such policies, trainings, and procedures help investigators understand pertinent ethical considerations, including, for example, obtaining informed consent from vulnerable populations such as those that may have some cognitive impairment, providing honorariums for study participation yet assuring this is not coercive, or protecting identifiable information of human participants.

Offices of research ethics and related policies and procedures also help investigators manage ethical dilemmas that might arise during the course of a study. For example, a wide range of issues unrelated to the research itself may be encountered such as physical or financial abuse of a participant, or hospitalization or death of a study participant, or home environmental problems (e.g., infestation, a hole in a roof), which impacts the health of participants. Similarly, a member of a research team may learn that a close colleague or another member of the team is violating ethical principles in an attempt to enhance recruitment efforts, or report better outcomes than the data suggest.

The topic of research ethics is complex and much has been written on ethical conduct in research. There is also a specialized discipline devoted to the study of research ethics—bioethics. The topic is dynamic—information and thinking in this area is continually evolving. For example, the widespread use of the Internet as a vehicle for data collection gives rise to new questions about the informed consent process and how use of the Internet impacts on issues related to privacy and confidentiality.

In this chapter, our goal is to provide an overview of the topic and highlight the critical issues that need to be considered in the conduct of behavioral intervention research. We begin with a brief overview of what falls within the umbrella of research ethics and some of the guidelines and requirements surrounding the ethical conduct of research in general. We then discuss in more detail specific aspects of importance to behavioral intervention research such as the informed consent process, IRBs, adverse events (AEs), and the role of Data and Safety Monitoring Boards (DSMBs).

FUNDAMENTALS OF ETHICAL CONDUCT IN RESEARCH

As discussed throughout this book, behavioral intervention research has multiple goals. First and foremost is to develop a meaningful intervention to address a targeted problem area and population at risk, to determine its efficacy and effectiveness, and to obtain the best outcomes for individuals, families, and/or their communities. Other goals include determining safety, cost-effectiveness, feasibility, and acceptability of an intervention and its implementation potential. Implicit in the conduct of intervention research is that ethical protocols are used to achieve these goals. A basic principle is that ethical goals do not justify unethical research practices to reach those goals even if the outcomes are beneficial in the long run. In fact, compromising ethics in any aspect when conducting a study to reach a larger ethical goal creates more ethical questions including whether the outcomes should be used or considered in decision making surrounding clinical practice or published in the literature (O'Mathúan, 2014). As noted by Beecher (1966) in his classic paper on ethics in clinical research, "An experiment is ethical or not at its inception; it does not become ethical post hoc—ends do not justify means. There is no ethical distinction between means and ends" (p. 372). This is a key point that needs to guide all actions related to behavioral intervention research.

As noted, there are numerous policies and guidelines governing research ethics, and a detailed discussion of these policies is beyond the scope of this chapter. International guidelines include the Declaration of Helsinki, The Council for International Organizations of Medical Sciences (CIOMS), International Ethical

Guidelines for Biomedical Research Involving Human Subjects, and the World Health Organization (WHO) and International Classification of Health (ICH) Guidelines for Good Clinical Practice. These guidelines are intended to facilitate and support ethical review worldwide and are intended to ensure that the dignity, rights, safety, and well-being of research participants are maintained and that the results of investigations are credible.

The Belmont Report (U.S. Department of Health and Human Services, 1979) is one of the most important documents guiding the ethical conduct of research in the United States. It is a statement of basic ethical principles and guidelines to assist in resolving the common and tricky ethical issues that arise during the conduct of research with human study participants. The report includes three important principles: (a) *Respect for Persons*: individuals should be treated as "autonomous agents," and those with diminished autonomy are entitled to protection; (b) *Beneficence*: do not harm individuals and maximize possible benefits and minimize possible harm; and (c) *Justice*: benefits to which an individual is entitled must not be denied without good reason or a burden being unnecessarily imposed.

This report was highly influential in the establishment of the current U.S. regulations for protection of human research participants (U.S. Department of Health and Human Services, 2009). These regulations include five subparts: subpart A, also known as the "Federal Policy" or the "Common Rule"; subpart B, additional protections for pregnant women, human fetuses, and neonates; subpart C, additional protections for prisoners; subpart D, additional protections for children; and (more recent) subpart E, registration of IRBs that conduct review of human research studies conducted or supported by Health and Human Services (HHS). The main elements of the Common Rule include requirements for assuring compliance by research institutions; requirements for researchers' obtaining and documenting informed consent; and requirements for IRB membership, function, operations, review of research, and record keeping. Investigators are typically introduced to, and receive training in, relevant policies when completing their institutional human subjects training.

Ethical Conduct in the Research Process

It is important to note that the ethical conduct of an intervention research study does not end with the informed consent, but must continue throughout the duration of the study no matter the stage of the pipeline. This means that the protection of the rights, interests, and safety of research participants, regardless of phase along the pipeline, must be considered during the recruitment process, data collection activities, handling of AEs, data storage activities, and data analysis and reporting. Most applications for federal, state, or foundation funding agencies require a dedicated section of a proposal that details the treatment of human subjects as part of the application process. This section of the application is also carefully evaluated within the NIH peer review process. Any infractions will require that the investigator address the issues raised prior for the proposal to be considered for funding.

There are several key reasons why it is important to adhere to ethical protocols in behavioral intervention research. Foremost, of course, is ensuring the protection of the rights, safety, and interests of research participants and the promotion of values such as social responsibility. Other reasons include the promotion of the general aims of research such as knowledge and truth and the avoidance of error; the promotion of values essential to collaborative work such as trust, accountability, and fairness; and the assurance that researchers are accountable to the public, which helps to build public support for research and adherence to regulations and guidelines (Resnik, 2011).

The ethical conduct of behavioral intervention research also encompasses honesty in scientific reporting; striving for objectivity; disclosure of personal or financial interests that may have an impact on a research project; respect for intellectual property such as patents and copyrights; protection of confidential information; responsible publication of research findings; and social responsibility and responsible mentoring (Shamoo & Resnik, 2009). In this regard, the U.S. government defines "fabrication, falsification, or plagiarism" as "misconduct." It is important to note that misconduct occurs only when a researcher intended to deceive or engage in what is considered to be unethical practice. Other examples of what is generally considered as misconduct within the scientific community include publishing the same paper in, or submitting the same paper to, two different journals without telling the editors; discussing confidential data with colleagues from a paper or grant that one is reviewing for a journal; trimming outliers from a data set without documenting the reasons in a publication; making significant deviations from the research protocol approved by the IRB; or failing to report an AE to the IRB (see Resnik, 2011 for a more complete list).

As noted by Resnik (2011), although codes, policies, and principles exist for the ethical conduct of research, they may not specifically cover every situation that arises. Thus, it is important to learn how to interpret and assess various situations. When in doubt, always consult the appropriate institutional office for assistance in resolving ethical issues. It is also useful to consult a trusted colleague or a more senior researcher who may have experience with the issue at hand.

Ethical Responsibilities of the Principal Investigator

A final comment relates to the responsibilities of a study's principal investigator (PI). Ultimately, the PI of an intervention study is responsible for assuring compliance with an institution's IRB policies, federal policies and regulations, oversight of the research, and the informed consent process. Although a PI may delegate tasks to other members of the research team, it is important to remember that the PI has the ultimate responsibility for the conduct of a study and is in charge of, and accountable for, all activities within a research project. Thus, a PI must be closely involved in the trial and directly interact with the research team. As we discuss in Chapter 22, the PI should have regular meetings with the research team to keep abreast of what is occurring within a trial and to discuss any issues or problems that arise.

INFORMED CONSENT

A critical component of the conduct of behavioral intervention research, regardless of phase along the pipeline, is the informed consent process. This involves preparing and administering an informed consent document to potential participants that has been preapproved by an IRB. The informed consent document operationalizes the principles described in the Belmont Report discussed previously. It describes what individuals need to know about their involvement in a behavioral intervention research study, including risks and benefits, in order to make an informed decision regarding consent to participate in the study. The informed consent document must include all essential information about the study, not be overly long or complex, and be written in lay language in an understandable way. In fact, most IRBs stress that an informed consent document must be written at an eighth-grade reading level or below. The Federal Government requirements for an informed consent document are presented in Table 13.1. In addition to these requirements, each institution usually has language that is required for an informed consent document. Therefore, it is always important to check with an institution's research or regulatory office prior to preparing an informed consent document. In addition, these documents must be approved by an institution's IRB before a study can commence.

The process of obtaining informed consent from potential study participants also needs careful consideration. It is critically important that participants understand what is contained in the document with respect to their involvement in the intervention study including the type of activities that they will be expected to perform, location of the study, time commitments, potential risks and benefits, and if there is compensation for participation. As an aside, compensation or an honorarium for participating in interviews or completing a study is common practice; however, the amount of compensation must be modest or reasonable and cannot appear to be or act as a form of coercion to participate. If there is any doubt that an individual is unable to comprehend what is in the document, it is advisable to read the document aloud to the person or ask him or her to summarize what is stated in the document. This might be accomplished by asking participants a series of questions. Common practice is to provide participants with a point-by-point verbal summary of the document before asking them to read and sign the form. Providing participants with the consent form prior to the face-to-face review can also facilitate the consenting process. In addition, as the PI's name and phone number are provided, he or she must always be available to answer any questions in person or by telephone. The member of the research team who has oriented and received the consent of the study participant must also sign and date the consent form. If the person is unable to speak English, the form should be in that person's preferred language and a team member who speaks that language should be available to answer questions. Consents that undergo translation into a language other than English need to be approved by the IRB and a certificate must be provided from a translational service indicating the methodology that was used.

In some studies, it may be necessary for a participant to sign a HIPAA (Health Insurance Portability and Accountability Act) Research Authorization form. Whereas the consent document reflects a participant's agreement to participate in a study, the authorization form allows an investigator to use or disclose the participant's protected health information (e.g., health status, birth date, address) to others delineated in the authorization form (e.g., funder, insurance company to obtain medical records). This form must also be signed and dated at the time that written consent for participation in the study is obtained.

TABLE 13.1   Federal Requirements for an Informed Consent Document

Eight Specific Areas That Must Be Addressed

1. A statement that the study involves research, an explanation of the purposes of the research and the expected duration of the subject's participation, a description of the procedures to be followed, and identification of any procedures which are experimental.

2. A description of any reasonably foreseeable risks or discomforts to the subject.

3. A description of any benefits to the subject or to others, which may reasonably be expected from the research.

4. A disclosure of appropriate alternative procedures or courses of treatment, if any, which might be advantageous to the subject including the alternative not to participate.

5. A statement describing the extent, if any, to which confidentiality of records identifying the subject will be maintained.

6. An explanation as to whether any compensation is provided and an explanation as to whether any medical treatments are available if injury occurs and, if so, what they consist of, or where further information may be obtained.

7. An explanation of whom to contact for answers to pertinent questions about the research and research subjects' rights and whom to contact in the event of a research-related injury to the subject.

8. A statement that participation is voluntary, refusal to participate will involve no penalty or loss of benefits, and the subject may discontinue participation at any time without penalty or loss of benefits to which the subject is otherwise entitled.

Additional Elements of Informed Consent When Appropriate

1. A statement that the particular treatment or procedure may involve risks to the subject (or to the embryo or fetus, if the subject is or may become pregnant), which are currently unforeseeable.

2. Anticipated circumstances under which the subject's participation may be terminated by the investigator without regard to the subject's consent.

3. Any additional costs to the subject that may result from participation in the research.

4. The consequences of a subject's decision to withdraw from the research and procedures for orderly termination of participation by the subject.

5. A statement that significant new findings developed during the course of the research which may relate to the subject's willingness to continue participation will be provided to the subject.

6. The approximate number of subjects involved in the study.

Source: U.S. Department of Health and Human Services (2009).

In addition, an IRB may require the use of an impartial third party to observe the consent process and verify that study participants fully understand a study; this procedure is typically used when enrolling vulnerable populations or for intervention protocols that are invasive or high risk. This might also be the case if a study involves participants with cognitive impairment or children. In general, vulnerable populations include children, prisoners, pregnant women and their fetuses, individuals with cognitive impairment or of lower socioeconomic status, students, or individuals in a subordinate role. In this case, the third-party person (a responsible party or proxy) must be someone who is independent of the potential participant and charged with protecting the individual's rights. A related point is that consideration should be given for re-consenting individuals with cognitive impairment or for those individuals who show cognitive decline over time in a study. Study participants may need to be re-consented to ensure that at each testing occasion there is an understanding of study procedures, that participating in the study is on a volunteer basis, and that the information they provide is confidential (Black, Kass, Fogarty, & Rabins, 2007; Black, Rabins, Sugarman, & Karlawish, 2010).

Finally, if there is a change in the research protocol or an investigator discovers new risks associated with study participation or that risks have increased or benefits decreased, it is usually necessary to re-consent study participants. In such cases, it is important to check with an institution's IRB office as to whether this is required and what procedures need to be used.

Federal requirements also state that study participants be given a copy of the signed consent document. The original informed consent documents must be stored in a secure location in the research office that is separate from the area where other study documents that contain de-identified participant information are filed (e.g., questionnaires, surveys, observation checklists, interview notes).

INSTITUTIONAL REVIEW BOARDS

For institutions engaging in funded research by HHS, such as the NIH, and involving human participants, the U.S. Federal Government requires such institutions to have an IRB. In addition, the HHS regulations require a written assurance from the performance-site institution that the institution will comply with the HHS regulations regarding protection of human subjects. The institution must also formally register the members and policies of the IRB. At most institutions, the IRB applies HHS regulations regarding human participation to all studies conducted at the institution whether or not they are funded by a federal agency. The HHS regulations also mandate minimal requirements for the composition of an IRB; an IRB must consist of at least five members and

> at least one member whose primary concerns are in scientific areas, at least one member whose primary concerns are in nonscientific areas . . . , and at least one member who is not affiliated with the institution and who is not part of the immediate family of a person who is affiliated with the institution. (U.S. Department of Health and Human Services, 2009)

Members of an IRB need to possess the professional competence necessary to review the specific research activities and ascertain the acceptability of proposed research in terms of institutional commitments and regulations, applicable law, and standards of professional conduct and practice. Therefore, at least some members of an IRB must have knowledge of, and be familiar with, existing guidelines, regulations, and policies.

The IRB is formally designated by the institution to review and monitor research involving human subjects and has the authority to approve, require modifications in (to secure approval), or disapprove research. The purpose of an IRB review of a research protocol is to ensure, both in advance and by periodic review, that appropriate steps are taken to protect the rights and welfare of humans participating in the research. The review encompasses research protocols and all related materials (e.g., informed consent documents, brochures, questionnaires/assessment instruments, recruitment materials). It is important to note that IRBs require that any changes to study materials or protocols must also be approved prior to using these materials or instituting these protocols. For example, if, during the early course of a study that is evaluating a new intervention for caregiver depression, an investigator decides that it would be helpful to include a short interview with the study participants during the 6-month outcome assessment, the protocol for doing so and any related documents would need to be submitted to the IRB for approval before these interviews could be conducted.

The type of review conducted by an IRB is also regulated according to specific criteria. For example, some minimal risk intervention research might be considered eligible for an "expedited review" in which the review of the protocol can be conducted by a smaller subgroup of a larger IRB or by the chair of the IRB or his or her designee. In the case of behavioral intervention research, this might occur for study designs such as focus groups, or surveys depending on the IRB and the content of the subject matter. For example, highly sensitive topics (e.g., sexual practices, substance abuse, HIV disclosure) typically would require full IRB review. The federal regulations include a list of expedited categories as well as categories of research that may be exempt from an IRB review such as studies that involve review of existing data that is publicly available. An intervention researcher may conduct a review of a public available database on the incidence of a particular disease at the "getting started phase" (see Chapter 3). In this case, it is likely that the protocol would likely be exempt from an IRB review. However, it is always necessary to consult with the institution's IRB office to make these determinations. As rules and guidelines that are followed differ from one institution to the next, a research team cannot make these determinations alone and must consult with the IRB to obtain appropriate guidance.

Investigators involved in intervention research will need to interact with the institution's IRB in the conduct of research at all phases of the pipeline and throughout their research career at that institution. Therefore, we recommend that investigators become familiar early on with the policies of the IRB and the IRB process. Many institutions offer training in these areas for new investigators or to inform seasoned investigators of changes in policies or protocols. Becoming familiar with the workings of an IRB will greatly facilitate the intervention research process. Lack of adherence to IRB submission requirements can significantly delay the start of a trial. It is generally a good idea to have a meeting with the IRB staff or chairperson prior to submitting an application. It is also prudent to document and keep records of all correspondence with the IRB in case there are questions or an audit of the study is conducted. Government agencies, the study sponsor, or the institution's IRB may sometimes request an audit of a study. This may occur for cause (e.g., the IRB receives complaints from study participants; there are a large number of AEs) or at random to ensure that the study is proceeding as approved and that there are no problems with respect to the research participants. This also underscores the importance of ensuring that all members of the research team are well versed in the study's goals, objectives, and protocols and well trained in the conduct of research. Finally, a good practice is for the investigator/team to periodically conduct their own internal audit in which all informed consent forms are reviewed to ensure proper signage, that all consents are available for enrolled study participants, and that signed informed consents reflect the most up-to-date approved IRB forms. Such internal audits and their outcomes should be documented and shared with the IRB with a description of any problems identified and their resolution. Self-audits represent ethical practice, can preempt external audits, and ensure continual compliance to these fundamental human protection procedures.

Interactions with an IRB can become more complex in the case of multisite trials or when an investigator is recruiting research participants at more than one institution. For example, if an investigator is recruiting participants for a cognitive intervention trial at the memory disorder clinic at his or her institution and from a memory disorder clinic at a local hospital, he or she would need IRB approval from both institutions. This can be time-consuming and can also create delays in the start of a trial. Therefore, when possible, it generally is a good idea for the investigators to work with the IRBs at their institutions to determine if an agreement can be set up so that their respective institutions can act as the primary IRB for the study and that consent forms approved by one can be used at another setting. The NIH is currently encouraging the use of single IRBs for multisite trials funded by an NIH Institute and, in fact, has a draft policy to promote the use of a single IRB in these circumstances (NIH Notice Number: NOT-OD-15-026). The goal of the policy is to enhance and streamline IRB review processes and reduce inefficiencies.

ADVERSE EVENTS

Investigators involved in behavioral intervention research also need to be aware of guidelines and policies regarding AEs and put into place specific procedures that are to be followed to identify, track, and resolve such events. This aspect of behavioral intervention research can be confusing as the definition of AEs varies across government and nongovernment agencies and DSMBs (described later), as well as institutions and types of studies. The guidelines provided by the U.S. Department of Health and Human Services (2007) defines AEs as

> any untoward or unfavorable medical occurrence in a human subject, including any abnormal sign (for example, abnormal physical exam or laboratory finding), symptom, or disease, temporally associated with the subject's participation in the research, whether or not considered related to the subject's participation in the research . . .

Importantly, these guidelines note that AEs encompass both physical and psychological harm. They also distinguish AEs from "unanticipated problems," which refers to incidents that meet the following criteria:

1. unexpected (in terms of nature, severity, or frequency) given (a) the research procedures that are described in the protocol-related documents, such as the

IRB-approved research protocol and informed consent document; and (b) the characteristics of the subject population being studied;

2. related or possibly related to participation in the research (in this guidance document, possibly related means there is a reasonable possibility that the incident, experience, or outcome may have been caused by the procedures involved in the research); and

3. suggests that the research places study participants or others at a greater risk of harm (including physical, psychological, economic, or social harm) than was previously known or recognized. (U.S. Department of Health and Human Services, 2007)

The NIH further distinguishes between serious AEs (SAEs) and other AEs. Using the Food and Drug Administration (FDA) definition, SAEs include AEs that result in death, require either inpatient hospitalization or the prolongation of hospitalization, are life-threatening, result in a persistent or significant disability/incapacity, or result in a congenital anomaly/birth defect. Other important medical events, based upon appropriate medical judgment, may also be considered SAEs if a trial participant's health is at risk. "Other AEs" are defined using the HHS guidelines (provided earlier).

An issue for those involved in behavioral intervention research is how to define AEs for a given intervention trial. As noted by Horigan and colleagues (Horigian, Robbins, Dominguez, Ucha, & Rosa, 2011), the process of defining, identifying, reporting, and monitoring AEs has received limited attention in behavioral intervention research. There is a lack of clear guidelines to aid investigators. In the Resources for Enhancing Alzheimer's Caregivers Health II (REACH II) multisite caregiver intervention trial (Belle et al., 2006), based on the consensus of the investigators, two categories of events were defined for both caregivers and patients: AEs and safety alerts. The definition of "AE" was consistent with the FDA and NIH definition of AEs and included events such as death, hospitalization, and emergency room visits. "Safety alerts" were events that were relevant to the study population and posed safety risks to study participants. Examples of safety alerts included caregivers having symptoms of depression or the care recipient driving (Table 13.2). Given that the intervention was based on a risk appraisal approach and the baseline assessment, which included measures of depression, quality of care, and care recipient problem behaviors, was administered prior to randomization, AEs and potential risks to the participants could be detected prior to the start of the intervention. Thus, a distinction was also made between events that were detected at baseline (baseline AEs and baseline safety alerts) versus those that occurred following randomization and the 6-month follow-up assessment (AEs and safety alerts) (Czaja et al., 2006).

Behavioral intervention researchers also need to be aware of the reporting processes for AEs. Reporting processes are somewhat confusing as existing policies vary across government and nongovernment agencies. Investigators who are engaged in an efficacy or effectiveness intervention trial generally need to develop an AE reporting form that includes information about the nature of the event, time

TABLE 13.2 Examples of the Adverse Events Protocol for the REACH II Trial

Baseline Adverse Events	Resolution	Adverse Event	Resolution
Caregiver emergency room visit	Not applicable	Caregiver emergency room visit	The PI or designee (e.g., clinical supervisor, project coordinator) contacted the caregiver to determine the reason for the emergency room visit and how the problem was handled (e.g., received treatment, is currently under treatment, and/or is being monitored by health care provider)
Care recipient institutionalization	Not applicable	Care recipient institutionalization	The PI or designee (e.g., clinical supervisor, project coordinator) contacted the caregiver to determine the reason and planned duration of the institutionalization
Care recipient death	Not applicable	Care recipient death	The PI or designee (e.g., clinical supervisor, project coordinator) obtained information regarding the circumstances of the event

Baseline Safety Alerts	Resolution	Safety Alerts	Resolution
Caregiver CESD score ≥15	The PI or designee (e.g., clinical supervisor, project coordinator) contacted the caregiver to discuss the seriousness of the situation and referred the caregiver to his or her primary care physician (or other health care or mental health professional) to discuss the symptoms	Caregiver CESD score ≥15	The PI or designee (e.g., clinical supervisor, project coordinator) contacted the caregiver to discuss the seriousness of the situation and referred the caregiver to his or her primary care physician (or other health care or mental health professional) to discuss the symptoms
Care recipient driving	The PI or designee (e.g., clinical supervisor, project coordinator) contacted the caregiver to discuss the safety implication of the care recipient driving and devise a plan of action to stop the care recipient from driving. Caregivers who were randomized to the control condition were sent the material on driving and dementia. Caregivers who were randomized to the intervention condition were encouraged to read the materials in the Caregiver Notebook related to driving	Care recipient driving	The PI or designee (e.g., clinical supervisor, project coordinator) contacted the caregiver to discuss the safety implication of the care recipient driving and devise a plan of action to stop the care recipient from driving. Caregivers who were randomized to the control condition were sent the material on driving and dementia. Caregivers who were randomized to the intervention condition were encouraged to read the materials in the Caregiver Notebook related to driving

(Continued)

TABLE 13.2   Examples of the Adverse Events Protocol for the REACH II Trial *(Continued)*

Baseline Safety Alerts	Resolution	Safety Alerts	Resolution
Care recipient has access to a gun	The PI or designee (e.g., clinical supervisor, project coordinator) contacted the caregiver to discuss the safety implications and devise a plan of action to block the care recipient's access to the gun. If the caregiver refused or was unable to block the care recipient's access, Adult Protective Services may have been contacted. If it appears that an assessor or interventionist was in danger, the caregiver's/care recipient's participation in the study was terminated	Care recipient has access to a gun	The PI or designee (e.g., clinical supervisor, project coordinator) contacted the caregiver to discuss the safety implications and devise a plan of action to block the care recipient's access to the gun. If the caregiver refused or was unable to block the care recipient's access, Adult Protective Services may have been contacted. If it appears that an assessor or interventionist was in danger, the caregiver's/care recipient's participation in the study was terminated

PI, principal investigator; CESD, Center for Epidemiologic Studies Depression Scale.

frame, action take, relationship to study treatment, and the severity of the event. An example of an AE form is provided in Figure 13.1.

A form for reporting SAEs typically requires additional information such as a brief description of the participant who experienced the event (Figure 13.2). It may be possible to combine these two forms for a study depending on the requirements of the IRB and the study monitoring committee if one exists (e.g., Data and Safety Monitoring Committee). These forms must be standardized for multisite trials. Protocols for resolution of the event must also be established and approved by the IRB and study-monitoring entities.

When reporting AEs, the PI of an intervention study is also responsible for determining the likely relationship between the AE and the intervention. The National Institute on Aging (NIA) has provided some guidance on this issue and provides the following scale:

Definitely Related: The adverse event is clearly related to the investigational agent/procedure—i.e. an event that follows a reasonable temporal sequence from administration of the study intervention, follows a known or expected response pattern to the suspected intervention, that is confirmed by improvement on stopping and reappearance of the event on repeated exposure and that could not be reasonably explained by the known characteristics of the subject's clinical state.

Possibly Related: An adverse event that follows a reasonable temporal sequence from administration of the study intervention, follows a known or expected response pattern to the suspected intervention, but that could readily have been produced by a number of other factors.

STUDY NAME

Site Number: _____

Pt_ID: _____

Has the participant had any Adverse Events during this study? ☐ Yes ☐ No *(If yes, please list all Adverse Events below)*

Severity	Study Intervention Relationship	Action Taken Regarding Study Intervention	Outcome of AE	Expected	Serious
1 = Mild 2 = Moderate 3 = Severe	1 = Definitely related 2 = Possibly related 3 = Not related	1 = None 2 = Discontinued permanently 3 = Discontinued temporarily 4 = Reduced dose 5 = Increased dose 6 = Delayed dose	1 = Resolved, no sequel 2 = AE still present-no treatment 3 = AE still present-being treated 4 = Residual effects present-not treated 5 = Residual effects present-treated 6 = Death 7 = Unknown	1 = Yes 2 = No	1 = Yes 2 = No (If yes, complete SAE form)

Adverse Event	Start Date	Stop Date	Severity	Relationship to Study Treatment	Action Taken	Outcome of AE	Expected?	Serious Adverse Event?	Initials
1.									
2.									
3.									

Figure 13.1 An example of an adverse event reporting form.
Source: The National Institute on Aging (2013).

Not Related: The adverse event is clearly not related to the investigational agent/procedure—i.e. another cause of the event is most plausible; and/or a clinically plausible temporal sequence is inconsistent with the onset of the event and the study intervention and/or a causal relationship is considered biologically implausible. (NIA, 2013, p. 5)

Serious Adverse Event (SAE) Report Form

Protocol Title:

Protocol Number: _____

Site Number: _____

Pt_ID: _____

1. SAE Onset Date: _____ (dd/mm/yyyy)

2. SAE Stop Date: _____ (dd/mm/yyyy)

3. Location of serious adverse event (e.g. at study site or elsewhere):
_____

4. Was this an unexpected adverse event?   ☐ Yes   ☐ No

5. Brief description of participant with no personal identifiers:
Sex: ☐ Female   ☐ Male   Age: _____

6. Adverse Event Term(s):
_____
_____

7. Brief description of the nature of the serious adverse event (attach description if more space needed):
_____
_____

8. Category of the serious adverse event:

☐ death – date _____(dd/mm/yyyy)   ☐ congenital anomaly / birth defect
☐ life-threatening   ☐ required intervention to prevent
☐ hospitalization - initial or prolonged   permanent impairment
☐ disability / incapacity   ☐ other:_____

Serious Adverse Event Report Form   1 of 2   Version 1.1

Figure 13.2 An example of serious adverse event reporting form. (*Continued*)

Serious Adverse Event (SAE) Report Form

9. Intervention type:

☐ Medication or Nutritional Supplement: specify_____
☐ Device: Specify: _____
☐ Surgery: Specify: _____
☐ Behavioral/Life Style: Specify: _____

10. Relationship of event to intervention:

☐ Unrelated (clearly not related to the intervention)
☐ Possible (may be related to intervention)
☐ Definite (clearly related to intervention)

11. Was study intervention discontinued due to event? ☐ Yes ☐ No

12. What medications or other steps were taken to treat serious adverse event?

_____
_____

13. List any relevant tests, laboratory data, history, including preexisting medical conditions

_____
_____

14. Type of report:

☐ Initial
☐ Follow-up
☐ Final

Signature of Principal Investigator: _____ Date: _____ (dd/mm/yyyy)

Serious Adverse Event Report Form   2 of 2   Version 1.1

Figure 13.2 (Continued) An example of serious adverse event reporting form.
Source: National Institute on Aging 2013.

While these guidelines are helpful, consideration also needs to be given to the characteristics of the study population and the contextual factors surrounding the intervention. For example, in a multisite trial that evaluated a psychosocial intervention for caregivers of persons with spinal cord injury (Schulz et al., 2009), a DSMB for the trial was established along with a protocol for tracking and reporting AEs. One of the AEs established for the study by the DSMB in collaboration with the PIs was the development of pressure ulcer sores in the patients. However, given that the onset of pressure ulcer sores is common among people with spinal cord injury, it was highly unlikely that the occurrence of this AE was related to the intervention. In contrast, if there were a significant number of caregivers who experienced symptoms of clinical depression since the trial onset (this in fact was not the case), this could potentially be linked to the intervention. However, depression is common among caregivers; so, if this in fact occurred, the causality would need careful examination by the PI, the research team, and the DSMB.

As noted, there are also requirements/guidelines for reporting AEs to the IRB, the monitoring entities established for the trial, and, in some cases, the funding agency. In general, the PI is responsible for reporting AEs to the IRB and the study monitoring entity within time windows agreed upon by the IRB and the monitoring entity. For example, in a current caregiver intervention trial, the DSMB agreed that quarterly reports would be sufficient unless significant issues arose within the trial—for example, a significant increase in the frequency of an AE or its high probability of occurrence due to the intervention. Unless otherwise specified in the protocol and approved by the IRB and monitoring entity, all SAEs require expedited reporting to the IRB and the monitoring entity as detailed in the approved Data and Safety Monitoring Plan (DSMP) (NIA, 2013).

Importantly, the PI must also establish an internal study-reporting protocol that encompasses the reporting structure and time windows for reporting and resolving the event. For example, in the intervention study targeted for caregivers and spinal cord injury patients (Schulz et al., 2009), for any AE identified by a member of the research team, the event needed to be reported to the PI or the designee of the PI within 24 hours and recorded on the AE form. In addition, the event needed to be resolved using the protocols established for the study within 3 days of learning of the event. A weekly review of SAEs and AEs should be conducted to ensure that they have been recorded properly, sufficiently resolved, and submitted to reporting bodies as required.

Finally, protocols must be established for resolution of AEs and SAEs, and these protocols must be approved by the IRB or the monitoring entity. Examples of the protocols used in the REACH II intervention trial (Belle et al., 2006) are provided in Table 13.2. The establishment of protocols for resolution of AEs can also be confusing for behavioral intervention trials. For example, in the REACH II trial, nursing home placement of persons with dementia was considered an AE. However, in question was determining its resolution. That is, should resolution be defined as the return of the person with dementia to the home setting or knowledge that placement occurred and the reason for the placement decision. Obviously, placement of patients who were permanently placed would never be "resolved" if the definition of resolution of this event was the person with dementia returning to home. Instead, it was agreed that the definition of "resolution" would be that the

PI or designee contact the caregiver to determine the reason for, and planned duration of, the placement of the person with dementia. This protocol was approved by the DSMB, which underscores the importance of educating the DSMB or any other monitoring entity about the nature of the intervention and the characteristics of the target population. It is also critical to ensure that all members of the research team are trained in the protocols for handling AEs and SAEs and that these protocols are included in the manual of operations developed for the study (see Chapter 6).

DATA AND SAFETY-MONITORING BOARDS

An additional question that arises in the conduct of behavioral intervention research is whether there is a need for a DSMB. Usually, this question is relevant at the later stages of the pipeline when the efficacy or the effectiveness of an intervention is being evaluated. As is the case with other aspects of research ethics, there is also some lack of consistency regarding the requirements for a DSMB across government-funding agencies. Other funding agencies such as foundations may also have requirements for the establishment of a monitoring entity for a trial. The NIH guidelines state that DSMBs are required for multisite clinical trials with interventions that entail risk(s) to participants and generally required for Phase III clinical trials (see Chapter 2). In addition, the guidelines state that a DSMB *may* be required for Phase I or Phase II clinical trials if it is blinded, involves a high-risk intervention, or includes vulnerable populations (National Institutes of Health, 2010). For example, a DSMB was required for the REACH II trial as it was a multisite test of an intervention and involved a vulnerable population—family caregivers and persons with dementia. However, the guidelines for when a DSMB is required are somewhat general. Thus, it is always important to review this issue with the funding official for an intervention study such as a program officer at the NIH since most institutes at the NIH have specific policies regarding the need for, and the actual structure and set of processes to follow for, a DSMB. For example, the NIA requires that all applications proposing interventions that involve humans such as behavioral interventions describe a DSMP, which includes information regarding how the study will be monitored and a plan for determination, monitoring, and a reporting system for AEs and SAEs as well as protocols for resolution of these events. In addition, the NIA may require the establishment of a DSMB depending on the characteristics of the study, and if so, will review the plan and approve its membership.

A DSMB is an independent group of experts who advise the funding agency and the investigators. That is, DSMB members must not be part of the investigative team of the study in question. Some funding agencies also insist that members are selected who are not affiliated with the institution in which the study is conducted. In general, the primary responsibilities of a DSMB are to: (a) review and approve the research protocol (including the selected outcome measures) and manual of procedures (MOPs) (see Chapter 6); (b) review and approve the safety data for the study participants and study conduct and progress (e.g., recruitment); and (c) make recommendations to the funding agency regarding continuation, modification, or termination of the trial. Generally, investigators do not nominate specific individuals for the DSMB in an application, but rather provide a list of prospective members to the funding officer (e.g., program officer) if a study is funded. The DSMB typically includes individuals with expertise in the research area and the target population, biostatistics, and research ethics. Once members are selected, the DSMB will work with the PI to determine the meeting schedule (typically twice per year) and the protocols (e.g., data table templates, what will be reported, frequency of reporting, and in-person vs. telephone vs. e-mail updates) for data reporting.

The initial meeting of the DSMB must take place at the beginning of a trial prior to entering the field or collecting data, as the DSMB is expected to review the entire IRB-approved study protocol and the MOP with regard to: subject safety, recruitment, randomization, intervention, data management, and quality control and analysis; the informed consent document with regard to applicability and readability; and protocols for identification, monitoring, reporting, and resolving AEs and SAEs (National Institute on Aging, 2015). At an initial meeting, the processes and data-reporting protocols are also determined and recommendations and/or requirements for any modifications to the protocol are provided to the PI. At subsequent meetings, the DSMB monitors the progress of the trial and the data related to the safety of the research participants. If the trial involves randomization, the committee will also review randomization outcomes. At midpoint assessment periods, they may also request to review the primary outcomes, blinded to condition. Although not typical in behavioral intervention research, they may recommend that the trial be stopped if there are significant numbers of AEs or the intervention is clearly causing harm; or the opposite, the intervention benefits are so dramatic that it is determined there is not a need to continue the study and that all participants should receive the intervention. The latter is, of course, rare.

For some intervention studies, a full DSMB may not be required and instead an independent safety monitor or Safety Monitoring Committee (SMC) is acceptable. An independent safety monitor is an "appropriate expert" who is available to review and recommend actions regarding safety events and other safety issues. An SMC is a small group of experts with at least two members who are independent of the protocol and can review the protocol and data for a study. Members of an SMC can usually be selected by the PI and research team and, of course, should have expertise relevant to the trial. A member with a strong background in biostatistics is highly recommended. As with the DSMB, a plan must be in place for the responsibilities, structure, and processes of a SMC.

CONCLUSION

In this chapter, we highlight and discuss issues related to the ethical conduct of research that are important to behavioral intervention researchers. Research ethics is a complex and dynamic question, especially for behavioral interventions. The existing regulations and guidelines are somewhat general and can be confusing, as they have been developed primarily for biomedical interventions. They also vary across governments and federal agencies. However, there are basic principles for the conduct of research with human participants that are essential to behavioral intervention research to ensure that the dignity, rights, safety, and well-being of research participants are maintained; the research is conducted in an ethical manner; and the results of the investigations are credible. As discussed in this chapter, important issues to consider are the informed consent process, the role of the IRB and safety monitoring bodies such as the DSMB, and protocols for handling potential AEs and SAEs. PIs need to be aware of existing regulations and guidelines regarding the protection of human subjects and research ethics, and should also be thoroughly familiar with the IRB and polices of their resident institutions. It is especially important now when research methodologies are changing as well as policies, regulations, and the literature in this area.

REFERENCES

Beecher, H. K. (1966). Ethics and clinical research. *The New England Journal of Medicine, 274*, 1354–1360.

Belle, S. H., Burgio, L., Burns, R., Coon, D., Czaja, S. J., Gallagher-Thompson, D., . . . Zhang, S. (2006). Enhancing the quality of life of dementia caregivers from different ethnic or racial groups. *Annals of Internal Medicine, 145*, P727–P738.

Black, B. S., Kass, N. E., Fogarty, L. A., & Rabins, P. V. (2007). Informed consent for dementia research: The study enrollment encounter. *IRB: Ethics & Human Research, 29*(4), 7–14.

Black, B. S., Rabins, P. V., Sugarman, J., & Karlawish, J. H. (2010). Seeking assent and respecting dissent in dementia research. *American Journal of Geriatric Psychiatry, 18*(1), 77–85.

Czaja, S. J., Schulz, R., Belle, S. H., Burgio, L. D., Armstrong, N., Gitlin, L. N., . . . Stahl, S. M. (2006). Data safety monitoring in social behavioral intervention trials: The REACH II experience. *Clinical Trials, 3*, 107–118.

Horigian, V. E., Robbins, M., Dominguez, R., Ucha, J., & Rosa, C. L. (2010). Principles for defining adverse events in behavioral intervention research: Lessons from a family-focused adolescent drug abuse trial. *Clinical Trials, 7*(1), 58–68.

National Institute on Aging. (2013). *Adverse events (AEs) and serious adverse events (SAEs) guidelines*. Retrieved July 1, 2015, from https://www.nia.nih.gov/research/dgcg/clinical-research-study-investigators-toolbox/adverse-events

National Institute on Aging. (2015). *Research & Funding. Division of Extramural Activities: Implementation of policies for human intervention studies*. Retrieved June 30, 2015, from https://www.nia.nih.gov/research/dea/implementation-policies-human-intervention-studies#ReqDSMB

National Institutes of Health. (2010). *Frequently asked questions from applicants: Human subjects research—Data and safety monitoring*. Retrieved June 30, 2015, from http://grants.nih.gov/grants/policy/hs/faqs_aps_dsm.htm#186

O'Mathuna, D. P. (2012). Ethical considerations in designing intervention studies. In B. M. Melnyk & D. Morrison-Beedy (Eds.), *Intervention research: Design, conduction, analyzing and funding* (pp. 7–79). New York, NY: Springer.

Resnik, D. B. (2011). What is ethics in research & why is it important? Retrieved July 1, 2015, from http://www.niehs.nih.gov/research/resources/bioethics/whatis/

Schulz, R., Czaja, S. J., Lustig, A., Zdaniuk, B., Martire, L. M., & Perdomo, D. (2009). Improving the quality of life of caregivers of persons with spinal cord injury: A randomized controlled trial. *Rehabilitation Psychology, 54*, 1–15.

Shamoo, A., & Resnik, D. (2009). *Responsible conduct of research* (2nd ed.). New York, NY: Oxford University Press.

U.S. Department of Health and Human Services. (1979). *The Belmont Report*. Retrieved July 1, 2015, from http://www.hhs.gov/ohrp/humansubjects/guidance/belmont.html

U.S. Department of Health and Human Services (2007). Guidance on reviewing and reporting unanticipated problems involving risks to subjects or others and adverse events. Retrieved July 14, 2015, http://www.hhs.gov/ohrp/policy/advevntguid.html

U.S. Department of Health and Human Services. (2009). *Code of federal regulations—Title 45, public welfare. Part 46: Protection of human subjects*. Washington, DC: U.S. Government Printing Office.

DOES THE INTERVENTION WORK? SELECTING OUTCOMES AND ANALYTICS

Behavioral interventions are intended to have an impact on specified outcomes. Thus, in Part III, we examine the role of measurement and data analyses in building the evidence for an intervention. Chapter 14 discusses the use of measures as outcomes, covariates, mediators, or moderators. Chapter 15 explores the relative advantages of objective measurement strategies and the challenge of demonstrating change in daily functioning, a key outcome for many behavioral interventions. We next discuss data analytic techniques and examine traditional and novel approaches (Chapter 16). Finally, we consider the importance of clinical significance (Chapter 17) and economic evaluations (Chapter 18) to optimize the impact of interventions.

The key "take home" points of Part III include the following:

- Measurement serves multiple purposes in behavioral intervention research including evaluation of treatment outcomes, mediators, moderators, covariates, and descriptors.
- Reliance on subjective measures alone has disadvantages whereas objective measures can enhance an understanding of important clinical benefits, particularly in the areas of cognition and daily function.
- Traditional and emerging novel analytic strategies are important to consider for evaluating intervention effects.
- Determining the clinical significance of an intervention is of critical importance and should be evaluated in addition to statistical significance.
- Interventions must also be evaluated for their economic value if they are to be implemented in community and clinical settings.

FOURTEEN

MEASUREMENT IN BEHAVIORAL INTERVENTION RESEARCH

SARA J. CZAJA AND DAVID L. LOEWENSTEIN

> *You can't fix what you don't measure.*
> —William Thomas Lord Kelvin (1893)

The selection of measures to include in a study is perhaps one of the most important, and often the most challenging, aspects of behavioral intervention research. Selection must be carefully planned at the inception stage of intervention development. Measures provide answers to questions regarding whether the intervention "works," for whom, and to what extent and provide evidence that is used for decision making regarding an intervention at all phases of the pipeline. A common source of misleading results from intervention trials often stems from inadequate attention to the choice of measures—a mismatch between the intent of the intervention and the measurement strategy.

Different measures can relay different stories about the impact of an intervention, so measures need to be carefully aligned with the research questions of interest and what the intervention intends to change, modify, or impact. Consider, for example, a study that is evaluating a new software tool to aid Internet searching. The new tool is being compared to the standard search tool available on the browser. The outcome measures include indices of user performance (e.g., time, errors) as well as user perceptions of usability. If the performance data indicated that the study participants performed an information search task more efficiently using the new tool, one might conclude that the tool is effective and should be adopted. However, if the usability ratings indicated the tool was cumbersome and difficult to use, decisions about implementation of the tool might be different as user perceptions of the usability of technology are strongly related to technology uptake.

In general, the type and quality of the measures included in an intervention research trial are critical to (a) answering questions related to the study goals and hypotheses, (b) detecting change attributable to the intervention, (c) one's ability to compare findings to previous research, (d) determining the type of statistical analyses that needs to be employed, (e) the internal validity of the study, and (f) furthering theoretical knowledge within the treatment domain area. The choice of measures influences other design considerations in a trial such as the frequency and length of assessments and needed sample size.

Consider an intervention research trial that involved a comparative analysis of the impact of training methodology on the ability of older adults to search the Internet to find credible health information. Two methods were compared: a standard classroom approach led by an instructor; and an interactive, multimedia approach where the instructor acted as a coach, provided one-on-one feedback, and the students completed online exercises. On the basis of the findings, the investigators claimed that the standard method was superior to the interactive method in terms of teaching older adults. However, the claim was based solely on the ratings of three instructors with respect to ease of implementation of the method; there were no indices of student learning or student evaluative ratings. Further, the method rated as easier was already in place in the senior community center where the training evaluation took place. Clearly in this case, it would be hard to make a convincing argument for adopting the new interactive method of training as compared to a scenario where there were findings favoring that method, which were based on student learning achievements and student evaluations.

In this chapter, we discuss (a) the role of measures in behavioral intervention research, (b) criteria for measure selection, (c) the types of measures available, (d) methods for collecting outcome data, and (e) the role of technology in measurement.

THE ROLE OF MEASURES IN BEHAVIORAL INTERVENTION RESEARCH

Measures can be used for different purposes within intervention research. Measures provide answers to questions regarding intervention efficacy and effectiveness, for whom the intervention works and under what conditions, and how an intervention impacts outcomes. Measures also provide insight into issues about the clinical significance (see Chapter 17) and cost-effectiveness of an intervention, and feasibility of implementing an intervention on a broader scale. Today, there is a myriad of measures available, and they are included in intervention trials that range from biomarkers to performance metrics and subjective evaluations.

Outcome measures generally provide evidence about the efficacy or effectiveness of an intervention. They are used as a barometer to judge the strength of the evidence supporting the impact of an intervention. They may also provide information about other aspects of an intervention such as feasibility, cost-effectiveness, and participant satisfaction with a treatment approach. Outcome measures also provide information about the clinical meaningfulness of the research findings or the impact an intervention has on an individual's functioning with respect to everyday activities. Studies may include a variety of outcome measures such as clinical outcomes, quality-of-life metrics, satisfaction or usability ratings, or cost or resource utilization metrics. The choice of outcome measures depends on the stakeholders, the research questions, the target population, and the intended use of the evidence. In all cases, outcome measures must be clearly defined and unambiguous; the manner in which a measure is operationalized has broad implications for how it is assessed.

In randomized controlled trials (RCTs), choices have to be made as to what constitutes primary versus secondary outcome measures. In the Resources for Enhancing Alzheimer's Caregivers Health II (REACH II) trial (Belle et al., 2006), the primary outcome measures were related to the five areas of caregiver risk/components of the intervention, but additional (secondary) measures were included that assessed variables such as use of formal support services, religiosity, and the caregiver's perception of the caregiving experience. Primary outcomes are generally considered the critical outcomes with respect to decision making and are few in number. Secondary outcomes are often used to gather effect size data for subsequent trials or used as mediating variables to help explain the effects of an intervention.

In addition, data are sometimes collected on measures that characterize treatment populations to examine moderator effects of an intervention. *Moderating variables* help explain for whom the intervention works and under what conditions. This provides information on the external validity of the intervention. One might gather data on the ethnic/culture affinity of the target population to examine if the effects or impacts of an intervention vary as a function of ethnicity or culture. For example, we found that religious coping mechanism and age moderated the effects of the REACH II intervention for African American and Hispanic dementia caregivers (Lee, Czaja, & Schulz, 2010).

Similarly, one might gather data on attitudinal variables or self-efficacy to determine if these variables mediate the relationship between a treatment and an outcome. *Mediating variables* help explain how or why an intervention results in a change in an outcome measure, the mechanism of change. For example, computer anxiety has been found to mediate the relationship between age and technology uptake (Czaja, Charness, Fisk, et al., 2006).

The literature also suggests that changes in self-efficacy mediate the relationship between physical activity interventions and changes in physical activity behaviors (Lewis, Marcus, Pate, & Dunn, 2002). Baranowski, Cerin, & Baranowski (2009) maintain that change in desired outcomes is contingent upon changes in mediator variables (e.g., self-efficacy) and that interventions will be "successful" to the extent that mediator variables are targeted by the intervention at the appropriate levels. However, the selection of the appropriate mediators is key and must be guided by theory (see Chapter 4).

Sometimes, measures are also used to screen study participants with respect to inclusion/exclusion criteria. *Screening measures* might be related to an individual's characteristics (e.g., age, gender, sexual preference), living conditions (e.g., community dwelling), health status, or relationship status (e.g., spouse). These types of measures are used to operationalize a study's inclusion/exclusion criteria. For example, if an exclusion criterion was cognitive impairment, the screening measure might be a score of 26 or less on the Mini–Mental State Examination (Folstein, Folstein, & McHugh, 1975), which is commonly used as a screen for general cognitive status.

Studies may also include *process measures* that evaluate aspects of the intervention that are related (or not) to an outcome such as therapeutic alliance or the ingredients of an intervention. Other types of measures, which are particularly relevant today with the emphasis on implementation of evidence-based treatments, are those related to treatment implementation such as staff-training requirements, delivery characteristics, and indices of treatment fidelity and clinical significance. As noted, most studies include a variety of measures (see Table 14.1 for examples). Sometimes, measures may be used as mediating variables (e.g., perceived social support) and in other studies as outcome variables depending on the goals of the study.

TABLE 14.1   Examples of Measures and How They Might Be Used in Behavioral Intervention Research

Role of Measure	Examples of Measures	Description of Measure
Screening Measures	■ Mini–Mental Status Examination (MMSE) (Folstein et al., 1975)	■ Cognitive status
	■ Wide Range Achievement Test (WRAT) (Wilkinson, 1993)	■ General reading level
	■ Snellen Test (Berson, 1993)	■ Basic visual acuity
Moderators	■ Demographic Questionnaire (Czaja et al., 2006a)	■ Age, education, occupational and socioeconomic status, culture ethnicity, living arrangements
	■ Technology Experience Questionnaire (Czaja et al., 2006b)	■ Use of general technology and use/breadth of experience with computer technology and the Internet
	■ General Health Perceptions Scale (Ware & Sherbourne, 1992)	■ Self-reported physical health
	■ Ten-Item Personality Inventory (TIPI) (Gosling, Rentfrow, & Swann, 2003)	■ Personality traits
Mediators	■ New General Self-Efficacy Scale (Chen, Gully, & Eden, 2001)	■ Belief in one's overall competence across a wide variety of situations
	■ Computer Attitudes (Jay & Willis, 1992)	■ Three dimensions of computer attitudes (comfort, efficacy, and interest)
	■ Family Caregiving Factors Inventory (Shyu, 2000)	■ Caregivers expectations of the caregiving role
	■ Perceived Stress Scale (Cohen, Kamarck, & Mermelstein, 1983)	■ Degree to which situations in one's life are perceived as stressful
Outcome Measures	**Self-Rating**	
	■ Center for Epidemiological Studies— Depression Scale (Radloff, 1977)	■ Depressive symptoms
	■ Functional Health and Well-Being (SF-36; Ware & Sherbourne, 1992)	■ Health-related quality of life
	■ Revised Memory and Behavior Problem Checklist (Teri et al., 1992; Zarit, Orr, & Zarit, 1985)	Caregiver burden
	■ The Community Health Activities Model Program for Seniors (CHAMPS) Questionnaire (Stewart et al., 2001)	■ Self-reported physical activity
	Informant-Rating	
	■ Instrumental Activities of Daily Living (Lawton & Brody, 1969)	■ Competence in higher order everyday activities (e.g., food preparation, money management)
	■ Katz Index of Independence in Activities in Daily Living (Katz ADL) (Katz, Ford, Moskowitz, Jackson, & Jaffe, 1963)	■ Competence in basic activities of daily living (e.g., bathing, toileting)

(Continued)

TABLE 14.1   Examples of Measures and How They Might Be Used in Behavioral Intervention Research   (Continued)

Role of Measure	Examples of Measures	Description of Measure
	■ Schizophrenia Cognition Rating Scale (SCoRs) (Keefe, Poe, Walker, Kang, & Harvey, 2006)	■ Ratings of cognitive function
	■ Independent Living Skills Inventory (ILSI) (Menditto et al., 1999)	■ Clinical rating scale of real-world, everyday functioning
	Performance-Based	
	■ Measures of task performance (task specific)	■ Task completion time, number and types of errors, accuracy
	■ Short Physical Performance Battery (SPPB) (Bean, Vora, & Frontera, 2004; Nelson et al., 2004)	■ Times measures of standing, balance, walking speed, and ability to rise from a chair
	■ Everyday Problem Solving Test (Marsiske & Willis, 1995)	■ Ability to solve problems in several domains (e.g., medication use, financial management, transportation)
	■ Measures of behavioral patterns (e.g., sensing data)	■ Sleep activity, communication patterns, movement patterns
	Physiological Indices	■ Weight, BMI, brain imaging, EEG, cortisol, heart rate, cholesterol
Cost Measures	■ Cost of Care Index (Kosberg & Cairl, 1980)	■ Perceived worthiness of providing care
	■ Health care costs	■ Number and type of insurance claims, medication costs, hospitalizations, outpatient visits, preventative health visits, use of services

Note: The role categories are not mutually exclusive—some measures may be used as mediators or outcome measures depending on the study goals.

For example, in a recently completed trial that examined the efficacy of a software application (PRISM) on outcomes related to social connectivity and quality of life among older adults at risk for social isolation (Czaja et al., 2015), the assessment battery included screening measures to evaluate cognitive status (Mini–Mental State Examination; Folstein et al., 1975), measures to characterize the sample/potential moderator variables (e.g., educational level), potential mediating variables (e.g., measures of component cognitive abilities), and primary (e.g., social support, loneliness) and secondary outcomes (e.g., computer proficiency). The trial also included measures of usability and perceived usefulness of the technology as well as interview data that captured more in-depth perceptions of the PRISM system.

Generally, the selection of the appropriate outcome measures for an intervention trial should be based on (a) the theoretical constructs or models guiding the intervention; (b) the research topic, questions, and hypotheses; (c) the psycho-metric properties of the measures; (d) the assurance that change in a measure is meaningful with respect to the target population and the intervention being evaluated; and (e) the previous literature. As noted in Chapter 4, the intervention evaluated in the REACH II trial was based on a stress process model that suggested multiple factors contribute to caregiver burden and distress. The intervention was multicomponent and addressed five areas of caregiver risk: depression and emotional well-being, burden, self-care and healthy behaviors, care recipient problem behaviors, and social support. The primary outcome measures chosen for the trial were also linked to these areas of risk and to the components of the intervention (Table 14.1).

Other important selection criteria for outcome measures are related to the feasibility and cost of collecting the data, the resources available with respect to data collection and analysis, and participant burden. For example, in cognitive aging research, the use of brain imaging is commonly employed to gather data on brain functioning or activity relative to behavior or cognitive operations. Collection of this type of data is feasible only if the appropriate imaging equipment is available, if there are sufficient funds available, and if someone on the research team has the requisite knowledge to collect and analyze the data. Finally, the choice of measures may vary according to stage in the intervention pipeline. In the initial development of an intervention, the measures may reflect responses from a focus group about the content of the intervention, whereas further in the pipeline, where a study is conducted to evaluate the efficacy of the intervention, the measures may reflect some psychosocial construct or change in behavior.

As noted, in behavioral intervention research, decisions must be made about outcome measures as well as measures that may be used for screening as mediating or moderator variables, and to assess issues relevant to treatment implementation and clinical significance. The selection of measures requires knowledge of (a) the relevant intervention literature and theories/models, (b) the psychometric properties (e.g., reliability and validity) of the measures, (c) the practical aspects/constraints of administering the measures, (d) the appropriateness of the measures for the target population (e.g., some measures may be culturally biased), (e) the currency of the measures (e.g., measures that assess attitudes toward technology may lose relevance if they ask questions about technology that is no longer available), and (f) associated effect sizes to help guide calculations about sample size and also guide understanding of the practical importance of a particular finding.

In the following sections, we provide a basic review of types of measures and the general criteria for measure selection. We proceed with a word of caution: the choice of measures for a study can be overwhelming; in most treatment domains, there are large numbers of measures available. It is also sometimes difficult to find consensus about which measure or measures are optimal with respect to answering a research question. For example, in the cognitive literature, there is a wide variety of measures and techniques available for measuring various aspects of cognition; however, researchers do not always agree on the best approach or how best to measure abilities such as working memory or attention. In this regard, there have been attempts to harmonize measures across studies such as in the United States, the National Institutes of Health (NIH) Toolbox for the Assessment of Neurological and

Behavioral Function (www.nihtoolbox.org), which includes a set of measures to assess cognitive, emotional, motor, and sensory functions.

The measurement literature is constantly evolving and advances in technology such as imaging techniques, sensing devices, and wearable technologies allow different ways to capture changes in behavior. As will be discussed a bit later in this chapter, developments in technology are also changing the way outcome data is collected. For example, computer adaptive testing (CAT) allows assessments to be specifically targeted to an individual, and computer-assisted telephone interviewing (CATI) is a telephone-interviewing technique in which the interviewer is guided by a software application. Measures can also become obsolete because they are cumbersome, no longer relevant, or there is an improved method for assessing the construct of interest. For example, in our Center for Research on Aging and Technology Enhancement (CREATE), we have to update our measure of technology experience to ensure that it is current with respect to current technologies; telephone answering machines are becoming obsolete whereas smartphones are becoming ubiquitous. This underscores the need to keep abreast of the current literature within any particular area.

CATEGORIES AND TYPES OF MEASURES

As noted, there is a myriad of measures available to evaluate the impact of a behavioral intervention, each with its associated strengths and weaknesses, as well as a variety of ways to assess intervention processes and implementation issues. There is also a number of ways to categorize these measures. A great deal of variability in terminology exists in the field of measurement. Measures can be classified according to measurement scale (e.g., ordinal vs. continuous); as subjective (e.g., observer ratings, participants evaluation of an intervention) or objective (biomarkers, errors on a task, or time to complete a task); or whether they are qualitative (e.g., responses in a focus group, interview data) or quantitative (e.g., responses to a standardized questionnaire or physiological indices); or according to stakeholder viewpoint (e.g., clinical/health outcomes or economic/cost outcomes). In addition, some measures are monotrait—they measure a single trait (e.g., the Center for Epidemiological Studies—Depression [CES-D] is used to measure depressive symptoms), whereas others are multitrait—they measure a variety of traits or aspects of behavior (e.g., the Symptoms Checklist-90-Revised (SCL-90-R) is used to measure nine primary symptoms). Recognizing these distinctions, we choose to discuss them according to method of assessment (e.g., self-report, performance indices) and, where possible, according to the target level of our socioecological intervention systems model (Chapter 1). These categories are not necessarily mutually exclusive. Our intent is not to provide a comprehensive list of measures, as this would be rather daunting and beyond the scope of this chapter, given the large number of domains included in behavioral intervention research. Instead, we provide examples of the types of measures that are commonly used in behavioral intervention research and the formats typically used for data collection (Table 14.2). Our focus is on highlighting issues that should be considered when selecting measures for a behavioral intervention study.

TABLE 14.2 Overview of the Primary Outcome Measures for the REACH II Trial in Relation to Intervention Component, Trial Objective, and Treatment Strategies

Intervention Component	Objective	Treatment Strategies and Techniques	Primary Outcome Measure
Self-care and healthy behaviors	Enhance caregiver's physical well-being and self-care behaviors	■ Provide educational materials on self-care and preventative health practices (Health Passport, Caregiver Notebook) ■ Demonstrate and review use of Health Passport ■ Instruct in healthy behaviors (e.g., nutrition, remembering medical appointments, adhering to medication schedule) ■ Refer to healthy living feature of computerized phone system	■ Self-Care Scale: The caregiver's diligence in looking after his or her health was assessed using 11 questions, such as getting enough rest when sick, seeing a doctor when you thought you should, and drinking or smoking more than usual (Belle et al., 2006).
Problem behaviors	Enhance the caregiver's ability to manage ADL/IADL and behavioral problems	■ Provide educational materials on symptoms of dementia and managing behaviors (Caregiver Notebook) ■ Engage in structured problem solving and brainstorming of strategies ■ Provide a written behavioral prescription that specifies step-by-step strategies to manage troublesome behaviors ■ Demonstrate and practice specific strategies using role-play ■ Refer to problem behavior feature of computerized phone system	■ Three questions assessing the primary domains of the Revised Memory and Behavior Problem Checklist (i.e., memory, depression, and disruption; Teri et al., 1992) were used to assess change in patient problem behaviors at baseline and follow-up.
Burden	Increase the caregiver's knowledge about the consequences of stress and enhance the caregiver's skills and strategies for managing the burden of care	■ Provide educational materials on safety, caregiving, and stress (Caregiver Notebook) ■ Instruct in and practice three stress management techniques (breathing exercise, music, stretching exercises) ■ Refer to stress management feature on computerized phone system	■ The brief (12-item) version of the Caregiver Burden Interview (Bédard et. al., 2001; Zarit et al., 1985) was used. However, because one of the questions was not appropriate for caregivers of care recipients who were institutionalized at the

(Continued)

TABLE 14.2   Overview of the Primary Outcome Measures for the REACH II Trial in Relation to Intervention Component, Trial Objective, and Treatment Strategies   (Continued)

Intervention Component	Objective	Treatment Strategies and Techniques	Primary Outcome Measure
			6-month follow-up (Do you feel that you don't have as much privacy as you would like because of [care recipient's name]?], caregiver burden was based on the sum of 11 questions (e.g., "Feel stressed between caring for CR and meeting other responsibilities?").
Depression	Enhance the caregiver's emotional well-being and skills for mood management	■ Provide education about importance of pleasant events and emotional well-being (Caregiver Notebook) ■ Instruct in and practice strategies for engaging in pleasant events ■ Instruct in and role-play strategies for mood management and use of Thought Record ■ Establish schedule of pleasant events	■ The 10-item version of the Center for Epidemiological Studies—Depression Scale (CES-D; Radloff, 1977) was used to assess depression.
Social support	Enhance the caregiver's emotional and social support, support with caregiving activities	■ Provide education about importance of social support (Caregiver Notebook) ■ Instruct in how to access community resources ■ Practice and role-play strategies to enhance communication with health care providers and family members ■ Reinforce participation in telephone support groups ■ Refer to resource guide; communication and respite features of computerized phone system	■ Social support was assessed using 10 items assessing three domains of support: (a) received support (3 items; Barrera, Sandler, & Ramsay, 1981; Krause, 1995); (b) satisfaction with support (3 items; Krause, 1995; Krause & Markides, 1990); and (c) negative interactions/support (4 items; Krause, 1995).

ADL, activities of daily living; IADL, instrumental activities of daily living.
Source: Adapted from Belle et al. (2006).

TYPES OF MEASURES

Individual-Level Measures

Measures at the individual level can target the study participant or an informant such as a caregiver or health care provider. They can include clinical outcomes (e.g., weight loss), physiological indices (e.g., heart rate) or biomarkers (e.g., blood proteins), or measures of emotional well-being (e.g., depression, anxiety). They may also include measures of cognition (e.g., working memory), functional performance (e.g., Activities of daily Living (ADL)/Instrumental Activities of Daily Living (IADL) performance), performance on a task or activity (e.g., Internet search), or some aspect of health behavior (e.g., amount of exercise, sleep patterns). Additional measures include psychosocial outcomes such as perceptions of social support, loneliness, burden, quality of life, or satisfaction. Measures of personality traits and personal beliefs or attitudes are also included in intervention trials as well as evaluation measures such as questionnaires that assess the value or acceptability of an intervention or some element of usability. These measures are sometimes used as indicators of the social validity of an intervention, which is also a marker of clinical significance (Chapter 17).

Community/Organization-Level Measures

Measures at the community or organizational level are typically gathered when an intervention is focused on implementation of an intervention in settings such as a school, clinic, hospital, housing units, or community. For example, housing conditions are related to childhood asthma and an intervention might be focused on educating residents within a housing unit or neighborhood about housekeeping practices, or building owners on building maintenance (e.g., water leaks, wall cracks) or rodent control. Alternatively, the intervention could be a community walking program or antismoking campaign within a neighborhood. These types of studies typically include measures targeted at the individual such as clinical outcomes (e.g., reductions in asthma prevalence), measures of health behaviors or activity patterns (e.g., decreased incidence of smoking or an increase in walking), or attitudes (e.g., attitudes toward the importance of health behaviors). However, other measures are also important such as those related to cost-effectiveness, resource utilization, changes in environments (e.g., better maintained housing units, safe walking paths in neighborhoods), changes in processes (e.g., reduced wait times in clinics), and measures related to treatment fidelity and sustainability of the intervention.

METHODS OF DATA COLLECTION

Measures can also be categorized according to the format used to gather the data. There is a variety of methods available for collecting data in behavioral intervention trials. These methods include self-reports, observer or informant reports, or group assessments and may involve the use of checklists, questionnaires, standardized assessment instruments, rating scales, surveys, interviews, or focus groups. They may also involve direct observation or direct measurement of some phenomena of interest (e.g., heart rate, brain activity, weight). Many studies include a variety of assessment methods. For example, one might obtain ratings of IADL performance for an individual as well as from his or her caregiver or measure stress using the Perceived Stress Scale and levels of catecholamine in the blood. One might also gather cost data or data regarding service utilization such as emergency room visits using an existing database.

Clearly, there are strengths and weaknesses associated with each of these methods. An advantage of self-report methods is that they allow individuals to describe their own feelings, perceptions, and experiences. Use of self-reports via standardized instruments can also be a relatively quick and inexpensive way to gather data; think of the stress measurement example alluded to earlier. However, potential weaknesses include things such as response biases (e.g., social desirability bias, extreme or acquiescent responding) or an individual may not respond truthfully, may not recall what is being assessed (e.g., "Did you have any difficulty doing XYZ in the past month?"), or may not understand the questions. Informant reports are often gathered as a way to verify or supplement self-report data or because an individual is not capable of accurately responding (e.g., someone with a cognitive impairment). Informants can offer a different perspective or enrich the data reported by an individual. Similar to self-reports data, informant reports are subject to biases; it may be difficult to identify informants and inclusion of informant data may add cost to a study. There may also be issues with informed consent and institutional review boards in cases where patients are unable to respond. In clinical assessments, there is often some degree of subjectivity.

Physiological indices or biomarkers are also increasingly being integrated into behavioral intervention research studies to enhance an understanding of the impact of an intervention. For example, it is common in cognitive intervention trials to include brain imaging to help unravel why an intervention results in a change in cognitive performance. Careful consideration needs to be given to the inclusion of physiological measures. The choice of these measures must be well justified and based on an understanding of the potential conceptual/empirical link between the biological/physiological process(es) and the intervention. It is also important to have updated and calibrated equipment, and members of the research team who are skilled in protocols for data collection and analysis. Other considerations in using these measurement approaches are related to data management and storage, cost of including these types of measures, and issues related to participant safety.

SELECTION CRITERIA

In this section, we discuss factors to consider when selecting measures for inclusion in a behavioral intervention research trial. It is not always possible to meet all criteria; however, having an understanding of the issues is important and will help guide the choice of measures. The relevance of some criteria also varies according to the stage in the pipeline.

Psychometric Properties and Scale of Measurement

The psychometric properties of a measure are important factors to consider in measurement selection. Psychometric properties influence the quality of the information gathered from a measure and include factors such as level of measurement, reliability, validity, and sensitivity.

Level of Measurement

The measurement properties or level of measurement of a measure is also an important consideration as it affects the selection of statistical techniques that can be used to analyze the data and the interpretation of the data. Nominal levels of measurement simply assign responses or individuals by category such as male versus female or married versus single. Nominal scales do not imply any ordering among the responses. Ordinal scales also involve mutually exclusive and exhaustive categories in terms of responses such as degree of agreement with a statement, but the categories do not have equal intervals. Interval level scales involve order and equal intervals between units of measurement such as the units on a Fahrenheit scale of temperature. However, there is not a true zero point on interval scales. Finally, ratio scales are interval scales with a true zero point that indicates presence or absence of a quality. As noted, the concern about scale of measurement in behavioral intervention research is the implications for the appropriate statistical analyses.

Reliability

Reliability refers to the consistency of a measure or the extent to which a score or outcome remains unchanged across assessments (if no change is expected) or among different assessors. For example, one would not expect a dramatic change in an individual's weight within an hour if the same scale was used or if different nurses in a clinic took the weigh measurement. Similarly one would not choose a scale that assessed depression if the data indicated that the same individuals had radically different scores throughout a day. Such a lack of consistency and stability over time would make this scale a poor choice as an outcome measure for a clinical intervention for depression as it would be difficult to assess whether changes in initial and follow-up scores on depression were related to the effects of the intervention or represent the intrasubject variability or lack of reliability of the scale. Lack of reliability, or the consistency of measurement of an instrument, introduces considerable error variance in statistical models and makes it virtually impossible to detect true effects as a function of treatment.

For behavioral intervention research, the most critical types of reliability include test–retest reliability, inter-rater reliability, parallel forms, and the internal consistency of a measure.

Test–retest reliability refers to the consistency or stability of the measure when the measure is administered over relatively short time intervals. For example, if an individual completes a measure assessing attitudes about weight loss, one would not expect large changes in these attitudes if the measure was administered later that same day.

Inter-rater reliability refers to consistency of measurement across assessors. For example, if an outcome measure involved independent clinician ratings of anxiety, one would anticipate a high degree of agreement on level of anxiety of an individual across two clinicians. Sometimes, use of a checklist can help ensure inter-rater reliability. Measures with high inter-rater reliability (usually measured by a statistic such as kappa) help ensure that the measure is structured so that different raters will obtain similar results. Similarly, intra-rater reliability refers to the degree to which an assessor administers and scores a measure consistently.

Parallel forms is another indicator of stability. It is obtained by administering different versions of a measure to the same group of individuals. The correlation between the two parallel forms is the measure of reliability. The measures should be administered in different orders to reduce error rates. The measures must have the same content. For example, one might develop two versions of a knowledge test. One issue, of course, is the need to generate lots of items to reflect the same content.

Internal consistency is an important aspect of validity if a measure is designed to assess one overall construct or there are specific subscales within a measure. For example, the Short Form Health Survey (SF36) (Ware & Sherbourne, 1992) includes eight subscales related to various aspects of quality of life (e.g., emotional health, physical health). Internal consistency reflects the degree to which the items in a measure "hang together" or are addressing the same underlying construct.

Validity

Validity is also an important factor in selection of outcome measures. At a global level, it is defined as the extent to which a measure is assessing what it is intending to measure; whether the measure actually captures the outcome of interest. It is important to recognize that the validity of a measure varies according to the population of interest. For example, a vocabulary test that is based on items related to current pop culture may not be a valid instrument for older adults or individuals from other cultures. Like reliability, there are various types of validity.

Face validity refers to the extent to which an item appears to measure what it is intended to measure. Of course, this is a subjective assessment. Importantly, this should be based on the perspective not only of the researcher but also of the intended responders.

Content validity refers to the extent to which a measure includes all of items or taps all of the issues that are important to the construct or outcome being assessed or the degree to which a measure accurately and comprehensively captures an outcome of interest. For example, a measure intended to broadly assess personality traits would have low content validity if it contained only items related to extroversion. This aspect of validity is particularly important if one is developing a new measure for a study. For example, in the PRISM trial, it was necessary to develop a measure that evaluated participants' computer proficiency. In this case, it was important that the items in the measure were current in terms of today's computer technology and also captured all of the aspects of proficiency (see Boot et al., 2015).

Concurrent validity refers to the degree to which a measure is correlated with or related to another established measure or indicator that taps the same construct. One might examine the correlation or degree of relationship between a scale assessing depression and clinical ratings of depression.

Predictive validity is the extent to which performance on a measure of interest is related to a later performance that the measure was designed to predict. A classic example is the degree to which performance on the SAT (a test taken by high school students) predicts future performance in college or performance on a cognitive measure is predictive of an individual's development of a future adverse outcome such as dementia.

Discriminative validity is an extremely important type of validity and refers to the extent to which a measure can discriminate among groups or individuals who vary on some dimension. An example might be a measure of cognition or functional performance that discriminates between noncognitively impaired older adults and older adults with mild dementia. It is usually discussed according to two dimensions: sensitivity and specificity. Sensitivity refers to the ability of a measure to correctly identify true cases (e.g., cognitively impaired) of some dimension whereas specificity refers to the ability to correctly identify nonaffected cases. It is important to remember that sensitivity and specificity are specific to a particular test. The utility of a test to discriminate in clinical populations is dependent on the base rate of particular disorders in the population. This gives rise to the terms *positive predictive power* and *negative predictive power.* Unfortunately, very low prevalence in a population (e.g., the number of completed suicides, number of patients with a rare illness) will result in poor positive predictive power for low occurrence outcome despite excellent sensitivity and specificity of a test. In general, low base rates result in lower positive predictive values whereas higher base rates result in lower negative predictive values. However, for the purposes of selecting outcome measures, techniques such as logistic regression, discriminant function analyses, and calculation of possible sensitivities and specificities under a receiver operator curve (ROC) will provide an investigator with the best means of determining discriminative validity.

Ecological validity is generally thought of as the ability to generalize results to natural or real-world situations and depends on capturing the critical elements of environments, tasks, and behaviors. In this case, ecological validity refers to the extent to which measures capture the relevant features of tasks and environments. For example, within the realm of cognition, there is a concern that, although standard neuropsychological measures provide important information regarding an individual's cognitive abilities, they have low ecological validity in the sense that they do not provide information relative to functioning in everyday activities. In this regard, our group has developed a battery of computer-based simulations of common everyday activities such as use of an ATM, refilling a prescription, using a ticket kiosk, and medication management. Preliminary data with diverse older adult populations suggest that the measures have test–retest reliability, face validity, and discriminant validity (Czaja, Harvey, & Loewenstein, 2014; see Chapter 15 for more discussion of this topic).

Sensitivity and Specificity

Sensitivity of a measure refers to the degree that a measure detects the presence of a characteristic in someone with the characteristics (e.g., cognitive impairment, high blood pressure, depression). Specificity refers to the likelihood that a measure will detect the absence of a characteristic in someone without the characteristic. The positive predictive value of a measure is the likelihood that someone with a positive result on a measure assessing a characteristic actually has the characteristic. The negative predictive value of a measure is the likelihood that someone with a negative result on a measure assessing a characteristic actually lacks the characteristic. Sensitivity and specificity may be combined to determine the positive likelihood ratio (LR) that describes the overall diagnostic properties of a measure (LR + = sensitivity/1 − specificity).

Additional Considerations

In addition to psychometric properties, there are other factors to consider such as the cost and feasibility associated with the measures of interest and the temporal relevance of a measure. It is important to ensure that the needed equipment and expertise for the administration of the measure and interpretation of the data gathered from the measure are available. Of course, available funding is also an important consideration. If one is interested in assessing both patients and their caregivers and participants are compensated for each assessment, the budget must include funds for both members of the dyads. Some types of measures such as physiological indices and biomarkers can be expensive and also require specialized types of expertise.

Other issues are related to floor and ceiling effects, both of which limit variability in responses. Ceiling effects occur when the items in a measure are "too easy" and floor effects occur when the opposite is true, the items in a scale or measure are "too difficult." Other considerations are timing of the assessment, number of assessments, and participant burden. As noted earlier, mode of administration is also important. Assessors must also be thoroughly trained and evaluated periodically to ensure that they are adhering to the assessment protocol. "Assessor drift" is not uncommon if assessors need to administer an assessment protocol for large numbers of individuals over long time periods. Additionally, it is important to consider the amount of data that is being collected as well as protocols for data management, storage, and security. All too often these issues are ignored or considered after the fact. Finally, it is critical to consider the characteristics of the population in terms of characteristics such as ability, prior knowledge of a domain, literacy, and culture/ethnicity. We highly recommend pilot testing measurement instruments and data collection protocols with representative participants prior to engaging in formal data collection.

THE ROLE OF TECHNOLOGY IN MEASUREMENT

As discussed in Chapter 7, developments in technology are affording new methods for data collection. For example, monitoring and sensing technologies are increasingly being used to monitor activities and track behaviors such as movement patterns or sleep behaviors. Wearable technologies such as smart watches that incorporate sensing and computing technologies are aimed at unobtrusively monitoring health indicators and providing feedback to the user. Advantages of these technologies are that they are for the most part unobtrusive and provide objective measurement of behavior in real time. However, there are also issues with privacy, data security and access, and data integration. For example, decisions need to be made about the schedule for data sampling (e.g., 24 hours/day; random times during a day). This has important implications for capturing relevant behavior patterns as well as for data management and analysis. Other important considerations are related to data coding and data integration. For example, in the PRISM trial, we collected real-time data on use of the PRISM software and had to make decisions about what constitutes actual use.

Other developments include the use of online data collection protocols and computer-assisted interviewing methods such as CATI. Use of CAT methods is also increasing, which allow assessments to be tailored to the level of the individual. The software program selects items that are relevant to the individual; the last response of the individual determines the next question that is asked. Items are selected from item banks that are assumed to represent the universe of potential items and levels of items for a particular construct or domain (e.g., health literacy). An example is the NIH-sponsored Patient-Reported Outcomes Measurement Information System (PROMIS) item bank for patient-reported health status for physical, mental, and social well-being (www.nihpromis.org). Potential benefits of these types of systems are efficiency (individuals are not asked questions that are irrelevant or beyond their ability level) and flexibility. Of course, use of these types of assessment techniques requires access to computer equipment, which can be costly. Development of item banks is also complex and time-consuming. Other concerns center around the psychometric properties of the assessment tool, determining branching protocols, and the content validity and currency of the item bank.

A CAUTIONARY NOTE: INCORRECT INTERPRETATIONS OF OUTCOME MEASURES

Sometimes even with diligence with respect to selection of outcome measures, the data collected from these measures can be misinterpreted. In intervention research, it is common practice to employ self-report measures because of time factors and ease of administration. One popular measure used with geriatric populations is the CES-D or the Geriatric Depression Scale. It certainly would be cost prohibitive to send trained geriatric psychiatrists into the homes of individuals for a 1-hour structured interview to assess depressive symptoms. However, it is important to recognize that these scales measure depressive symptoms and a high score, though certainly a reason for caution, does not necessarily indicate that a person is clinically depressed. There are many factors in geriatric populations that will elevate scores on depression measures including anxiety, general psychiatric distress, or physical symptoms related to medical illness. This is particularly true of scores in the lower clinical and subclinical ranges. Another problem with self-report is inherent reporter biases. Many older men may also underreport on depression inventories because of fear of revealing weakness (Eisdorfer et al., 2003). In published papers, one often reports decreased scores of several points on depression inventories as indicating reduced "depression." What is forgotten is that self-report measures are generally indices of reported depression or psychological distress. Just because a measure is called a depression or anxiety inventory does not imply that it is always capturing clinical depression or anxiety. There are many factors that may account for increases and decreases in these measures, which may have to do with other psychological processes other than clinical depression or clinical anxiety. Therefore, it is always prudent to report self or informant-based measures of depression and anxiety for what they are, self and proxy reports. Overall, it is important to understand the characteristics of a measure and its strengths and limitations.

CONCLUSION

In any behavioral intervention study including development to trial-type studies, decisions must be made about the type of outcome data that will be gathered and the instruments, measures, and methods that will be used for data capture. Decisions must also be made about other types of measures such as screening measures or measures that might be used to characterize a sample or serve as mediating variables. Measurement decisions are a critical aspect of behavioral intervention research and important at all phases of the pipeline. As discussed in this chapter, there are a myriad of measures available and a variety of ways to gather outcome data. The choice of measures must be guided by relevant theories and models, the current literature, the research questions of interest and hypotheses, the interests of stakeholders, characteristics of the target population, and the stage in the intervention pipeline. There are also a number of practical considerations such as cost, convenience, and participant burden. There is no simple answer to the question: Which measures should I use? Equally important is being able to comprehend, integrate, and interpret data that is yielded from the measures chosen. It is also important to recognize that measurement is not perfect and all measures are subject to error. An error can be random, or caused by chance, or be systematic resulting from the measure itself (e.g., confusing questions), method of administration (e.g., untrained assessors), or environmental influences (e.g., noise). It is important to be aware of the sources of measurement errors so that steps can be taken to minimize them such as pilot testing measures and training assessors.

REFERENCES

Baranowski, T., Cerin, E., & Baranowski, J. (2009). Steps in the design, development and formative evaluation of obesity prevention-related behavior change trials. *International Journal of Behavioral Nutrition and Physical Activity, 6*, 6. doi:10.1186/1479-5868-6-6

Barrera, M., Sandler, I., & Ramsay, T. (1981). Preliminary development of a scale of social support: Studies on college students. *American Journal of Community Psychology, 9*, 435–441.

Bean, J. F., Vora, A., & Frontera, W. R. (2004). Benefits of exercise for community-dwelling older adults. *Archives of Physical Medicine and Rehabilitation, 85*, 31–42.

Bédard, M., Molloy, D. W., Squire, L., Dubois, S., Lever, J. A., & O'Donnell, M. (2001). The Zarit Burden Interview: A new short version and screening version. *The Gerontologist, 41*(5), 652–657.

Belle, S. H., Burgio, L., Burns, R., Coon, D., Czaja, S. J., Gallagher-Thompson, D., & Zhang, S. (2006). Enhancing the quality of life of dementia caregivers from different ethnic or racial groups. *Annals of Internal Medicine, 145*(10), 727–738.

Berson, G. G. (1993). *Basic ophthalmology for medical students and primary care residents* (6th ed.). San Francisco, CA: American Academy of Ophthalmology.

Boot, W. R., Charness, N., Czaja, S. J., Sharit, J., Rogers, W. A., Fisk, A. D., . . . Nair, S. (2015). Computer proficiency questionnaire: Assessing low and high computer proficient seniors. *The Gerontologist, 55*(3), 404–411. doi:10.1093/geront/gnt117

Chen, G., Gully, S. M., & Eden, D. (2001). Validation of a new general self-efficacy scale. *Organizational Research Methods, 4*(1), 62–83.

Cohen, S., Kamarck, T., & Mermelstein, R. (1983). A global measure of perceived stress. *Journal of Health and Social Behavior, 24*, 385–396.

Czaja, S. J., Boot, W. R., Charness, N., Rogers, W. A., Sharit, J., Fisk, A. D., . . . Nair, S. N. (2015). The personalized reminder information and social management system (PRISM) trial: Rationale, methods, and baseline characteristics. *Contemporary Clinical Trials, 40*, 35–46.

Czaja, S. J., Charness, N., Dijkstra, K., Fisk, A. D., Rogers, W. A., & Sharit, J. (2006a). *Demographic and background questionnaire.* CREATE Technical Rep. No. CREATE-2006-02.

Czaja, S. J., Charness, N., Dijkstra, K., Fisk, A. D., Rogers, W. A., & Sharit, J. (2006b). *Computer and technology experience questionnaire.* CREATE Technical Rep. No. CREATE-2006-01.

Czaja, S. J., Charness, N., Fisk, A. D., Hertzog, C., Nair, S. N., Rogers, W., & Sharit, J. (2006). Factors predicting the use of technology: Findings from the Center for Research and Education on Aging and Technology Enhancement (CREATE). *Psychology and Aging, 21*, 333–352.

Czaja, S. J., Harvey, P., & Loewenstein, D. (2014). *A novel technology-based functional outcomes assessment.* Invited presentation at the 4th Annual Schizophrenia International Research Society Conference, Florence, Italy.

Eisdorfer, C., Czaja, S. J., Loewenstein, D. A., Rubert, M. P., Arguelles, S., Mitrani, V. B., & Szapocznik, J. (2003). The effect of a family therapy and technology-based intervention on caregiver depression. *The Gerontologist, 43*(4), 521–531.

Folstein, M. F., Folstein, S. E., & McHugh, P. R. (1975). Mini-mental state: A practical method for grading the cognitive state of patients for the clinician. *Journal of Psychiatric Research, 12*(3), 189–198.

Gosling, S. D., Rentfrow, P. J., & Swann, Jr., W. B. (2003). A very brief measure of the big-five personality domains. *Journal of Research in Personality, 37*(6), 504–528.

Jay, G. M., & Willis, S. K. (1992). Influence of direct computer experience on older adults' attitude toward computers. *Journal of Gerontology Psychological Sciences, 47*(4), P250–P257.

Katz, S., Ford, A. B., Moskowitz, R. W., Jackson, B. A., & Jaffe, M. W. (1963). Studies of illness in the aged: The index of ADL: A standardized measure of biological and psychosocial function. *Journal of the American Medical Association, 185*, 914–919.

Keefe, R. S. E., Poe, M., Walker, T. M., Kang, J. W., & Harvey, P. D. (2006). The schizophrenia cognition rating scale: An interview-based assessment and its relationship to cognition, real-world functioning, and functional capacity. *The American Journal of Psychiatry, 163*(3), 426–432.

Kosberg, J. I., & Cairl, R. E. (1986). The cost of care index: A case management tool for screening informal care providers. *The Gerontologist, 26*(3), 273–278.

Krause, N. (1995). Negative interaction and satisfaction with social support among older adults. *Journal of Gerontology Series B: Psychological Science and Social Science, 50*, P59–P73.

Krause, N., & Markides, K. (1990). Measuring social support among older adults. *International Journal of Aging and Human Development, 30*(1), 37–53.

Lawton, M. P., & Brody, E. (1969). Self-maintaining and instrumental activities of daily living. *The Gerontologist, 9*(3), 179–186.

Lee, C. C., Czaja, S. J., & Schulz, R. (2010). The moderating influence of demographic characteristics, social support, and religious coping on the effectiveness of a multicomponent psychosocial caregiver intervention in three racial ethnic groups. *The Journal of Gerontology Series B: Psychological Sciences, 65*(2), 185–194.

Lewis, B. A., Marcus, B. H., Pate, R. R., & Dunn, A. L. (2002). Psychosocial mediators of physical activity behavior among adults and children. *American Journal of Preventive Medicine, 23*(2), 26–35. doi:10.1016/S0749-3797(02)00471-3

Marsiske, M., & Willis, S. L. (1995). Dimensionality of everyday problem solving in older adults. *Psychology and Aging, 10*(2), 269–283.

Menditto, A. A., Wallace, C. J., Liberman, R. O. P., Vander Wall, J., Toumi Jones, N., & Stuve, P. (1999). Functional assessment of independent living skills. *Psychiatric Rehabilitation skills, 3*(2), 200–219.

Nelson, M. E., Layne, J. E., Bernstein, M. J., Nuernberger, A., Castaneda, C., Kaliton, D., . . . Singh, M. A. F. (2004). The effects of multidimensional home-based exercise on functional performance in elderly people. *The Journal of Gerontology Series A: Biological Science & Medical Science, 59*(2), M154–M160.

Radloff, L. (1977). The CES-D scale: A self-report depression scale for research in the general population. *Applied Psychological Measurement, 1*(3), 385–401.

Shyu, Y. I. L. (2000). Development and testing of the family caregiving factors inventory (FCFI) for home health assessment in Taiwan. *Journal of Advanced Nursing, 32*(1), 226–234.

Stewart, A. K., Verboncoeur, C. J., McLellan, B. Y., Gillis, D. E., Rush, S., Mills, K. M., . . . Bortz, W. M. (2001). Physical activity outcomes of CHAMPS II: A physical activity promotion program for older adults. *The Journal of Gerontology Series A: Biological Science & Medical Science, 56*(8), M465–M470.

Teri, L., Truax, P., Logsdon, R., Uomoto, J., Zarit, S., & Vitalino, P. P. (1992). Assessment of behavioral problems in dementia: The revised memory and behavioral problems checklist. *Psychology and Aging, 7*(4), 622–631.

Ware, J. E., & Sherbourne, C. D. (1992). The MOS 36-item short form health survey (SF-36). *Medical Care, 30*(6), 473–483.

Wilkinson, G. (1993). *Wide range achievement test—Third revision.* Wilmington, DE: Jastak Associates.

Zarit, S. H., Orr, N. K., & Zarit, J. M. (1985). *The hidden victims of Alzheimer's disease: Families under stress.* New York, NY: New York University Press.

FIFTEEN

COGNITIVE AND FUNCTIONAL OUTCOMES: THE ROLE OF OBJECTIVE MEASUREMENT

PHILIP D. HARVEY

To understand how [people] really think and feel, it is vital to go beyond words.
—Katja Bressette

Many behavioral intervention studies are aimed at increasing cognitive and functional skills, with the eventual goal of improving everyday functioning, subjective quality of life, and lessening care needs. Target populations may include healthy older adults, older adults with chronic conditions and impairments, and individuals with disabling conditions such as neuropsychiatric disorders (e.g., schizophrenia). The focus of this chapter is on measures specific to intervention studies that are designed to impact cognitive and functional domains of everyday living. A focused discussion on these two domains of outcomes is warranted as there is a vast and emerging literature on this topic and cognition and functional independence is of increasing concern, particularly with the aging of the population.

As noted in Chapter 14, the choice of outcome measures for behavioral intervention trials is an important issue as it has a significant influence on many aspects of the study design and the evidence regarding the impact of the intervention. Researchers conducting intervention trials aimed at cognitive and functional performance are faced with a myriad of choices as there are several different strategies for collecting outcomes data for these types of intervention studies. These strategies include informant reports, self-reports, standardized neuropsychological tests, observational strategies, and objective indices of functional performance. Each of these measures provides different insights into the impact of an intervention and has associated strengths and weaknesses. Although a brief overview of the myriad of measures used is provided, the emphasis in this chapter is on objective performance-based measures.

We begin the chapter with rationale for the importance of performance-based measures and the shortcomings of self-report, followed by a brief overview of the construct of cognition and how it is distinct from functional performance. We then briefly discuss the strengths and weaknesses of self-report and informant-based measures as this topic was covered in the prior chapter. In the sections that follow, we describe the different types of objective performance-based assessments, the distal targets of these interventions, and the strengths and limitations of each approach. Finally, strategies for obtaining optimal assessment data are presented.

WHY USE PERFORMANCE-BASED MEASURES?

The primary reason for using objective performance-based measures, as opposed to other measurement strategies such as self-report or informant-report, is that they afford a less biased assessment of performance. In addition, they can be adapted to the unique needs of a population and task/behavior in question. For example, the difficulty level of the tasks, or the language, or contextual cues can be adjusted. The skills required for different aspects of everyday functioning (e.g., work, school, everyday activities of living, social activities) generally differ depending on the functional domain assessed (e.g., social vs. employment).

The types of performance-based assessments that are available vary considerably, and include standardized tests of cognitive abilities (that are related to but do not directly assess functional skills), paper-and-pencil simulations of everyday tasks, and realistic, virtual-reality performance scenarios that directly model real-world functional activities. They also include observational strategies and physiological indices. Obviously, these types of measures vary considerably in terms of issues such as administration requirements, scoring algorithms, the nature of the data collected, and the type of data required for validation. With respect to the latter, novel realistic computer-based simulations have the least demands for assessment of convergent validity, and performance-based neuropsychological tests have the best data in terms of psychometric properties and alternate forms.

THE LIMITATIONS OF SELF-REPORT AS AN OUTCOME MEASURE

Objective outcome measures are important because self-reports in several domains of functioning are often unreliable. This is the case for both healthy and impaired populations. These domains include self-assessment of cognitive abilities, functional capacity, and some elements of everyday outcomes. Self-reports of previous experiences, such as health care and medical conditions, can be accurate in some circumstances, but even these reports become somewhat challenging if a long duration of time has passed since the experience. Healthy individuals often tend to overestimate their competence, and mood state variation can also impact the accuracy of self-assessment. Further, the discrepancy between self-reported functioning and objective outcome measures can provide valuable information about the response styles of an individual, with overestimation and underestimation of functioning having considerably different implications.

Often, people become candidates for interventions aimed at cognitive or functional enhancement interventions because of their subjective experience of cognitive change or difficulty performing everyday activities or because of concerns of a family member. Thus, self-reported measures of cognitive functions have been explored as an assessment strategy (Keefe, Poe, Walker, Kang, & Harvey, 2006; Ventura et al., 2013). Self-report measures of everyday functioning are often included in behavioral intervention studies aimed at improving cognitive or functional performance. An example of this type of measure is the Lawton and Brody Instrumental Activities of Daily Living (IADL) scale (Lawton & Brody, 1969), which requires participants to provide self-reported ratings on their ability to perform IADL tasks. The IADL domains included in this questionnaire consist of telephone use, shopping, meal preparation, housekeeping, laundry, transportation, medication responsibility, and finances. Another example is the Independent Living Skills Survey (ILSS) (Wallace, Liberman, Tauber, & Wallace, 2000), which assesses basic functional living skills and is typically used with patients with psychiatric disorders. Informants can also complete the ILSS.

Although these measures provide important insights into functional abilities and intervention outcomes, they obviously have both strengths and limitations. Overall, these measures are relatively quick and easy to administer and inexpensive. In addition, people have important insights into certain aspects of their behavior that are not accessible to outside observers. However, these types of measures are also subject to biases. As noted in Chapter 14, one type of bias is social desirability bias where people tend to report what they think the assessor or researcher wants to hear. In addition, people who are healthy with severe mental illness and those with other neuropsychiatric conditions all tend to overestimate their abilities (Bowie et al., 2007; Carone, Benedict, Munschauer, Fishman, & Weinstock-Guttman, 2005; Kruger & Dunning, 1999; Spikman & van der Naalt, 2010). Additionally, people with moderate or more severe depression tend to underestimate their functioning (Bruce & Arnett, 2004). Individuals who are experiencing subjective distress will often index their functioning in terms of their distress level and rate their functioning accordingly (Kaye et al., 2014). Furthermore, sometimes individuals have incomplete or inaccurate memories of their performance abilities.

At the same time, self-reported cognitive ability is typically unrelated to objective performance and the opinions of others (Durand et al., 2015; Keefe, Poe, et al., 2006). It was recently shown (Keefe et al., 2015) that self-reports of cognitive functioning in people with schizophrenia were not sensitive to pharmacological cognitive enhancement, whereas both observer ratings and objective test performance were sensitive. Studies that have relied on patient self-report have also consistently found minimal correlation between reports of functional skills and objective indices of performance (Bowie et al., 2007; Durand et al., 2015; Sabbag et al., 2011). A reasonable conclusion is that the type of person who is targeted for cognitive or functional enhancement interventions is unlikely to be an adequate reporter of either his or her baseline functioning or his or her improvements from that baseline. Performance-based assessments are not prone to any of these limitations and have been shown, even in impaired populations, to be correlated with the achievement of functional milestones.

DEFINING THE CONSTRUCTS OF COGNITION AND FUNCTIONAL PERFORMANCE

The scientific construct of cognition generally refers to a broad range of functions including perception; attention and concentration; learning; and various aspects of memory, reasoning, and problem solving; as well as crystalized knowledge and speed of processing (Harvey, 2012). Attempts to enhance or improve these different aspects or domains of cognition require very different intervention strategies, which in turn have different potential levels of benefit. For instance, certain pharmacological compounds have demonstrated benefits in transmitter systems with specific cognitive benefits (acetylcholine and episodic memory; Risacher et al., 2013). Other compounds, such as amphetamine, have wide-ranging cognitive benefits that are not specifically related to the primary pharmacological effects of the compound (see Sostek, Buchsbaum, & Rapoport, 1980 for a classic early study). Behavioral interventions can either be targeted toward a particular cognitive domain, multiple domains (e.g., Fisher, Holland, Merzenich, & Vinogradov, 2009), or global cognition (McGurk, Mueser, Feldman, Wolfe, & Pascaris, 2007), and the assessment strategy chosen must be commensurate with the goal of the intervention in terms of the domain or domains targeted by the treatment.

It is beyond the scope of this chapter to fully describe the ranges of functioning that can be considered cognitive in nature. However, we subscribe to the idea that cognition is a broad construct that can be conceptualized in terms of separable cognitive domains, which are then amenable to measurement with specialized assessments (Nuechterlein et al., 2004). Traditional domains of cognitive functioning (e.g., sensation, perception, sustained attention, selective attention, working memory, episodic memory, executive functioning, processing speed) are differentially affected in healthy aging and various neuropsychiatric conditions and have been the target of cognitive enhancement interventions.

More recent conceptualizations of cognitive performance are focused on networks, which can affect an array of cognitive abilities (Callicott et al., 1999). For instance, impairments in striatal regions, such as those induced by Huntington's disease and related conditions, impact an array of cognitive functions. These include processing speed, concentration and attention, and learning and memory (Paulsen et al., 1995). The notion of separable versus highly related cognitive domains may influence strategies for selecting measures for interventions aimed at enhancing cognition. First of all, if measures of different cognitive domains are highly intercorrelated, it may be challenging to develop interventions that are selective in their measured cognitive benefits. Certain interventions can have specific effects on a limited set of cognitive domains (Fisher et al., 2009), but global functioning is also likely to improve. Second, research on the correlates of real-world functioning has consistently suggested that specific measures from individual cognitive domains are much less strongly related to real-world outcomes than composite measures that summarize global performance (Green, 1996; McClure et al., 2007). Thus, the typical distal goal of improving functional outcomes may be better facilitated by interventions that are effective across multiple cognitive domains (Bowie, McGurk, Mausbach, Patterson, & Harvey, 2012). As a result, treatments with broad cognitive benefits may be the best ways to improve everyday functioning.

In recent years, there has been an emphasis on performance of functional everyday skills, often referred to as "functional capacity." This generally refers to skills involved in everyday living and important to independence and includes tasks such as managing finances and medications; preparing meals; scheduling; driving; and activities related to way-finding. Generally, the literature shows that standardized measures of cognition do not capture the complexity of these tasks and therefore are considered to have low "ecological validity" (see Chapter 14). As a result, prediction of the ability to perform complex everyday activities is improved when a combined strategy of cognitive and functional capacity assessment is employed.

MEASUREMENT STRATEGIES FOR EVALUATING COGNITIVE AND FUNCTIONAL PERFORMANCE

As discussed earlier in this chapter, indexing the impact of various behavioral interventions aimed at improving aspects of cognition or functional performance is a complex and multidimensional task and requires many decisions on the part of the researcher. These decisions are related to the type of measures to use, the number of measures, the timing of measurement, and staffing. Thus, measurement requires a careful conceptualization of the goals of the intervention and the possible benefits. There are multiple assessment strategies that can be employed and which vary in complexity, associated strengths and weaknesses, and challenges with respect to indexing the treatment goals and populations targeted by the treatment (Nuechterlein et al., 2004). In the section that follows, we briefly review the use of self-report and informant measures.

Informant Measures

Informants are often queried about functioning, particularly in pathological conditions where the observer may have a long history of interacting and observing the cognitively relevant behaviors of the individual in question (Morris, McKeel, & Storandt, 1991). Similar to self-reports data, informant reports are subject to biases; it may be difficult to identify informants for all cases; and inclusion of informant data may add cost to a study. In some cases, it might be useful to gather data from several informants (e.g., clinician, caregiver, teacher) to gain insight into someone's functional ability from different perspectives. Although this approach is useful, it can add to the cost and logistic constraints of the project and it may be difficult to integrate discordant ratings. Finally, another approach, which is based on observation, is to use informants who are unaware of the results of other assessment data and unmotivated to generate ratings that support either greater impairment (in search of disability) or reduced impairment (to reduce stigma). As described later, we have shown that only certain informants can provide information that meets suitable validity standards.

Overall, the strategies discussed earlier have different strengths and weaknesses regarding their reliability, validity, and practicality. A detailed discussion of these aspects of measurement is provided in the previous chapter. These strengths and weaknesses tend to be reciprocal in many instances; for example, more practical strategies may have some weaknesses with respect to validity. Thus, the selection of outcomes assessment strategies may be very different depending on the goals of the study and the populations to be assessed. The general criteria for selection of outcome measures are presented in Chapter 14. The focus of the remainder of our discussion is on performance-based assessment strategies.

PERFORMANCE-BASED ASSESSMENTS

Performance-based assessments do not rely on the opinion of an observer and are typically highly standardized. Further, these assessments have been refined over time and their psychometric characteristics can be easily quantified and have been investigated in detail over time (Nuechterlein et al., 2008). Thus, these measures will have known ranges of scores and have often been normed in the healthy population. As a result, performance can immediately be interpreted, and improved performance can be quantified with ease. These tests are often administered together as described later in this chapter, and the administration of these tests can be taught to people without advanced degrees, if the interpretation of the scores is performed statistically. Interpretation of the pattern of scores and their clinical meaning usually requires an advanced degree in psychology or at least certification.

History of Performance-Based Assessment Measures

For the past 90 years, performance-based assessment has been a mainstay of measuring the outcomes or impact of interventions aimed at increasing the cognitive functional skills of target populations. Starting with Binet in the early 1900s, performance-based tests were developed to characterize abilities and attempted to match intervention outcomes (in the case of Binet, special education) with individuals. Neuropsychological assessment had its origins in the evaluation of injured soldiers after the First World War when performance-based testing was implemented in order to identify the deficits in function associated with various localized lesions caused by missile wounds (Goldstein, 1995). The history of clinical neuropsychology, which is the origin of many of the assessments that are used today to generate outcome measures in cognitive enhancement research, was partially based on the assessment of individuals with focal brain injuries or strokes as described earlier (Harvey, 2012). Thus, tasks were developed to be sensitive to deficits in specific brain regions when performance is preserved in other regions of the brain. These assessment methods have persisted to this day and are widely used to measure decline after injury or illness (Adams & Grant, 2009) and, recently, gains after cognitive enhancement therapy (Fisher et al., 2009).

After the development of performance-based assessment of cognition, the vocational rehabilitation domain began to use performance-based testing for individuals who had experienced an injury or illness to assess their ability to perform critical vocational, residential, and self-care skills. These assessments range from elaborate laboratories, which contain full-scale simulations of a home or work environment (Menditto et al., 1999), to paper-and-pencil simulations of everyday tasks (Patterson, Goldman, McKibbin, Hughs, & Jeste, 2001). These assessment strategies have been applied as well in other clinical settings, including individuals who have lifelong neuropsychiatric conditions that led to decrements in their functional performance (Harvey, Velligan, & Bellack, 2007).

Standard Neuropsychological Tests of Cognition

The standard way to measure cognition in clinical practice and intervention trials is with standardized neuropsychological tests. The tradition in clinical neuropsychological assessment has been to perform a detailed assessment aimed at examining a variety of cognitive domains to document level of abilities or changes in abilities (Heaton, Grant, & Matthews, 1991; Reitan & Wolfson, 1993). These measures are also sometimes used as mediating variables to describe how changes in a targeted outcome measure (e.g., some aspect of functional performance) observed after the implementation of an intervention are mediated by changes in cognition (see Chapter 13).

There is a wide variety of neuropsychological measures available and they are generally linked to a specific cognitive domain/ability (e.g., working memory, attention). It is beyond the scope of this chapter to review the comprehensive and somewhat unyielding list of available measures. Although these specific cognitive domains can be defined and measured with neuropsychological tests, there are two important points to consider. First, the neuropsychological tests that are targeted at different domains of functioning are often highly intercorrelated (Dickinson, Ramsey, & Gold, 2007), and the best fitting factor structure is a single, global factor (Keefe, Bilder, et al., 2006). On the other hand, scores on tests measuring similar cognitive domains, such as elements of intelligence, are often somewhat discrepant from each other in healthy people (Zakzanis & Jeffay, 2011), indicating that variability in performance across domains is not abnormal.

Further, there is often disagreement among researchers about which measures are optimal for each domain and population of interest (e.g., minority vs. nonminority). In this regard, the National Institutes of Health (NIH) Toolbox includes a set of brief measures that can be used to assess cognitive, emotional, motor, and sensory functions in individuals aged 3 to 85. The intent of the development of the NIH Toolbox was to harmonize measurement of functions across diverse study designs and settings (www.nihtoolbox.org).

Factors to Consider in Selecting a Cognitive Assessment Battery

There are numerous factors to consider in the selection of a cognitive measure or an assessment battery for an intervention trial. Of most importance are the measurement characteristics and the psychometric properties of the selected measures (see Chapter 14). Most of the available neuropsychological measures have been used with a wide variety of populations and have established norms, known psychometric properties, and sensitivity to change. Many are also available in languages other than English. Other important factors to consider when selecting these measures include the breadth of the battery with respect to domains assessed, number of measures, duration of the battery, frequency of assessments, and mode of administration as well as, of course, whether the assessment reflects the domain being targeted by the intervention. Each of these issues is discussed in turn.

Breadth of the Assessment Battery

In many intervention trials, the use of an extensive assessment battery that contains multiple measures of multiple domains is not needed. In some conditions where performance is highly intercorrelated across tests, a carefully selected, briefer assessment battery may provide the same amount of information as a much longer assessment (Keefe et al., 2004; Keefe, Poe, et al., 2006). A briefer battery may also be appropriate in situations where the intervention is targeted at a specific cognitive domain. Also, in some instances, a condition can be identified through the presence of a single salient deficit. For instance, diagnostic exclusion of possible Alzheimer's disease can be accomplished through a very abbreviated assessment of delayed recall memory (Welsh, Butters, Hughes, Mohs, & Heyman, 1991), with this deficit leading to substantial separation from the performance of various other diagnostic groups, including even patients with schizophrenia (Davidson et al., 1996).

An advantage of a more detailed assessment is that the identification of multiple effects of a cognitive enhancing intervention is possible only with a wide-ranging assessment. Such an assessment would likely be undertaken in the early development phases of an intervention, as regulatory agencies require investigators to declare their primary outcome measure prior to the initiation of a trial (Buchanan et al., 2011) or an experimental intervention is being developed with no clear understanding of the breadth of its benefit. An additional use of a more detailed assessment in early phase studies is that of the detection of any possible adverse effects of a treatment. For example, if a cognitive remediation procedure is designed to improve problem solving but induces anxiety or distractibility, this could not be detected unless an assessment of all of these domains was employed. Regulatory agencies may require relatively comprehensive cognitive batteries so that any deleterious effects of a new treatment on cognition can be detected (Buchanan et al., 2011).

Duration of the Assessment

Some formal neuropsychological assessment batteries can take 6 to 12 hours or more to complete. Duration of the assessment is generally correlated with level of detail, but an assessment of episodic memory can take an hour itself while an abbreviated but wide-ranging assessment of cognition often used in clinical trials can take as little as 20 minutes (Keefe et al., 2004). It depends on the measures selected for the assessment.

Longer assessments pose challenges from two directions. If an intervention trial has multiple assessments other than cognition, then a cognitive assessment with a long duration may increase the length of a study visit to the point that it is not practical. The other point is that some populations are challenged by long assessments. For instance, it is not a surprise to see that children who have difficulty sustaining their attention in school have similar problems tolerating long psychological assessments, which can lead to misleading results. Older adults can also become fatigued. In general, however, even patient populations such as those with schizophrenia can provide valid data with cognitive batteries requiring approximately 75 minutes of assessment time (Keefe et al., 2011; Neuchterlein et al., 2008).

The take-home principles from this discussion are that the shortest possible assessment that evaluates important aspects of cognition is the best strategy; however, attention must be paid to important psychometric characteristics of the data collected, such as the psychometric qualities of the assessment (see Chapter 14) and most importantly whether enough information is being collected to allow meaningful conclusions about the impact of an intervention. There are no generic answers for how long and how broad the assessment should be. It depends on the nature of the intervention strategies, targeted outcomes, and target populations.

Format of the Assessment

Cognitive measures are available in paper-and-pencil or computerized formats. Although computerized assessments would seem to ensure greater fidelity (see Chapter 12) and validity, the results are clearly divided. For populations with significant impairments that may lead to problems in cooperation or effort, there have been several studies showing that computerized assessments generate data that are less complete and possibly less reliable than standard administration procedures (Iverson, Brooks, Ashton, Johnson, & Gualtieri, 2009; Keefe, Bilder et al., 2006; Silver et al., 2006), and computerized assessment can serve to mask invalid performance. Some recently developed assessment strategies can detect invalid performance (Harvey, Siu, et al., 2013), but the message here is clear: Testers need to be as active, observant, and involved in the administration of computerized assessments as they are in the administration of paper-and-pencil assessments.

Frequency of Assessments and Practice Effects

In a cognitive or functional enhancement intervention study, an estimate of treatment-related cognitive change requires assessment before and after treatment. As we have noted before, there are several situations where repeated assessments pose challenges. One is the retest improvement, or "practice," effect, which can be due to exposure to testing, familiarity with the materials, and increased comfort levels. There are several solutions to this problem (Goldberg, Keefe, Goldman, Robinson, & Harvey, 2010). One is the use of alternate forms, but alternate forms can be remarkably poorly correlated with each other in certain populations, which can significantly weaken the reliability of assessing cognitive change. Another is the use of a parallel research design, which allows for comparison of changes in performance over time across active and inactive treatments. As long as participants do not perform at the ceiling of a measure such that improved performance cannot be detected, the difference between active and inactive conditions can index the effect of the treatment minus the effects of repeated testing alone.

Practice effects are challenging, because few measures will have information from normative studies that examined practice effects beyond two or three reassessments in the population of interest and even fewer in healthy individuals for normative comparison. While it is generally believed that practice effects habituate after a few assessments, leading to stable performance over time, some other data suggest small but incremental effects across numerous assessment sessions. However, in the absence of ceiling effects, practice effects are preferable over poorly correlated alternate forms, which will prevent the identification of a treatment effect.

Interview-Based Assessments of Cognition

Interview-based assessments of cognition are appealing as a supplement to neuropsychological assessments, because they are easy to administer, score, and interpret. Some conditions cannot be diagnosed without a subjective cognitive complaint (i.e., Mild Cognitive Impairment [MCI]). An example of this type of measure is the Cognitive Assessment Interview (CAI) (Ventura et al., 2013), a brief, 10-item, interview-based measure of cognitive functioning that is often used in patient populations such as patients with schizophrenia.

Measures of Functional Skills/Performance

The real target of cognitive enhancement is to improve functioning in real-world situations, whether it is the workplace, school, or managing one's life with more efficiency. However, the assessment of real-world outcomes differs substantially in the context of ongoing clinical studies of some pharmacological agent versus behavioral intervention studies. A 12-week clinical trial is very different because some functional changes require time or may not be benefitted by a pharmacological agent alone.

Assessment of real-world functioning might seem to be a trivial task, in that it would be expected that most people would know where they live, what they do for work, and how many friends they have, and how they manage their finances and medications. However, some of the subpopulations targeted for cognitive enhancement and other skills training programs may present challenges in these areas. Further, for individuals who have experienced challenges and are functioning suboptimally, there may be a complex array of factors, other than skills, that contribute to real-world functioning. These include disability compensation, opportunities in the local area for intervention programs, and the complex interaction between environments, care systems, families, and the patients (Harvey et al., 2009; Rosenheck et al., 2006). Many people can perform skilled acts with person support, even minimal support, but are unable to do so without this assistance. While many of these issues are related to assessments with data collected from various observers or informants, there are technology-based assessments of real-world functioning, including ecological momentary assessment (EMA), which are evolving (especially with developments in technology) and are important in addressing these issues.

Importance of Milestones and Consideration of Subthreshold Performance to Assessment

In a largely healthy population, achievement of functional milestones such as full-time work, living independently, and having friends, family, and social network are expected. Individuals who have achieved these milestones and are seeking cognitive or functional enhancement may be trying to increase their level of functioning. In these individuals, the real-world outcome would be school grades, promotions, and other indicators of greater functional success. In impaired populations, however, these milestones often present major challenges. Further, their lack of experience with successfully or optimally meeting functional demands may prohibit individuals from being able to accurately evaluate their own functioning.

For instance, in a recent study of ours, people with severe mental illness who had never had a job in their lives rated themselves as more socially, vocationally, and residentially capable than other individuals who were employed full time (Harvey et al., 2012). As many populations seeking cognitive or functional enhancement may have a lack of functional success to date and even lack experience with efforts to attain functional success, modification of the typical assessment strategy may be required. As a result, previous achievement needs to be an ongoing index to which to compare both current functioning and improvements from the initiation of the intervention. There may be a large difference between regaining some elements of previous functioning that were impaired or lost owing to illness or injury or normative age-related changes in cognition, and aspects of functioning, though a normative part of healthy experience, that were never fully learned due to early-onset neuropsychiatric or other illness conditions. Thus, it is important to be aware of an individual's baseline threshold when establishing treatment goals or assessing change related to an intervention program.

For example, if one is currently unemployed and has not held a job for an extended time period, there are a variety of functional acts that are preparatory to employment that are positive from the perspective of vocational outcomes. For instance, preparing a resume, applying for jobs, and going on job interviews are positively valenced vocational activities. Similarly, obtaining independent residential functioning has a number of similar subthreshold steps. However, they do not equate to having a full-time job or living as the head of a household. For a variety of populations where there are long-term aspects of disability and the assessment of job performance or residential independence is not possible, we are limited to collecting information about the preparation and background activities aimed at real-world functioning. However, these subthreshold milestones can be positively affected by skills training and cognitive enhancement interventions and are relevant measures related to eventual real-world successes.

Subthreshold milestones are particularly amenable to performance-based assessments. There are a variety of performance-based assessments that measure the specific skills associated with residential and vocational achievement that are the building blocks of obtaining and sustaining employment or obtaining and sustaining independent living, but are not the same as working full time or living independently.

Ecological Momentary Assessment Techniques

EMA is a sound alternative to informant ratings of functional performance. Though not technically a performance-based assessment and actually akin to ongoing in-person observation, EMA shares several critical features with performance-based assessments. Participants are assessed in real time while performing activities. They are queried as to their current activities and with whom they are in contact. They are occasionally asked to provide rating information regarding their mood, current behavior, and level of autonomy. This strategy involves sampling of behavioral activities in real time, either with diary methods (Stone et al., 2000), paging strategies (Swendson et al., 2000), or with smartphone assessments (Freedman, Lestor, McNamara, Millby, & Schumacher, 2006). These strategies have many advantages in adherent populations, including the ability to use smartphone GPS technology to identify the locations of respondents and their speed and trajectory of motion. As noted later, these technological strategies have the advantage of contemporaneous assessment while not requiring participants to engage in burdensome reporting activities. As noted earlier, measures of functional performance have also been evolving, which attempt to assess an individual's ability to perform everyday activities.

EMA was initially delivered with paper-and-pencil logs based on timers, pagers, or other notifications (Stone et al., 2000). With the advent of personally available high technology (e.g., PDAs, smartphones), EMA is now much more highly automated. This automated technology allows for several critical pieces of information to be obtained. For example, a momentary assessment allows for assessment of where one is, what he or she is doing, with whom, with what level of satisfaction, and with what level of assistance. Current smartphone technology allows for use of the GPS feature on the phone, which makes it possible to see where a person is and at what rate he or she is moving, if not stationary. There are several benefits of this strategy.

The first benefit is an intrinsic validity assessment. If the participants say that they are on a bus and they are not moving or say that they are at home while moving 65 miles per hour, then critical validity information is collected. If a participant who is impaired is on the bus going to a medical appointment on his or her own, then that would generally be a good outcome unless he or she is going with his or her mother who has to accompany him or her, which would be a less significant functional achievement, unless, of course, that was the intention or intervention goal.

The second benefit is also related to validity, in the domain of response bias. With EMA, a strategy can be developed to avoid bias, in that participants can be sampled for their behavior prior to being assessed with other, reporting-based, methods, which allows for an additional assessment of self-report accuracy and validity. Thus, both recollection accuracy and any response biases can be evaluated through comparison of the data collected before the self-report assessment and the self-reported functioning after the intervention.

Functional Capacity Measures

Because of our increased knowledge that real-world outcomes are affected by an array of factors other than cognitive abilities, interest has grown in the area of direct assessment of functional skills. Referred to as "functional capacity," this is the process of assessing the ability to perform critical everyday living skills in simulation settings (Harvey et al., 2007). The ability to perform skilled acts can be contrasted with the actual likelihood of performing those acts (Depp et al., 2010; Mausbach et al., 2011) in real-world settings. Similar to standard neuropsychological measures, functional capacity measures do not rely on self-report, and can be evaluated for their psychometric and validity properties.

There is an array of performance-based measures of everyday functioning skills aimed at assessing skills in the domains of residential, social, and vocational functions (Mausbach, Harvey, Goldman, Jeste, & Patterson, 2007; Patterson et al., 2001; see Moore, Palmer, Patterson, & Jette, 2007 for a review). The majority of these procedures use realistic assessments of functional activities such as shopping, cooking, managing money, and social interactions. These are generally administered as interactive tests, with systematic administration of the stimuli, systematic scoring procedures, and normative standards. Thus, much like performance-based cognitive tests, they provide a repeatable index of skills competence that can be used as an outcome measure in behavioral intervention trials.

Other investigators have developed ecologically valid simulations of common technology-based work tasks (e.g., Czaja, Sharit, Ownby, Roth, & Nair, 2001; Sharit

& Czaja, 1999) and have also shown that while cognitive abilities are important to task performance, other factors such as prior technology experience and amount of task practice are also important predictors of performance. More recently, our group has developed a battery of computer-based simulations of common everyday activities such as use of an ATM, refilling a prescription, using a ticket kiosk, and medication management. Preliminary data indicate that these tasks are reliable and have construct and discriminant validity. They are also "ecologically valid" (Czaja, Harvey, & Lowenstein, 2014). However, like neuropsychological measures of cognition, issues associated with comprehensiveness, duration of the assessment, and practicality need to be considered. Also similar to cognitive assessments, the same caveats and concerns need to be applied to the computerized versions of functional capacity measures (Ruse et al., 2014).

Some Unique Considerations

There are several special issues related to cognitive and functional assessment that are important for the design of behavioral intervention trials and assessment of outcomes in these studies.

Cognition or Capacity as the Outcome

The high correlation between assessments of cognitive performance and functional capacity has led to the question (Leifker, Patterson, Bowie, & Harvey, 2010), partially supported by data: Are these actually different assessments of the same general ability domain (Harvey, Raykov, et al., 2013)? Future research will need to determine the differential suitability of these indices for outcomes assessment in treatment studies. Given that abbreviated assessments of both cognition and functional capacity are available, it would seem prudent to invest the time to assess both of these domains. This issue may change with the continued development of computerized functional capacity assessments, as highly validated functional capacity assessments may lead to increased validity and practicality.

What Defines Improvement?

The definition of improvement in performance following cognitive or functional skills-enhancing interventions depends on the goal of the assessment. Clinical treatment will have a very different set of standards from a regulatory efficacy trial. Further, improvement can be indexed in several ways. These improvements can be defined, in hierarchical order of rigorousness, as statistically significant, clinically meaningful, definitely nonrandom, and normalization of functioning,

Statistically Significant. Statistically significant is the criterion for demonstrating differences between active treatments and control conditions. This is the lowest bar for empirically defined improvement, because it is largely dependent on the sample size of the study. This criterion does not depend in any way on the level of baseline performance and does not require any predetermined end of study level of performance. Although the lowest of the bars that we are discussing, it is still important. Any intervention that does not separate from an inactive treatment cannot be seen to provide reliable improvements. This criterion is also required for an intervention to receive regulatory approval.

Clinically Meaningful. Clinically meaningful is a higher bar than statistical significance. This threshold would imply a certain average degree of improvement in performance for the populations treated. Required as part of this criterion is some notion of what the size of such a change would be and this requires information obtained from other sources other than statistics such as actual indices of functioning in everyday settings. Embedded within this concept is the expectation that a certain amount of improvement in cognition or functional skills would be associated with a certain amount of improved everyday functioning. For instance, several different studies of functional measures have identified threshold levels of cognitive performance consistent with achievement of functional milestones such as independence in residence, or ability to manage finances or medications, or improvements in driving skills. Intervention-related improvements that reach these thresholds would be possible indices of clinically meaningful change (see Chapter 17 for a more detailed discussion of this issue).

Definitely Nonrandom. When a group of participants receives treatment, even if the benefit is statistically or clinically significant for the group, there is likely to be variation in response among the people treated. The assessment of improvement for individuals differs from that for groups in that to be certain that an individual has improved to a level greater than chance, a host of influences on performance such as practice effects requires consideration. The "reliable change index" has been developed in order to quantify whether an improvement in one person exceeds what is expected based upon general influences (Heaton et al., 2001). The reliable change index statistic incorporates the test–retest reliability of the measure and establishes a range of scores that exceeds this level of change. The confidence interval of the reliable change index is typically set at 90%, meaning that there is only a 1 in 10 chance that the threshold amount of change would have occurred by random factors alone.

With commonly used outcome measures for clinical trials in humans, the typical level of change required to define a definitely nonrandom change is in the range of about 1.0 standard deviation (SD) (Leifker et al., 2010). This is a fairly high bar, but in several previous cognitive treatment studies, the group improvements in cognitive outcomes have been as great as 0.8 SD (Bowie et al., 2012; Fisher et al., 2009). This could mean that a number of people treated in those studies manifest individual improvements that are definitely nonrandom.

Normalization of Functioning. This is the highest bar and is not necessarily a goal of every intervention study. Normalization of functioning would imply two things: substantial improvement in functioning that is entirely within the normal range, or improvement on the part of individuals to at least their pre-illness level of functioning if not better. The normal range of functioning is typically defined as within 1.0 SD of the population mean or higher. Further, if an individual's performance was within that range prior to illness, then their posttreatment functioning should be within that range as well. Normalization is a high bar because many individuals whose performance is slightly below the cutoff for normal cognitive functioning (−1.0 SD) are functioning adequately in their lives.

Practical Concerns

One of the issues that is at the forefront of interventions aimed at enhancing cognitive or functional performance is whether behavioral and computerized interventions can be self-administered at home (Fisher et al., 2015). Like pharmacological interventions, behavioral interventions can be delivered outside the clinic setting. As these interventions transition toward wider use, with the anticipated approval of drugs or medical devices for cognitive remediation treatment, assessments may also need to be performed outside of the clinic. This would require the ability to use remotely deliverable cognitive and functional assessment strategies, with the same reliability and validity standards that are conventionally applied to paper-and-pencil and other in-person testing procedures.

Cognitive tests and functional capacity measures have already been developed for remote administration. The issues associated with computerization and remote delivery of these assessments are the same as in-person assessments. There needs to be considerable evidence supporting the psychometric characteristics of the instruments, and a match between the content of the instrument and clinically relevant community outcomes. Questions related to the usability of these techniques are also important. This is likely to be a major area for future technology development, and these procedures will be more successful if they are flexibly adapted across emerging technology.

Realistic Assessment Strategies

As noted previously, EMA allows for the momentary assessment of functional activities. However, in cases where an individual is not spontaneously performing these activities, a functional capacity assessment in the real-world may be an important assessment strategy. Several such strategies have been developed in the past, targeting both aging and neuropsychiatrically impaired samples.

As noted earlier, realistic Virtual Reality (VR) variants of functional tasks have been developed. These tasks examine a variety of everyday functional skills, including shopping, banking, bill paying, using the Internet for health information, and other health management activities (e.g., prescription refill, doctor's visit). These assessment strategies have several advantages over paper-and-pencil functional capacity assessments. First, a structured simulation of an everyday task already performed on the computer, such as bill paying or ATM interaction, does not have to be examined for criterion-referenced validity, as the task is identical. Second, there is no need to infer from cognitive limitations that there would be a functional skills deficit, as the functional skills are assessed directly. Third, these realistic assessments are more amenable to targeted intervention than more general skills deficits. One does not need to determine which cognitive abilities underlie the skills deficits and then train them; the training can be directed at the functional skills alone. Thus, in a way, these outcome measures can "bootstrap back" to intervention development because they are directly related to critical daily activities and poor performance directly results in functional deficits.

CONCLUSION

Objective outcome measures span performance-based and interview-based assessments. They can focus on cognition, the ability to perform everyday living skills, or on real-world functional outcomes. These measures vary in their comprehensiveness and in their practicality, with some being quite extensive and others intentionally abbreviated. Performance-based assessments have several advantages to self-report and informant-report measures when cognition and functioning is concerned, it is important to recognize that they do not capture subjective elements of functioning such as quality of life. Depending on the population, the treatment intervention, and the goals of the research program, it is possible to select outcome measures well matched to the research design and practical for purposes of the study. New advances in technology are leading to rapid changes in the measurement of functional outcomes, and computerized assessment will be the rule for many studies in the immediate future.

REFERENCES

Adams, K. M., & Grant, I. (2009). *Neuropsychological assessment of neuropsychiatric and neuromedical disorders* (3rd ed.). New York, NY: Oxford University Press.

Bowie, C. R., McGurk, S. M., Mausbach, B. T., Patterson, T. L., & Harvey, P. D. (2012). Combined cognitive remediation and functional skills training for schizophrenia: Effects on cognition, functional competence, and real-world behavior. *American Journal of Psychiatry, 169*(7), 710–718.

Bowie, C. R., Twamley, E. W., Anderson, H., Halpern, B., Patterson, T. L., & Harvey, P. D. (2007). Self-assessment of functional status in schizophrenia. *Journal of Psychiatric Research, 41*(12), 1012–1018.

Bruce, J. M., & Arnett, P. A. (2004). Self-reported everyday memory and depression in patients with multiple sclerosis. *Journal of Clinical and Experimental Neuropsychology, 26*(2), 200–214.

Buchanan, R. W., Keefe, R. S., Umbricht, D., Green, M. F., Laughren, T., & Marder, S. R. (2011). The FDA-NIMH-MATRICS guidelines for clinical trial design of cognitive-enhancing drugs: What do we know 5 years later? *Schizophrenia Bulletin, 37,* 1209–1217.

Callicott, J. H., Mattay, V. S., Bertolino, A., Finn, K., Coppola, R., Frank, J. A., . . . Weinberger, D. R. (1999). Physiological characteristics of capacity constraints in working memory as revealed by functional MRI. *Cerebral Cortex, 9*(1), 20–26.

Carone, D. A., Benedict, R. H., Munschauer, F. E., Fishman, I., & Weinstock-Guttman, B. (2005). Interpreting patient/informant discrepancies of reported cognitive symptoms in MS. *Journal of the International Neuropsychological Society, 11*(5), 574–583.

Czaja, S. J., Harvey, P. D., & Loewenstein, D. (2014). *Development and evaluation of a novel technology-based functional assessment package.* Paper presented at Society of Biological Psychiatry 69th Annual Scientific Meeting, New York, NY.

Czaja, S. J., Sharit, J., Ownby, R., Roth, D., & Nair, S. (2001). Examining age differences in performance of a complex information search and retrieval task. *Psychology and Aging, 16,* 564–579.

Davidson, M., Harvey, P. D., Welsh, K., Powchik, P., Putnam, K. M., & Mohs, R. C. (1996). Cognitive impairment in old-age schizophrenia: A comparative study of schizophrenia and Alzheimer's disease. *America Journal of Psychiatry, 153,* 1274–1279.

Depp, C. A., Mausbach, B. T., Harvey, P. D., Wolyniec, P. S., Thornquist, M. H., Luke, J. R., & Pulver, A. E. (2010). Social competence and observer-rated social functioning in bipolar disorder. *Bipolar Disorders, 12*(8), 843–850.

Dickinson, D., Ramsey, M., & Gold, J. M. (2007). Overlooking the obvious: A meta-analytic comparison of digit symbol coding tasks and other cognitive measures in schizophrenia. *Archives of General Psychiatry, 64*(5), 532–542.

Durand, D., Strassnig, M., Sabbag, S., Gould, F., Twamley, E. W., Patterson, P. T., & Harvey, P. D. (2015). Factors influencing self-assessment of cognition and functioning in schizophrenia: Implications for treatment studies. *European Neuropsychopharmacology, 25*(2), 185–191.

Fisher, M., Holland, C., Merzenich, M. M., & Vinogradov, S. (2009). Using neuroplasticity-based auditory training to improve verbal memory in schizophrenia. *American Journal of Psychiatry, 166*(7), 805–811.

Fisher, M., Loewy, R., Carter, C., Lee, A., Ragland, J. D., Niemdam, T., . . . Vinogradov, S. (2015). Neuroplasticity-based auditory training via laptop computer improves cognition in young individuals with recent onset schizophrenia. *Schizophrenia Bulletin, 41*, 250–258.

Freedman, M. J., Lestor, K. M., McNamara, C., Millby, J. B., & Schumacher, J. E. (2006). Cell phones for ecological momentary assessment with cocaine-addicted homeless patients in treatment. *Journal of Substance Abuse Treatment, 30*, 105–111.

Goldberg, T. E., Keefe, R. S. E., Goldman, R., Robinson, D. G., & Harvey, P. D. (2010). Circumstances under which practice does not make perfect: A review of the practice effect literature in schizophrenia and its relevance to clinical treatment studies. *Neuropsychopharmacology, 35*, 1053–1062.

Goldstein, K. (1995). *The organism* (reprinted from 1939 ed.). Cambridge, MA: MIT Press-Zone Books.

Green, M. F. (1996). What are the functional consequences of neurocognitive deficits in schizophrenia? *American Journal of Psychiatry, 153*, 321–330.

Harvey, P. D. (2012). Clinical applications of neuropsychological assessment. *Dialogues in Clinical Neuroscience, 14*, 91–99.

Harvey, P. D., Helldin, L., Bowie, C. R., Heaton, R. K., Olsson, A., Hjärthag, F., . . . Patterson, T. L. (2009). Performance-based measurement of functional disability in schizophrenia: A cross-national study in the United States and Sweden. *American Journal of Psychiatry, 166*, 821–827.

Harvey, P. D., Raykov, T., Twamley, E. W., Vella, L., Heaton, R. K., & Patterson, T. L. (2013). The factor structure of neurocognition and functional capacity in schizophrenia: A multidimensional examination of temporal stability. *Journal of the International Neuropsychological Society, 19*, 656–663.

Harvey, P. D., Sabbag, S., Prestia, D., Drurand, D., Twalmey, E. W., & Patteson, T. L. (2012). Functional milestones and clinician ratings of everyday functioning in people with schizophrenia: Overlap between milestones and specificity of ratings. *Journal of Psychiatric Research, 46*, 1546–1552.

Harvey, P. D., Siu, C., Hsu, J., Cucchiaro, J., Maruff, P., & Loebel, A. (2013). Effect of lurasidone on neurocognitive performance in patients with schizophrenia: A short-term placebo- and active-controlled study followed by a 6-month double-blind extension. *European Neuropsychopharmacology, 11*, 1373–1382.

Harvey, P. D., Velligan, D. I., & Bellack, A. S. (2007). Performance-based measures of functional skills: Usefulness in clinical treatment studies. *Schizophrenia Bulletin, 33*, 1138–1148.

Heaton, R. K., Grant, I. S., & Matthews, C. G. (1991). *Comprehensive norms for an expanded Halstead-Reitan battery: Demographic corrections, research findings, and clinical applications.* Odessa, FL: Psychological Assessment Resources.

Heaton, R. K., Temkin, N., Dikmen, S., Avitable, N., Taylor, M. J., Marcotte, T. D., & Grant, I. S. (2001). Detecting change: A comparison of three neuropsychological methods, using normal and clinical samples. *Archives of Clinical Neuropsychology, 16*(1), 75–91.

Iverson, G. L., Brooks, B. L., Ashton, V. L., Johnson, L. G., & Gualtieri, C. T. (2009). Does familiarity with computers affect computerized neuropsychological test performance? *Journal of Clinical and Experimental Neuropsychology, 31,* 594–604.

Kaye, J. L., Dunlop, B. W., Iosifescu, D. V., Mathew, S. J., Kelley, M. E., & Harvey, P. D. (2014). Cognition, functional capacity, and self-reported disability in women with post-traumatic stress disorder: Examining the convergence of performance-based measures and self-reports. *Journal of Psychiatric Research, 57,* 51–57.

Keefe, R. S. E., Bilder, R. M., Harvey, P. D., Davis, S. M., Palmer, B. W., Gold, J. M., . . . Lieberman, J. A. (2006). Baseline neurocognitive deficits in the CATIE schizophrenia trial. *Neuropsychopharmacology, 31,* 2033–2046.

Keefe, R. S. E., Davis, V. G., Spagnola, N. B., Hilt, D., Dgetluck, N., Ruse, S., . . . Harvey, P. D. (2015). Reliability, validity and treatment sensitivity of the Schizophrenia Cognition Rating Scale. *European Neuropsychopharmacology, 25*(2), 176–184.

Keefe, R. S. E., Fox, K. H., Harvey, P. D., Cucchiaro, J., Siu, C., & Loebel, A. (2011). Characteristics of the MATRICS consensus cognitive battery in a 29-site antipsychotic schizophrenia clinical trial. *Schizophrenia Research, 125,* 161–168.

Keefe, R. S. E., Goldberg, T. E., Harvey, P. D., Gold, J. M., Poe, M., & Coughenour, L. (2004). The brief assessment of cognition in schizophrenia: Reliability, sensitivity, and comparison with a standard neurocognitive battery. *Schizophrenia Research, 68,* 283–297.

Keefe, R. S. E., Poe, M., Walker, T. M., Kang, J., & Harvey, P. D. (2006). The schizophrenia cognition rating scale: An interview-based assessment and its relationship to cognition, real-world functioning, and functional capacity. *American Journal of Psychiatry, 163,* 426–432.

Kruger, J., & Dunning, D. (1999). Unskilled and unaware of it: How difficulties in recognizing one's own incompetence lead to inflated self-assessments. *Journal of Personality and Social Psychology, 77*(6), 1121–1134.

Lawton, M. P., & Brody, E. M. (1969). Assessment of older people: Self-maintaining and instrumental activities of daily living. *The Gerontologist, 9,* 179–186.

Leifker, F. R., Patterson, T. L., Bowie, C. R., & Harvey, P. D. (2010). Psychometric properties of performance-based measurements of functional capacity. *Schizophrenia Research, 119,* 246–252.

Mausbach, B. T., Depp, C. A., Bowie, C. R., Harvey, P. D., McGrath, J., Thornquist, M., . . . Patterson, T. L. (2011). Sensitivity and specificity of the UCSD performance-based skills assessment (UPSA-B) for identifying functional milestones in schizophrenia. *Schizophrenia Research, 132*(2), 165–170.

Mausbach, B. T., Harvey, P. D., Goldman, S. R., Jeste, D. V., & Patterson, T. L. (2007). Development of a brief scale of everyday functioning in persons with serious mental illness. *Schizophrenia Bulletin, 33*(6), 1364–1372.

McClure, M. M., Bowie, C. R., Patterson, T. L., Heaton, R. K., Weaver, C., Anderson, H., & Harvey, P. D. (2007). Correlations of functional capacity and neuropsychological performance in older patients with schizophrenia: Evidence for specificity of relationships? *Schizophrenia Research, 89*(1), 330–338.

McGurk, S. R., Mueser, K. T., Feldman, K., Wolfe, R., & Pascaris, A. (2007). Cognitive training for supported employment: 2–3 year outcomes of a randomized controlled trial. *American Journal of Psychiatry, 164*(3), 437–441.

Menditto, A. A., Wallace, C. J., Liberman, R. P., Vander Wal, J., Jones, N. T., & Stuve, P. (1999). Functional assessment of independent living skills. *Psychiatric Rehabilitation Skills, 3,* 200–219.

Moore, D. J., Palmer, B. W., Patterson, T. L., & Jeste, D. V. (2007). A review of performance-based measures of everyday functioning. *Journal of Psychiatric Research, 41,* 97–118.

Morris, J. C., McKeel, D. W., & Storandt, M. (1991). Very mild Alzheimer's disease: Informant-based clinical, psychometric, and pathologic distinction from normal aging. *Neurology, 41*(4), 467–478.

Nuechterlein, K. H., Barch, D. M., Gold, J. M., Goldberg, T. E., Green, M. F., & Heaton, R. K. (2004). Identification of separable cognitive factors in schizophrenia. *Schizophrenia Research, 72,* 29–39.

Nuechterlein, K. H., Green, M. F., Kern, R. S., Baade, L. E., Barch, D., Cohen, J. D., . . . Marder, S. R. (2008). The MATRICS consensus cognitive battery: Part 1. Test selection, reliability, and validity. *American Journal of Psychiatry, 165*(2), 203–213.

Patterson, T. L., Goldman, S., McKibbin, C. L., Hughs, T., & Jeste, D. V. (2001). UCSD performance-based skills assessment: Development of a new measure of everyday functioning for severely mentally ill adults. *Schizophrenia Bulletin, 27*(2), 235–245.

Paulsen, J. S., Salmon, D. P., Monsch, A., Butters, N., Swenson, M. R., & Bondi, M. W. (1995). Discrimination of cortical from subcortical dementias on the basis of memory and problem-solving tests. *Journal of Clinical Psychology, 51,* 48–58.

Reitan, R. M., & Wolfson, D. (1993). *The Halstead-Reitan neuropsychological test battery: Theory and clinical interpretation* (2nd ed.). Tucson, AZ: Neuropsychology Press.

Risacher, S. L., Wang, Y., Wishart, H. A., Rabin, L. A., Flashman, L. A., McDonald, B. C., . . . Saykin, A. J. (2013). Cholinergic enhancement of brain activation in mild cognitive impairment during episodic memory encoding. *Frontiers in Psychiatry, 4,* 105. doi:10.3389/fpsyt.2013.00105

Rosenheck, R., Leslie, D., Keefe, R., McEvoy, J., Swartz, M., Perkins, D., . . . CATIE Study Investigators Group. (2006). Barriers to employment for people with schizophrenia. *American Journal of Psychiatry, 163,* 411–417.

Ruse, S. A., Davis, V. G., Atkins, A. S., Krishnan, K. R. R., Fox, K. H., Harvey, P. D., & Keefe, R. S. E. (2014). Development of a virtual reality assessment of everyday living skills. *Journal of Visual Experiments,* (86), e51405. doi:10.3791/51405

Sabbag, S., Twamley, E. M., Vella, L., Heaton, R. K., Patterson, T. L., & Harvey, P. D. (2011). Assessing everyday functioning in schizophrenia: Not all informants seem equally informative. *Schizophrenia Research, 131*(1), 250–255.

Sharit, J., & Czaja, S. J. (1999). Performance of a complex computer-based troubleshooting task in the bank industry. *International Journal of Cognitive Ergonomics and Human Factors, 3,* 1–22.

Silver, J. M., Koumaras, B., Chen, M., Mirski, D., Potkin, S. G., Reyes, P., . . . Gounay, I. (2006). The effects of rivastigmine on cognitive function in patients with traumatic brain injury. *Neurology, 67,* 748–755.

Sostek, A. J., Buchsbaum, M. S., & Rapoport, J. L. (1980). Effects of amphetamine on vigilance performance in normal and hyperactive children. *Journal of Abnormal Child Psychology, 8,* 491–500.

Spikman, J. M., & van der Naalt, J. (2010). Indices of impaired self-awareness in traumatic brain injury patients with focal frontal lesions and executive deficits: Implications for outcome measurement. *Journal of Neurotrauma, 27,* 1195–1202.

Stone, A. A., Turkkan, J. S., Jaylan, S. Jobe, J. B., Kurtzman, H. S., & Cain, V. S. (Eds.). (2000). *The science of self-report: Implications for research and practice.* Mahwah, NJ: Lawrence Erlbaum Associates.

Swendsen, J., Tennen, H., Carney, M. A., Affleck, G., Willard, A., & Hromi, A. (2000). Mood and alcohol consumption: An experience sampling test of the self-mediation hypothesis. *Journal of Abnormal Psychology, 109*(2), 194–204.

Ventura, J., Reise, S. P., Keefe, R. S., Hurford, I. M., Wood, R. C., & Bilder, R. M. (2013). The cognitive assessment interview (CAI): Reliability and validity of a brief interview-based measure of cognition. *Schizophrenia Bulletin, 39*(3), 583–591.

Wallace, C. J., Liberman, R. P., Tauber, R., & Wallace, J. (2000). The independent living skills survey: A comprehensive measure of the community functioning of severely and persistently mentally ill individuals. *Schizophrenia Bulletin, 26*, 631–658.

Welsh, K. A., Butters, N., Hughes, J., Mohs, R. C., & Heyman, A. (1991). Detection of abnormal memory decline in mild cases of Alzheimer's disease using CERAD neuropsychological measures. *Archives of Neurology, 48*, 278–281.

Zakzanis, K. K., & Jeffay, E. (2011). Neurocognitive variability in high-functioning individuals: Implications for the practice of clinical neuropsychology. *Psychological Reports, 108*, 290–300.

SIXTEEN

STATISTICS IS NOT A SUBSTITUTE FOR SOLID EXPERIMENTAL METHODOLOGY AND DESIGN

JYOTI SAVLA AND DAVID L. LOEWENSTEIN

> *Statistics are no substitute for judgment.*
> —Henry Clay

Scientific research is a process of arriving at a dependable solution to a problem through planned and systematic collection, analysis, and interpretation of data. The study design and data analysis are thus a fundamental aspect of all research studies and especially behavioral intervention research in that they provide investigators the means by which to determine whether the obtained results show reliable differences between one or more treatment or control groups, or are merely obtained as a matter of chance. In many ways, however, the design of a research study is more important than the analysis as no amount of sophisticated data analytic approaches will be able to compensate for the lack of methodological rigor in study design and measurement. Therefore, it is always imperative to obtain input on the study design when evaluating a behavioral intervention research and before a study commences. Consideration of research design is also important because the design of a study will govern how the data are to be analyzed.

In this chapter, we describe a few key issues to consider when designing a research study to evaluate a behavioral intervention. Through examples, we show how research design and analytical techniques are intrinsically tied such that a good study design will lend itself to better analytic techniques and, therefore, yield a better understanding of the phenomenon under study. Most of the issues discussed are relevant to an evaluation of an intervention at any stage of its development along the pipeline, but may be particularly relevant to Phase III efficacy and Phase IV effectiveness studies in which an intervention is compared to a comparison group.

SELECTION OF RELIABLE AND VALID STUDY VARIABLES

One of the most fundamental decisions that investigators must make in a prospective study is to select and carefully distinguish between independent variables (IVs) and dependent variables (DVs). This process is guided by both the nature of the research questions that are being posed and previous scientific literature in the area. In a classical experimental design, the IV often represents variables or factors that the investigator may manipulate such as those randomly assigned to receive Treatment A, Treatment B, or some type of control condition. IVs may also be factors that cannot be experimentally manipulated such as gender or ethnic/language group.

In contrast, DVs are measures of outcomes that one might be interested in measuring to answer the scientific questions or shown change as a consequence of exposure to a treatment or intervention. Proper selection of DVs is essential in comparing the results of a study to previous literature in the field. It is also essential that DVs be both reliable (can be measured with consistency) and valid (the test measures what it was intended to measure). Identification of IVs and DVs can occur early on in constructing an intervention as discussed in Chapter 3 in the prephase of discovery.

Equally important is the need to employ measures that have adequate reliability and validity (Campbell, Stanley, & Gage, 1963; Trochim, 2000). A common problem in the literature is the use of measures that may actually not have sufficiently high test–retest reliabilities (stability of measurement over time) or high interrater reliabilities (high agreement for a measure when used on the same study participant by different raters established by a coefficient of agreement such as a weighted kappa). "Validity" refers to the degree to which an instrument measures what it is supposed to measure. Many instruments may have face validity based on item content or event content validity as designated by expert consensus opinion, but this is not a substitute for concurrent validity (examining the association of the proposed measure with established valid measures in the field), factorial validity (the proposed measures load on a predicted construct using traditional factor analytic techniques or linear structural equation modeling [SEM]), or discriminant validity (the proposed measure discriminates among well-defined groups identified by an accepted "gold standard," using techniques such as discriminant function analysis [DFA], logistic regression, or receiver operator curve [ROC]).

Careful selection of measures that have high levels of reliability and validity can greatly enhance the internal validity of a study, or, in other words, heighten the ability to conclude that outcomes are a consequence of an intervention versus other confounding factors. However, equally important is external validity, which is the generalizability of a measure or finding to a real-world population (Rothwell, 2005). This construct is of critical importance since the goal of inferential statistics is to generalize from a given sample to a population (see Chapter 9 on sampling). One limitation of much of the current research is that samples for intervention studies may be randomly assigned to groups, but the participant pool may not adequately reflect the population as a whole. Research participants are often brighter, more highly motivated, and differ in important characteristics from the population as a whole. Further, in double-blind drug trials or nonpharmacological interventions, inclusion and exclusion criteria may not reflect real clinical populations that may have many more comorbid conditions than the sample included in an initial test of an intervention.

Another issue related to measurement choice is that there is an unfortunate tendency for some investigators to venerate or reify a measure based on the name of a scale or its historical usage. For example, the Center for Epidemiological Studies-Depression (CES-D) (Radloff, 1977) scale is often used as a measure of depression in caregiver research. However, the actual diagnosis of depression requires an extensive structured interview by a well-trained clinician using standard diagnostic criteria such as the *DSM-5*. The CES-D can be described as a self-report scale of depressive symptoms, but may indicate depression in those without a clinical diagnosis of depression or fail to identify true depression when a person refuses to disclose or underreport symptoms. Further, measures of depression such as the CES-D may not be specific to depression, but may reflect anxiety or generalized psychological distress. As a result, there is a potential world of difference between a measure of reported depressive symptoms and the actual presence of clinical depression (Breslau, 1985).

Another issue to consider for intervention studies in which there is long-term follow-up is to ensure that the same construct is being measured across occasions and groups, referred to as longitudinal or measurement invariance (Schaie, Maitland, Willis, & Intrieri, 1998). This issue is especially important in studies where the scales that were used to assess a construct are changed or a new scale is added to refine the measurement of the construct. Other threats to validity include the effects of history, reactivity to testing, statistical regression, experimental mortality or attrition, and developmental processes (Schaie, 1988).

Scales of Measurement

The analysis of data is dependent on the scale of measurement that is employed in the study design and data collection. At the most basic level, the form of measurement is nominal or categorical. A good example is the numbers that professional athletes such as football players wear on their uniforms. A higher or lower number has no bearing on the skill level or performance, but rather merely identifies a certain player. Therefore, categorical data do not have to confer rank although they sometimes do in the illustration that follows. As an example, one might arbitrarily classify those persons over 5 feet 6 inches or more as "tall" and those less than 5 feet 5 inches or less as "short." These same persons might be classified by gender as male or female. These are categorical variables and if one wanted to examine males and females by whether they were classified as tall or short, one would conduct a 2×2 chi-square analysis that would test the null hypotheses that there are no differences in the distribution of tall versus short persons among the two genders. (*Note*: In any 2×2 chi-square analysis, the Yate's correction for discontinuity would be applied whereas such a correction is not required for any other type of chi-square analyses.) If one wanted to determine if a particular set of variables (e.g., age, gender, height of father) would predict a dichotomous categorical outcome such as those who are classified as tall or short, one could employ techniques such as DFA or logistic regression (which does not require a multivariate normality assumption as is seen with DFA).

Of course, the problem with arbitrarily categorizing participants into dichotomous categories is the loss of information. If we categorized persons in terms of their actual height without classifying them as tall or short, we would have a scale that is interval in that there is a range of higher and lower scores and equal intervals between measures, which would be scaled by inches or feet. One could argue that height might even be categorized as a ratio' scale since there is hypothetically an absolute zero point such as on a thermometer. However, since no human being is without height, this would be a specious argument and an interval versus a ratio scale would actually have no impact on choice of analyses. A simple correlation between height and weight could be conducted using the Pearson product–moment correlation coefficient, or height might be predicted by a number of IVs (linear regression). If we wanted to determine how those with high SES (socio-economic status), medium SES, or low SES differed in terms of standardized test scores, one could conduct a one-way analysis of variance (ANOVA) with standardized test scores serving as an outcome measure. Following a statistically significant F test (typically $p < .05$), comparisons between means could be conducted using a post hoc test such as the Student–Neuman–Keuls procedure or Tukey's honestly significant difference (Tukey's HSD) test. This is a compromise between liberal post hoc tests such as independent t tests and conservative procedures such as the Bonferroni correction.

It should be noted that many scales that seem like they are interval do not have equal intervals between measurements. For example, in a horse race, the difference in length between the first place horse and the second place horse may be quite different than that of the third and fourth place horses or the fifth place and the sixth place horses. Unequal intervals between numbers on a scale constitute an ordinal scale, which must be analyzed using statistics that examine the differences between ranks. These nonparametric tests in the case of correlation coefficients may be a Spearman rank–order correlation test rather than a Pearson product–moment test for interval or ratio data. Instead of an independent t test for interval- or ratio-level data, investigators might consider a Mann–Whitney U. Instead of a classic ANOVA with an F test, ordinal data for three or more groups may be analyzed using a non-parametric distribution-free Kruskal–Wallis Test.

Establishing Causality

Correlation does not imply causation even though this mistake continues to be repeatedly made in the discussion section of some published studies (William, Shadish, Cook, & Campbell, 2002). To illustrate, there is a strong association between the number of earthworms on a road in a certain county in Florida and the number of automobile accidents. Let's hypothetically assert that the strength of association is .6 ($p < .001$). This means that the number of earthworms could account for 36% of the variability in automobile accidents on the road. Does this mean that the earthworms on the road caused the automobile accidents? Certainly not! It turns out that rain brings out the earthworms and also makes the roads slick. Thus, a third unaccounted for factor (rain) is the causal mechanism underlying the association between the other two variables. Confusing association with causation has resulted in a number of faulty scientific conclusions that were rectified by further research. For example, it was once thought that aluminum caused Alzheimer's disease (AD) since there were high levels of aluminum in the plaques found in the brains of AD patients upon autopsy. However, aluminum was not the cause of the disease but a result of other pathological processes that occurred in the brain after the disease started. The beating of drums after an eclipse is always associated with the sun coming out. However, this association is spurious and certainly not causal.

In experimental design when testing a behavioral intervention, the way in which causality is assessed is by randomly assigning participants to different experimental and control groups (Imai, Tingley, & Yamamoto, 2013). It is assumed that random assignment will minimize group differences and, if other variables are held constant or carefully controlled or accounted for, the temporal change among groups may be attributable to the experimental condition to which a participant was assigned. In pharmacological studies, it is easy to use double-blind procedures in which both the experimenter and the subject cannot differentiate the active drug from the placebo. However, in behavioral intervention research, experimenters conducting interventions and participants are often not blind to the condition to which they are assigned. As a result, it is imperative for independent raters who are blind to condition to obtain baseline and outcome measures (referred to as a "single-blind trial"). Issues such as expectancy effects of the participant and experimenter, or disappointment that one may feel when assigned to an "inactive group," make it imperative to design evaluations of behavioral interventions with control groups that can be equated to the intervention in terms of the interventionist's time and attention (see Chapter 8 for a discussion on selecting control groups). Although this is not feasible in all types of studies, and particularly for early tests of the intervention for proof of concept, failure to have adequate control groups raises the question as to whether obtained results were due to the active ingredients of the intervention or merely nonspecific aspects of the treatment that differed from the control condition.

MEDIATING AND MODERATING EFFECTS

Another statistical method that researchers use to understand the mechanism through which IVs affect the DVs is the moderation and mediation tests. A classic discussion of moderator and mediator analyses can be found in Baron and Kenny (1986), which has recently been expanded upon by Fairchild and MacKinnon (2014). A moderator variable is one that affects the strength of the relationship between two other variables. The moderator variable can either be qualitative in nature (e.g., gender) or quantitative (e.g., level of reinforcement) that influences the association between two other variables and points to why these effects might hold and its inclusion changes the strength of association between the two other variables.

In contrast, a mediator variable explains the mechanism or process that underlies the relationship between the two variables. For example, level of education might be seen as a mediator variable if it explained the relationship between SES and health-related behaviors. In many cases, mediators may describe underlying psychological processes (e.g., beliefs, emotions) and may explain the relationship between two variables. Trauma might affect someone's ability to return to work after a natural disaster. However, this effect may be mediated by autonomic reactivity that may explain the effect of trauma on the ability to return to work. With the help of newer statistical software, we are now able to test more complicated hypotheses that test the simultaneous influence of multiple mediators and moderated mediation effects as well as mediated moderation effects (see Preacher, Rucker, & Hayes, 2007). For example, a home-based intervention study used SEM techniques to simultaneously model multiple mediators and found that identification of personal goals, enhanced depression knowledge, and reduced anxiety each independently mediated the effects of the intervention program on depression (Gitlin, Roth, & Huang, 2014).

STATISTICAL SIGNIFICANCE VERSUS PRACTICAL IMPORTANCE

The role of significance testing is to determine whether a particular result is obtained as a result of chance or the result is so unusual that it would occur only by chance on rare occasions. Statistics were first employed in agricultural research and a statistical result so uncommon that it would occur by chance less than 1 time out of 20 (or 5 times in 100) led to the widespread adoption of a criterion of significance set at $p < .05$. There is nothing that precludes the investigator from being more conservative. For example, a p value of $<.01$ reflects that a chance result or a Type I error (falsely rejecting the null hypothesis or, for example, accepting that an intervention has a positive effect when it does not) would occur less than 1% of the time. In classic between-groups t tests, a group mean would be calculated for each of the groups and then the group mean would be subtracted from each individual's score in the group. Unfortunately, unless one squares the difference scores, they add up to zero. Thus, the sum of squared deviations is calculated for each group, and then divided by the number of scores in each group. This results in a measure of variability that can be calculated by taking a square root of the sum of squares divided by n (although $n - 1$ is used in most inferential statistical equations). This results in a standard deviation that can be calculated for each group that provides a measure of how the group average or mean is representing the central tendency of the data. In the case of a t test, the difference between means over the pooled average standard deviation results in a ratio that, if sufficiently large given the number of study participants (and resultant degrees of freedom), will reach statistical significance. A one-way ANOVA or an F test is simply the variance of group means around a grand mean (the mean of the means) divided by the pooled standard deviation. Thus, the ratio provided by a t test or an F test can be a result of a large difference between means (the between-group effect) or a small standard deviation (the within-group effect).

Since the number of study participants affects the formula for standard deviation and a large number of participants requires a smaller t ratio or F ratio for statistical significance, groups with very large numbers of subjects can achieve statistical significance without an actually large effect. A statistically significant effect means that a researcher can trust the reliability of his or her results at a specific p value. However, in the cases of a large n, statistically significant results do not necessarily mean that a result is practically important. For example, there may be an experiment in which there are 1,000 persons in each of three different groups. One could calculate the effect size for a t test or an ANOVA F by dividing the explained sum of squares total over the total sum of squares in the model and obtain a value equivalent to R^2, the proportion of variance explained by the model. In this case, an effect size of less than 6% of the explained variability might produce a statistically significant result but a trivial finding. This is why it is essential that investigators a priori specify a clinically meaningful effect size that is suggested by existing literature or that can be argued to have clinical significance (see Chapter 17 for a discussion on clinical significance). On the other hand, one may have very large group differences but may not achieve statistical significance because of a small number of subjects. One cannot tout this finding because, if it does not reach statistical significance, it is not considered reliable. However, such a large effect size would likely prompt the experimenter to conduct a larger experiment with a greater number of subjects.

PLANNED COMPARISONS VERSUS POST HOC COMPARISONS

Generally speaking, experiments (and particularly tests of behavioral interventions in a Phase II pilot randomized trial, Phase III efficacy trial, or Phase IV effectiveness trial) are usually conducted with a specific hypothesis in mind. These planned analyses are derived from theory and are pivotal and essential tests. Even so, the more comparisons or analyses conducted, the more Type I error will be made when the null hypothesis is true. Although everyone agrees that planned comparisons should be limited in number, there is no real agreement on what this number should be. One suggestion is to restrict the number of comparisons to the number of degrees of freedom associated with the treatment source of variances. Other researchers suggest a special correction such as the Bonferroni or Dunn test to compensate for the Type I error. Researchers who pursue post hoc comparisons often use Tukey's tests, for example, which will help generate planned comparisons for subsequent experiments.

Measurement Over Time

So far we have addressed issues related to cross-sectional designs where one might want to evaluate the effects of a treatment versus an active placebo condition (e.g., attention control) in three different, older, ethnic/cultural groups. Longitudinal data analyses are different from cross-sectional designs in that each subject has a set of observations measured repeatedly over time and these observations are intercorrelated. As a result, standardized regression methods ignoring such a correlation would render an insufficient estimate of the beta weights and potentially inaccurate conclusions.

One of the most common experimental designs is a "pre–post" two-group study in which a single health status measurement is obtained, an intervention is administered to the treatment group but not to the placebo group, and a single follow-up measurement is collected once again from participants in both groups. In this design, change in the outcome(s) is associated with the intervention exposure and the two groups can be compared to see if the change in the outcome is different for those subjects who are actively treated as compared to control group participants. In other longitudinal designs, follow-up measurements could be made at more time points, for example, at baseline, and then at 6, 12, and 18 months after the intervention exposure. This would necessitate a 3 (Groups) × 2 (Intervention) × 4 (Time) design. If there were multiple measures for the DV (e.g., depression, social isolation), multivariate approaches such as Multivariate analysis of variance (MANOVA) would be employed. Some investigators might also consider transforming and standardizing

the individual depression measures on the same scale to create an average composite measure. This analysis would generate an F value for group, intervention, and
time. Although a statistically significant F value of $p < .05$ or $p < .01$ would provide
overall main effects for the group and intervention across all measurement time as
well as general changes in all scores over time, this would provide little information
on whether there was an effect of the intervention by group and how these differences might manifest themselves over time. Thus, the Intervention × Time F value
(two-way) interaction term would provide a reliable estimate that either the intervention produced differed general effects over time or there were group differences
in the intervention effect over time (a three-way interaction). Following a statistically significant interaction, one could look at actual mean differences and control
for multiple comparisons by using procedures such as the Tukey's HSD test, Scheffe
procedure, or the more conservative Bonferroni procedure.

Let's suppose that a researcher is collecting interview data and, owing to the
limited number of interviewers, not all participants could be interviewed on the
same day or week. Thus, there would be unequal spacing between measurement
occasions for participants in the study (e.g., Person A was followed up at 6 months
after the baseline measurement; Person B was followed up at 7 months after the
baseline measurement). This is a common scenario in field-based intervention
research in which follow-up assessments cannot be controlled. Participants may not
be able to schedule follow-ups at the precise moment an investigator desires owing
to personal issues (e.g., hospitalization, work demands, busy schedules) or practical issues (e.g., weather-related conditions interfering with testing conditions).
Let's also say that each day participants would get better at using the intervention
material; thus, the amount of time each participant has access to the intervention
material is important. In these instances, where there are three or more measurement occasions, growth curve model, which is a special case of multilevel models,
may be a useful framework for analyzing change with longitudinal data. In contrast
to approaches such as repeated-measures ANOVA, growth curve models make use
of all available data from an individual, correct for unreliability of measurement,
and, most importantly, emphasize each individual's trajectory, rather than average
group values at each occasion (Duncan, Duncan, & Strycker, 2013). Simulation
studies have found growth curve models to be statistically more powerful in detecting group differences in change than Analysis of covariance (ANCOVA) models.
Conceptually, these models involve estimating individual regressions of the DV over
time and adding at the next level predictors of the regression parameters of individual trajectories.

Growth or change trends within individuals, including polynomial trends, can
be modeled over time, which is not possible in classic models that use average
trends. For instance, in the Personalized Reminder Information and Social Management System (PRISM) study, an online platform was designed to decrease social
isolation in older adults; if we were interested in determining the effect of the intervention from the time beginning at the initiation of intervention (i.e., installation
of the PRISM system in the participant's home or one-on-one training session of
how to use the "folder" of information for the control group), then time could be
coded as a continuous variable. In this case, growth curve models could be used to
estimate the average rate of change in the DV, as well as individual trajectories of

the rate of change for each participant in the study. Next, residence type could be utilized as predictors or moderators of the intervention effect on the DV.

The benefits of longitudinal designs are not without costs. Some challenges of longitudinal studies include proper accounting of covariates that also change at each occasion of measurement, also known as "time-varying" covariates. For instance, researchers may use baseline measures of a health indicator as a covariate in their analyses. The activities of daily living (ADLs) skills, which refer to the basic tasks of everyday life, such as eating, dressing, toileting, are often used as covariates. However, older adults may show steep declines in ADLs during the study span, which in turn may impact outcomes such as social isolation and depression. It is thus necessary to make informed decisions on which variables to collect at each data collection wave.

Multilevel Modeling

It is hard to ignore the importance of context when considering any scientific inquiry that is of social or health interest. Context is particularly critical as we move an intervention from a randomized trial to implementation phase. At a more simplistic level, we can account for contextual factors as main effects in our models, for instance, examining informal care in urban versus rural settings. This approach disaggregates group-level information to the individual level so that all predictors in the regression model are tied to the individual unit of analysis. This approach can be problematic as all of the unmodeled contextual effects are pooled into a single error term at the individual level. It is also problematic because individuals from the same context will presumably have correlated errors. Traditional techniques such as ANOVA and ANCOVA ignore the random variability associated with group-level characteristics. Newer analytic methods such as multilevel models allow for more rigorous approaches to testing contextual and structural effects taking into account the nonindependent observation. In these multilevel models, sampling errors are simultaneously appropriated at each level of analysis, which is often not possible using ordinary least squares approaches (see Kenny, Bolger, & Kashy, 2002). Multilevel models are also more flexible in handling missing data and unbalanced designs. Of importance is identifying the contextual factors vis-à-vis a particular intervention and how such factors will be measured.

Missing Data

Missing data are a ubiquitous aspect of behavioral intervention research. There are a number of reasons why data could be missing, some of which are controllable by the researcher and some that are not, and each prompting a different inference. For instance, researchers who study rural populations often employ community-based participatory research techniques to get a buy-in from the community they are studying. Stakeholders and community advocates are mobilized to collect data and to ensure that participants regularly attend all of the intervention sessions and also come back for follow-up visits. However, often even after much effort, researchers can collect follow-up data on only a subset of the initial study sample. Although list-wise deletion continues to be offered in popular software programs, in recent years there is growing recognition that failure to address issues of missing data can lead to biased parameter estimates and incorrect standard errors. Researchers have now been relying on a multitude of techniques for dealing with missing or incomplete data that are currently available to behavioral interventionists and run the full gamut of sophistication and effectiveness, with full-information maximum likelihood and multiple imputation methods deemed to be the most effective strategies for analysis with incomplete data (Little & Rubin, 2014). However, there is no consensus as to which methods should be used in managing missing data, and the best policy is to try to minimize this occurrence as much as possible.

Another issue specific to all randomized trials is the issue of compliance. Intention to treat (ITT) utilizes the data of every participant who was randomly assigned to condition, essentially ignoring what treatment the participant actually received. This approach provides a conservative estimate of treatment effect, but eliminates bias from protocol deviations when persons drop out, for example, because of their lack of response to treatment (Gupta, 2011). Complier-average causal effect (CACE) estimation is an alternative approach that provides robust estimates of a treatment effect among compliant patients (Little & Rubin, 2000) and is becoming increasingly acceptable as an accompaniment to ITT to more fully understand treatment effects.

CACE analysis builds upon Rubin's causal modeling framework to yield causal estimates of the effects of intervention for individuals who comply with treatment (Little & Yau, 1998). The main challenge in CACE modeling is identifying the proportion of individuals who fall under the four compliance subgroups in the study population, namely, compliers, always-takers, never-takers, and defiers. These compliance subgroups are defined on the basis of how participants would comply with an assigned treatment under random assignment. *Compliers* are those who will use the treatment if they are assigned to the intervention arm of the study, but not if they are assigned to the control arm of the study. *Always-takers* will use the treatment irrespective of their intervention assignment. *Never-takers* will never use the treatment even if it is provided to them in the intervention arm, and *defiers* will do the opposite of their assigned treatment. Once researchers are able to account for the sample proportions for each of the four subgroups and verify necessary assumptions, they could determine an unbiased estimate of the difference in outcomes for compliers in the intervention group with those in the control group who would have complied with treatment given the opportunity to do so.

Structural Equation Modeling

Often, researchers are interested in variables that cannot be directly observed or measured (e.g., beliefs, intelligence). These unobserved variables are known as "latent" constructs or factors. We try to measure these unobserved constructs through observable variables. For example, there are underlying memory, language, perceptual organization, speed of processing, and executive functions among all human beings that underlie their performance on a wide range of neuropsychological observed performance tests. SEM is a family of analytical methods that are designed to specify relations between latent constructs and the underlying observed indicators (measurement model) as well as test the causal relations between latent constructs (structural models). These techniques include confirmatory factor analysis (CFA), path analysis, full structural models, latent growth models, and many other variations of these techniques.

CFA is a special form of factor analysis and is used to test the a priori hypothesis that certain observed variables capture or measure a latent construct. An advantage of factor analysis, in general, is that five different measures assessing well-being can be reduced into a latent variable of well-being that has less error and more reliability than any of the individual variables that it comprises.

Path analysis or causal modeling tests, at the simplest level, use linear modeling techniques to examine the casual relationships between manifest variables (observed variables), latent variables (unobserved variables), or a combination of the two. While we have already discussed the premise that correlation does necessarily mean causation, one can examine the logical flow of relationships. As an example in Figure 16.1, we examine the effects of age, presence of an ApoE+ blood genotype, accumulation of abnormal amyloid levels in the brain, volume of the hippocampus on brain MRI, and resultant memory performance on the Auditory Verbal Learning Test Delayed Recall (AVLTDEL) among subjects with mild cognitive impairment. By using regression models and standardized beta weights that simultaneously adjust for the effect of each variable on each other, we discover that having a positive ApoE4+ blood genotype is related to increases in abnormal amyloid levels in the brain as well as reduced hippocampal volume. However, this increase in amyloid does not seem to relate to poorer AVLTDEL performance. Rather, it seems that there are direct effects of reduced hippocampal volume as well as direct effects of ApoE4+ status on AVLT-DEL performance, as well as an indirect effect of ApoE4+ status on hippocampal volume, which in turn is related to cognitive performance. This model controls for the direct and nondirect effects of age on AVLTDEL performance. Because ApoE4 status is genetically determined at birth, and age cannot be caused by any of the biological measures, and cognition cannot cause biological changes in the brain, this type of modeling provides clues as to how different risk factors may affect each other and the resultant effect on cognitive performance. Please note that *e1*, *e2*, and

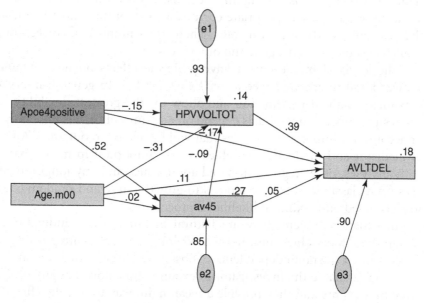

Figure 16.1 A graphical representation of a path analysis model.

$e3$ within the oval shapes refer to the error terms in the model. All of the variables in the model are in boxes because they are directly observed variables. Latent variables, if added to the model, would be denoted by oval shapes.

In SEM, a series of simultaneous equations is assessed using path-tracing rules. The discrepancy between data-derived covariance matrix and the model-derived covariance matrix forms the basis for estimating how well the conceptual model or tested model fits the data. On the basis of this discrepancy function, a wide variety of fit measures are being used; however, there is little consistency in choice of fit indexes or criteria for their evaluation. Regardless of the fit index that is being used, researchers should not forget the most fundamental rule that there is no *true* model, and the best model is the one that is most parsimonious, substantively and theoretically meaningful, and that can be cross-validated and replicated reasonably well in another population (MacCallum & Austin, 2000).

CONCLUSION

We have described the importance of considering a number of issues before embarking upon an evaluation of a behavioral intervention. The most important consideration is determining how one's specific research questions and hypotheses will contribute to knowledge in the existing scientific literature. One of the most important tasks for the investigator is to carefully construct a priori hypotheses, select reliable and valid dependent measures, and to specify an effect size that would have to be achieved to be considered clinically meaningful and practically important. Statistical significance merely refers to the confidence that obtained results are reliable and not a function of chance. While a nonreliable result is not worth pursuing, it is equally improper to present a trivial (albeit reliable) result as important. Before the results of a study are analyzed, investigators should have a clear indication as to their criterion for statistical significance, distinguish primary analyses from secondary analyses, and use appropriate corrections for multiple post hoc tests that raise the possibility of Type I error rates. There are a number of correction procedures available, some very stringent and others less so.

The levels of measurement have profound effects on how obtained data are analyzed and interpreted (see as well Chapter 14). In general, interval-level data maximize obtained information and allow for the greatest flexibility in analyzing test results. Since many models depend on measures of fit, it is imperative to include or account for important variables that will be related to outcome. An appreciation of mediator and moderator variables is very important in many analyses such as path analyses, other regression-based approaches, and any longitudinal data analyses from classic least square models to growth curve and random effects mixture models based on maximum likelihood procedures.

In situations where there are natural hierarchies and individuals are nested within these hierarchies, multilevel modeling approaches are powerful approaches to account for the nonindependence of observations. Growth curve and growth mixture models enable the investigator to examine trajectories of growth over three or more time points and they provide a meaningful way to test the effects of different variables on the individual trajectories of change over time.

Despite the plethora of newer statistical approaches, an old adage is true. No amount of sophisticated data analytic approaches will be able to compensate for the lack of methodological rigor in study design and measurement. Random assignment and blinding raters to expected outcomes are vitally important as are the expectancies of the research participants themselves. In any treatment study, those who drop out of studies are often those who are different from completers and may be the ones who did not derive actual treatment benefit. As a result, ITT and CACE approaches must be strongly considered.

Finally, despite our attempts to recruit research participants who are representative of a particular population, those who volunteer for research studies may differ in many critical ways from target clinical populations, and efficacy in a particular trial may not generalize to effectiveness with clinical groups that do not closely resemble the sample in which a study is based. This points to two pressing needs in the field: (a) independent replication studies (unfortunately, negative results are not often published) and (b) meta-analyses where effect sizes can be pooled across a number of studies to arrive at a conclusion as to the efficacy of a specific set of interventions. Despite our attempts to examine effects at a group level, individuals have complex and varied responses owing to unique and individual characteristics. Recent attempts to more fully incorporate individual-level participant data in our analytic models may result in better tailored interventions that can be appropriately targeted to those in need.

REFERENCES

Baron, R. M., & Kenny, D. A. (1986). The moderator–mediator variable distinction in social psychological research: Conceptual, strategic, and statistical considerations. *Journal of Personality and Social Psychology, 51*(6), 1173–1182.

Breslau, N. (1985). Depressive symptoms, major depression, and generalized anxiety: A comparison of self-reports on CES-D and results from diagnostic interviews. *Psychiatry Research, 15*(3), 219–229.

Campbell, D. T., Stanley, J. C., & Gage, N. L. (1963). *Experimental and quasi-experimental designs for research* (pp. 171–246). Boston, MA: Houghton Mifflin.

Duncan, T. E., Duncan, S. C., & Strycker, L. A. (2013). *An introduction to latent variable growth curve modeling: Concepts, issues, and application*. New York, NY: Routledge Academic.

Fairchild, A. J., & MacKinnon, D. P. (2014). Using mediation and moderation analyses to enhance prevention research. In Z. Sloboda & H. Petras (Eds.), *Defining prevention science* (pp. 537–555). New York, NY: Springer.

Faul, F., Erdfelder, E., Lang, A. G., & Buchner, A. (2007). G*Power 3: A flexible statistical power analysis program for the social, behavioral, and biomedical sciences. *Behavior Research Methods, 39*(2), 175–191.

Gitlin, L. N., Roth, D. L., & Huang, J. (2014). Mediators of the impact of a home-based intervention (beat the blues) on depressive symptoms among older African Americans. *Psychology and Aging, 29*(3), 601–611.

Gupta, S. K. (2011). Intention-to-treat concept: A review. *Perspectives in Clinical Research, 2*(3), 109–112.

Imai, K., Tingley, D., & Yamamoto, T. (2013). Experimental designs for identifying causal mechanisms. *Journal of the Royal Statistical Society: Series A (Statistics in Society), 176*(1), 5–51.

Kenny, D. A., Bolger, N., & Kashy, D. A. (2002). Traditional methods for estimating multilevel models. In D. S. Moskowitz & S. L. Hershberger (Eds.), *Modeling intraindividual variability with repeated measures data: Methods and applications* (pp. 1–24). New York, NY: Psychology Press.

Little, R. J., & Rubin, D. B. (2014). *Statistical analysis with missing data.* Hoboken, NJ: Wiley.

Little, R. J., & Yau, L. (1998). Statistical techniques for analyzing data from prevention trials: Treatment of no-shows using Rubin's causal model. *Psychological Methods, 3,* 147–159.

MacCallum, R. C., & Austin, J. T. (2000). Applications of structural equation modeling in psychological research. *Annual Review of Psychology, 51*(1), 201–226.

Preacher, K. J., Rucker, D. D., & Hayes, A. F. (2007). Addressing moderated mediation hypotheses: Theory, methods, and prescriptions. *Multivariate Behavioral Research, 42*(1), 185–227.

Radloff, L. S. (1977). The CES-D scale: A self-report depression scale for research in the general population. *Applied Psychological Measurement, 1*(3), 385–401.

Rothwell, P. M. (2005). External validity of randomised controlled trials: "To whom do the results of this trial apply?" *The Lancet, 365*(9453), 82–93.

Schaie, K. W. (1988). Internal validity threats in studies of adult cognitive development. In M. L. Howe & C. J. Brainerd (Eds.), *Cognitive development in adulthood: Progress in cognitive development research* (pp. 241–272). New York: Springer-Verlag.

Schaie, K. W., Maitland, S. B., Willis, S. L., & Intrieri, R. C. (1998). Longitudinal invariance of adult psychometric ability factor structures across 7 years. *Psychology and Aging, 13*(1), 8–20.

Shadish, W. R., Cook, T. D., & Campbell, D. T. (2002). *Experimental and quasi-experimental designs for generalized causal inference.* Boston, MA: Wadsworth Cengage Learning.

Trochim, W. (2000). *The research methods knowledge base* (2nd ed.). Cincinnati, OH: Atomic Dog Publishing.

SEVENTEEN

CLINICAL SIGNIFICANCE

> *. . . and when is enough proof enough?*
> —Jonathan Safran

In clinical and community practices, there is an increased emphasis on evidence-based treatments for physical, emotional, and social issues. Generally, the term "evidence" refers to data or information, relevant to a question or issue, obtained from experience, or observational or experimental trials (Jenicek, 2010). Evidence is not necessarily correct, complete, satisfactory, or useful. The strength or utility of evidence depends upon the process used to gather the data, the sample and outcome measures on which the data are based, and the context in which the data were collected. In behavioral intervention research, the outcomes of a study or evidence for a treatment can be evaluated according to different criteria: effectiveness with respect to important outcomes, relevance, feasibility, cost versus benefit, equivalence to usual care, and sustainability. Many interventions have empirical evidence from a randomized clinical trial to indicate if they are efficacious with respect to specified outcomes. However, a question that often arises with respect to the translation and then widespread implementation of the treatment is: What type and level of evidence is sufficient, adequate, and generalizable to community settings and clinical practices?

For example, consider a skills-training intervention for spousal caregivers of persons with dementia that is compared to an educational/information provision control group. Assume that 120 caregivers were randomly assigned to either the skills-training group ($n = 60$) or the education/information group ($n = 60$). After the 6-month intervention period, caregivers who received the skills group experienced on average a 2-point drop in depression (as measured by the Center for Epidemiologic Studies Depression scale (CES-D)) as compared to those who received education/information, which was statistically significant ($p < .05$). Although the data provide reliable evidence that there was a difference in change in depression between the groups and suggest that providing caregivers with skills training is efficacious in terms of reducing depressive symptoms, statistical significance does not necessarily imply that the caregivers demonstrated improvements in their mood that is meaningful to their everyday lives. Similar comments can be made for the effect size statistic, which is a measure of the strength of the relationship between a treatment and an outcome. Even large effect sizes do not necessarily mean that the results are clinically meaningful or of practical importance with respect to everyday living. Thus, overall, there are some shortcomings associated with implementing treatments that are based solely on statistical findings related to differences between treatment groups.

In response to the limitations of statistical tests, researchers have been focusing on developing methods for identifying practically or clinically meaningful outcomes (Kazdin, 2008). To date, much of the discussion of clinical significance has been within the realm of psychotherapy or clinical medicine. For example, Schulz and colleagues (2002) conducted a review of intervention studies aimed at improving the lives of caregivers with dementia. They found that, although many studies reported small-to-moderate statistically significant effects on a broad range of caregiver outcomes, only a small portion of studies reported clinically significant outcomes. The authors concluded that the assessment of clinical significance in addition to statistical significance is needed in the domain of caregiver intervention research.

In this regard, the topic of clinical significance is receiving more attention in the broader intervention literature, given the increased emphasis on evidence-based treatments and the higher bar that is being established for evidence—achieving outcomes that are not only statistically significant but also meaningful and practically relevant. As discussed by Kazdin (2008), apart from statistical issues, other concerns related to the choices of outcome measures are the extent to which they are sensitive to change and capture functioning in everyday life. We also discuss this issue in Chapter 15 as it relates to the objective measurement of cognition and daily function. The essential question is: To what extent are changes in standardized measures of cognition related to changes in an individual's ability to perform everyday activities such as managing medication and financial management tasks?

There is increasing recognition of the importance of evaluating the clinical meaning of statistically significant changes brought on by an intervention. It is no longer good enough, so to speak, to find statistical group differences and attribute them to a treatment. Thus, the objectives of this chapter are to (a) define the construct of clinical significance, (b) review the currently available methods for measuring clinical significance, and (c) discuss strategies for maximizing clinical significance. Our overall goal is to extend our understanding of methods for evaluating the effectiveness of interventions in order to advance the quality of intervention research; enhance the likelihood that treatments are implemented in community and clinical settings; and, perhaps most importantly, ensure that intervention programs are improving lives of individuals, families, and communities in meaningful ways.

THE MEANING AND MEASUREMENT OF CLINICAL SIGNIFICANCE

Defining Clinical Significance

"Significance" generally refers to the quality of being important (Merriam-Webster, 2014). In behavioral intervention research, we are generally concerned with two types of significance: statistical significance and clinical significance. Statistical significance is based on probability likelihood and is typically operationalized at an alpha level of .05 or .01. Observing a significant difference between two treatment groups means that there is a reliable difference between two groups on a chosen outcome measure or only a 5% ($\alpha = .05$) or a 1% ($\alpha = .01$) likelihood that the difference was due to chance. Statistical significance is influenced by factors other than the relationship between the independent and dependent variables such as sample size and variability in the data. In addition, statistical significance does not indicate the magnitude of the difference. The effect size statistic is an indication of the magnitude of a treatment effect and often thought of as a measure of practical significance. Effect sizes are often calculated using Cohen's "d" (the difference between the means, $M_1 - M_2$, divided by the standard deviation of either group) and sometimes interpreted as small (0.0–0.2), medium (0.3–0.5), or large (0.6–0.8), but as cautioned by Cohen (1988), there is some risk in using these operational guidelines given the diversity of behavioral research.

Clinical significance has evolved as a means to determine the impact of an intervention or treatment and refers to the *importance* of the effect of an intervention and whether it makes a difference in the lives of individuals (Kazdin, 1999). For example, in the case of an intervention to treat individuals with severe depression—has the treatment moved the patient to remission or a more functional level? Measures of clinical significance are usually used as a supplement to measures of statistical significance and are intended to address the issue of impact of an intervention. For individuals, this is clearly important, as an intervention should effect a change on some outcome that is impactful in their lives. Among caregivers, this might include reduced burden, better coping skills, enhanced social support, or the ability to keep the person they live with at home with life quality. Among overweight adults, this might be weight loss, enhanced mobility, or lower cholesterol. Clinical significance is also pivotal to health care professionals and social agencies/policy makers. Clinicians who are faced with choosing among available treatments are often faced with a dearth of information regarding the impact or practical relevance of research findings for individuals. Social agencies and policy makers are also increasingly asking for evidence about real-world effects of treatments when making decisions about investing in intervention programs. Generally, tests of statistical significance are not sufficient to yield evidence that a treatment is worthwhile. Thus, assessment of clinical significance adds a critical dimension to the evaluation of treatment effectiveness that is not captured by standard statistical evaluation methods.

It is important to recognize that what constitutes clinical significance depends upon the problem or issue that is being addressed and the goals of the intervention or treatment (Kazdin, 1999). For example, in the case of a cognitive training intervention directed at schizophrenic patients, it would not be reasonable to assume that patients would obtain normative levels of cognitive functioning. Instead, in this case, improvements in quality of life (QoL) and/or the ability to perform everyday activities could be markers of clinical significance.

Measuring Clinical Significance

Clinical significance can be assessed or measured in different ways. Each method answers a somewhat different question about clinical significance. A summary of these approaches is provided in Table 17.1.

TABLE 17.1 Summary of Approaches for Measuring Clinical Significance

Approach	Examples of Method/Measures
Comparison approaches: Comparison of individuals who receive an intervention with other individuals (e.g., normative samples)	■ *Change score approach (Jacobson and Truax method)*: People who receive the intervention are compared on a measure (e.g., depressive symptoms) with individuals who did not receive the treatment but had a similar level of symptoms pretreatment (Jacobson & Truax, 1991) ■ *Normative comparison*: The behavior or symptoms of individuals at posttreatment are compared to a sample of peers who are functioning well or without significant problems on the outcome measure of interest (Kendall, Marrs-Garcia, Nath, & Sheldrick, 1999)
Number needed to treat (NNT); number needed to harm (NNH)	■ NNT and NNH reflect two helpful metrics that can help clinicians, in particular, determine whether a treatment is worth the risk for its relative benefits
Subjective evaluations: Determination of the importance of the outcome of an intervention through subjective ratings by the targeted individual, family members/ friends, or clinicians who have contact with the individual	■ *Social validity*: Subjective ratings of acceptability, usability, value, and benefits/impact of an intervention ■ *Quality of life (QoL)*: Ratings of physical well-being, social well-being, and emotional well-being as well as behavioral competence 　■ QoL: WHOQOL-BREF (World Health Organization, 1996) 　■ Satisfaction with Life Scale (Diener, Emmons, Larsen, & Griffin, 1985) ■ *Health-related QoL (HRQoL)*: Ratings of the impact of health status on aspects of QoL (e.g., social, emotional, physical functioning) 　■ Short-Form Health Survey (SF-36) (Ware & Sherbourne, 1992) 　■ Sickness Impact Profile (Bergner, Bobbitt, Carter, & Gilson, 1981) 　■ PROMIS (www.nihpromis.org)
Social impact measures: The impact an intervention has on communities and society as a whole	■ Patient placement ■ Rehospitalization ■ Use of respite services

PROMIS, Patient Reported Outcomes Measurement Information System.

Comparison Approaches

As noted, the measurement of clinical significance has received considerable attention in the psychotherapy literature. The focus in this field is typically on measuring clinical significance in terms of symptom change (e.g., changes in level of depression, anxiety, social phobia). In this scenario, methods have been derived that focus on changes in symptomatology in specific clinical populations. However, clearly measures of symptoms also apply to other interventions and populations beyond those found in the field of psychotherapy. For example, caregiver intervention studies often include measures of symptoms such as indices of depression, anxiety, and health symptoms in which symptom reduction as a clinical significant outcome would be relevant.

A classic example of a measure of symptom reduction that has clinical meaning is the Patient Health Questionnaire-9 (PHQ-9) scale, a screen for depression that is widely used in trials. This scale yields a symptom severity score, and, in turn, scores can be categorized as no symptomatology, to mild, moderate, moderate severe, and severe depression, mapping on to *DSM-5* classifications of depression. Interventions designed to reduce depressive symptoms and which use the PHQ-9 as an outcome measure can demonstrate clinical significance by showing the percentage of individuals who entered remission, who changed diagnostic categories, or who reduced symptomatology by 10 points—all approaches identified as having clinical relevance (Gitlin et al., 2013; Kroenke & Spitzer, 2002).

Comparison methods, which involve comparisons of individuals who receive an intervention with other individuals (e.g., normative samples, dysfunctional samples), are commonly used to determine the clinical significance of changes in symptoms. These methods can also be used with other measures if comparative norms are available. A widely used comparison approach is the method developed by Jacobson and Truax (1991) (Jacobson, Roberts, Berns, & McGlinchey, 1999), which is based on a change score approach where intraindividual comparisons are made on an outcome measure pre- and posttreatment. Participants who receive the treatment are compared posttreatment with the untreated sample that has a similar level of dysfunction prior to treatment. The idea is that, following treatment, individuals will be significantly different from that group. The method assumes that there are two distributions for the outcome measure of interest: a functional distribution and a dysfunctional distribution. Using this method, there are two criteria for establishing clinically significant change. First, a cutoff point must be established for the outcome measure of interest that a person must cross (their posttest score must cross this cutoff point) to move from the dysfunctional to the functional group. The cutoff is typically a weighted midpoint between the means of the two distributions. For example, a depressed caregiver who is involved in a coping skills–training intervention must have a CES-D score following treatment that is more similar to a CES-D score for the general population than to a score of a depressed caregiver who has not received the intervention. Different criteria can be used to determine if the change in the treated individual is significantly different from the untreated dysfunctional group.

Second, the change from pre- to posttest must be large enough to be reliable and not due to measurement error. Reliability is assessed by calculation of the Reliable Change Index (RCI), which is based on the pretreatment score, the posttreatment score, and the standard error of the difference between the two scores. For example, a common criterion that is used as an RCI greater than ± 1.96 standard deviation units indicates reliable change. Using this method, one can determine the percentage of individuals who improved but did not recover, the percentage of individuals who are no longer depressed, and the percentage of individuals who remain unchanged or who have gotten worse. These percentages can then be compared between groups (e.g., treatment vs. control) using contingency table analyses to determine whether the observed differences between the groups in symptom improvement are statistically significant.

There are limitations to this approach. Of course, the method works best when adequate norms are available for chosen outcome measures for both the dysfunctional and functional populations. It is also difficult to make comparisons about the clinical significance of a given treatment across studies if different outcome measures are used (e.g., the CES-D [Radloff, 1977] vs. the Beck Depression Inventory [Beck, Ward, Mendelson, Mock, & Erbaugh, 1961]). The method is also limited to the extent that return to normal functioning is a feasible goal of the intervention. There may be some populations for which return to normal functioning is not possible (e.g., schizophrenics) or for whom other outcomes such as better coping skills or QoL may be more reasonable or of greater practical value. In addition, the method does not address a person's level of functioning at the end of an intervention. A significant change in the level of a symptom does not necessarily mean that a person is functioning at a "normal" level. As noted by Kazdin (1994), using statistical criteria to determine a clinically important change is problematic as is the reliance on assessing symptoms with paper and pencil tests as this may not adequately capture a person's level of functioning.

Several alternatives to the Jacobson and Truax (JT) method have been proposed, which represent statistical refinements to the JT method and are designed to improve sensitivity in detecting clinically meaningful change. The Edwards–Nunnally method (McGlinchey, Atkins, & Jacobson, 2002) derives reliable change by observing an individual's posttest score relative to an established confidence interval, which is intended to reduce problems with measurement error and misclassification of individuals. Hierarchical Linear Modeling (HLM) method (Speer, 2001) is useful for studies that have missing data points. Studies (McGlinchey et al., 2002; Speer & Greenbaum, 1995) have been conducted to compare the predictive utility of these methods. The results indicate that there is little evidence to suggest that these refinements yield different information or are superior to the JT approach.

An alternative comparison approach for estimating clinically significant change is based on normative comparison (Kendall et al., 1999), where the behavior or symptoms of individuals at posttreatment are compared to a sample of peers who are functioning well or without significant problems on the outcome measure of interest. In essence, normative comparisons are used to determine if treated individuals are indistinguishable from "well-functioning" individuals on the outcome measure(s) of interest. Clinical significance is defined as end-state functioning that falls within normal range on the critical dependent measures.

For example, Kazdin and colleagues (Kazdin, Siegel, & Bass, 1992) evaluated three interventions for children with aggression and antisocial behavior patterns: a problem-solving skills training (PSST) intervention, parent management training (PMT), and PSST + PMT. Treatment was provided to the children and/or their parents, and the outcome measures included standardized scales that were completed by both the children and parents and had available normative data. The investigators identified that the using the 90th percentile cutoff on the measures from the normative sample best separated the clinical from community samples. In addition, in the intervention study, scores at this percentile were used to define the upper limit of the range of problematic behaviors. They defined clinically significant change as scores that fell below this cutoff. Overall, they found that, although the statistical evaluation of change was evident across many measures, when considering clinical significance (return to normative levels of function), the findings were more modest. For example, using the parent evaluation measure, 33% of the PSST group, 39% of the PMT, and 64% of the combined treatment group returned to "normative" levels of performance.

Typically, equivalence testing is employed to determine if an intervention group performs in a manner that is statistically equivalent to a functional sample. The use of equivalence testing requires the availability of a normative nonpatient sample that is comparable to the treatment group on key dimensions (e.g., age, ethnicity, socioeconomic status). Thus, careful consideration must be given to the selection of the normative group in terms of sample representativeness and sampling equivalence. For example, if the study is concerned with a weight loss intervention for obese adults, it is important that the normative data used for comparison are based on adults with similar characteristics as the obese sample included in the study (e.g., age, gender, height). Decisions about which group will serve as the reference group have a large impact on conclusions regarding clinical significance. It is also important that the normative data is current as norms for various metrics can change. Another potential shortcoming with this approach is that there may be a lack of normative data for the outcome of interest.

One general issue with the comparison approaches relates to the clinical relevance of the measures used to evaluate treatment outcomes. For example, the Revised Memory and Behavior Problem Checklist (RMBPC) (Teri et al., 1992) is often used in caregiver intervention studies to assess the extent and severity of behavior problems in persons with dementia. A significant reduction in ratings of behavior problems by caregivers following an intervention does not necessarily equate with real changes in behavioral occurrences, a change in the caregiver's level of distress, or an improvement in the quality of his or her life. Also, what constitutes a meaningful change in certain measures is unclear; for example, there is no agreed-upon cutoff score for many psychosocial measures such as burden or well-being. Furthermore, some people may experience a change in functioning that is not within normative limits, but the change makes a significant improvement in their everyday functioning. A caregiver may experience a reduction in the frequency of behavioral symptoms although the behaviors still persist. Nevertheless, the reduction in the frequency or severity of their occurrence may be of importance to the caregiver. A person who is severely depressed might experience a reduction in symptoms sufficient to allow a return to work even though he or she is still more depressed at the end of treatment than someone in the normative range.

Second, most measures are unidimensional and tap constructs such as depression, anxiety, or burden. Yet, many intervention studies target multidimensional problems. Thus, one issue is determining the measure or measures that best reflect that an intervention has achieved a clinically significance impact. This problem is compounded if there is discordance among measures. For example, a caregiver may not show any change in symptoms of depression, but report a decrease in burden and better coping skills.

As noted, domains other than symptoms also hold importance in defining clinical significance. Thus, symptoms are not the sole criteria for making judgments about clinical significance. There are other key constructs along which clinical significance could be evaluated depending on the goals of the intervention. For example, the intervention goals might be aimed at increasing mobility or amount of exercise, or enhancing knowledge about a topic or coping skills.

Number Needed to Treat and Number Needed to Harm

The number needed to treat (NNT) and the number needed to harm (NNH) are two useful metrics for understanding an intervention's clinical potential (Cook & Sackett, 1995; Zapletal, LeMaitre, Menard, & Degoulet, 1996). NNT refers to the number of patients or participants who would have to receive a treatment for a particular benefit to occur or to prevent a particular negative outcome such as a death; conversely, NNH refers to the number of patients who would have to receive a treatment for a particular harmful outcome to occur. NNT is a simple measure of the impact of an intervention on one person. For example, if an intervention has an NNT of 10, it means that 10 persons would have to receive the treatment for one person to benefit or to prevent one additional negative outcome. As not all persons will benefit from a treatment and some may be harmed or not affected, the NNT offers a measurement of how many persons are needed for each scenario. To calculate NNT, the absolute risk reduction (ARR) needs to be determined; the NNT is the inverse of ARR (NNT = 1/ARR). NNT and NNH are associated with effect sizes. A small effect size may reflect statistical but not clinical significance. In order for an intervention to be worth implementing, a trial must yield more than a trivial effect to also reflect a clinically meaningful difference. NNH is an important metric particularly for high-risk interventions. As most behavioral interventions report adverse events and are of low risk, NNH may not be as relevant as NNT.

Subjective Evaluations

Subjective evaluation methods involve determining the importance of the outcome of an intervention through ratings or assessments from the targeted individual, family members/friends, or clinicians who have contact with the individual. The issue that is assessed is whether the individual or those in contact with the individual detect a meaningful change in some outcome measure—for example, an individual feels that he or she has better coping skills if the treatment or intervention is valuable and acceptable. The need to show that a treatment is feasible and acceptable within community settings is becoming increasingly important given the current emphasis on translational research within the social and behavioral sciences. Interventions have little chance of succeeding in the community if the target population finds them cumbersome or is unwilling to accept or implement them or if the outcomes are not perceived as important.

Social Validity. In this regard, measures of social validity have been discussed as important indicators of clinical significance. Social validity is a multidimensional construct that includes both acceptability and importance (Foster & Mash, 1999). There are three distinct but related elements of intervention programs that can be assessed for social validity: (a) the goals of treatment (e.g., enhancement of problem-solving skills), (b) the treatment procedures (e.g., home-based intervention approach), and (c) the outcomes produced by the treatment (e.g., reduction in the frequency of disruptive behaviors). Generally, treatment goals are assessed for both their importance and acceptability; treatment procedures are assessed for their acceptability; and treatment outcomes are assessed for their importance (Is the outcome meaningful to the individual?) and derived benefits.

Assessment of social validity is typically achieved by using subjective evaluations, which involve having study participants rate interventions in terms of their overall value, the extent to which the intervention was helpful or beneficial, the acceptability of the intervention protocols, and whether they would recommend the intervention to others in similar circumstances. In the review of caregiver intervention studies conducted by Schulz and colleagues (2002), 14 of the 43 reviewed studies included measures of social validity. The typical finding was that the majority of participants rated the intervention as helpful, beneficial, or valuable. However, the authors warned that the results should be interpreted with caution with respect to generalizability as they are based on rating of participants who choose to remain in the study. In addition, respondents may have been biased in their ratings in a desire to please the study interventionists, and they may have felt a need to provide positive ratings to bring value to their efforts in participating in the study.

It is also important to note that subjective ratings may not necessarily correlate with actual behavior—a caregiver may indicate that increasing support from other family members is an important outcome, but they may choose not to participate in conference calls with other family members. There may also be a lack of congruence between ratings of importance and ratings of acceptability, so decisions may have to be made regarding the relative importance of these criteria. Careful attention also needs to be paid to the selection of individuals chosen to do the evaluations. For example, health care professionals may have different ideas from caregivers about the importance of intervention goals.

When choosing how to measure social validity, it is important to consider the purpose of the assessment and the phase of the pipeline. The intervention development phase might involve the use of focus groups or pilot testing to evaluate the contents of the intervention protocol. At all phases of the pipeline, it is important to identify relevant aspects of the intervention to be included in the evaluation. For example, in an evaluation of the Personalized Reminder Information and Social Management (PRISM) system (see Chapter 14), an evaluation was included that assessed the value of the overall system and each of the features with respect to whether they improved the ability to perform various everyday activities; the usefulness of the system and the features; and the adequacy of the training protocol. Also included were measures of system usability and acceptability.

Finally, when assessing the goals of an intervention, it is important to distinguish between ultimate or distal goals (e.g., reduced stress, improved relationship with a spouse) and more instrumental goals (e.g., enhanced problem-solving skills, improved communication skills). Instrumental goals are outcomes that are hypothesized to be related to ultimate outcomes. The distinction between ultimate and instrumental intervention goals has important implications for defining the clinical significance of an intervention. Of course, all measures of social validity should be pilot tested with representatives of the target population.

Quality of Life

QoL has recently emerged as an important indicator of clinical significance. Health care providers and funding agencies are increasingly requiring that indexes of QoL be incorporated in assessments of treatment effectiveness. One difficulty with including measures of QoL in studies of behavioral intervention is identification of the appropriate metric. There is no agreed-upon strategy for measuring QoL as it represents a multidimensional construct that includes a broad range of life domains and it is shaped by both objective and subjective factors. Generally, QoL includes physical well-being, social well-being, and emotional well-being as well as behavioral competence or the ability to effectively engage in valued life activities. Definitions of QoL have included a number of concepts including life satisfaction, social support, psychological well-being, social and emotional functioning, and standard of living. Lawton (1983) eloquently defined QoL as a multidimensional evaluation, by both personal- and social-normative criteria, of the person–environment system of an individual in time past, current, and anticipated. In essence, QoL is a type of umbrella construct that includes health states and satisfaction with a number of life domains.

An aspect of QoL that is particularly relevant to behavioral intervention studies is health-related QoL (HRQoL), where QoL is considered in the context of health and disease. HRQoL is also a multidimensional construct that includes domains related to physical, emotional, and social functioning and focuses on the impact of health status on QoL or the QoL consequences of health status.

There is a wide variety of QoL measures that have been used in studies assessing treatment effects. These measures generally fall into two categories: measures of generic QoL and measures of HRQoL. Generic measures can be applied to both healthy and ill individuals and tend to cut across a broad range of domains. Measures of well-being, social support, and life satisfaction are typically placed in this category (e.g., the Satisfaction With Life Scale; Diener et al., 1985). The World Health Organization (WHO) has developed what is intended to be an international, cross-culture measure of QoL—WHOQOL-BREF, a 26-item instrument, which measures physical health, psychological health, social relationships, and the environment (WHO, 1996).

There are numerous HRQoL measures (e.g., Short-Form Health Survey [SF-36], Sickness Impact Profile [Bergner et al., 1981]; Quality of Well-Being Scale [Kaplan & Bush, 1982; Ware & Sherbourne, 1992]) available. Haywood, Garratt, and Fitzpatrick (2005) provide a review of the measurement properties of many of these instruments for older people. Generally, HRQoL measures are intended to assess the impact of illness on QoL. Although these measures may include some items related to overall QoL or life satisfaction, their primary emphasis is on symptoms, impairment, function, and disability. The Patient Reported Outcomes Measurement Information System (PROMIS; www.nihpromis.org) includes a 10-item global health measure, which assesses global physical, mental, and social HRQoL. PROMIS is part of the National Institutes of Health (NIH) Roadmap initiative that was designed to develop an electronic system to collect HRQoL from diverse populations.

More recently, an emphasis has been placed on Quality-Adjusted Life Years (QALYs), which is a single index that combines quality of remaining life years with survival data. QALYs have two basic components: the quantity and quality of life. It is used to measure the extent of health gains from a health care intervention related to the cost associated with the intervention to assess the worth of an intervention from an economic prospective. Of course, there are shortcomings associated with using QALYs as outcome measure. For example, QALY represents a single index and excludes other health-related consequences, has limitations with respect to sensitivity, and does not give sufficient weight to emotional and mental health issues. In addition, QALY does not appear to work well with complex interventions (Normand, 2009; Phillips, 2009).

When selecting a measure of QoL, it is important to establish an operational definition of QoL relevant to the intervention being evaluated and the target population (e.g., burden associated with caregiving). In some cases, it might be advisable to include more than one measure of QoL in an assessment battery. It is also important to recognize that, for many of the QoL instruments, it is difficult to interpret scores and magnitude of change in terms of clinical relevance. Of course, the general criteria for selection of outcome measures outlined in Chapter 14 need to be considered.

Social Impact Measures

Social impact refers to the impact of an intervention on communities and society as a whole. Measures of social impact assess outcomes that go beyond an individual and are important to society, and outcomes that are more global in nature. These measures might include patient placement, rehospitalization, emergency room use, recidivism, or use of some social program or resource such as respite services. Including these measures as indices of clinical significance needs to be done with caution. One issue is that these are gross measures and subject to other influences such as changes in policy or budget cuts. The psychometric properties of these types of measures are also problematic as errors can result from inconsistencies in data-reporting or data-capture techniques. In essence, it is often difficult to link changes in these types of measures with an intervention; absence of change on these measures may not necessarily imply that a program is not impactful (Kazdin, 1994).

The Reach Effectiveness Adoption Implementation Maintenance (RE-AIM) Framework (Glasgow, Vogt, & Boles, 1999) can be conceptualized as an evaluation framework that can be used to assess the social impact of interventions. This framework assesses five dimensions: *reach*, the percentage and risk characteristics of persons who receive or are affected by a program; *efficacy*, positive and negative outcomes associated with a program; *adoption*, the proportion and representativeness of settings that adopt a program; *implementation*, the extent to which the program is delivered as intended; and *maintenance*, the extent to which the program becomes ingrained or routine and part of the everyday culture of a community or organization. Some limitations with this approach are that all of the components of the framework may not have equal weight or be needed for a particular program. There also needs to be a strategy for combining the components or indices that represented the combined impact of or interactions among the components. Further, the optimal time points for measurement need to be established.

STRATEGIES FOR MAXIMIZING THE CLINICAL SIGNIFICANCE OF INTERVENTION PROGRAMS

A clear goal of behavioral intervention research is to develop and implement intervention programs that are clinically significant and effect a change that is meaningful to an individual and society. One strategy for achieving this goal is to design interventions that place individuals "at risk" and target factors that are amenable to change. For example, the Resources for Enhancing Alzheimer's Caregiver Health II (REACH II) intervention (Chapters 2, 4 and 14) targeted five areas that place caregivers who are at risk (e.g., care recipient target behaviors, lack of social support). Although the cognitive status of the person with dementia could not be changed, family caregivers could be instructed in concrete strategies for managing behavior problems, one of the most challenging aspects of caregiving. Also, in REACH II, caregivers in most need were targeted in the intervention. This is not to suggest that studies should "stack the deck" by including only individuals who exhibit extreme levels of dysfunction. Rather, it suggests that intervention programs are more likely to be successful if they target populations who are most in need of the intervention.

Intervention programs are also more likely to achieve clinically significant outcomes if they are congruent with the beliefs, attitudes, values, and needs of target populations. Thus, it is important to conduct a needs assessment prior to the development of an intervention program to obtain information on the needs, goals, and preferences of relevant populations (e.g., caregivers, family members, social service agencies). This can be accomplished through techniques such as focus groups, interviews, or questionnaires. As noted earlier in the chapter, evaluations of social validity should occur at different points during the intervention process—at the beginning, during the course of treatment, or at follow-up. Using community-based participatory approaches and including a community advisory board as part of the intervention team (see Chapter 10) are effective strategies to help achieve these goals.

It is also important to choose measures of clinical significance that are relevant and sensitive to treatment-related goals (Chapter 14). Some measures, such as measures of social impact, may not be sensitive to detect change that results from treatment effects. This issue is further complicated when multiple measures of clinical significance are employed—some measures may change and others may not, or some may change in the reverse direction. This makes it difficult to evaluate the overall impact of the treatment program and determine if clinically significant outcomes have been achieved. A criterion needs to be established for defining clinical significance such as a small improvement on multiple outcomes, a large improvement on a few outcomes, or meeting the absolute standard on a few key outcomes. The criterion chosen will vary with the goals of the program and the stakeholders invested in program outcomes. For example, in caregiver intervention research, the stakeholders are likely to include health care providers, insurers, payers, care recipients, other family members, and, of course, the caregiver. For the caregiver, a meaningful effect may be a reduction in burden and increase in caregiving skills; for other family members, an important outcome may be the physical health of the caregiver; whereas for health care providers, insurers, and payers, cost-effectiveness may be the most important outcome. It is important to be aware of the concerns of the stakeholders during the design and implementation of an intervention program.

CONCLUSION

The assessment of clinical significance is an important aspect of behavioral intervention research. Measures of clinical significance should be included in the evaluation of intervention programs, especially at the later phases of the pipeline (efficacy, effectiveness, translation/implementation studies). Evaluation of an intervention program needs to extend beyond statistical significance and assess the practical value or the importance of an intervention for the targeted population and/or stakeholders. Understanding the clinical significance of programs has important implications for the implementation of a program (Part IV) and public policy. When making programmatic decisions, public policy makers generally consider effectiveness (Did the intervention result in outcomes or benefits that are important?), efficiency (program benefits vs. costs), and equity (number of people likely to benefit from the program) and cost.

We recommend that multiple measures of clinical significance be included in intervention assessment batteries, of course without adding to participant burden (Table 17.1). However, as noted throughout this chapter, there are a number of challenges associated with the measurement of clinical significance and thus these measures need to be carefully chosen. An initial consideration is operationalizing the construct of clinical significance—what constitutes meaningful change? This might include a reduction in symptoms, lessened impairment, enhanced coping skills, or QoL. It also might mean maintaining people at moderate levels of impairment or preventing further deterioration. The costs of achieving practically important outcomes also need to be considered. A program may be effective; however, the costs associated with program implementation in terms of staff resources may outweigh the benefits.

Other challenges associated with the assessment of clinical significance are the lack of normative data for some measures and identification of cutoff points that equate to "normal" functioning. Strategies also need to be identified for combining data for multiple measures and for handling the overlap that is likely to exist among measures.

Clearly, the study of clinical significance is a fruitful and important area of investigation. To the extent that we reach the goal of achieving reliable and clinically significant outcomes, we will not only make a meaningful difference in solving health and social problems and improving the lives of individuals and families, but we will also advance the field of behavioral intervention research.

REFERENCES

Beck, A. T., Ward, C. H., Mendelson, M., Mock, J., & Erbaugh, J. (1961). An inventory for measuring depression. *Archives of General Psychiatry, 4*, 561–571.

Bergner, M., Bobbitt, R. A., Carter, W. B., & Gilson, B. S. (1981). The sickness impact profile: Development and final revision of a health status measure. *Medical Care, 19*, 787–805.

Cohen, J. (1988). *Statistical power analysis for the behavioral science* (2nd ed.). Hillsdale, NJ: Lawrence Erlbaum Associates.

Cook, R. J., & Sackett, D. L. (1995). The number needed to treat: A clinically useful measure of treatment effect. *British Medical Journal, 5*, 452–454.

Diener, E., Emmons, R. A., Larsen, R. J., & Griffin, S. (1985). The satisfaction with life scale. *Journal of Personality Assessment, 49*, 71–75.

Foster, S. L., & Mash, E. J. (1999). Assessing social validity in clinical treatment research: Issues and procedures. *Journal of Consulting and Clinical Psychology, 67*, 308–319.

Gitlin, L. N., Harris, L. F., McCoy, M. C., Chernett, N. L., Pizzi, L. T., Jutkowitz, E., . . . Hauck, W. W. (2013). A home-based intervention to reduce depressive symptoms and improve quality of life in older African Americans. *Annals of Internal Medicine, 159*(4), 243–252.

Glasgow, R. E., Vogt, T. M., & Boles, S. M. (1999). Evaluating the public health impact of health promotion interventions: The RE-AIM framework. *American Journal of Public Health, 89*, 1322–1327.

Haywood, K. L., Garratt, A. M., & Fitzpatrick, R. (2005). Quality of life in older people: A structured review of generic self-assessed health instruments. *Quality of Life Research, 14*, 1654–1668.

Jacobson, N. S., Roberts, N. S., Berns, S. B., & McGlinchey, J. B. (1999). Method for defining and determining the clinical significance of treatment effects: Description, application, and alternatives. *Journal of Consulting and Clinical Psychology, 67*, 300–307.

Jacobson, N. S., & Truax, P. (1991). Clinical significance: A statistical approach to defining meaningful change in psychotherapy research. *Journal of Consulting and Clinical Psychology, 59*, 12–19.

Jenicek, M. (2010). *Foundations of evidenced-based medicine.* New York, NY: Informa Healthcare.

Kaplan, R. M., & Bush, J. W. (1982). Health-related qualify of life measurement for evaluation research and policy analysis. *Health Psychology, 1*, 61–80.

Kazdin, A. E. (1994). Methodology, design, and evaluation in psychotherapy research. In A. E. Bergen & S. L. Garfield (Eds.), *Handbook of Psychotherapy and Behavior Change* (4th ed., pp. 19–71). New York, NY: Wiley.

Kazdin, A. E. (1999). The meanings and measurement of clinical significance. *Journal of Consulting and Clinical Psychology, 67*, 332–339.

Kazdin, A. E. (2008). Evidence-based treatment and practice: New opportunities to bridge clinical research and practice, enhance the knowledge base, and improve patient care. *American Psychologist, 63*, 146–159.

Kazdin, A. E., Siegel, T., & Bass, D. (1992). Cognitive problem-solving skills training and parent management training in the treatment of antisocial behavior in children. *Journal of Consulting and Clinical Psychology, 60*, 733–744.

Kendall, P. C., Marrs-Garcia, A., Nath, S. R., & Sheldrick, R. C. (1999). Normative comparisons for the evaluation of clinical significance. *Journal of Consulting and Clinical Psychology, 67*, 285–299.

Kroenke, K., & Spitzer, R. L. (2002). The PHQ-9: A new depression diagnostic and severity measure. *Psychiatric Annals, 32*(9), 1–7.

Lawton, M. P. (1983). Environment and other determinants of well-being in older people. *The Gerontologist, 23*, 349–357.

McGlinchey, J. B., Atkins, D. C., & Jacobson, N. S. (2002). Clinical significance methods: Which ones to use and how useful are they? *Behavioral Therapy, 33*, 529–550.

Merriam-Webster. (2014). Significance. Retrieved March 3, 2015, from www.merriam-webster.com

Normand, C. (2009). Measuring outcomes in palliative care: Limitations of QALYs and the road to PalYs. *Journal of Pain and Symptom Management, 38*, 27–31.

Phillips, C. (2009). *What is a QALY?* Retrieved March 5, 2015, from http://www.medicine.ox.ac.uk/bandolier/painres/download/whatis/qaly.pdf

Radloff, L. (1977). The CES-D scale: A self-report depression scale for research in the general population. *Applied Psychological Measurement, 1*, 385–401.

Schulz, R., O'Brien, A., Czaja, S. J., Ory, M., Norris, R., Martire, L. M., . . . Stevens, A. (2002). Dementia caregiver research intervention: In search of clinical significance. *The Gerontologist, 42,* 589–602.

Speer, D. C. (1991). Clinically significant change: Jacobson and Truax (1991) revisited. *Journal of Consulting and Clinical Psychology, 60,* 402–408.

Speer, D. C., & Greenbaum, P. E. (1995). Five methods for computing clinical significance individual client change and improvement rates: Support for an individual growth curve approach. *Journal of Consulting and Clinical Psychology, 63,* 1044–1048.

Teri, L., Truax, P., Logsdon, R., Uomoto, J., Zarit, S., & Vitaliano, P. P. (1992). Assessment of behavioral problems in dementia: The revised memory and behavior problems checklist. *Psychology and Aging, 7,* 622–631.

Ware, J. E., & Sherbourne, C. D. (1992). The MOS 36-item short form health survey (SF-36). *Medical Care, 30*(6), 473–483.

World Health Organization. (1996). *WHOQOL-BREF. Introduction, administration, scoring and generic version of the assessment* (Field Trial Version). Geneva, Switzerland: World Health Organization's Qualify of Life Group.

Zapletal, E., LeMaitre, D., Menard, J., & Degoulet, P. (1996). The number needed to treat: A clinically useful nomogram in its proper context. *British Medical Journal, 312,* 426–429.

EIGHTEEN

ECONOMIC EVALUATIONS OF BEHAVIORAL INTERVENTIONS

LAURA T. PIZZI, ERIC JUTKOWITZ, AND JOHN A. NYMAN

> The chronically ill and those toward the end of their lives are accounting
> for potentially 80% of the total health care bill. There is going to have
> to be a very difficult democratic conversation that takes place.
> The decision is not whether or not we will ration care. The decision
> is whether we will ration with our eyes open.
> —Donald Berwick, Former Administrator of the
> U.S. Centers for Medicare and Medicaid Services

Economic evaluations are emerging as a critical component to the conduct of behavioral intervention research and are important for several reasons. They provide an understanding of what it costs to deliver a behavioral intervention in relationship to specified outcomes such as clinical effectiveness and health utility; and they enable a comparison of an intervention to usual care and/or other treatments as to expended resources and benefits. Any intervention requires resources for its implementation, and these resources can be measured in terms of their costs. Interventions also have specified outcomes, which may be positive (e.g., improved health) or negative (e.g., adverse events). An economic evaluation will involve the measurement of both costs and outcomes.

The relationship between resources and cost is an important one to consider and can be illustrated by the Tailored Activity Program, which is a home-based occupational therapy intervention designed to reduce behavioral symptoms in participants with dementia and burden in caregivers (Gitlin et al., 2009). The resources used to implement the Tailored Activity Program included the cost of employing the interventionists (occupational therapists), interventionist travel, and intervention supplies (Gitlin, Jutkowitz, Hodgson, & Pizzi, 2010). Benefits of this intervention included the reduction in behavioral symptoms and improved quality of life of the person with dementia as well as time saved by caregivers in providing hands-on care. The cost of delivering the Tailored Activity Program is critical to informing stakeholders who are considering adopting the intervention. Cost information informs planning for the need and allocation of resources, and whether the intervention is feasible to implement given an existing budget.

This chapter examines the importance of economic evaluations of behavioral interventions and introduces the basic methods for conducting economic evaluations and the key scientific issues involved in costing behavioral interventions. As analyzing the costs of interventions draws upon fundamental terminology that may be new to readers, Table 18.1 provides a summary of brief terms and serves as a reference point throughout this chapter.

WHY COSTING INTERVENTIONS IS IMPORTANT

A variety of factors has transpired to bring the economic evaluation of behavioral interventions to the forefront of analytic considerations. One primary reason is the reorganization of health care. In the United States, the health care marketplace is increasingly cost conscious, with system-level initiatives being implemented to improve health care value. In this context, "value" is defined by interventions that achieve desired patient outcomes at a cost lower than the current standard of care, or interventions that achieve better outcomes than the standard of care but cost more. It is no longer sufficient to accept treatment just on the basis of an efficacy trial and positive outcomes alone. At a minimum, a treatment must also have demonstrated value. This change in focus to value presents a challenge for behavioral intervention researchers. The challenge is that the evidence necessary for adopting a behavioral intervention has been expanded from efficacy and effectiveness (demonstrated against a control group) to also include comparative effectiveness (demonstrated vs. a usual care comparison) and cost-effectiveness.

It could be argued that, given these contextual factors, economic evaluations are relevant for any intervention whether it be medical, drug, or behavioral. Yet, economic evaluations of behavioral interventions are particularly important since traditional medical approaches (e.g., pharmaceuticals) may have limited effectiveness and/or be contraindicated—and cannot address alone the array of major public health concerns such as mental illness, health disparities, obesity, and disabilities (see Chapter 1). In addition, medical approaches alone may result in negative consequences such as polypharmacy and medication-related problems. Added to this, the aging of the population is resulting in an increase in persons with physical, cognitive, or financial limitations or complex health conditions that need ongoing self-care management. Behavioral strategies have the potential to address these issues, thereby meeting an urgent and growing population health need.

Nevertheless, there is little evidence about what behavioral interventions actually cost and what their value is compared to traditional practices. In order for behavioral interventions to be adopted, health care decision makers from both government and private health care payers (particularly health plans), as well as health care providers, will need credible information about the costs of these interventions in terms of the human and nonhuman resources required for training persons and delivering these programs. Unlike traditional medical approaches where the price is set by the innovator, behavioral interventions often do not have a clear market established and/or enter the marketplace without having an established price or reimbursement mechanism. Therefore, behavioral researchers must be proactive in measuring costs, for example, by embedding cost measures during the efficacy and

TABLE 18.1   Key Terms

Term	Definition	Source
Value	A balance of economic, humanistic, *and* clinical outcomes	Dipiro et al. (2011)
Adopter	The person or institution who decides whether to invest in a new treatment alternative	Dearing (2009)
Perspective	The point of view taken (i.e., participant, provider, payer, or society) when determining the value of a treatment alternative	Dipiro et al. (2011)
Societal perspective	The broadest perspective of an economic evaluation that considers the benefits to society as a whole and includes both direct (health care) and indirect (non–health care) costs	Dipiro et al. (2011)
Piggybacking	The term used to describe an economic study that is added onto a clinical trial that originally focused on clinical issues	Berger, Bingefors, Hedblom, Pashos, and Torrance (2003)
Prospective studies	Studies that involve the collection of data on endpoints, treatments, and related measures forward in time	Berger et al. (2003)
Economic model	A simplified framework that mathematically represents a population, with outputs (e.g., effectiveness measures) that respond to changes in inputs (e.g., participant characteristics) in a realistic way	Berger et al. (2003)
Retrospective studies	Studies that analyze outcomes on the basis of currently available data and are typically collected from medical claims, electronic medical records, hospital discharge data, and managed care encounter data	Berger et al. (2003)
Economic evaluations	An evaluation that compares the costs of two or more alternatives without regard to outcome	Dipiro et al. (2011)
Partial economic evaluations	See "Economic Evaluations"	
Cost-minimization studies	Evaluations comparing two or more treatment alternatives with an assumed or demonstrated equivalence in safety and efficacy to determine the least costly alternative	Dipiro et al. (2011)
Return-on-investment studies	Studies that examine the health care investments made, in relation to financial savings	Authors
Cost-of-illness studies	Evaluations that identify and estimate the overall cost of a particular disease for a defined population by measuring the direct and indirect costs attributable to the specific disease	Dipiro et al. (2011)

(Continued)

TABLE 18.1 Key Terms *(Continued)*

Term	Definition	Source
Cost-effectiveness analysis	A systematic method of comparing two or more alternative programs by measuring the costs and consequences of each	Berger et al. (2003)
Incremental cost-effectiveness ratio (ICER)	The difference between program costs divided by the difference between program outcomes	Berger et al. (2003)
Cost-utility analysis	A method for comparing two or more treatment alternatives in terms of both costs and outcomes that integrates participant preferences and utility	Dipiro et al. (2011)
Quality-adjusted life years (QALYs)	A universal measure of disease burden (including quality and quantity of life) applicable to all individuals and all diseases	Berger et al. (2003)
Cost-benefit analysis	An evaluation that allows for the identification, measurement, and comparison of the costs to provide a program or treatment alternative and the benefits to be realized from it	Dipiro et al. (2011)
Intervention costs	The expenses that are required to implement an intervention. Examples of intervention costs include materials/supplies, personnel training, and personnel time delivering intervention	Authors
Health care costs	The costs incurred for medical products and services used to prevent, detect, and/or treat a disease. Examples include but are not limited to medications, medical supplies, hospitalizations, and physician visits	Dipiro et al. (2011)
Non–health care costs	Costs for nonmedical services (e.g., transportation or childcare) and reduced work productivity that result from illness/disease	Dipiro et al. (2011)
Gross costing	A method of collecting cost data by using cost estimates for units of input or output that are large relative to the intervention being analyzed	Gold et al. (1996)
Microcosting	A method of collecting cost data that calls for the "direct enumeration and costing out of every input consumed in the treatment of a particular participant" (Gold et al., 1996). Examples of microcosting include documenting personnel time to complete tasks, or collecting travel data of participants or personnel	Gold et al. (1996)
Health status questionnaires	Survey instruments used to assess participant outcomes. Examples commonly used in economic evaluation include quality-adjusted life, productivity, functional status	Authors

(Continued)

TABLE 18.1 Key Terms *(Continued)*

Term	Definition	Source
Preference-based quality-of-life weights	A degree of preference individuals or society has for living in a particular health state or condition. Weights typically vary between 0 (interpreted as "deceased") and 1 (interpreted as "perfect health")	Neumann, Goldie, and Weinstein (2000)
Health utility	Refers to the preferences individuals or society place on any specific health outcome relative to other possible outcomes	Pizzi and Lofland (2006)
Sensitivity analysis	A way to analyze the impact of uncertainty on an economic evaluation or decision	Berger et al. (2003)
One-way sensitivity analysis	The simplest form of sensitivity analysis by which the value of one variable is varied within a range of plausible values while the other variables are kept constant	Berger et al. (2003)
Threshold analysis	A method of investigating the impact of uncertainty upon payoffs and decisions by identifying the levels of one or more parameters, assumptions, or methods at which the decision switches	Berger et al. (2003)
Two-way sensitivity analysis	A form of sensitivity analysis by which the value of two variables are varied within a range of plausible values while the other variables are kept constant	Berger et al. (2003)
Probabilistic sensitivity analysis	A method of investigating the impact of uncertainty in all parameters simultaneously, assuming that each parameter has a range of possible values	Wang, Salmon, and Walton (2004)
Base case	In reference to a cost model, the expected case of a model using an initial set of assumptions	Authors
Statement of benefits	Statement sent by the health plan explaining what medical treatments and/or services were paid	"Glossary" (2015)
Out-of-pocket costs	The portion of a payment paid for by an individual with his or her own money (copayments and deductibles) as opposed to the portion paid for by the insurer	Berger et al. (2003)

effectiveness phases of research, or possibly before when demonstrating proof of concept as part of a Phase II study. It is only when the cost of the intervention is established that it can be examined in relation to its effectiveness.

STEPS IN AN ECONOMIC EVALUATION

Economic evaluations serve as a formal approach for comparing competing interventions from which to make decisions concerning the allocation of scarce resources. For example, when a new technology or intervention has been developed, a government or health plan must decide if it is willing to reimburse or pay for it. An economic evaluation provides important information by which to make a decision regarding reimbursement. There are six basic steps for completing a health economic evaluation of a behavioral intervention as shown in Figure 18.1.

Step 1: Determine the Primary Adopter of the Intervention

The first step in conducting an economic evaluation is to decide who is the primary adopter of the intervention. The adopter is the stakeholder (individual, organization, or collective group of organizations) that holds the primary responsibility for deciding whether to implement the treatment and whose *perspective* is used to evaluate costs. Typically, the adopter bears financial responsibility for the management of health care. There are different perspectives that can be assumed.

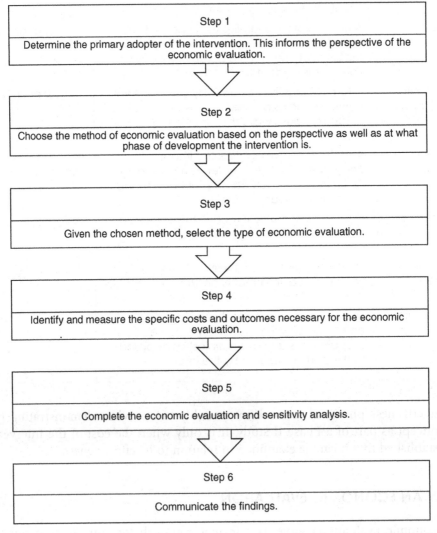

Figure 18.1   Steps to conduct economic evaluations of behavioral interventions.

Perspectives that are commonly chosen for economic evaluations include health care payer (including public payers such as Medicare and Medicaid, as well as private payers such as employers or employer coalitions), health care plan, health care delivery system, individual provider (e.g., physician or other health care provider), participant (or participant-family unit), health sector, or society as a whole (referred to as "societal perspective"). The *health sector* perspective includes health care costs paid by health plans but also participants' out-of-pocket costs. The *societal perspective* encompasses all costs and benefits to society. The Panel on Cost-Effectiveness in Health and Medicine recommends the societal perspective as a primary perspective for an analysis (Gold, Siegel, Russell, & Weinstein, 1996). Although the societal perspective is the gold standard (Gold et al., 1996) in the United States, many studies have also adopted health care plan, health care payer, or health care delivery system perspectives. In contrast, countries with national health care systems such as the United Kingdom, Australia, and Canada tend to apply broader perspectives (e.g., health sector or societal perspective) to economic evaluations. Defining the perspective early on in the analytic process is important as it frames the subsequent steps in conducting the economic evaluation. As the perspective broadens (i.e., from individual/participant to societal), more costs and benefits will need to be captured or collected and then included in the analysis.

Step 2: Choose the Method of Economic Evaluation

The next step is to decide which economic method best fits the chosen perspective and phase of intervention development. There are three main methods of economic evaluation: prospective, retrospective, and modeling approaches as described in Table 18.2.

Here we focus on approaches for establishing the costs of an intervention. Costs of an intervention should be considered early on as one is developing the delivery characteristics of a behavioral intervention and then more formally as one evaluates the intervention. That is, cost data should be collected prospectively, which is typically accomplished by integrating economic evaluations within efficacy and effectiveness studies. This is referred to as "piggybacking" economic evaluations alongside *prospective studies*. While the main goal of such trials is to establish the efficacy or effectiveness of the behavioral intervention, secondary goals should include an economic evaluation. Piggybacking allows the investigator to collect all relevant cost data. One important piece of cost data is the actual cost of delivering the intervention. As there is often little to no data available on the cost of delivering novel behavioral programs, this is an important endeavor. Piggybacking also has some disadvantages; it can increase respondent burden, and with small sample sizes, there may be insufficient power to analyze the cost data.

A *retrospective economic evaluation* is performed using historical data (e.g., claims data) with the goal of determining what the cost or cost-effectiveness of the treatment is compared to usual care or a relevant comparator. Retrospective economic evaluations are generally less expensive to conduct and can include large sample sizes. However, many retrospective data (e.g., health care claims or medical records) lack data on the cost of delivering behavioral interventions.

TABLE 18.2 Summary of Three Methods of Economic Evaluation

Method of Economic Evaluation	Question Intended to Answer	Description	Example(s)
Prospective study	What *is* the financial impact of the intervention, when actually measured in a defined population?	Economic measures are included within study variables and *actually measured* during the course of the study Sometimes referred to as "piggybacking" when economic measures are added to studies that are primarily being conducted to test efficacy or effectiveness	Prospective observational study; randomized clinical trial
Retrospective study	What *was* the financial impact of the intervention, based on costs and effectiveness actually observed, and considering investments made in the intervention?	An examination of health care investments made, in relation to financial savings (in other words, calculating the net financial benefit of the intervention, or return on investment) and/or in relation to the effectiveness achieved	Health care claims analysis; chart or electronic medical record review
Economic model	What *might be* the financial impact of the intervention, given reasonable assumptions about its costs and effects?	Retrospective data from credible sources are scientifically analyzed to *estimate* costs with versus without the treatment, or costs per unit of effectiveness, with versus without the treatment	Decision analysis; Markov model; budget impact model

Modeling is performed using data from multiple sources (e.g., meta-analysis, published clinical trial results, registries, and databases). Modeling is often used when all the necessary components of an economic evaluation cannot be collected in a single study, hence necessitating simulation on the basis of available literature and existing data. Examples of modeling approaches commonly used in health care include decision analyses and Markov models. These models synthesize results from multiple sources to estimate cost and cost-effectiveness. Yet, in the case of behavioral interventions, data on costs and effectiveness are still emerging, so at the present time, models may be difficult to accurately inform.

For the purposes of this chapter, we discuss modeling as an approach suited for conducting sensitivity analysis of piggybacked economic evaluations. In this case, modeling serves as a vehicle for performing sensitivity analysis on trial-based cost studies to account for potential real-world uncertainty resulting from restrictive inclusion criteria and/or inadequate sample size.

Step 3: Select the Appropriate Type of Analysis

Once the method of economic evaluation has been chosen (e.g., prospective, retrospective, or modeling), the next step is to choose an appropriate type of health economic evaluation. Here we provide a brief overview of basic health economic evaluation types and refer the reader to other sources for more detailed discussions (see e.g., *Methods for the Economic Evaluation of Health Care Programs*; Drummond, Sculpher, Torrance, O'Brien, & Stoddart, 2005; Russell, Gold, Siegel, Daniels, & Weinstein, 1996; Siegel, Weinstein, Russell, & Gold, 1996; Weinstein, Siegel, Gold, Kamlet, & Russell, 1996).

The five main types of health economic evaluations are summarized in Table 18.3 and include cost studies, cost-effectiveness analysis, cost-utility analysis, and cost-benefit analysis.

TABLE 18.3   Types of Economic Evaluation

Type of Evaluation	Measures Needed	When to Use
Cost study 1. Return on investment 2. Cost of illness 3. Budget impact	Cost	1. To determine if an intervention reduces cost in the long run 2. To calculate the total cost burden of a disease 3. Cost to a payer for implementing an intervention
Cost-effectiveness analysis	Cost and a measure of clinical effectiveness	Comparing competing interventions where effectiveness can be measured using the same clinical endpoint (e.g., cognitive score, depressive symptoms, functional status, blood pressure, hemoglobin A1c)
Cost-utility analysis	Cost and health utility	A type of cost-effectiveness analysis where effectiveness of the competing interventions can be measured using quality of life and/or quantity of life (e.g., survival)
Cost-minimization analysis	Cost	A type of cost-effectiveness analysis where the competing interventions have equivalent effectiveness; therefore, the preferred intervention is that which has lower cost
Cost-benefit analysis	Cost and benefits measured in dollars	When effectiveness can be valued in monetary terms (e.g., dollars), therefore the goal is to examine whether the treatment results in a net financial benefit or a net financial loss

Cost Study

In a *cost study*, costs are measured without consideration of the intervention's efficacy or effectiveness. There are three subtypes: (a) return on investment, (b) cost-of-illness analyses, and (c) budget impact analyses. Return-on-investment studies are generally performed to demonstrate the financial savings to a business from implementing an intervention, and results are often expressed as savings per dollar spent. These analyses often monetize the benefits of interventions. For example, a company may want to know the savings it achieved from implementing a workplace wellness program to help employees manage chronic conditions. Cost-of-illness studies are used to demonstrate the total and relative burden of a disease (e.g., the total cost of dementia). Cost-of-illness studies have also been used to demonstrate potential savings from adopting interventions. Finally, a budget impact analysis is used to determine the additional cost of implementing a new intervention from the perspective of the payer (e.g., a health plan).

Cost-Effectiveness Analysis

Although the aforementioned approaches are used, the most common type of economic evaluations in practice is *cost-effectiveness analysis*. Cost-effectiveness evaluations are used to compare competing interventions to determine the additional cost per unit of effectiveness when competing interventions are not equally effective. An example of a cost-effectiveness study would be comparing a behavioral intervention to manage problem behaviors in dementia (e.g., the Tailored Activity Program) to the use of antipsychotics for the management of behaviors in dementia. Although not always the case, more effective interventions are also generally more costly, and cost-effectiveness studies help to understand the additional cost per unit of benefit gained from implementing the more effective intervention. In cost-effectiveness studies, the benefit is measured in terms of natural units or intermediate endpoint (e.g., depression cases identified, or percentage reduction in blood pressure). Intermediate endpoints are often appealing to use because most clinical studies report results in natural units. Although intermediate endpoints are easy to use, there are several drawbacks. Foremost, in cost-effectiveness analyses, only one intermediate endpoint can be evaluated at a single time; yet, many interventions are multidimensional and impact multiple intermediate endpoints. In addition, intermediate endpoints may be surrogate in that they are a short-term proxy for effectiveness but fall short of actual effectiveness. For example, a stress reduction program aimed at reducing cardiovascular events might employ blood pressure readings as an intermediate measure of effectiveness owing to the design challenges of measuring cardiovascular events (e.g., need large sample size and a much longer observation period).

Cost-Utility Analysis

Cost-utility analyses represent a special case of a cost-effectiveness analysis where effectiveness is measured in terms of *quality-adjusted life years* (QALYs). QALYs represent years of life weighted by the quality of life in those years. QALYs have some special properties that are discussed in greater detail in the Outcome Measures section of this chapter. Cost-utility analyses have several additional advantages over cost-effectiveness analyses. Foremost, any medical intervention can be measured in terms of QALYs. Therefore, QALYs represent a standard outcome measure that can be used to compare a variety of medical treatments. Comparing across medical interventions is important for policy and budgetary planning (e.g., a dementia caregiver intervention can be evaluated against a depression intervention). In addition, QALYs combine all outcomes of an intervention into one single measure. This overcomes the challenge associated with cost-effectiveness studies in that multiple cost-effectiveness ratios may be evaluated. For these reasons, cost-utility analysis is considered the gold standard for health economic evaluations. However, QALYs are not without limitations, such as limited movement in this measure during short duration trials (i.e., those lasting <6 months), differences in the precision of QALY measurement instruments, and debates as to whether the weighting values obtained from the instrument development process accurately represent the preferences of the population being studied.

The statistic of interest in cost-effectiveness and cost-utility analyses is the incremental cost-effectiveness ratio (ICER). The ICER represents the price of an additional unit of effectiveness achieved from a new treatment compared to the standard of care. The ICER can also be graphically represented on a Cartesian plane. Figure 18.2 shows a graphical representation of the ICER. In the graph, the x-axis represents the difference in effectiveness between two interventions, and the y-axis represents the difference in cost between two interventions. The graph is divided

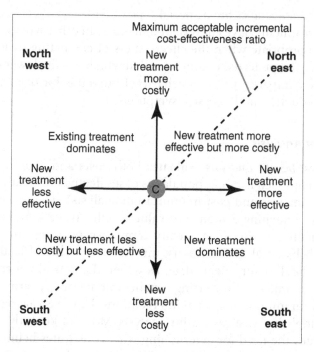

Figure 18.2 Cost-effectiveness plane reproduced from economic analysis alongside randomized controlled trials: design, conduct, analysis, and reporting.

Source: Reprinted from Petrou and Gray (2011), with permission from BMJ Publishing Group Ltd.

into four regions (Northeast, Southeast, Southwest, and Northwest). If the ICER of a new treatment compared to the standard of care falls in the Northeast region, then the new treatment is more costly but also more effective. If the ICER falls in the Southeast region, then the new treatment is less costly and more effective than the comparator. ICERs that fall in the Southeast region are said to dominate. If the ICER falls in the Southwest region, then the new treatment is less effective and less costly than the comparator. Finally, ICERs that fall in the Northwest region indicate the new treatment is less effective and more costly than the standard of care.

Importantly, cost-effectiveness does not imply cost savings. A cost-effective intervention can cost more yet be more effective than the comparator (Northeast region, Figure 18.2). However, not all ICERS that fall in the Northeast region are cost-effective. In order for an intervention to be considered cost-effective (Northeast region, Figure 18.2), it must have an ICER that is less than the decision makers' maximum acceptable ICER (i.e., is the extra cost of the benefit worth it?). The main drawback of cost-effectiveness analysis is a lack of consensus as to what is considered cost-effective or whether the extra cost of the benefit is worth it. In the United States, there is no established societal threshold for determining cost-effectiveness; however, studies typically use $50,000 to $150,000 as a threshold. This range represents the value of a QALY from a societal perspective, and decision makers from different payers or care delivery settings may value a QALY differently (Gold et al., 1996).

Cost-Minimization Analysis

Cost-minimization studies are a special type of cost-effectiveness analysis where the competing treatments have equivalent outcomes. In other words, cost-minimization analysis is appropriate when the effectiveness of competing treatments is equal. In this situation, the preferred treatment is that which has the lower cost. One example of this is the comparison of two behavioral programs for depression that result in equivalent reduction in depressive symptoms.

Cost-Benefit Analysis

Finally, a *cost-benefit analysis* evaluates both costs and effectiveness in monetary terms. This approach is not as popular as cost-effectiveness analysis or related types (cost-utility analysis and cost-minimization analysis). This is due primarily to the challenges of attaching a monetary value to effectiveness measures. Effectiveness can be difficult to value in monetary terms because there may be nonmarketed benefits to behavioral interventions; thus the true value of health or a behavioral change may be difficult to elucidate. However, theoretically, a cost-benefit analysis has several advantages. Converting benefits into monetary terms helps to aggregate outcomes from multidimensional interventions. However, aggregation of outcomes is also accomplished in a cost-utility analysis. More importantly, a cost-benefit analysis eliminates the need for determining what constitutes being cost-effective. In a cost-benefit analysis, the decision rule is simply benefits − costs. If benefits − costs > $0, then the intervention generates net financial benefits—in other words, a net savings—and should be implemented. On the other hand, if the benefits − costs

< $0, then the intervention results in net costs. In this case, rejection of the intervention may be warranted, if costs are the main factor determining its adoption. The intervention may be adopted despite its net costs if there are other factors in its favor (e.g., improved participant satisfaction or adherence compared to treatment alternatives).

Step 4: Identify and Measure Specific Costs and Outcomes

All economic evaluations incorporate cost estimates. However, the perspective (e.g., societal or public payer) of the study defines the costs that should be included in the analysis. As the perspective of the study narrows, fewer costs will be included. For example, the societal perspective is the broadest perspective and captures all costs incurred to society from implementing an intervention. This includes the cost of medical care, cost of time in receiving care, formal caregiving cost, informal caregiving cost, transportation/other nonmedical cost, and administrative costs (Gold et al., 1996). In contrast, the payer perspective is much narrower and would include only the cost of covered services, and would not take into account any of the other costs (i.e., informal care, transportation). Regardless of the perspective, it is helpful to think of costs as multidimensional. That is, costs can come from various sources (e.g., the intervention, morbidity associated with disease, and side effects from treatment), and each source can have multiple types of costs (e.g., health care resources, non–health care resources, informal care resources) (Gold et al., 1996; Weinstein & Stason, 1977). Importantly, there are several theoretical debates about the inclusion of survivor and unrelated medical costs (Braithwaite, Meltzer, King, Leslie, & Roberts, 2008; Gold et al., 1996; Hunink & Glasziou, 2001; Meltzer, 1997; Nyman, 2004; Owens, Qaseem, Chou, & Shekelle, 2011). For practical purposes, most studies do not include survivor costs.

Intervention Costs

Often, the first step in costing is to determine the *intervention costs*. For interventions that already receive reimbursement or are sold on the market, this is easy to obtain (i.e., reimbursement amount or out-of-pocket cost). However, since behavioral interventions are often not reimbursed and/or are not available on the market, defining the cost of the intervention can be more challenging.

For example, Get Busy Get Better is a novel nonpharmacological home-based intervention designed to reduce depression in older African Americans (Gitlin et al., 2012). Get Busy Get Better is not currently reimbursed by health care payers and is not available on the market. To determine the cost of implementing Get Busy Get Better, the components of the intervention were decomposed into its various parts detailed in Table 18.4. The cost-effectiveness analysis of Get Busy Get Better was planned during the original study design to enable a prospective approach, and therefore many of the necessary cost components were included in the data collection instruments so that costs could be captured prospectively. However, in many cases, cost-effectiveness is evaluated post hoc or after data collection has been completed. In such cases, it is necessary to estimate the cost of delivering the intervention retrospectively.

TABLE 18.4   Cost Framework for the Get Busy Get Better Intervention Trial

Microcost	Description	Measurement
Screening cost	Screener's time spent screening participants	Time spent screening potential participants multiplied by screener's wage rate + fringe benefit costs divided by sample size
Intervention delivery	Interventionists' time spent with subjects	Time conducting intervention multiplied by wage rate of interventionist + fringe benefit costs divided by sample size
Participant contact outside of intervention delivery	Interventionists' time spent in communication with subjects outside of designated intervention visits	Time spent in contact outside of intervention multiplied by wage rate + fringe benefit costs of interventionist divided by sample size
Travel time	Interventionists' time spent traveling to and from appointments with subjects	Wage rate + fringe benefit costs of interventionist multiplied by time spent in travel divided by sample size
Mileage reimbursement	Reimbursement for interventionists' auto expenses	Miles traveled multiplied by mileage reimbursement rate divided by sample size
Supervision cost	Supervisors' time spent supervising interventionists as well as reviewing recordings of intervention visits	Wage rate + fringe benefit costs of supervisor and interventionist multiplied by time spent supervising employee then divided by sample size
Training	Cost of training the interventionists	Wage rate + fringe benefit costs of screeners why screeners? and trainers, multiplied by time spent in training divided by sample size
Materials	Materials needed for the study included GPS devices, electronic recorders, educational pamphlets, and paper encounter forms	Cost of materials used for screening and during the intervention divided by sample size
Alerts	Time spent by MD responders to alerts	Supervisor wage rate + fringe benefit costs, multiplied by time spent dealing with adverse events divided by sample size

Note: Originally published in *BMC Geriatrics* (Gitlin et al., 2012).

Health Care and Non–Health Care Costs

In addition to the cost of the intervention, there are other important cost-related considerations. *Health care costs* correspond to health care resources used. For example, if an individual experiences an adverse event and is hospitalized, then the cost of the hospitalization represents a health care cost. *Non–health care costs* are the cost of any non–health care resource that may be impacted by the intervention. Examples of non–health care resources include transportation to and from a doctor's office, home modifications (e.g., wheel chair ramp), or an overnight stay in a hotel in order to receive care. Participant time in travel, treatment, and recovery includes time spent missing work due to care and time in treatment and recovery. There is little consensus on how to value participant time, and, in applied work, participant time in travel, treatment, and recovery is seldom included in analyses (Drummond et al., 2005). However, if these represent significant costs, then they should be included. Finally, the cost of informal care represents care delivered by friends and family. Informal caregiving can be monetized either by applying the cost of purchasing similar care on the market or by using the wage rate of the informal care provider.

Sources of Cost Data

Understanding where costs come from (e.g., the intervention, morbidity associated with disease, and side effects from treatment) and the types of costs helps to frame the collection of cost data. Cost data can be obtained in several different ways. Most clinical trials do not directly include cost endpoints nor are they powered to detect differences in costs. For clinical trials that do capture costs, statistical modeling may be needed to detect significant differences (Briggs, Sculpher, & Claxton, 2006). If a cost-effectiveness analysis is being planned alongside a clinical trial, identifying the types of costs is an important first step. In the planning phase of the study, it is often helpful to think of all of the different types of costs that can be incurred (e.g., hospitalizations). When identifying resources, it is important to include those resources that are expensive (e.g., hospitalizations) or that are not expensive but are used by a large number of people (e.g., screenings). For cost-effectiveness, cost-utility, and cost-benefit analyses, if resource utilization is the same in all groups tested, then these categories of costs can be ignored.

A limited number of instruments are available for assessing health care utilization. One such tool is the research utilization and dementia (RUD) questionnaire, which includes a comprehensive set of questions regarding the participants' use of inpatient care, outpatient medical care, home health, formal caregiving, and social services (Wimo & Winblad, 2003). RUD also captures health care utilization and work loss experienced by the informal caregiver. Another relevant tool is called the Service Use and Resources Form (SURF), which includes detailed questions on health care utilization, social services, caregiving, and medical supplies (Schneider et al., 2001). In addition to existing survey tools, an investigator can implement his or her own survey questions to capture utilization (Mahoney et al., 2003). For example, an investigator may include the following question to capture hospitalizations (health utilization): How many times were you hospitalized in the past month owing to your condition?

Converting Health Care Utilization to Health Care Costs

If health care utilization variables are used to inform cost measures, they must be monetized post hoc. Health care utilization can be evaluated in the aggregate (i.e., *gross costing*) or at a microlevel (referred to as *microcosting*). *Gross costing* applies aggregate costs accounting for all the components required to deliver the health care service. A common approach to gross costing is to apply published reimbursement rates to the utilization that was reported. For example, in a study, an individual may visit the doctor's office for an evaluation. To evaluate the cost of this visit using the gross costing approach, the cost of this service would be based on the reimbursement for the visit, using the appropriate physician billing code (e.g., current procedural terminology [CPT] code 99211, which applies to a low-level visit for evaluation and management). Gross costing can be completed in the analysis phase of the project by applying reimbursements to the health care services utilized. Determination of the appropriate billing codes and, consequently, reimbursement rates can be difficult and subjective, but is considered a reasonable proxy for health care costs where the perspective of the analysis is the health plan, health care payer, or a societal perspective. Billing codes and associated reimbursements can be obtained from published sources such as the U.S. Agency for Healthcare Research and Quality Healthcare Utilization Project Network (HCUPnet) and the *National Fee Analyzer* (2014).

Microcosting consists of disaggregating the utilization into all its parts. For example, to determine the cost of a hospitalization, an evaluation of all of the resources used during the hospitalization (e.g., the hospital bed, staff time, meals, medication, surgical equipment, diagnostic tests and procedures performed) would need to be performed. Although the microcosting method more closely approximates the true costs of delivering an intervention, this method requires a considerable amount of time and effort for the researcher, since each cost item must be captured and monetized.

Gross costing and microcosting can be used to evaluate separate components in a single analysis. For example, in the Get Busy Get Better cost-effectiveness study, microcosting was used to determine the cost of the intervention, and gross costing was used to determine health care utilization (Gitlin et al., 2012).

Discounting Future Costs

The last issue regarding costs involves timing. Costs occurring in future years (i.e., beyond the first year of analysis) should be discounted at a rate of 2% to 5% per year. This is particularly important when evaluating interventions that have differential timings related to costs. Furthermore, if it is assumed that costs will increase over time, then they should be adjusted for inflation. More detail on discounting and inflation can be found in *Methods for the Economic Analysis of Health Care Programs* (Drummond et al., 2005).

Outcome Measures

All economic evaluations require evaluating costs. However, inclusion of outcome measures depends on the type of study being conducted. Cost-effectiveness, cost-utility, and cost-benefit analyses employ a ratio examining cost per outcome achieved. A good economic evaluation will incorporate high-quality outcome (effectiveness) data. Effectiveness data can come from a variety of sources; however, not all sources are equal. Obtaining quality effectiveness data can be challenging. As with any critical analysis, effectiveness data should be carefully scrutinized on the basis of the study designs (Drummond et al., 2005). The U.S. Preventive Service

Task Force has listed randomized controlled trials as the gold standard of evidence. This is followed by observational data (e.g., cohort, case-control, and cross-sectional studies), uncontrolled experiments, descriptive series, and expert opinion (Gold et al., 1996). Prior to using data, its quality should be considered.

Cost-effectiveness studies use physical measures of effectiveness. Ideally, long-term outcomes are used (e.g., life-years gained, or deaths avoided). However, cost-effectiveness studies also use intermediate outcomes as that is what is available in the literature (e.g., depression cases identified, or percentage reduction in blood pressure). When intermediate outcomes are used, they should be linked to long-term outcomes (e.g., survival or long-term care placement). Linking intermediate outcomes to long-term outcomes is challenging and can be accomplished through additional modeling (Briggs et al., 2006; Hunink & Glasziou, 2001). For a detailed discussion of linking intermediate to long-term outcomes, please see *Methods for the Economic Evaluation of Health Care Programs* (Drummond et al., 2005).

Cost-effectiveness studies sometimes employ outcomes from health status questionnaires (e.g., the Medical Outcomes Study Short Form, 36-item; SF-36). *Health status questionnaires* are appealing to use because they capture many dimensions of health and provide a single summary score. However, many health status questionnaires arbitrarily weigh responses to provide summary scores. These health status instruments are not preference based, and summary scores are often not interpretable.

Quality-of-life weights use preference-based methods to evaluate the importance of each response levels, questions, and dimensions in a health status questionnaire. *Preference-based quality-of-life weights* produce a single summary score that represents the quality of life associated with a given health state for an individual. Preference-based quality-of-life weights are sometimes referred to as "health utility" values and have several important mathematical properties that make them ideal for statistical analysis. Foremost, quality-of-life weights are based on an interval scale and scored from 0 to 1, where 0 represents dead and 1 represents perfect health. The properties of an interval scale are important because they allow for evaluating the difference between values, and the difference between values represents an interpretable magnitude. This property does not hold for many general health status instruments.

In addition, quality-of-life weights can be used to determine QALYs, a measure which combines morbidity and mortality into a single measure of effectiveness. Mortality is measured in life years, and morbidity is measured by the quality-of-life weights. The quality-of-life weights are used to assess morbidity over the years of life. Studies that use QALYs as the outcome measure are referred to as cost-utility analyses.

Several off-the-shelf health status questionnaires exist that can be used to derive quality-of-life weights. The most common questionnaire is the EuroQol-5 Dimensions (EQ-5D). The EQ-5D consists of five domains (mobility, self-care, usual activities, pain/discomfort, and anxiety/depression) and each question has three responses (no problems, some problems, and extreme problems) (Shaw, Johnson, & Coons, 2005). Another popular health status questionnaire is the Health Utility Index Mark III (HUI-III). The HUI-III is more complex than the EQ-5D, and consists of eight domains (vision, hearing, speech, ambulation, dexterity, emotion, cognition, and pain) and five or six response levels for each dimension (Horsman,

Furlong, Feeny, & Torrance, 2003). Finally, the Quality of Well-Being Index represents another health status questionnaire that can be used to derive quality-of-life weights (Kaplan, 1998). Any of these instruments can be included as part of a prospective study design. Unfortunately, many large national surveys (in the United States) have not included these instruments as part of their design. However, there are published studies that report quality-of-life weights for common instruments for individuals with various conditions. For example, the Beaver Dam study provides an inventory of quality-of-life weights for individuals with and without various chronic conditions (Fryback et al., 1993).

Step 5: Complete the Economic Evaluation and Sensitivity Analysis

Economic evaluations are complex and often require assumptions regarding costs and effectiveness where gaps exist. Complexities are compounded by lack of guidance regarding key assumptions. *Sensitivity analysis* is used to determine whether the results are robust to differences that arise from uncertainty (i.e., conclusions do not change when different assumptions are used in the analysis) and for this reason sensitivity analyses are a fundamental component of any health economic evaluation. Examples of uncertainty include uncertainty regarding the true value of a cost or effectiveness parameter, uncertainty regarding the generalizability of effectiveness results, and uncertainty regarding the structure of the model (Hunink & Glasziou, 2001). Various methods exist for testing uncertainty; however, in cost-effectiveness analyses, hypothesis testing is normally not done because negative and positive ICERs can have two meanings. For example, in Figure 18.2, an ICER is negative when it is in Southwest or Northeast regions. Yet, the interpretation of the ICER is different in Southwest region compared to Northeast region. Furthermore, the ICER is a ratio statistic and ratios are not normally distributed.

One-way sensitivity analysis is the most common type of sensitivity analysis. In a one-way sensitivity analysis, an individual parameter is varied between a low and high value and all other parameters are held constant. In turn, this generates a low and high value for the ICER (in the case of a cost-effectiveness analysis) and indicates the relative impact of a parameter. The range can be based on a confidence interval, clinical opinion, or a best- and worst-case scenario. A *threshold analysis* is a form of a one-way sensitivity analysis. In a threshold analysis, a parameter is changed until a condition is met. For example, a parameter may be changed to find the point at which the ICER rises above $50,000 per QALY. One-way sensitivity analysis will generally understate uncertainty if there is uncertainty in multiple parameters. A *two-way sensitivity analysis* can be used to vary two parameters at the same time. Finally, a probabilistic sensitivity analysis can be used to account for multiple parameters changing simultaneously. A *probabilistic sensitivity analysis* takes into account uncertainty by assuming there is a distribution around each parameter. The distribution around parameters in turn can be used to generate a distribution of ICERs. Distributions of ICERs can be generated from bootstrapping (if parameters are based on participant-level data) or Monte Carlo simulation (if a decision analytic model is used). The distribution of ICERs can then be used to determine the probability that an ICER will be less than a given cost-effectiveness threshold.

Step 6: Communicate the Findings

Dissemination of findings is an important objective of economic evaluation, but one that requires careful planning. It can be difficult to determine which publications to target for economic evaluations. The decision as to where to publish findings is perhaps best made by considering the perspective of the study, since journals or other publications which target that perspective would be a logical priority. For example, evaluations taking the health plan perspective could be targeted toward managed care or health care benefit–focused journals. Evaluations taking a health system perspective may be best targeted toward journals that target health systems. Evaluations taking societal perspectives may be best suited for population health–focused journals, where the broad costs and effects of treatment are of interest. Newsletters, blogs, social media, and trade magazines are other potential outlets for cost research.

If pursuing publication in an academic journal, careful consideration should be given as to which journal best fits the material. The journal should either indicate that economic evaluations are of interest or have a submission category specific to health economic studies. Table 18.5 provides a short list of criteria that can be used to evaluate a journal's fit for the economic evaluation. Additionally, a number of credible checklists can serve as a guide to developing a cost-related publication (Drummond & Jefferson, 1996; Husereau et al., 2013a, 2013b; Siegel et al., 1996). Most recently, the Consolidated Health Economic Evaluation Reporting Standards (CHEERS) checklist was developed and jointly published by several journals (Husereau et al., 2013a, 2013b). Recommendations are summarized in a 24-item checklist that guides the authors on the key elements of cost papers, including the title, abstract, introduction, objective, methodological aspects (e.g., the comparators included, time horizon, cost and effectiveness measures, assumptions, and presentation of results).

While these checklists are helpful in guiding the content of health economic papers, crafting these manuscripts is very much an art. Assuming the necessary information is contained, it must be packaged well, by incorporating graphical depiction of Consolidated Standards of Reporting Trials (CONSORT) statements (for clinical trials), and assumptions must be detailed and referenced (including for the sensitivity analysis, a table specifying base case assumptions, ranges tested, distribution of the ranges tested, and source of the ranges tested). Often, the word count of health economic manuscripts exceeds journal limits, necessitating placement of selected methods and results in an appendix.

Finally, the importance of a clear and compelling discussion in economic papers cannot be underestimated. The meaning of findings must be clearly articulated

---

TABLE 18.5   Factors to Consider When Identifying Where to Submit Economic Evaluations

- Cost or cost-effectiveness is stated in the journal's scope of interest.
- Instructions for authors include a submission type that fits cost papers.
- Examination of the journal's publication history indicates a track record of publishing cost papers.
- The journal allows submitters to recommend reviewers.

on the basis of the perspective chosen for the economic evaluation. The discussion section should answer the following questions: For cost-effectiveness studies, is the treatment cost-effective on the basis of expected willingness to pay values? Should the treatment be adopted? If so, for all or for select subgroups? How do the cost findings compare to other studies? Are the limitations completely and candidly acknowledged, in particular, limitations posed by the data sources and assumptions? Finally, conclusions should be consistent with the results presented, without presumption.

CHALLENGES IN CONDUCTING ECONOMIC EVALUATIONS

There are multiple challenges in conducting economic evaluations including the time frame chosen and statistical power.

Time Horizon

The time horizon of the analysis is determined when defining the perspective, and represents how far out into the future costs and benefits should be evaluated. The appropriate time horizon depends on the clinical problem. Interventions designed for acute problems may not require long-term time horizons. In contrast, economic evaluations of interventions for chronic conditions will require longer time horizons. Importantly, the time period chosen should not produce misleading results. Several studies have shown that over short periods of time there may be differences in costs; however, over time, cost differences may disappear (Drummond et al., 2005; Gold et al., 1996). Practically, the time horizon generally corresponds to the length of time for which data are available. For example, studies using participant-level data collected in randomized trials will generally have shorter time horizons than studies using data from long-term cohort studies. However, decision analytic methods (e.g., Markov models) can be combined with participant-level data to extrapolate beyond the data (Briggs et al., 2006; Hunink & Glasziou, 2001). Extrapolating beyond the data is important when it is believed that there are important long-term outcomes associated with the intervention and there are only short-term data available.

Statistical Power

Economic evaluations conducted alongside clinical trials often suffer from inadequate statistical power. Trials are generally powered to detect a significant difference in the main efficacy or effectiveness outcome, not powered to detect a significant difference in cost. Even if the trials were powered to detect a statistically significant difference in costs, this may not translate into what a decision maker considers a meaningful difference in costs. While a trial could be powered on the basis of cost aims, there are practical challenges to doing so. The first challenge is that sample size requirements for cost aims tend to be much larger than efficacy/effectiveness aims. Reasons for this include a high-level of variation typical to health care costs owing to some participants being high utilizers of care with others being low utilizers of care. This manifests as wide standard deviations in cost measures, therefore making it harder to detect statistically significant differences between groups. In addition, the magnitude of cost differences between study groups may be small, particularly if the behavioral intervention being researched is not designed to specifically affect health care use such as hospital care, outpatient care, and/or medications prescribed. These scientific issues essentially translate to very large sample size requirements for cost studies. Obviously, sample size requirements in the thousands would require much larger study budgets than what is typically available for behavioral research, and may not be possible if the recruitment pool is limited.

To address sample size considerations, it is advisable, if possible, to power the study on the basis of the cost measure. The method used to determine sample size depends on the type of economic evaluation. One approach is to complete traditional power calculations for the cost measure, and then, if a cost effectiveness analysis, conduct a separate power calculation for the effectiveness measure (Gafni, Walter, Birch, & Sendi, 2008). Glick and colleagues as well as the International Society for Pharmacoeconomics and Outcomes Research provide useful guidance on this subject (Glick, 2011; Ramsey et al., 2005).

In many cases, it will not be feasible to power the study on the basis of cost measures. In this situation, an economic model can be developed to estimate costs and/or cost-effectiveness. In the model, initial assumptions, sometimes referred to as the "base case", can be obtained from the study. Then sensitivity analyses (previously discussed in this chapter) can be performed to test the impact of modifying base case assumptions in accordance with the ranges expected in real-world settings. These ranges can be informed by available literature, external data, variation observed in the trial, or expert opinion.

DATA COLLECTION CONSIDERATIONS

Using Self-Reported Data

When designing economic evaluations, a common question is what data sources should be used for specific cost measures. One option is to capture health care utilization via self-reported data (i.e., health care utilization is added to the data collection forms). The recall period for cost measures should ideally be the past 7 days; however, in practice this may encompass up to a month. In some instances, health care experiences which are more memorable, such as overnight hospital stays, could potentially be reported using an even longer recall (i.e., up to a year), depending on the frequency of the service used, availability of records to verify the service used, and cognitive abilities of the individual reporting the data.

Using Health Care Statements or Claims Data

One alternative to obtaining health care costs via self-report is to collect participants' health plan statements. It is standard process for both private and public (i.e., Medicare, Medicaid) health plans to mail (or e-mail) a statement of benefits following the use of inpatient and outpatient health care services. The *statement of benefits* typically states the dates of service, provider name, billing codes, allowable amount (the contracted amount that the provider will be paid), the amount paid by the plan, and the amount that must be paid by the individual who is insured (commonly referred to as "out-of-pocket costs"). The information provided on the statements can in turn be collected alongside the study; hence, it can have the potential to be a reliable source of information regarding health care costs. However, it should be noted that individuals might be prone to forget to retain these statements for study purposes, and thus, should be reminded (perhaps even provided a clearly labeled folder). In addition, such statements exclude health care services that are not reimbursed (e.g., massage therapy, acupuncture, caregiver support, over-the-counter medications, and nutritional supplements).

A third potential approach to costing health care services is to use administrative claims. Table 18.6 shows variables that are typically included in administrative inpatient (hospital), outpatient (provider visits), and pharmacy (prescription)

TABLE 18.6   Data Elements in Administrative Health Care Claims Databases

Data Element	Inpatient Hospital Claims	Outpatient Medical Claims	Pharmacy Claims
Participant name	Not usually	Not usually	Not usually
Participant identification number	X	X	X
Gender	X	X	X
Date of birth	X	X	X
Diagnoses (ICD-9 or ICD-10[a] codes for primary and other conditions)	X	X	
Date of service	X	X	X
Diagnosis-related group (DRG) reimbursement code	X		
Current procedural terminology (CPT) reimbursement code	X[b]	X	
Drug(s) dispensed		X[c]	X
Days' supply of medication			X
Quantity of medication dispensed			X
Plan name	Sometimes	Sometimes	Sometimes
Amount charged for the service ($)	X	X	
Amount ($) reimbursed for the service	Sometimes	Sometimes	X

[a]International Classification of Diseases, 9th and 10th revisions.
[b]Hospital claims include CPT codes if procedures such as diagnostic tests or surgeries are performed during the inpatient stay.
[c]Prescription medications are included only in outpatient claims databases when the drug is administered in the physician's office.

claims databases. Claims are considered a reasonable measure of the amount reimbursed by health plans for health care services, but it may be difficult to obtain these data if obtaining the data is expensive and/or if the data are "siloed" (e.g., inpatient claims may be in one data set, and outpatient and pharmacy in other data sets, each of which may have its own nuances and take considerable time and planning to properly analyze). The main limitation of using claims to complement clinical trial data is that the number of different payers represented by trial participants may pose significant practical challenges to obtaining data use agreements, with the potential that some payers may not agree to provide data.

CONCLUSION

In summary, this chapter provides a context for using economic evaluations for behavioral interventions, summarizes the approach for conducting an economic evaluation, and discusses some of the key methodological challenges in doing so. Given the complexities of conducting economic evaluations, it is best to add a health economic researcher to behavioral intervention studies early on to help identify the most appropriate perspective, cost method, and required measures. In addition, research staff will typically need training in finding the most appropriate design for the economic evaluation, as well as in data collection procedures and measures. A cost researcher should also be in routine communication with an intervention team to troubleshoot data collection challenges. In turn, the cost researcher will need to vet findings from the economic evaluation with the research team and stakeholders to craft key discussion points and messaging that can be presented to potential adopters of the interventions studied.

REFERENCES

Berger, M. L., Bingefors, K., Hedblom, E. C., Pashos, C. L., & Torrance, G.W. (2003). *Health care cost, quality, and outcomes: ISPOR book of terms*. Lawrenceville, NJ: International Society for Pharmacoeconomics and Outcomes Research.

Braithwaite, R. S., Meltzer, D. O., King, J. T., Leslie, D., & Roberts, M. S. (2008). What does the value of modern medicine say about the $50,000 per quality-adjusted life-year decision rule? *Medical Care, 46*(4), 349–356. doi:10.1097/MLR.0b013e31815c31a7

Briggs, A., Sculpher, M., & Claxton, K. (2006). *Decision modelling for health economic evaluation*. Oxford, England: Oxford University Press.

Dearing, J. W. (2009). Applying diffusion of innovation theory to intervention development. *Research on Social Work Practice, 19*(5), 503–518. doi:10.1177/1049731509335569

Dipiro, J. T., Talbert, R. L., Yee, G. C., Matzke, G. R., Wells, B. G., & Posey, L. M. (2011). *Pharmacotherapy: A pathophysiologic approach* (8th ed.). New York, NY: McGraw-Hill.

Drummond, M. F., & Jefferson, T. O. (1996). Guidelines for authors and peer reviewers of economic submissions to the BMJ. The BMJ economic evaluation working party. *British Medical Journal, 313*, 275–283.

Drummond, M. F., Sculpher, M. J., Torrance, G. W., O'Brien, B. J., & Stoddart, G. L. (2005). *Methods for the economic evaluation of health care programs* (3rd ed.). Oxford, England: Oxford University Press.

Fryback, D. G., Dasbach, E. J., Klein, R., Klein, B. E., Dorn, N., Peterson, K., & Martin, P. A. (1993). The beaver dam health outcomes study: Initial catalog of health-state quality factors. *Medical Decision Making, 13*(2), 89–102.

Gafni, A., Walter, S. D., Birch, S., & Sendi, P. (2008). An opportunity cost approach to sample size calculation in cost-effectiveness analysis. *Health Economics, 17*(1), 99–107.

Gitlin, L. N., Harris, L. F., McCoy, M., Chernett, N. L., Jutkowitz, E., & Pizzi, L. T. (2012). A community-integrated home-based depression intervention for older African Americans: Description of the beat the blues randomized trial and intervention costs. *BMC Geriatrics, 12*(4), 1–11. doi:10.1186/1471-2318-12-4

Gitlin, L. N., Jutkowitz, E., Hodgson, N., & Pizzi, L. (2010). The cost-effectiveness of a nonpharmacologic intervention for individuals with dementia and family caregivers: The tailored activity program. *American Journal of Geriatric Psychiatry, 18*(6), 510–519. doi:10.1097/JGP.0b013e3181c37d13

Gitlin, L. N., Winter, L., Vause Earland, T., Adel Herge, E., Chernett, N. L., Piersol, C. V., & Burke, J. P. (2009). The tailored activity program to reduce behavioral symptoms in individuals with dementia: Feasibility, acceptability, and replication potential. *Gerontologist, 49*(3), 428–439. doi:10.1093/geront/gnp087

Glick, H. A. (2011). Sample size and power for cost-effectiveness analysis (part 1). *PharmacoEconomics, 29*(3), 189–198. doi:10.2165/11585070-000000000-00000

Glossary. (2015). Retrieved from http://www.cigna.com/glossary

Gold, M. R., Siegel, J. E., Russell, L. B., & Weinstein, M. C. (1996). *Cost-effectiveness in health and medicine.* New York, NY: Oxford University Press.

Horsman, J., Furlong, W., Feeny, D., & Torrance, G. (2003). The health utilities index (HUI): Concepts, measurement properties and applications. *Health and Quality of Life Outcomes, 1*, 54. doi:10.1186/1477-7525-1-54

Hunink, M. G. M., & Glasziou, P. P. (2001). *Decision making in health and medicine: Integrating evidence and values.* Cambridge, England: Cambridge University Press.

Husereau, D., Drummond, M., Petrou, S., Carswell, C., Moher, D., Greenberg, D., . . . Loder, E. (2013a). Consolidated health economic evaluation reporting standards (CHEERS) statement. *PharmacoEconomics, 31*(5), 361–367. doi:10.1007/s40273-013-0032-y

Husereau, D., Drummond, M., Petrou, S., Carswell, C., Moher, D., Greenberg, D., . . . Loder, E. (2013b). Consolidated health economic analysis reporting standards (CHEERS) statement. *Value in Health, 16*(2), e1–e5. doi:10.1016/j.jval.2013.02.010

Kaplan, A. (1998). *The conduct of inquiry: Methodology for behavioral science.* Township, NJ: Transaction Publishers.

Mahoney, D. F., Jones, R. N., Coon, D. W., Mendelsohn, A. B., Gitlin, L. N., & Ory, M. (2003). The caregiver vigilance scale: Application and validation in the resources for enhancing Alzheimer's caregiver health (REACH) project. *American Journal of Alzheimer's Disease and Other Dementias, 18*(1), 39–48.

Meltzer, D. (1997). Accounting for future costs in medical cost-effectiveness analysis. *Journal of Health Economics, 16*(1), 33–64.

National fee analyzer. (2014). West Valley City, UT: Ingenix.

Neumann, P. J., Goldie, S. J., & Weinstein, M. C. (2000). Preference-based measures in economic evaluation in health care. *Annual Review of Public Health, 21*, 587–611.

Nyman, J. A. (2004). Should the consumption of survivors be included as a cost in cost-utility analysis? *Health Economics, 13*(5), 417–427.

Owens, D. K., Qaseem, A., Chou, R., & Shekelle, P. (2011). High-value, cost-conscious health care: Concepts for clinicians to evaluate the benefits, harms, and costs of medical interventions. *Annals of Internal Medicine, 154*(3), 174–180. doi:10.7326/0003-4819-154-3-201102010-00007

Petrou, S., & Gray, A. (2011). Economic evaluation alongside randomised controlled trials: Design, conduct, analysis, and reporting. *BMJ, 342,* 2.

Pizzi, L. T., & Lofland, J. H. (2006). *Economic analysis in US healthcare: Principles and applications.* Sudbury, MA: Jones and Bartlett.

Ramsey, S., Willke, R., Briggs, A., Brown, R., Buxton, M., Chawla, A., . . . Reed, S. (2005). Good research practices for cost-effectiveness analysis alongside clinical trials: The ISPOR RCT-CEA task force report. *Value in Health, 8*(5), 521–533. doi:10.1111/j. 1524-4733.2005.00045.x

Russell, L. B., Gold, M. R., Siegel, J. E., Daniels, N., & Weinstein, M. C. (1996). The role of cost-effectiveness analysis in health and medicine. *Journal of the American Medical Association, 276*(14), 1172–1177. doi:10.1001/jama.1996.03540140060028

Schneider, L. S., Tariot, P. N., Lyketsos, C. G., Dagerman, K. S., Davis, K. L., Davis, S., . . . Lieberman, J. A. (2001). National Institute of Mental Health Clinical Antipsychotic Trials of Intervention Effectiveness (CATIE): Alzheimer disease trial methodology. *American Journal of Geriatric Psychiatry, 9*(4), 346–360. doi:10.1097/00019442-200111000-00004

Shaw, J. W., Johnson, J. A., & Coons, S. J. (2005). US valuation of the EQ-5D health states: Development and testing of the D1 valuation model. *Medical Care, 43*(3), 203–220.

Siegel, J. E., Weinstein, M. C., Russell, L. B., & Gold, M. R. (1996). Recommendations for reporting cost-effectiveness analyses. *Journal of the American Medical Association, 276*(16), 1339–1341. doi:10.1001/jama.1996.03540160061034

Wang, Z., Salmon, J. W., & Walton, S. M. (2004). Cost-effectiveness analysis and the formulary decision-making process. *Journal of Managed Care Pharmacy, 10*(1), 48–59.

Weinstein, M. C., Siegel, J. E., Gold, M. R., Kamlet, M. S., & Russell, L. B. (1996). Recommendations of the panel on cost-effectiveness in health and medicine. *Journal of the American Medical Association, 276*(15), 1253–1258. doi:10.1001/jama.1996.0354015 0055031

Weinstein, M. C., & Stason, W. B. (1977). Foundations of cost effectiveness analysis for health and medical practices. *New England Journal of Medicine, 296*(13), 716–721. doi:10.1056/NEJM197703312961304

Wimo, A., & Winblad, B. (2003). Resource utilization in dementia: "RUD lite." *Brain Aging, 3*(1), 48–59.

INTO THE REAL WORLD: IMPLEMENTATION AND DISSEMINATION

In Part IV, we examine the challenges of moving proven interventions into the real-world and how the implementation experience can help inform the development of the next generation of behavioral interventions. Chapter 19 examines emerging theoretical and conceptual frameworks in implementation science that are helpful to consider even when developing and evaluating an intervention. Chapter 20 delves deeper into the implementation experience to identify lessons learned from moving proven behavioral interventions into different settings for their everyday use. This section concludes with a discussion of dissemination (Chapter 21), a phase along the pipeline involving purposively moving interventions from the randomized trial environment into community and clinical settings.

The key "take home" points of Part IV include the following:

- Knowledge of the "end game" or having a vision for one's intervention in terms of its future implementation should inform the actual development of an intervention.
- A myriad of theories and conceptual frameworks concerning implementation processes are evolving and can guide intervention development and evaluation.
- A key lesson from the implementation experience includes the importance of understanding "context" in which interventions are to be delivered and the characteristics of the target population upfront when developing the intervention.
- To effectively disseminate interventions for adoption by a setting, organization, community, or an individual, a purposeful plan of action is necessary and this should be established early on in the pipeline.

NINETEEN

THE ROLE OF IMPLEMENTATION SCIENCE IN BEHAVIORAL INTERVENTION RESEARCH

NANCY A. HODGSON AND LAURA N. GITLIN

. . . looking inside the "black box" of implementation.

Behavioral interventions hold the promise of improving life expectancy, quality of life, health outcomes, and health care for vulnerable populations including older adults, family caregivers, and those with chronic health problems. Nevertheless, the impact of proven programs ultimately depends upon their adoption and sustained implementation by an agency or practice setting, clinician, patient, consumer, participant, and/or his or her caregivers. Only a fraction of effective behavioral interventions are fully implemented and their benefits are only partially, or not at all, realized (Rahman, Surkan, Cayetano, Rwagatare, & Dickson, 2013). This has proven to be the case for every area of investigation into health and human service problems. For example, hundreds of original studies and systematic reviews concerning the effectiveness of behavioral interventions to improve the health and care of vulnerable populations exist (Ebrahim et al., 2011).

Although many effective interventions are theory-based, have been tested using randomized clinical trial methodologies, and have yielded strong evidence for their effectiveness, few, if any, have been implemented in practice settings. It has been estimated that up to 40% of patients do not receive care according to current scientific evidence, or receive potentially harmful care (Ewing, Selassie, Lopez, & McCutcheon, 1999; Grimshaw et al., 2004). In the area of dementia caregiving, there are over 200 proven behavioral interventions for family caregivers, yet less than 3% of these interventions have been submitted for translation into real practice settings and only 4,566 caregivers have participated in a translational effort representing 0.0003% of the 15+ million caregivers in the United States (Gitlin & Hodgson, 2015; Gitlin, Marx, Stanley, & Hodgson, 2015).

Given the challenges of moving successful behavioral interventions from research into practice, new approaches to designing, evaluating, and implementing programs need to be pursued (hence this book). One approach is to understand the challenges of implementation or to begin with the end in mind, a premise introduced in Chapter 1 and explored in more depth in Part IV and specifically this chapter. Implementation science—the discipline that studies the processes of translating, implementing, disseminating, and sustaining research evidence into routine care—can provide insight into, and help understand, the "endgame."

The purpose of this chapter is to provide an introduction to implementation science and specifically how understanding theoretical frameworks for implementation can inform intervention development. First, we examine in more detail the reasons why the gap between research and implementation exists. We then define implementation science and its commonly used terminology and summarize existing implementation frameworks that can be useful when developing an intervention and evaluating an intervention. Finally, we identify key steps to advance the field of behavioral intervention research in light of the contributions of implementation science. We seek to show how understanding and using implementation science and specifically its emerging frameworks may maximize the likelihood for effective translation/implementation and long-term adoption of behavioral interventions into clinical practice, social service, and/or community settings.

WHY IS PUTTING EVIDENCE INTO PRACTICE SO DIFFICULT?

One reason why putting evidence into practice is difficult is due to the type of evidence that is generated. Stakeholders, ranging from providers to patients/participants, increasingly seek high-quality evidence in decision making concerning which behavioral interventions and evidence-based strategies to use to improve health or maximize quality of life of clients or communities that are served. Yet, the way in which interventions are developed and tested do not typically address the questions that decision makers or key stakeholders pose (Tunis, Stryer, & Clancy, 2003). For example, whereas the Centers for Medicare and Medicaid Services is concerned about cost savings and reduction of harm and hospitalizations, most behavioral interventions do not examine these types of outcomes in the efficacy or even effectiveness trial phases. Thus, outcomes critical to a stakeholder may not necessarily be addressed, leaving a gap in the evidence that is produced and the evidence that would be more valued and subsequently used.

Another reason for the persistent research-to-practice gap is related to the approaches used to enhance research uptake in practice settings. Traditional approaches to enhance the uptake of research findings have focused on improving the way in which the evidence is presented. Thus, efforts have been directed at identifying, synthesizing, and then disseminating evidence in practical and accessible formats such as producing clinical practice guidelines, Cochrane reviews, and systematic and meta-analytic approaches. Professional societies and some government agencies (Agency for Health Research and Quality [AHRQ]) fund researchers to produce practice guidelines to assist clinicians, patients, and their families in making intervention decisions. Although these are helpful tools, the process by which the evidence or the intervention actually becomes adopted, operationalized, and put into practice remains a "black box" (Brownson & Jones, 2009). Implementation science has revealed that the dissemination of research findings via practice guidelines is only one potential factor influencing uptake of evidence. Other factors such as clinician experience, patient characteristics, reimbursement, and financial considerations, as well as organizational climate, have also all been shown to influence whether an intervention is adopted, implemented, and sustained.

Yet another reason for the research-to-practice gap is that it is challenging for clinicians or health and human service professionals to use evidence-based programs and guidelines. Most clinicians can barely keep pace with the rapid advances in health care knowledge. There are thousands of published papers on how to develop clinical guidelines across health care issues; yet, there are relatively few on how to actually implement such guidelines into routine practices in care settings and to do so cost-effectively (Thompson, Estabrooks, Scott-Findlay, Moore, & Wallin, 2007).

Furthermore, a consistent finding from the practice guideline literature is that the available evidence is missing important details essential for its ultimate translation into practice (Glasgow & Emmons, 2007). For example, a recent review of dementia caregiving interventions concluded that few studies provided data on the long-term effectiveness of interventions in typical care settings, the specific disease stage or etiology of people with dementia who are most likely to respond, or the outcomes of most relevance to families and decision makers (e.g., quality of life, symptom reduction, costs, reduction in hospitalizations; Maslow, 2012). This scenario is the same for most areas of health care as well; few behavioral intervention studies have examined long-term outcomes, outcomes relevant to decision makers, the cost, cost-benefit or cost-effectiveness, and who benefits most and why.

Thus, the challenge of improving clinically important outcomes such as quality of life, health, and costs of care for culturally diverse populations is, in large part, a consequence of difficulties in disseminating and implementing effective interventions. It is not, however, due to a dearth of innovative behavioral intervention research. Behavioral intervention research has yielded a multitude of proven programs. Still, the issue remains the mismatches between: the design and methodological decisions by researchers (and what funders support); and the interests, values, and needs of key stakeholders and end users; and restrictions or realities of practice and community settings. Research design and methodological decisions may initially be appropriate for the research endeavor and for developing a competitive grant proposal, but may not meet the needs and interests of potential end users and stakeholders. As a result, the "knowledge gap," also referred to as the "implementation gap" or "quality chasm," as illustrated in Figure 19.1, persists despite best efforts to date.

WHAT IS IMPLEMENTATION SCIENCE?

Implementation science holds the promise of disentangling the challenges of dissemination and implementation and helping to solve knowledge–practice gaps by

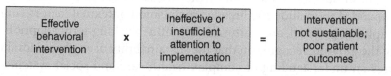

Figure 19.1 The implementation gap.

informing research decision making early on in the developmental process of an intervention (Brownson, Colditz, & Proctor, 2012). A relatively new discipline, implementation science has emerged in part in response to knowledge–practice gaps and to systematically move evidence to action. The primary goal of implementation science is to develop, test, and evaluate specific strategies for translating, implementing, and sustaining evidence into practice environments. Given that the effectiveness of embedding evidence into practice is influenced by multiple contextual factors (see Chapter 1, Figure 1.2), implementation science represents the domain of studies that examine these factors.

Numerous definitions of implementation science have been posited. The National Cancer Institute defines implementation research as "the use of strategies to adopt and integrate evidence-based health interventions and change practice patterns within specific settings" (National Institutes of Health [NIH], 2013). Dearing and Kee (2012) provide a more restrictive definition and suggest that it is "the study of what happens after adoption occurs, especially in organizational settings. Implementation is one stage (after awareness and adoption, and before sustained use) in the over-time process diffusion" (p. 56).

We use as our referent point Eccles and Mittman's (2006) approach, which defines implementation science as the scientific evaluation of methods to promote the systematic uptake of research findings or other evidence-based practices into routine practice and, hence, to improve the quality and effectiveness of health services and care. Implementation represents the transition period in which the ultimate end user becomes skilled, consistent, and committed to using a proven intervention.

Although implementation science has only recently gained wide recognition and is in an early developmental stage of its science, its roots are grounded in decades of research that have focused on the factors influencing sustained adoption of an effective innovation. In 1962, Rogers posed his breakthrough Diffusion of Innovations Theory. He suggested that an s-shaped innovation curve reflected the diffusion process in which a small minority group becomes early adopters of an innovation followed by rapid adoption by a majority of the population and then a period in which holdouts finally adopt. Diffusion of an innovation is influenced by the characteristics of the innovation itself, an adopter's level of innovativeness, and social system, adoption, and diffusion processes. Similarly, medical sociology (Burt, 1973), communication studies (Rogers & Kincaid, 1981), and marketing research (Bass, 1969) produced important findings on factors that influence the adoption of innovations. However, this early work primarily focused on individual-level factors that influenced adoption such as characteristics of adopters of an intervention versus understanding the larger context such as organizational culture in which such changes occurred.

During the past two decades, the focus has shifted from diffusion to dissemination and implementation, reflecting the need for more active processes to foster long-term or sustained adoption of the research evidence. Additionally, the focus has expanded to include the broader social and contextual factors (organizational, geographical, political, and cultural) that influence long-term adoption. This is a result of the growing recognition that the sustainability of any behavioral intervention requires an understanding of complex health care and social systems and coordinated behavioral and organizational mechanisms to invoke change. Implementation is the gateway between deciding to adopt an intervention and the routine use (or the sustainability or maintenance, Phase VII) of that intervention. It therefore requires attention to the specific factors that may influence implementation of evidence in practice settings such as the culture of care, leadership, facility size, staffing support and training, organizational innovativeness, workload, resistance to change, and available resources (money and time). These factors may vary by location, type of setting, resources, and other related factors.

The shift in focus from diffusion of knowledge to dissemination and implementation into practice has revealed the lack of a common language and standard terminology. For example, dissemination and implementation research is also variably defined and referred to as "knowledge translation" or "scaling up." The NIH defines dissemination as "the targeted distribution of information and intervention materials to a specific public health or clinical practice audience" (NIH, 2007) and is the focus of Chapter 21. Conversely, implementation is defined as "the use of strategies to adopt and integrate evidence-based health interventions and change practice patterns within specific settings" (NIH, 2007). Dissemination and implementation are closely related, but not synonymous, and represent a continuum of the translation of evidence into a practice setting. For example, whereas the publication of the Centers for Disease Control and Prevention Physical Activity Guidelines of Americans (U.S. Department of Health and Human Services, 2008) can be considered dissemination of evidence, the process by which the guidelines are subsequently adopted into routine practice is considered implementation. Table 19.1 provides brief definitions of the key terms commonly used in implementation science and can serve as a quick reference.

FRAMEWORKS IN IMPLEMENTATION SCIENCE

Along with the rapid growth and interest in implementation science has been the development of theories and models to guide this field of inquiry. There are currently over 61 diffusion and implementation models (Tabak, Khoong, Chambers, &

TABLE 19.1 Common Lexicon in Implementation Science

Term	Definition
Innovation	The object of the implementation process. It captures a broad range, including cognitive behavioral or psychoeducational interventions, a policy, a program, guidelines, educational material, and behaviors. It has multiple attributes that might influence its ability to diffuse and to be adopted. Innovation "is the implementation of a program and infrastructure that supports evidence-based practice" (Newhouse, 2007, p. 23). Innovation is defined "as a novel set of behaviours, routines and ways of working, which are directed at improving health outcomes, administrative efficiency, cost-effectiveness, or the user experience, and which are implemented by means of planned and coordinated action" (Greenhalgh et al., 2004, p. 6).

(Continued)

TABLE 19.1 Common Lexicon in Implementation Science *(Continued)*

Term	Definition
Diffusion	The passive spread of an innovation. Diffusion "refers to the spread and use of new ideas, behaviors, practices, or organizational forms, which may include unplanned or spontaneous spread, as well as dissemination" (Mendel, Meredith, Schoenbaum, Sherbourne, & Wells, 2008, p. 25).
Dissemination	The active spread of an innovation, usually through specific distribution channels and plans. Dissemination is "the targeted distribution of information on evidence-based health interventions" (Mendel et al., 2008, p. 22). Dissemination "is the purposive distribution of information and intervention materials to a specific public health or clinical practice audience. The intent is to spread information and the associated evidence-based interventions. Research on dissemination addresses how information about health promotion and care interventions is created, packaged, transmitted, and interpreted among a variety of important stakeholder groups" (NIH, 2011).
Implementation	The process of incorporating an intervention—ideally an evidence-based one—to a specific setting. Implementation "is the constellation of processes intended to get an intervention into use within an organization; it is the means by which an intervention is assimilated into an organization. Implementation is the critical gateway between an organizational decision to adopt an intervention and the routine use of that intervention; the transition period during which targeted stakeholders become increasingly skillful, consistent, and committed in their use of an intervention" (Damschroder et al., 2009, p. 3). Implementation is defined as "a specified set of activities designed to put into practice an activity or program of known dimensions. According to this definition, implementation processes are purposeful and are described in sufficient detail such that independent observers can detect the presence and strength of the 'specific set of activities' related to implementation. In addition, the activity or program being implemented is described in sufficient detail so that independent observers can detect its presence and strength" (Fixsen, Naoom, Blase, Friedman, & Wallace, 2005, p. 5).
Implementation strategy	The collection of systematically organized resources, processes, and activities that are deployed to achieve a successful implementation. "Implementation strategies can be defined as methods or techniques used to enhance the adoption, implementation, and sustainability of a clinical program or practice" (Proctor, Powell, & McMillen, 2013, p. 2).
Adoption	The active decision of an individual, an organization, or a community to incorporate an innovation.

(Continued)

TABLE 19.1   Common Lexicon in Implementation Science   (Continued)

Term	Definition
Sustainability	An attribute of an innovation that reflects its ability to be adopted, and to produce beneficial effects, for longer periods of time and after the stimulus or support from an external agency is over. Schell et al. (2013) "define sustainability capacity as the existence of structures and processes that allow a program to leverage resources to effectively implement and maintain evidence-based policies and activities" (p. 2). Scheirer (2005) enumerates three operational defintions: "(a) continuing to deliver beneficial services (outcomes) to clients (an individual level of analysis); (b) maintaining the program and/or its activities in an identifiable form, even if modified (an organizational level of analysis); and (c) maintaining the capacity of a community to deliver program activities after an initial program created a community coalition or similar structure (community level of analysis)" (p. 341).
Translation	Translation is defined as "the process of applying ideas, insights, and discoveries generated through basic scientific inquiry to the treatment or prevention of human disease" (as cited in Fang & Casadevall, 2010, p. 563). The second definition "concerns research aimed at enhancing the adoption of best practices in the community" (Stevens, 2013, p. 7).
Replication	Replication is the "process of repeating services and/or program model undertaken by someone else using the same methodology. Commonly the location and participants will be different. Replication results either support earlier findings or question the accuracy of earlier results."
Context	Horner, Blitz, and Ross (2014) "define contextual fit as the match between the strategies, procedures, or elements of an intervention and the values, needs, skills, and resources available in a setting" (p. 1). Context "is the set of circumstances or unique factors that surround a particular implementation effort. Examples of contextual factors include a provider's perception of the evidence supporting the use of a clinical reminder for obesity, local and national policies about how to integrate that reminder into a local electronic medical record, and characteristics of the individuals involved in the implementation effort. In this paper, we use the term context to connote this broad scope of circumstances and characteristics. The 'setting' includes the environmental characteristics in which implementation occurs. Most implementation theories in the literature use the term context both to refer to broad context, as described above, and also the specific setting" (Damschroder et al., 2009, p. 3).

Brownson, 2012), suggesting an increasingly robust conceptual grounding for this area of science. Theories and models are used to guide implementation studies and to explain how, why, and when a proven intervention is adopted (see Chapter 4). Table 19.2 provides a summary of 13 key and commonly used implementation theories and models that have high relevance to the conduct of behavioral intervention research. Familiarity with these models is an important first step in helping to advance the

TABLE 19.2   Implementation Science Models and Frameworks

Theory and Key Citation	Brief Description
Reach, Efficacy, Adoption, Implementation, and Maintenance (RE-AIM) Glasgow, Vogt, & Boles (1999)	Each letter of the acronym represents one construct of the theory, which collectively aims to explain the public health impact of a given intervention using individual and organizational domains. *Reach* refers to who received the intervention—in terms of numbers, demographic characteristics, biopsychosocial history, and set of risk and protective factors. *Efficacy* refers to reporting on both the positive and negative outcomes of an intervention, as well as measuring the physiologic, behavioral, and quality of life metrics of both the participant and the interventionist. *Adoption* refers to the setting(s) that carries out the intervention. *Implementation* refers to participant adherence and interventionist fidelity, both of which help determine if the intervention was delivered as intended. *Maintenance* refers to the extent to which individuals relapse (cf. attrition) and if programs continue an intervention as part of an enduring policy.
Promoting Action on Research Implementation in Health Services (PARiHS) Model Kitson et al. (2008)	To explain the complexities of implementation, the PARiHS model has three core elements—(1) evidence, (2) context, and (3) facilitation—that all have subelements. *Evidence* includes research (e.g., is there sufficient evidence?), clinical experience (e.g., does experience fit the data?), patient experience (e.g., are we gathering patient opinions?), and information from local context (e.g., are the key messages tailored to the environment?). *Context* includes receptive contact (e.g., are professional networks and human resources in place?), culture (e.g., does the organization value collaborative partnerships?), leadership (e.g., are the roles clear?), and evaluation (will data be collected that will routinely improve and change practice?). *Facilitation* includes the skills, knowledge, and expertise of the facilitator(s) designated to carry out the implementation goal.
PRECEDE-PROCEED Model Green & Krueter (1999)	PRECEDE-PROCEED is a heuristic framework that can help guide the development of an intervention. Importantly, the target population is included in the planning processes, as an underlying tenet is that health behavior change is voluntary and interventions are most effective if the community context is considered. It is divided into two components: (1) PRECEDE (an "educational diagnosis" or description of the problem) and (2) PROCEED (an "ecological diagnosis" or consideration of the environmental factors necessary for health change). Each arm of the model contains sub elements: PRECEDE (*Predisposing, Reinforcing, and Enabling Constructs in Educational Diagnosis and Evaluation*) and PROCEED (*Policy, Regulatory, and Organizational Constructs in Educational and Environmental Development*).

(Continued)

TABLE 19.2 Implementation Science Models and Frameworks *(Continued)*	
Theory and Key Citation	**Brief Description**
CFIR (Consolidated Framework for Implementation Research) Damschroder et al. (2009)	CFIR was the result of a comprehensive review (Damschroder et al., 2009) that aimed at consolidating various implementation frameworks. This model consists of five themes: intervention characteristics, outer setting, inner setting, characteristics of the individuals, and process. Each theme is also composed of additional constructs related to the theme. For example, the intervention characteristics theme contains the intervention source, evidence strength, relative advantage, adaptability, trialability, complexity, design quality, and cost.
Technology Acceptance Model (TAM) Legris, Ingham, & Collerette (2003)	TAM is a model that aims to explain why individuals use (or reject) information technology. The core tenet is that external variables impact individual beliefs and intentions through two core-mediating constructs: perceived usefulness and perceived ease of use. *Perceived usefulness* includes the perception that a given technology increases productivity, performance, and effectiveness. *Perceived ease of use* includes the perception that learning to operate the technology is easy and that it is learnable and flexible.
Normalization Process Theory (NPT) May (2006); May et al. (2007, 2009); May & Finch (2009)	A theory that aims to explain the sociological mechanisms that lead to (or inhibit) the implementation, embedding, and integration of an intervention or policy. The most recent iteration of the theory (May & Finch, 2009) has four core constructs: coherence, cognitive participation, collective action, and reflexive monitoring. *Coherence* asks, "what is the work?" *Cognitive participation* asks, "who does the work?" *Collective action* asks, "how does the work get done?" *Reflexive monitoring* asks, "how is the work understood?"
General Theory of Implementation May (2013)	Building on NPT, the General Theory of Implementation has four interactive core constructs: potential, capacity, capability, and contribution. *Potential* includes individual intentions and collective commitment. *Capacity* includes material resources, social roles, social norms, and cognitive resources. *Capability* includes workability and integration. *Contribution* includes coherence, cognitive participation, collective action, and reflexive monitoring.
Theoretical Domains Framework (TDF) Michie et al. (2005); Cane, O'Connor, & Michie (2012); French et al. (2012)	In response to the large body of theories seeking to explain behavior change, the TDF was created to provide an organizational heuristic of the extant theories. Overall, 33 theories encompassing a total of 128 core constructs were distilled into 12 theoretical domains that explain behavior change and inform implementation efforts. The 12 domains identified include (1) knowledge; (2) skills; (3) social/professional role identify; (4) belief about capabilities; (5) beliefs about consequences; (6) motivation and goals; (7) memory, attention, and decision processes; (8) environmental context and resources; (9) social influences; (10) emotion regulation; (11) behavior regulation; and (12) nature of the behavior.

(Continued)

TABLE 19.2   Implementation Science Models and Frameworks *(Continued)*

Theory and Key Citation	Brief Description
Diffusion of Innovations Theory Rogers (2003); Greenhalgh, Robert, Macfarlane, Bate, & Kyriakidou (2004)	Proposes that four elements account for an idea being spread throughout a system or a society and among members of each group: (1) innovation (i.e., a novel idea); (2) communication channels (i.e., transmitting messages to one another); (3) time (i.e., how fast a given system or society adopts the new practice); and (4) social system (i.e., the stakeholders).
Social Constructivist Theory Thomas, Menon, Boruff, Rodriguez, & Ahmed (2014)	A sociological theory that proposes that knowledge is created ("meaning-making") in the context of other human beings—that is, it is a collectivist, rather than individualist, effort.
Replicating Effective Programs Kilbourne, Neumann, Pincus, Bauer, & Stall (2007)	Four steps: (1) *preconditions* (identify the need, identify an effective intervention, identify barriers, draft a package for training and assessment purposes); (2) *preimplementation* (orient community groups in core elements, customize delivery, plan logistics, train staff, provide technical assistance); (3) *implementation* (continue partnership with community organization, provide booster trainings, perform process evaluations, provide feedback and refinement of intervention package/training); and (4) *maintenance and evolution* (make organizational and financial changes to sustain intervention, prepare package for national dissemination, recustomize delivery as needed).
Translating Evidence into Practice (TRIP) Model Pronovost, Berenholtz, & Needham (2008)	Four components: (1) summarize the evidence; (2) identify barriers to implementation at the local level; (3) measure performance; and (4) ensure all patients receive the interventions. The fourth component is further broken down into the "four Es": engage (explain why the interventions are important), educate (provide evidence as to the interventions' efficacy), execute (design a toolkit), and evaluate (provide ongoing assessment for performance measures).
PRISM (Practical, Robust Implementation and Sustainability Model) Feldstein & Glasgow (2008)	PRISM establishes a basic and practical approach to define the elements that influence a successful implementation. This model states that the factors are the program (or intervention), which has an organizational and a patient perspective, the recipients (with also an organizational and a patient perspective), the external environment, and the implementation and sustainability infrastructure.

development of an intervention when the ultimate goal is its implementation, dissemination, and wide-scale adoption in a real-world setting. Understanding downstream (e.g., implementation) considerations, as expressed in these theories/models upfront in the developmental process for an intervention, may ultimately positively impact the implementation potential of an intervention once it is proven to be effective. Common frameworks that have been used to inform behavioral intervention research include but are not limited to RE-AIM, PRECEDE-PROCEED, PARiHS, and Rogers's Diffusion of Innovations Theory (see Table 19.2 for others).

Normalization Process Theory

A recent approach, Normalization Process Theory (NPT) (Murray et al., 2010), can be helpful in developing an intervention and purposively involving clinical or community teams or when using a pragmatic or embedded trial design. NPT identifies four factors to evaluate and those which indicate whether an intervention has potential to ultimately be implemented and normalized in a practice setting. Its first factor "coherence" refers to "sense-making" or whether an intervention is easy to describe, distinguishable from other interventions, fits with organization goals, and its benefits clearly understood. Evaluating coherence in the developmental phase of an intervention can provide immediate feedback to the investigative team as to how the intervention is perceived, how best to describe the intervention, and/or how to modify its delivery characteristics to enhance its acceptability.

The second NPT indicator is "cognitive participation," which refers to whether users of a program consider the intervention as a good idea and has the potential of making a positive difference. This serves as an indicator of whether stakeholders and interventionists will be invested in the program and motivated to make it work. If the intervention is perceived as too time-consuming and not particularly beneficial or not providing added value to a practice, then commitment to it will be low and implementation and sustainability threatened.

The third NPT factor is "collective work," or how the program will affect the work of agency or clinical staff, whether the program promotes or impedes their work, whether extensive training is required, and whether the program is compatible with existing work flow. As most interventions will require a practice setting to change its practices and/or work flow, understanding the demands of an intervention would be important to identify and articulate upfront in developmental and testing phases. For example, changes might need to include the establishment of screening, referral, and follow-up mechanisms, supervision, and adherence to fidelity of the intervention.

The fourth consideration is "reflexive monitoring" or how users of the program will perceive it: what kind of supports will be needed for its integration into a context and/or what booster trainings may be needed.

Evaluating an intervention along these dimensions early on when developing the delivery characteristics or evaluating its outcomes can help inform how best to tweak the design of the intervention, and the type of training and supportive structures that will be necessary for the successful integration of the program in a practice setting.

Table 19.2 lists only a few of the many available frameworks in implementation science that can provide guidance in developing behavioral intervention studies that have as the goal to facilitate and maximize translation into practice. It is essential to have some familiarity with the elements of these models since one model may not encompass the entire process and impact of implementation or be relevant across all interventions. For example, the PARiHS model does not specify how implementation should be planned, organized, or scheduled (Helfrich et al., 2010). Rogers's (1962) Diffusions of Innovations model emphasizes collaborative learning across an organization, but does not specify the process for accomplishing this aim. Therefore, it may be necessary to draw upon different but complementary theories or models or to select elements from relevant models to guide an implementation project.

THE BLACK BOX OF IMPLEMENTATION

Although there are a sufficient range and number of implementation theories/models for guiding implementation of behavioral intervention research, there is a lack of measures to evaluate readiness of stakeholders, the process of uptake, and actual implementation of an intervention. Two areas, in particular, warrant measurement development, organizational readiness, and contextual fit. As features of an organization (team, department, organization) affect adoption of an evidence-based program, gauging the level of readiness could help guide what organizations to target first and how to better prepare and support a setting for changing their practices (Shea, Jacobs, Esserman, Bruce, & Weiner, 2014). Similarly, the successful implementation of a proven intervention depends upon the fit with the context (Horner et al., 2014). A measure of "contextual fit" would provide critical information even early on in the development of an intervention as to its potential for implementation. This is discussed in more depth in Chapter 20.

As a consequence of the lack of adequate measures, there is still a "black box" regarding the mechanisms that may influence intervention "uptake" (e.g., the optimal timing of dose and duration of the intervention) and there remains a critical need to develop and test measures of implementation outcomes (e.g., barriers assessment, knowledge use, impact, sustainability). Nevertheless, even in the initial steps in designing an intervention, it is important to consider the ultimate end user(s) and to document the contextual factors and the characteristics of an organization that could use the intervention in order to boost the potential for adoption of an intervention, if proven to be effective.

A formative evaluation that is designed to elicit the organizational culture and the perceptions of the end user is an important initial step that can be accomplished early on in the developmental phase of the intervention pipeline. Intervention projects targeted at evaluating obstacles to change using one or more of the theories of implementation may be more effective than intervention efforts that do not follow this approach. If resources permit, early examination of processes and outcomes at every level (e.g., targeted person as well as practitioner and organizational level) could be helpful. Data could be used to answer questions such as: What aspects of the intervention were successful in promoting improvements in practice, in what environments, and why? and What are the barriers to overcome? Process information collected early on using mixed methodologies (see Chapter 11) on how the intervention has effected or changed the standard of practice and whether this is associated with measurably improved patient outcomes could potentially shorten the elongated pipeline of bringing interventions to practice.

Since most behavioral interventions are complex and multicomponent, it is essential to identify the delivery characteristics (see Chapter 5) of the intervention that are absolutely necessary for treatment benefits to occur and those elements that are potentially modifiable (e.g., the scheduling of treatment sessions, or whether a session can be shorter or longer).

Consideration of the cost and potential cost savings of behavioral interventions is another important requisite in intervention development (see Chapter 18). What can be scalable or generalized, and at what cost? Rigorous evaluations of behavioral interventions increasingly need to include measurement of costs to argue that insurance programs should cover such interventions and thus are able to be implemented on a large scale.

CONCLUSION

In summary, the past 50 years of intervention research have yielded important findings that have yet to be fully disseminated and implemented. There are numerous behavioral interventions for which we have sufficient existing evidence to warrant "scaling up" through the application of rigorous dissemination and implementation processes. At the same time, there are many available frameworks in implementation science that can provide guidance in designing behavioral interventions to facilitate and maximize translation of these programs into practice settings.

Dissemination and implementation of evidence should be critical considerations in the early stages of behavioral intervention design and not simply an afterthought at the completion of the testing phase of an intervention study. It is essential that behavioral intervention researchers obtain both expertise in and partner with dissemination and implementation science investigators to apply relevant theories and methods to guide intervention development. Pragmatic efficacy and effectiveness trials (see Chapter 2) are examples of intervention study designs that may optimize dissemination and implementation potentiality by building in research questions about stakeholder values that may facilitate translation of evidence into a designated practice environment more efficiently and effectively.

With the emergence of a science for implementation, funding agencies and grant reviewers are beginning to explicitly and implicitly expect and/or require that proposals consider the implementation potential of proposed interventions. This represents a paradigm shift in the way in which funders are considering behavioral intervention research.

Implementation science will help to create generalizable knowledge that can be applied across care settings to answer central questions of importance for behavioral intervention researchers. This line of inquiry will yield understandings of why established behavioral interventions may lose their effectiveness over time or when transferred to other settings, why well-tested behavioral interventions may exhibit unintended effects when introduced in new settings, or how an intervention can maximize cost-effectiveness with strategies for effective adoption. The challenges of implementation should be of concern and significance to behavioral intervention researchers.

The emergence of implementation science calls for researchers and practitioners to carefully examine how to refine current practices in developing behavioral interventions and to design new and innovative strategies for their advancement that reflects a better understanding of contextual factors that support or hinder eventual program adoption.

At a minimum, behavioral interventions have to be designed and tested "with the end in mind," and to do so, implementation theories and models may be helpful to consider. Additionally, the inclusion of stakeholder groups early on to ensure appropriate selection of process and outcome variables may help to advance implementation. Interventions then need to be pilot tested and retested recognizing that implementation efforts require: detailed assessment of contextual characteristics of the settings in which the targeted populations are served; evaluation of the changes in primary and secondary outcomes that are of clinical importance to stakeholders; and a consideration of implementation, maintenance, and cost at both the individual and organizational levels. Implementation science provides working tools in the form of theories, conceptual frameworks, and empirical evidence that can assist in the thinking and action processes of behavioral intervention researchers.

REFERENCES

Brownson, R., Colditz, G., & Proctor, E. (Eds.) (2012). Dissemination and implementation research in health: Translating science to practice, New York, NY: Oxford University Press.

Bass, F. M. (1969). A new product growth model for consumer durables. *Management Science, 13*(5), 215–227.

Brownson, R. C., & Jones, E. (2009). Bridging the gap: Translating research into policy and practice. *Preventive Medicine, 49*(4), 313–315.

Burt, R. S. (1973). The differential impact of social integration on participation in the diffusion of innovations. *Social Science Research, 2*(2), 125–144.

Cane, J., O'Connor, D., & Michie, S. (2012). Validation of the theoretical domains framework for use in behavior change and implementation research. *Implementation Science, 7*(37), 1–17.

Damschroder, L. J., Aron, D. C., Keith, R. E., Kirsh, S. R., Alexander, J. A., & Lowery, J. C. (2009). Fostering implementation of health services research findings into practice: A consolidated framework for advancing implementation science. *Implementation Science, 4*(50), 1–15.

Dearing, J. W., & Kee, K. F. (2012). Historical roots of dissemination and implementation science. In R. Brownson, G. Colditz, & E. Proctor (Eds.), *Dissemination and implementation research in health: Translating science to practice* (pp. 55–71). New York, NY: Oxford University Press.

Ebrahim, S., Taylor, F., Ward, K., Beswick, A., Burke, M., & Davey Smith, G. (2011). Multiple risk factor interventions for primary prevention of coronary heart disease. *Cochrane Database of Systematic Reviews,* (1), CD001561. doi:10.1002/14651858.CD001561.pub3

Eccles, M. P., & Mittman, B. S. (2006). Welcome to implementation science. *Implementation Science, 1*(1), 1–3.

Ewing, G. B., Selassie, A. W., Lopez, C. H., & McCutcheon, E. P. (1999). Self-report of delivery of clinical preventive services by US physicians: Comparing specialty, gender, age, setting of practice, and area of practice. *American Journal of Preventive Medicine, 17*(1), 62–72.

Fang, F. C., & Casadevall, A. (2010). Lost in translation—Basic science in the era of translational research. *Infection and Immunity, 78*(2), 563–566.

Feldstein, A. C., & Glasgow, R. E. (2008). A practical, robust implementation and sustainability model (PRISM). *Joint Commission Journal on Quality and Patient Safety, 34*(4), 228–243.

Fixsen, D. L., Naoom, S. F., Blase, K. A., Friedman, R. M., & Wallace, F. (2005). *Implementation research: A synthesis of the literature* (FMHI Publication No. 231). Tampa, FL: University of South Florida, Louis de la Parte Florida Mental Health Institute, National Implementation Research Network.

French, S. D., Green, S. E., O'Connor, D. A., McKenzie, J. E., Francis, J. J., Michie, S., . . . Grimshaw, J. M. (2012). Developing theory-informed behavior change interventions to implement evidence into practice: A systematic approach using the Theoretical Domains Framework. *Implementation Science, 7*(38), 1–8.

Gitlin, L. N., & Hodgson, N. (2015). Caregivers as therapeutic agents in dementia care: The evidence-base for interventions supporting their role. In J. Gaugler & R. Kane (Eds.), *Family caregiving in the new normal.* London, England: Elsevier.

Gitlin, L. N., Marx, K., Stanley, I., & Hodgson, N. (2015).Translating evidence-based dementia caregiving interventions into practice: State-of-the-science and next steps. *Gerontologist, 55*(2), 210–226. doi:10.1093/geront/gnu123

Glasgow, R. E., & Emmons, K. M. (2007). How can we increase translation of research into practice? Types of evidence needed. *Annual Reviews of Public Health, 28,* 413–433.

Glasgow, R. E., Vogt, T. M., & Boles, S. M. (1999). Evaluating the public health impact of health promotion interventions: The RE-AIM framework. *American Journal of Public Health, 89,* 1322–1327.

Green, L. W., & Kreuter, M. W. (1999). *Health promotion planning: An educational and ecological approach.* Mountain View, CA: Mayfield Publishing Company.

Greenhalgh, T., Robert, G., Bate, P., Kyriakidou, O., Macfarlane, F., & Peacock, R. (2004). *How to spread good ideas: A systematic review of the literature on diffusion, dissemination and sustainability of innovations in health service delivery and organization.* Report for the National Co-ordinating Centre for NHS Service Delivery and Organisation. R & D 1-424. Retrieved from http://nets.nihr.ac.uk/__data/assets/pdf_file/0017/64340/FR-08-1201-038.pdf

Greenhalgh, T., Robert, G., Macfarlane, F., Bate, P., & Kyriakidou, O. (2004). Diffusion of innovations in service organizations: Systematic review and recommendations. *Milbank Quarterly, 82,* 581–629.

Grimshaw, J. M., Thomas, R. E., MacLennan, G., Fraser, C., Ramsay, C. R., Vale, L., . . . Donaldson, C. (2004). Effectiveness and efficiency of guideline dissemination and implementation strategies. *Health Technology Assessment, 8*(6), 1–72.

Helfrich, C. D., Damschroder, L. J., Hagedorn, H. J., Daggett, G. S., Sahay, A., Ritchie, M., . . . Stetler, C. B. (2010). A critical synthesis of literature on the promoting action on research implementation in health services (PARIHS) framework. *Implementation Science, 5*(1), 82.

Horner, R. H., Blitz, C., & Ross, S. W. (2014). *The importance of contextual fit when implementing evidence-based interventions.* ASPE Issue Brief. Retrieved from http://aspe.hhs .gov/hsp/14/iww/ib_contextual.pdf

Kilbourne, A. M., Neumann, M. S., Pincus, H. A., Bauer, M. S., & Stall, R. (2007). Implementing evidence-based interventions in health care: Application of the replicating effective programs framework. *Implementation Science, 2*(42), 1–10.

Kitson, A. L., Rycroft-Malone, J., Harvey, G., McCormack, B., Seers, K., & Titchen, A. (2008). Evaluating the successful implementation of evidence into practice using the PARiHS framework: Theoretical and practical challenges. *Implementation Science, 3*(1), 1–12.

Legris, P., Ingham, J., & Collerette, P. (2003). Why do people use information technology? A critical review of the technology acceptance model. *Information & Management, 40*(3), 191–204.

Maslow, K. (2012). *Translating innovation to impact: Evidence-based interventions to support people with Alzheimer's disease and their caregivers at home and in the community. A white paper.* Retrieved from http://www.aoa.gov/AoA_Programs/HPW/Alz_Grants/docs/ TranslatingInnovationtoImpactAlzheimersDisease.pdf

May, C. (2006). A rational model for assessing and evaluating complex interventions in health care. *BMC Health Services Research, 6*(86), 1–11.

May, C. (2013). Towards a general theory of implementation. *Implementation Science, 8*(18), 1–14.

May, C., & Finch, T. (2009). Implementing, embedding, and integrating practices: An outline of normalization process theory. *Sociology, 43,* 535–554.

May, C., Finch, T., Mair, F., Ballini, L., Dowrick, C., Eccles, M., . . . Heaven, B. (2007). Understanding the implementation of complex interventions in health care: The normalization process model. *BMC Health Services Research, 7*(148), 1–7.

May, C. R., Mair, F., Finch, T., MacFarlane, A., Dowrick, C., Treweek, S., . . . Montori, V. M. (2009). Development of a theory of implementation and integration: Normalization Process Theory. *Implementation Science, 4*(29), 1–9.

Mendel, P., Meredith, L. S., Schoenbaum, M., Sherbourne, C. D., & Wells, K. B. (2008). Interventions in organizational and community context: A framework for building evidence on dissemination and implementation in health services research. *Administration and Policy in Mental Health and Mental Health Services Research, 35*(1/2), 21–37.

Michie, S., Johnston, M., Abraham, C., Lawton, R., Parker, D., & Walker, A. (2005). Making psychological theory useful for implementing evidence-based practice: A consensus approach. *Quality and Safety in Health Care, 14,* 26–33.

Murray, E., Treweek, S., Pope, C., MacFarlane, A., Ballini, L., Dowrick, C., . . . May, C. (2010). Normalisation process theory: A framework for developing, evaluating and implementing complex interventions. *BMC Medicine, 8*(63), 1–11.

National Institutes of Health. (2007). NIH Conference on *Building the science of dissemination and implementation in the service of public health.* Retrieved from www.obssr.od.nih.gov/di2007/about.html

National Institutes of Health. (2011). 4th Annual NIH Conference on the *Science of dissemination and implementation: Policy and practice.* Retrieved from http://obssr.od.nih.gov/scientific_areas/translation/dissemination_and_implementation/DI2011/abstracts.html

National Institutes of Health. (2013). *Dissemination and implementation research in health* (PAR 10-038). Retrieved from http://grants.nih.gov/grants/guide/pa-files/PAR-10-038.html

Newhouse, R. P. (2007). Creating infrastructure supportive of evidence-based nursing practice: Leadership strategies. *Worldviews on Evidence-Based Nursing, 4*(1), 21–29.

Proctor, E. K., Powell, B. J., & McMillen, J. C. (2013). Implementation strategies: Recommendations for specifying and reporting. *Implementation Science, 8*(39), 1–11.

Pronovost, P., Berenholtz, S., & Needham, D. (2008). Translating evidence into practice: A model for large-scale knowledge translation. *British Medical Journal, 337,* 963–965.

Rahman, A., Surkan, P. J., Cayetano, C. E., Rwagatare, P., & Dickson, K. E. (2013). Grand challenges: Integrating maternal mental health into maternal and child health programmes. *PLoS Medicine, 10*(5), 1–7. doi:10.1371/journal.pmed.1001442

Rogers, E. M. (1962). *Diffusion of innovations.* New York, NY: The Free Press.

Rogers, E. M. (2003). *Diffusion of innovations* (5th ed.). New York, NY: The Free Press.

Rogers, E. M., & Kincaid, D. L. (1981). *Communication networks: Toward a new paradigm for research.* New York, NY: The Free Press.

Scheirer, M. A. (2005). Is sustainability possible? A review and commentary on empirical studies of program sustainability. *American Journal of Evaluation, 26*(3), 320–347.

Schell, S. F., Luke, D. A., Schooley, M. W., Elliott, M. B., Herbers, S. H., Mueller, N. B., & Bunger, A. C. (2013). Public health program capacity for sustainability: A new framework. *Implementation Science, 8*(15), 1–9.

Shea, C. M., Jacobs, S. R., Esserman, D. A., Bruce, K., & Weiner, B. J. (2014). Organizational readiness for implementing change: A psychometric assessment of a new measure. *Implementation Science, 9:*7. doi:10.1186/1748-5908-9-7

Stevens, K. (2013). The impact of evidence-based practice in nursing and the next big ideas. *OJIN: The Online Journal of Issues in Nursing, 18*(2), 1–13.

Tabak, R. G., Khoong, E. C., Chambers, D. A., & Brownson, R. C. (2012). Bridging research and practice: Models for dissemination and implementation research. *American Journal of Preventive Medicine, 43*(3), 337–350.

Thomas, A., Menon, A., Boruff, J., Rodriguez, A. M., & Ahmed, S. (2014). Applications of social constructivist learning theories in knowledge translation for healthcare professionals: A scoping review. *Implementation Science, 9*(54), 1–20.

Thompson, D. S., Estabrooks, C. A., Scott-Findlay, S., Moore, K., & Wallin, L. (2007). Interventions aimed at increasing research use in nursing: A systematic review. *Implementation Science, 2*(15), 1–16.

Tunis, S. R., Stryer, D. B., & Clancy, C. M. (2003). Practical clinical trials: Increasing the value of clinical research for decision making in clinical and health policy. *JAMA, 290*(12), 1624–1632.

U.S. Department of Health and Human Services. (2008). *Physical Activity Guidelines for Americans.* Washington, DC: Author. Retrieved from http://www.health.gov/PAGuidelines/pdf/paguide.pdf

TWENTY

LESSONS LEARNED FROM IMPLEMENTING PROVEN INTERVENTIONS INTO REAL-WORLD CONTEXTS

LAURA N. GITLIN AND BRUCE LEFF

> . . . *start with the end in mind.*
> —Covey (1989)

Many behavioral interventions are designed and evaluated in a context external to, or independent of, a health or social service system or community agency. As such, a translational phase (see Chapter 2) is often required in which adaptations to the proven intervention are needed to optimize delivery in a particular setting and to facilitate implementation, dissemination, and adoption on a broad scale.

In this chapter, we examine some of the key challenges that are encountered when moving a proven intervention from its developmental and evaluative phases to its translation and implementation in real-world settings. We draw upon three of our own interventions that vary in their purposes, delivery characteristics, and levels of evidence and contexts for delivery to illustrate key lessons learned from the implementation experience.

Building on the discussion of implementation science constructs in Chapter 19, we start with the primary lesson learned—the importance of understanding "context" for implementation of interventions. We then consider how characteristics of interventionists can impact implementation potential. Finally, we discuss the need to derive the value alignment or the "just right fit" between the benefits of an intervention and stakeholder interests. Drawing upon our case examples, we highlight the relative strengths and limitations of the delivery characteristics of these exemplar interventions as related to their implementation potential in different real-world contexts.

Reflecting upon the lessons learned from attempts to move interventions from their test phase to real-world contexts can inform the next generation of intervention development work. Specifically, our purpose is to explicitly link intervention delivery characteristics and approaches to their evaluation, to the unique challenges encountered when implementing these interventions in practice and community settings. Our goal is to shed light on the trade-offs in decision making that may need to occur early on when designing delivery characteristics of an intervention (discussed in Chapter 5) and when choosing evaluative approaches (see Part III) to prove intervention effectiveness. Familiarity with potential future implementation challenges can enable investigators/teams to proceed more knowledgeably in the construction of interventions and evaluation approaches.

THE CHALLENGE OF CONTEXT

A key challenge when introducing a new intervention into a setting concerns the characteristics of that setting, which may or may not support the adoption of the intervention (Burke & Gitlin, 2012; Gitlin, 2013). As previous research has shown, the fit between an intervention (e.g., its delivery characteristics, purpose, targeted population) and the values and goals of a practice or social service setting is associated with the dissemination potential of the intervention (discussed in Chapter 21) and whether the intervention is adopted; the better or stronger the fit, the greater the potential for adoption to occur and for the new intervention to be sustained (Fixsen, Naoom, Blase, Friedman, & Wallace, 2005; Horner & Blitz, 2014). Unfortunately, most researchers lack a clear understanding of the "contexts" in which their interventions may eventually be implemented, the aspects of contexts that may impact implementation, and the degree of "fit" between their interventions and these contexts (Fixsen et al. 2005; Wilson, Brady, & Lesesne, 2011).

Although there is no doubt as to the importance of "context," the term does not have a clear conceptual and operational definition or measurement approach—what do we mean by "context" and how should we measure it? Undoubtedly, context should be considered as a multifaceted construct. Many aspects of context have been identified as potentially influencing the implementation, dissemination, and wide-scale adoption of proven interventions (Greenhalgh, 2005). These include but are not limited to contextual characteristics such as staffing, resources, payment structures, beliefs and long-held routines, habits or practices, perceptions of benefits, and so forth (Jacobs, Weiner, & Bunger, 2014). Central to the development of a conceptual and measurement approach to context are the questions: Are there specific aspects of contexts that are more important than others to understand, identify, and measure? Are contextual considerations global and do they transcend any type of intervention? Are contextual factors of importance intervention-specific? These are important questions for which more research and measurement development are warranted and very much needed.

One approach to understanding context is reflected in the construct of "implementation climate," which refers to the perceptions and expectations of an organization concerning the rewards and supports that might be derived from a new intervention. As measurement of this construct is in development, it is not clear if one factor, such as support, is more important than another factor, say rewards, for the implementation of an intervention by an organization (Jacobs et al., 2014). A related question is whether perceptions or behaviors of an organization or both drive the "climate" of implementation.

Fixsen and colleagues (2005) have tackled this issue by identifying six core components of interventions that enhance their implementation potential. These include having a clear description of the who, what, when, and where of the intervention; a practical measure of fidelity; a fully operationalized intervention (e.g., what to say and when); and an intervention that has been field tested and revised and which can be contextualized or fit a system of care or organization and be perceived as effective (e.g., it is worth the effort). Despite the identification of these core components, the construct of "context" itself is not fully articulated nor its measurement properties discerned. An intervention that possesses these core components also enhances its dissemination potential for distribution and wide-scale adoption by organizations, as discussed in Chapter 21.

Other approaches for understanding context are embedded in more than 60 implementation theories or conceptual frameworks that have been developed to examine implementation processes (see Chapter 19 for a discussion of select theories). Although critical for guiding translation/implementation efforts, most of these conceptual frameworks do not provide an explicit operational framework for, nor clearly delineate, this notion of context.

Contextual Fit

An emerging and important construct is that of "contextual fit." This refers to "the match between the strategies, procedures, or elements of an intervention and the values, needs, skills, and resources available in a setting" (Horner & Ross, 2014, p. 1). On the basis of a systematic review of implementation studies, their outcomes, and lessons learned, Horner and Ross (2014) suggest that there are eight essential elements that need to be considered to establish whether there is an adequate fit between an intervention and a setting (e.g., an adopter, social service agency, community organization, clinical practice) for its delivery. These include (a) "need" or extent to which the intervention addresses a perceived need by stakeholders of a setting; (b) "precision" or the extent to which the features of the intervention and delivery approach for an intervention are clear and replicable; (c) the "evidence base" or whether the intervention has demonstrated efficacy/effectiveness for a targeted population; (d) "efficiency" or the extent to which the intervention is practical; (e) "skills/competencies" or the skills needed by implementers and how they are acquired and sustained; (f) "cultural relevance" or the fit of the intervention with the values and preferences of implementers, administrators, and those who may benefit; (g) "resources" or the time, funding, and materials needed for adoption and maintenance; and (h) "administrative and organizational support" or extent to which adoption is supported by key leaders and if fidelity can be maintained. Horner and Ross have urged for the development and testing of a global contextual fit measure that captures these eight elements, which can then be used to guide and systematically evaluate the implementation potential of a proven intervention.

These eight elements of contextual fit can also serve diagnostically to pinpoint the particular aspects of a context that may pose as a challenge for the implementation of a proven intervention. Knowing which elements may be challenging for implementation can inform and alert an investigator/team to the need to develop strategies to address specific areas of contextual difficulties.

It should be noted that these eight elements focus on the immediate characteristics of a context (e.g., a service organization or practice setting) and do not include considerations related to the large "context" of policy, social trends and values in which a service or practice setting is in turn embedded (see Chapter 1, Figure 1.2). The perspective(s) from which an evaluation of fit should occur is also unclear. For example, these eight elements reflect the perspective of an organization or setting; other criteria are not addressed such as the extent to which a context/setting/ organization itself is malleable and can be modified to fit the requirements for delivery of a particular intervention. In this respect, the contextual fit construct appears to be one-directional—how the intervention fits or needs to be modified to match a context versus the other way around. Other related concepts that may be important to consider in an equation of fit include the "readiness" of an organization to adopt an intervention, or the extent to which it has or could develop appropriate supervisory, payment, and other infrastructures as well as whether it values evidence-based interventions. Another unknown is what constitutes "context" for interventions delivered via technology such as Web-based applications (see Chapter 7).

Case Examples

Keeping the aforementioned caveats in mind, we evaluate three interventions along Horner and Ross's eight elements to explore how an intervention's characteristics drive contextual fit. In the absence, however, of a quantitative global measure of contextual fit, we examine each element qualitatively. We also impose a rating of 'high,' 'medium,' or 'low' congruence for each element with "high" reflecting a better fit. We recognize the need for future research to establish clear and tested evaluative criteria and response formats. As described in Table 20.1, the three interventions we use as cases have different purposes, target different populations, and were designed for, and tested in, different contexts. Thus, they serve to highlight the nuances of contextual fit along these eight elements.

Skills$_2$Care^R. Skills$_2$Care^R is a six-session intervention designed to provide family caregivers with education and skills to manage the daily challenges of caring for individuals with dementia (Gitlin et al., 2003). Delivered by occupational therapists, it was tested in a Phase III efficacy trial as one of the test sites of the National Institutes of Health (NIH) Resources for Enhancing Alzheimer's Health (REACH) initiative. It was shown to reduce caregiver distress and behavioral symptoms of persons with dementia. The intervention was tested by enrolling families in the community that volunteered to participate; thus, it was evaluated independent of any health care or payment system or agency structure. Nevertheless, it was initially designed with the vision that it might be able to be embedded in a home care delivery system of care. Through a translational study, the intervention was shown that it could be embedded in home care practices and be reimbursed through Medicare Part A and B payment mechanisms (Gitlin, Jacobs, & Earland, 2010; Gitlin et al., 2003).

Occupational therapists were designated as the interventionists to deliver the intervention. They were chosen as interventionists because of their professional background and expertise in activity analysis, and ability to assess and integrate knowledge about cognitive status, physical function, psychosocial and environmental considerations. These considerations form the basis from which strategies are developed to help families address various care challenges including functional decline, behavioral symptoms and a caregiver's own stress and upset. Families are then trained in the use of these strategies.

TABLE 20.1 Basic Characteristics of Three Interventions

Intervention/Target Population	Type of Evaluation	Interventionists	Training Requirements	Intervention Characteristics	Potential Delivery Contexts and Payment Mechanisms
Skills₂Care[R]: Dementia caregivers who are stressed and need skills training	Phase III efficacy trial tested outside of service delivery context	Occupational therapists	■ One-week training including readings, online modules, and one day of face-to-face practice sessions followed by three coach documentation	■ Flexible number and scheduling of sessions ■ Up to six home sessions of 60 to 90 minutes delivered between 2 and 6 months ■ Tailored to caregiver needs ■ Specific strategies to improve skills to manage functional decline, behaviors, and reduce caregiver stress	■ Home care agencies through Medicare Parts A and B reimbursements ■ Private pay
Get Busy Get Better: African Americans 55+ with depressive symptoms	Phase III efficacy tested in senior center and homes	Tested with licensed social workers but any health professional could deliver	■ One-week training including readings, and face-to-face practice sessions ■ Ongoing supervision needed	■ Up to 10 1-hour sessions at home (telephone calls can replace home visit)	■ Aging service network ■ Senior centers but no designated budget line ■ Behavioral health departments ■ Medicare reimbursement
Hospital at Home: Acutely ill older adults in need of hospitalization	Quasi-experimental design Three Medicare-managed care health systems at two sites and a Veterans Administration medical center	Physicians and nurses	■ Training in the model and care coordination needed whereas health care protocol followed per patient reflect medical/nursing best practices		■ Managed care health systems

TABLE 20.2 Evaluation of Contextual Fit of Four Interventions Along Eight Characteristics as High, Medium, or Low

Intervention (Context)	Need Addressed	Precision	Evidence Base	Efficiency (Practicality)	Skills	Cultural Relevance	Resources	Organization Support
Skills$_2$Care^R (home care)	■ High ■ Family education and skills training on dementia unaddressed in home care ■ Increasing number of dementia patients in home care	■ Medium ■ Set number of sessions and content tailored to family needs ■ High level of clinical reasoning needed	■ Medium to high ■ One RCT conducted but its components have been tested in other trials	■ Medium ■ Can be integrated within traditional home care session ■ Not practical for agencies without occupational therapists	■ High ■ Training and coaching program established and available	■ High ■ Matches professional values and caregiver needs ■ However, approach differs from traditional practice and may not be immediately acceptable	■ Medium ■ Resources needed include funding for training, supervision, and fidelity monitoring	■ High ■ Can be reimbursed through Medicare Parts A and B, or private pay
Get Busy Get Better (senior centers)	■ High	■ Medium ■ Up to 10 1-hour sessions ■ Five treatment components	■ Medium to high ■ One RCT but each component tested in other trials	■ High ■ Any health and human service professional can deliver making it very practical	■ Low ■ Training and coaching programs being established but not currently available	■ High ■ Matches values of targeted population and service provider	■ Low ■ Resources needed include funding for training and staffing and travel to homes	■ Low ■ May be reimbursed through Medicare with licensed staff

(Continued)

TABLE 20.2 Evaluation of Contextual Fit of Four Interventions Along Eight Characteristics as High, Medium, or Low (Continued)

Intervention (Context)	Need Addressed	Precision	Evidence Base	Efficiency (Practicality)	Skills	Cultural Relevance	Resources	Organization Support
	■ Depressive symptoms in African Americans underdetected and undertreated in aging network services	■ Tailored to needs of participants		■ Tested only with home visits, which adds cost to its delivery				■ Costs would have to be absorbed by existing budgets of aging services
Hospital at Home (managed care health systems)	■ High ■ Can reduce adverse events associated with hospitalization	■ Medium-to-high variability dependent upon local resources and patient needs	■ Medium to high ■ One quasi-experimental test at three sites with some variability by site	■ High ■ Can be integrated in health care system and delivered by local practitioners	■ Medium ■ Training mechanisms currently under development	■ High ■ Matches desire of older adults to remain at home; reduced costs	■ High ■ Minimal resource needs; reflects reorganization of existing resources	■ High with value-based care ■ Low with capitated fee-for-service care

RCT, randomized controlled trial.

As shown in Table 20.2, and with regard to the first contextual fit criteria, Skills$_2$Care^R addresses a critical unmet "need" of dementia caregivers. The intervention provides education and skills tailored to the specific daily care challenges families identify as most difficult for them and which would not otherwise be addressed in current home or health care systems. As such, Skills$_2$Care^R can be scored as "high" on the dimension of need. However, this characteristic may negatively impact its "precision," which we rate as "medium." Also its flexible visit schedule and approach to delivery increase its fit with dynamic clinical settings; yet, its tailoring feature (e.g., developing strategies specific to a caregiver's home context and working with families differentially on the basis of their level of "readiness") introduces less precision as it relies upon a high level of clinical reasoning and decision making by interventionists. As one strategy does not fit all families, interventionists must derive specific approaches by applying the principles of the intervention (e.g., client-centered, culturally relevant strategies, tailoring). This increases the acceptability and cultural relevance of the intervention to families, yet simultaneously decreases its precision in the delivery of the intervention. Thus, not all therapists may feel comfortable or feel they are able to deliver this intervention. It can also be challenging to practically evaluate treatment fidelity (see Chapter 12).

We rate its effectiveness as "high" as Skills$_2$Care^R was tested using a single-blind, prospective randomized trial followed by a translational or pre–post preimplementation study (Gitlin et al., 2010). Its various components have been tested further in different combinations in other trials contributing in part to support of its evidence base. Nevertheless, there are some elements of effectiveness that are missing. The intervention was tested with African American and Caucasian caregivers and it was found that women tended to benefit more than men. Thus, its effectiveness with other caregiver groups is unknown and the mechanisms or why this approach results in reduced distress is not clear. Also, a formal economic evaluation (see Chapter 18) has not been conducted.

For "efficiency" or practicality, Skills$_2$Care^R can be rated as "mixed" or "medium." Given that it must be delivered by occupational therapists, this may not be a practical intervention for all agencies in the United States or in other countries that do not have access to or the resources to support delivery by this professional group. However, for home care agencies involving occupational therapists, this is a highly practical intervention in that the intervention can be embedded into traditional home care therapeutic practices. With respect to "skills," there are clearly articulated competencies, an established training program, and certification process with follow-up coaching available (see information about training at www.jefferson.edu/university/health_professions/elder_care/jec_team.html); thus, Skills$_2$Care^R receives a "high" rating for this contextual element. Nevertheless, at the time of this writing, training is dependent upon a handful of individuals, thus limiting its potential for large-scale dissemination (see Chapter 21) and scaling up, although a master train-the-trainers program is currently being designed. The intervention also has high "cultural relevance"; therapists often comment that, given its family-centered approach, Skills$_2$Care^R enables them to practice the way they would like to and also to be creative in applying strategies. Families equally value the education and skills they acquire and testify that the intervention makes a difference in their own lives and the care they are able to provide. For "resources," the intervention receives a "low" to "medium" rating as funding is needed for training therapists and there must be an organizational commitment to ongoing supervision and fidelity monitoring. Also, it is highly recommended that a guide book be purchased, which details the strategies offered to families; thus, this represents a potential ongoing cost to either agencies or families (Gitlin & Piersol, 2014). Finally, with regard to "organizational support," Skills$_2$Care^R can be rated as "medium." The intervention can be reimbursed through Medicare Parts A and B; however, reimbursement levels do not cover the actual costs of intervention delivery, thus requiring a large volume of participants to be enrolled in the program for it to have economic value to a home care agency to invest in training its therapists.

Taken as a whole, this intervention has potential for scalability in the home care delivery context. Its essential contextual challenge is: advancing its training approach to be self-sustaining versus being dependent upon a few trainers; developing a dissemination infrastructure (see Chapter 21) that effectively markets widely to home care agencies; and possibly developing a derivative of the intervention that can be delivered by other health and human service professionals to broaden its adoption potential by organizations and hence reach to family caregivers. This case also highlights the evolution that occurs through the implementation process. As an increasing number of organizations have gained interest in adopting the intervention, a train-the-trainers program now must be put into place to enable continued training activities and sustainability.

Get Busy Get Better. Our second example is the Get Busy Get Better (GBGB) intervention (also discussed in Chapter 4). GBGB (Table 20.1) involves up to 10, 1-hour home-based sessions delivered by licensed social workers. The intervention, having five treatment components (care management, referral/linkage, stress reduction, depression education, behavioral activation), is designed to reduce depressive symptoms, improve daily function, and enhance engagement in meaningful activities of African Americans with depressive symptoms and also to be provided by senior center staff (Gitlin et al., 2013). Rigorously tested in a Phase III efficacy trial, it was shown to reduce depressive symptoms and improve daily functioning. In this efficacy trial, staff at the test site—a large senior center—screened individuals by telephone or on site for depressive symptoms, and for those who were eligible (PHQ-9 score $\geq$5), deliver the home-based intervention. Analyses revealed that all groups (men vs. women, young vs. old, those with high or low financial strain) benefited (Gitlin et al., 2013; Szanton, Thorpe, & Gitlin, 2014). Also, mediation analyses provided guidance as to the mechanisms by which the intervention reduced depressive symptoms and suggested that each of its treatment components contributes to reductions in depressive symptoms (Gitlin, Roth, & Huang, 2014; Gitlin, Szanton, Huang, & Roth, 2014). A formal cost-effectiveness analysis also demonstrated the economic value of GBGB (Pizzi et al., 2014). The intervention was designed with the intent of having senior centers implement the intervention, but it was tested only in one site and there is not a viable payment mechanism to support its implementation. As grant funds supported its evaluation, the senior center that served as the test site has not been able to continue with the home visit portion owing to its associated costs and lack of reimbursement avenues at this point in time.

As to contextual fit (Table 20.2) with senior centers, GBGB receives a high score for addressing an identified unmet need (Gitlin et al., in press). Similar to

Skills$_2$Care^R, GBGB has prescribed assessments and clearly articulated treatment components; yet, the tailoring of each component to the specific needs of participants adds complexity to its delivery. The tailoring aspect of the intervention makes its delivery dependent upon skilled interventionists who can apply clinical reasoning, and thus it has medium precision.

As to effectiveness, we give GBGB a "medium" to "high" rating. It was rigorously tested but only in one randomized controlled trial (RCT) with 208 participants. Its efficacy for populations other than African Americans and delivery in other senior centers or aging network service settings is unknown. This limits its contextual fit with settings providing mental health services to other minority groups such as behavioral health departments that seek evidence-based home depression programs for highly diverse communities. It is unclear whether and what types of adaptations may be needed for diverse linguistic and cultural groups. GBGB, however, can be rated as having high efficiency or practicality. Although it was tested with licensed social workers as interventionists, the investigative team believes any health and human service professional with some psychosocial background (e.g., psychiatric nurse, occupational therapist with psychosocial training) could be trained to deliver the intervention. For skills, it receives a "low" rating; while a well-designed training and certification approach was followed during the trial, a translational phase would be needed to modify the training program and manuals and these are not yet available on a larger scale, although they are under construction. Whereas cultural relevance to agencies targeting African American communities and to African Americans with depressive symptoms themselves can be rated as "high," GBGB receives "low" ratings for resources and organizational support as there are no existing funding mechanisms that are available to support this highly efficacious program. Also, low-resourced agencies may not have access to skilled service providers who have the comfort level to deliver a behavioral activation form of mental health treatment.

Thus, the essential contextual challenge for this program is identifying or creating funding mechanisms to support its delivery in the aging network and specifically in senior centers in the United States (Gitlin et al., in press). This may entail policy changes, improving reimbursement mechanisms through Medicare, or determining how to operationalize opportunities that may become available as a consequence of the Mental Health Parity Act. Secondarily, its manuals and an infrastructure for training would have to be secured to enhance its contextual fit prior to implementing a full-blown dissemination plan.

Hospital at Home. Our final case example is the Hospital at Home program (Leff & Burton, 1996; Leff et al., 1999, 2005). Designed to provide hospital-level care to acutely ill older adults in their homes, this program was tested in three health care organizations in a prospective quasi-experimental design (Table 20.1). The program was found to be feasible, efficacious, and safe and reduced length of stay and cost.

As to its contextual fit (Table 20.2), Hospital at Home receives a "high" score for addressing a critical unmet need: medical care for acutely ill vulnerable older adults, which minimizes risk associated with hospitalizations. It offers acutely ill older adults the opportunity to heal in their home, yet with the intense medical attention they may need. Similar to the other case examples, the approach is necessarily specific to the needs of patients adding a level of complexity to its delivery; hence, we suggest precision is at a "medium" level. As to effectiveness, Hospital at Home shows very positive outcomes and was tested in three distinct health care systems, thus providing knowledge of implementation challenges under differing payment and organizational care systems. Its components and approach have also been tested in other settings and countries, and meta-analyses support its effectiveness (Caplan et al., 2013; Shepperd, et al., 2009). The level of acceptability of the program by patients varied across programs such that continued evaluation is warranted along with identifying strategies to address patient and/or practitioner concerns that prevent participation. The program, however, is rated as having "high" efficiency or practicality as any health care system has the necessary resources to adopt the program. The program uses indigenous medical staff of hospitals but organizes the way in which they deliver acute medical care. For skills, it receives a "medium" rating as training would involve multiple personnel (administrators, physicians, nurses). However, the skill level and knowledge needed to conduct this program are well articulated, and training manuals and programs are available.

Whereas currently the cultural relevance and organizational support for Hospital at Home are "high," this has not always been the case. The program's cost savings were initially perceived as a threat to the revenue streams of hospitals; however currently, Hospital at Home aligns well with a value-based system of health care. Thus, its implementation (and dissemination) potential has dramatically increased with recent changes in policy and payment mechanisms.

The essential contextual challenge for this program is refining and standardizing delivery components such that they can fit with a wide variety of hospital organizational systems. The model program may be implemented differently based upon the adopting organization's areas of strength. For example, if an adopter hospital system has a strong competency in providing home-based care, then that component of the model may be delivered more easily, efficiently, and effectively. The challenge is to enable an organization without that competency to be able to fulfill the program's goals and implement all of its components. Thus, training in the model is necessarily context specific and varies on the basis of the relative strengths and weaknesses of the adopter organization. Other related challenges include advancing training strategies to meet context-specific needs, and developing a dissemination infrastructure for deploying the model rapidly.

In summary, a comparison of these three interventions affords an understanding of the way in which specific delivery characteristics of the interventions affect contextual fit. Each program has unique challenges along the eight dimensions of context, thus highlighting how the characteristics of an intervention drive in part future implementation potential or are at least associated with distinct challenges that will be encountered in different contexts. We can also conclude that there is no right or wrong way of designing the characteristics of an intervention (discussed in Chapter 5). Also, it may not be possible for any intervention to have a "high" score across all eight dimensions of contextual fit. However, "low" fit across all elements may preclude moving forward with dissemination and implementation (discussed as well in Chapter 21).

Caveats in Attending to Context Early On

While we have posited that interventions should be designed with the end in mind, there are a few caveats. Designing an intervention for existing contexts and stakeholder values may in fact shortchange innovation by confining intervention development to fit current inadequate or ineffective practice realities. Take for example, Hospital at Home—while it draws upon prevailing resources (physicians, nurses, existing medical treatments, best practices and protocols), it was designed as a different mechanism than prevailing hospital models for delivering acute medical care. At the time of its development, hospitals sought revenue through encouraging hospitalizations and greater lengths of stay and thus the approach threatened the culture and value context of hospitals. Hospital at Home also illustrates how the broader sociohistorical and political contexts (see Chapter 1, Figure 1.2) influence implementation potential. When it was initially shown to be an effective alternative to hospitalizing vulnerable older adults, it was not viewed favorably by stakeholders. With changes in U.S. health care and policy, the model now is a better fit and health care organizations seek to adopt it.

Similar to the Hospital at Home program, it may be that, with policy and contextual changes, GBGB will be able to be adopted more easily in the future in senior centers. If GBGB was designed for delivery in existing mental health systems, it would not have had the same positive impact on the population it targeted, older African Americans, or have the potential to address health disparities that continue to persist in existing mental health delivery approaches. Nevertheless, an understanding of its current implementation challenges helps to frame the evidence needed for policy change. It may be that GBGB will not be adopted at this point in time, but its evaluation demonstrates the feasibility of addressing depressive symptoms in a practice and cost-efficient manner. With policy change, the implementation potential of GBGB may be more feasible, similar to Hospital at Home.

Thus, timing, policy, and societal fit are equally important contextual factors to understand and consider. Some interventions may be designed for current contexts whereas others need to be designed in such a way as to push for change in contexts.

How Much Evidence Is Sufficient?

These cases also implicitly raise the issue: What constitutes sufficient evidence for an intervention/program/service model to warrant moving forward with its implementation? There is no consensus as to how much evidence is enough for implementation to be considered. In drug studies, multiple tests for safety, efficacy, and delineating underlying mechanisms are required prior to U.S. Federal Drug Administration (FDA) approval and adoption. Once FDA approval has been achieved, there is a tendency not to require more trials for the drug for the indication for which it was approved.

There are, however, no parallel pipeline and approval mechanisms for behavioral interventions. Most stakeholders of practice settings are seeking at a minimum the following forms of evidence: benefit for a targeted population; some understanding as for whom the intervention is most effective; and its cost, cost–benefit and/or cost-effectiveness. As behavioral interventions address many important and pressing needs with few adverse events, adoption may occur on the basis of findings from only a single randomized trial. Nevertheless, while ongoing evaluation of an intervention in new contexts is always warranted, the question is the rigor and design of such evaluations; that is, can the intervention be evaluated within, for example, a quality indicator framework or is a new RCT required? Take for example GBGB; the essential question is whether we need to wait another 3 to 5 years to complete a randomized trial that evaluates the intervention's outcomes for low-income minority populations not included in the original trial. Alternately, GBGB could be implemented with populations that loosely fit the criteria of the original trial (e.g., low income, having depressive symptoms, amenable to an activity-oriented behavioral approach) and evaluated within the context of its delivery. Although we favor the latter approach, this is an issue that needs careful consideration, empirical evidence regarding cultural adaptations to interventions to guide decision making. It remains a hotly debated issue among funders and researchers.

A related question is how intervention programs should be evaluated in order to improve their implementation potential. Chapter 2 discussed the potential role of hybrid and pragmatic designs as one way of rigorously addressing efficacy-, effectiveness-, and/or implementation-type questions in a trial or multisite study. As discussed earlier, Hospital at Home was evaluated in the actual context in which it is intended to be delivered. As shown, this affords distinct advantages including obtaining immediate knowledge as to its implementation challenges, the modifications or refinements to the intervention that need to occur or which work best in a particular setting, and the resources needed for successful implementation of this model in different hospital organizations. On the basis of the program's evaluation in three different settings, Hospital at Home may not need a translational phase in which tweaks to the program are implemented and evaluated—rather it may now be ready for broad implementation.

In contrast, as Skills$_2$Care^R was not tested within a home care organizational context, a translational phase was necessary in which manuals, training, and intervention protocols were redesigned to fit work flow, supervisory structures, and referral mechanisms (Gitlin et al., 2010). Similarly, as GBGB was tested within only one senior center, it is unclear as to whether other senior centers with varying levels of resources and staffing could effectively implement the program. Thus, GBGB still needs to be evaluated on a much larger scale in multiple senior center settings that differ with regard to staffing, staff-member ratios, and so forth.

These cases also highlight the tension between testing interventions in rigorous yet static protocol-driven randomized trials versus other evaluative frameworks that allow for immediate program refinements such as in quality improvement (QI) evaluations or using some of the emerging design strategies mentioned in Chapter 2. Different design strategies may facilitate more rapid research responses and provide critical insights as to the contextual challenges that occur in implementation (Riley et al., 2013; Szanton, Leff, & Gitlin, 2015), thus easing the implementation tension.

The take-home message is this: Understanding contextual factors that impinge upon implementation is a worthy research goal early on in the pipeline when developing an intervention and evaluating its effectiveness.

INTERVENTIONIST CHARACTERISTICS

Although each of the eight elements that form a composite understanding of contextual fit are important to consider, we would like to highlight in particular the role of "skills/competencies" of interventionists. Identifying who can deliver an intervention is an important consideration and decision that typically occurs early on in the pipeline when developing a program (see Chapter 5). As these cases illustrate, the availability of interventionists with the requisite skills and competencies is an important challenge impacting implementation potential.

In classic Phase III efficacy trials, tradition has it that "super" clinicians or interventionists are selected for intervention delivery as the goal at this phase is to optimize internal validity and the potential for treatment benefits. However, this practice has significant downstream consequences with respect to wide-scale program implementation. If only certain professional groups can deliver the intervention, and within that group, only elite clinicians, then the replication potential of a proven program may be significantly reduced. Also, training in a proven program will then need to be adjusted to account for greater variation in skills and competencies that exist in the larger population of potential interventionists.

As illustrated by both Skills$_2$Care^R and GBGB, dependence upon highly skilled personnel drives up the cost of an intervention and may limit its potential reach and adoption in settings that do not have access to such personnel. This is not to say, however, that interventions should be designed for delivery only by interventionists who reflect a common denominator or simplified skill set; clearly, the competencies of interventionists must reflect the needs and purposes of an intervention. However, knowledge of the potential challenges presented by the skill sets needed should be noted early on in intervention development as it will affect downstream issues related to the potential reach of an intervention, its ease of adoption by agencies and organizations, and the scope and nature of training that may be necessary.

Still, concern with using highly skilled and costly personnel for intervention delivery and also the need to reach populations not traditionally included in behavioral intervention research have promoted an interest among researchers in examining the role of community health workers (CHWs) and/or peers. CHWs are indigenous workers who share similar backgrounds (ethnicity, language, or geography) as the population being targeted by an intervention (Han et al., 2015). In this respect, they may be uniquely qualified ethnically, linguistically, socioeconomically, culturally, and/or experientially to deliver an intervention. This may be the case in particular when designing interventions for underserved and diverse populations that have limited access to present health and human services owing to economics, culture, and language. Use of peers and CHWs may appear to be cost-effective, although as use of this group would necessitate potentially more intensive training, oversight, and monitoring, cost efficiencies may not be fully realized as initially expected. Interventions delivered by peers/CHWs for chronic disease self-management, cancer detection, and depression demonstrate preliminary support for this approach (Han et al., 2015). Clearly, however, the CHW model for interventions would not be appropriate when highly skilled health and human service professionals are needed such as in Skills$_2$Care^R or the Hospital at Home model; nevertheless, the delivery of elements of each of these approaches may be possible. For example, some portions of the Hospital at Home model may be delivered by CHW such as patient education, assistance with self-care needs, and so forth. For Skills$_2$Care^R, once an action plan has been established by a skilled interventionist (an occupational therapist), peer mentors may be able to practice the strategy with family caregivers. However, such deviations to these evidence-based programs would need careful evaluation.

In summary, a highly manualized intervention (see Chapter 6) may require a less skilled interventionist, which may in turn enhance precision and implementation potential. Interventions requiring a high level of skill and/or clinical reasoning may be necessary, but they may drive up cost and potentially limit adoption by organizations with limited resources and/or access to staff with the needed competencies. These are the trade-offs that need to be thoughtfully considered early on when developing an intervention in the crucial period of discovery as discussed in Chapter 3.

VALUE ALIGNMENT

Another element of contextual fit that is important to highlight is "cultural relevance" or the fit of the intervention with the values and preferences of implementers, administrators, and those who may benefit. When initially evaluating an intervention (e.g., Phase I, II, III, or IV, Chapter 2), the concern is with its proof of concept, safety, and treatment benefits. The outcome measures selected (see Chapters 14 and 15) should be closely aligned with intervention intent and the proximal and global benefits that may be afforded by exposure to a treatment. However, the outcomes of interest at these phases may not be those of importance to stakeholders and end users downstream at the implementation phase. Thus, striking the right balance and considering ways to align outcomes with a broad range of potential stakeholders are an important challenge to consider early on when developing an intervention.

Value alignment or deriving a fit between the intervention and the values and outcomes sought by different stakeholders is critical to an organization's willingness to adopt and then implement an intervention. First, it is important to identify all potential stakeholders. Stakeholders may include policy makers, administrators, payers, interventionists, and/or end users or beneficiaries (e.g., individuals and families). Second, it is important to discern each stakeholder's particular perspective, needs, and values. For example, an agency may be interested in a particular intervention for the following reasons: it addresses an unmet need of the community served; it enhances capacity to deliver needed services; it would provide a market advantage; it may generate a new revenue stream; and/or, it enables the agency to "do the right thing." Alternately, an interventionist or clinician may be interested in an intervention because it expands and/or enhances his or her own professional skills, or enables him or her to practice in a way that is different from and less confining than his or her traditional practices. Individuals or family members may value an intervention because of the immediate benefits that they experience, such as an improvement in quality of life. Furthermore, policy makers may value only the cost savings generated from an intervention, for example, if it results in fewer hospitalizations or nursing home placements. Identifying each stakeholder's values leads to what is referred to as a "value proposition" or a concise statement as to why an intervention should be adopted (see Chapter 21).

As noted earlier, in the evaluation phases of an intervention, typically the focus is solely on one form of value—the impact of the intervention on an individual/

family/community (Table 20.3). However, identifying early on the value perspectives of other stakeholders will yield important information that can subsequently inform implementation as one moves forward through the pipeline from testing to implementing an intervention. Obtaining the perspectives of various stakeholders can occur early on in the development of an intervention through, for example, key informant interviews or focus groups.

As illustrated by Hospital at Home, knowledge of stakeholder values and the settings for delivery does not guarantee easy implementation. Other factors including timing, existing payment structures, societal priorities, and trends and policies form the larger context influencing implementation. Also noteworthy is that stakeholder values are dynamic and may change in response to broader policy and societal trends.

CONCLUSION

In accordance with the premise of this book, the key theme of this chapter is that behavioral intervention researchers should develop and evaluate interventions keeping the end or big picture in mind, whether that be to change policy, construct new care systems, or change current practices to address a pressing public health priority. Having a vision of where an intervention might be located in a specific setting and payment structure, or in a future health and human service world, can inform intervention development work. In addition, understanding a particular setting, where an intervention might be situated in a work flow as well as how

TABLE 20.3 Exemplar Value Propositions From the Individual, Interventionist, Agency, and Societal Perspectives

Intervention	Individual	Interventionist	Organization	Society
Skills₂Care[R]	Improves indicators of objective and subjective burden and behavioral symptoms	Embraces a person-centered treatment approach	■ Brings in revenue; training dollars immediately recouped	■ May reduce health care costs but not proven
Get Busy Get Better	Improves symptomatology and activity engagement	Embraces a person-centered treatment approach	■ Links care to senior center activities ■ Addresses an unmet need of community	■ Shown to be cost-effective
Hospital at Home	Improves health, reduces risks	Embraces a person-centered treatment approach	■ Reduces risk to patients and costs ■ Fulfills mission of improved health care and cost efficiencies	■ Reduces length of stay; reduces cost

individuals/end users might access an intervention, can inform evaluation plans. In other words, having some type of vision of where an intervention may be located in the future may ultimately lead to more purposeful intervention development and evaluation when the ultimate goal is for the intervention to be made widely available, if shown to be effective (e.g., clinically, statistically, and from a cost perspective). We also note that contexts themselves are fluid and dynamic, thus adding complexity to deriving the just right fit between an intervention and a setting.

Implementing a proven intervention into a practice setting and promoting its wide-scale adoption involve considerable effort and a different kind of "know-how" than developing and evaluating the intervention for its efficacy and effectiveness. Much can be learned from implementation science and its theories as well as from the experiences of moving proven programs forward. Finally, to advance an understanding of implementation potential, development of measures that capture the nuances of contextual fit is very much needed.

It should also be noted that the eight elements we applied to our three cases reflect "fit" from the perspective of an organization. It may be that practice contexts also need to be evaluated as to their ability to be modified to adopt an intervention. As such, other aspects such as an organization's readiness and willingness to modify various practices or "de-implement" its ineffective practices, and its malleability to adapt to the characteristics of an intervention may be equally important and necessitate conceptual and measurement development.

Finally, in applying these eight elements, we observe that some of the strengths of an intervention (tailoring to a targeted population's need) also present as weaknesses for its contextual fit (imprecision in delivery). For example, a clear strength of our three exemplars is that they address unmet needs unique to participant populations and use the principle of tailoring to optimize treatment benefits; yet, that approach precludes prescripting every interaction and treatment session. Rather, on-the-ground decision making by interventionists who are well trained in the principles and parameters of the intervention is required. This has important implications for choice of interventionists and their training. It also suggests that contextual fit may vary by setting and availability of interventionists as well as by the delivery characteristics of the intervention itself.

REFERENCES

Burke, J. P., & Gitlin, L. N. (2012). How do we change practice when we have the evidence? *American Journal of Occupational Therapy, 66*(5), e85–e88. doi:10.5014/ajot.2012.004432

Caplan, G. A., Sulaiman, N. S., Mangin, D. A., Ricauda, N. A., Wilson, A. D., & Barclay, L. (2013). A meta-analysis of "hospital in the home." *The Medical Journal of Australia, 198*(4), 195–196. doi:10.5694/mja12.11841

Fixsen, D. L., Naoom, S. F., Blase, K. A., Friedman, R. M., & Wallace, F. (2005). *Implementation research: A synthesis of the literature.* Tampa, FL: University of South Florida, Louis de la Parte Florida Mental Health Institute, The National Implementation Research Network (FMHI Publication #231).

Gitlin, L. N. (2013). Introducing a new intervention: An overview of research phases and common challenges. *American Journal of Occupational Therapy, 67*(2), 177–184. doi:10.5014/ajot.2013.006742

Gitlin, L. N., Harris, L. F., Mccoy, M. C., Chernett, N. L., Pizzi, L. T., Jutkowitz, E., . . . Hauck, W. W. (2013). A home-based intervention to reduce depressive symptoms and improve quality of life in older African Americans. *Annals of Internal Medicine, 159*(4), 243. doi:10.7326/0003-4819-159-4-201308200-00005

Gitlin, L., Harris, L., McCoy, M., Hess, E., & Hauck, W. (in press). Delivery characteristics, acceptability and depression outcomes of a home-based depression intervention for older African Americans: The Get Busy Get Better program. *The Gerontologist, Practice Concepts.*

Gitlin, L. N., Jacobs, M., & Earland, T. V. (2010). Translation of a dementia caregiver intervention for delivery in homecare as a reimbursable Medicare service: Outcomes and lessons learned. *The Gerontologist, 50*(6), 847–854. doi:10.1093/geront/gnq057

Gitlin, L. N., & Piersol, C. V. (2014). *A caregiver's guide to dementia: Using activities and other strategies to prevent, reduce and manage behavioral symptoms.* Philadelphia, PA: Camino Books.

Gitlin, L. N., Roth, D. L., & Huang, J. (2014). Mediators of the impact of a home-based intervention (beat the blues) on depressive symptoms among older African Americans. *Psychology and Aging, 29*(3), 601–611.

Gitlin, L. N., Szanton, S. L., Huang, J., & Roth, D. L. (2014). Factors mediating the effects of a depression intervention on functional disability in older African Americans. *Journal of the American Geriatrics Society, 62*(12), 2280–2287. doi:10.1111/jgs.13156

Gitlin, L. N., Winter, L., Corcoran, M., Dennis, M. P., Schinfeld, S., & Hauck, W. W. (2003). Effects of the home environmental skill-building program on the caregiver–care recipient dyad: 6-month outcomes from the Philadelphia REACH Initiative. *The Gerontologist, 43*(4), 532–546.

Greenhalgh, T. (2005). *Diffusion of innovations in health service organisations: A systematic literature review.* Malden, MA: Blackwell.

Han, H., Kyounghae, K, Choi, J. S., Choi, E., Nieman, C. L., Joo, J. J., Lin, F. R., & Gitlin, L. N. (2015). Do community health worker interventions improve chronic disease management and care among vulnerable populations? A systematic review. Manuscript submitted for publication.

Horner, R., & Blitz, C. (2014, September). *The importance of contextual fit when implementing evidence-based interventions* (ASPE Issue Brief). Washington, DC: U.S. Department of Health and Human Services. Office of Human Services Policy. Office of the Assistant Secretary for Planning and Evaluation.

Jacobs, S. R., Weiner, B. J., & Bunger, A. C. (2014). Context matters: Measuring implementation climate among individuals and groups. *Implementation Science, 9*, 46. doi:10.1186/1748-5908-9-46

Leff, B., & Burton, J. R. (1996). Acute medical care in the home. *Journal of the American Geriatrics Society, 44*(5), 603–605. doi:10.1111/j.1532-5415.1996.tb01452.x

Leff, B., Burton, L., Guido, S., Greenough, W. B., Steinwachs, D., & Burton, J. R. (1999). Home hospital program: A pilot study. *Journal of the American Geriatrics Society, 47*(6), 697–702. doi:10.1111/j.1532-5415.1999.tb01592.x

Leff, B., Burton, L., Mader, S. L., Naughton, B., Burl, J., Inouye, S. K., . . . Burton, J. R. (2005). Hospital at home: Feasibility and outcomes of a program to provide hospital-level care at home for acutely ill older patients. *Annals of Internal Medicine, 143*(11), 798-808. doi:10.7326/0003-4819-143-11-200512060-00008

Pizzi, L. T., Jutkowitz, E., Frick, K. D., Suh, D., Prioli, K. M., & Gitlin, L. N. (2014). Cost-effectiveness of a community-integrated home-based depression intervention in older African Americans. *Journal of the American Geriatrics Society, 62*(12), 2288–2295. doi:10.1111/jgs.13146

Riley, W. T., Glasgow, R. E., Etheredge, L., & Abernethy, A. P. (2013). Rapid, responsive, relevant (R3) research: A call for a rapid learning health research enterprise. *Clinical and Translational Medicine, 2*(1), 10. doi:10.1186/2001-1326-2-10

Shepperd, S., Doll, H., Angus, R. M., Clarke, M. J., Iliffe, S., Kalra, L., . . . Wilson, A. D. (2009). Avoiding hospital admission through provision of hospital care at home: A systematic review and meta-analysis of individual patient data. *Canadian Medical Association Journal, 180*(2), 175–182. doi:10.1503/cmaj.081491

Szanton, S. L., Leff, B., & Gitlin, L. N. (2015). Improvement interventions. *Annals of Internal Medicine, 162*(8), 596–597. doi:10.7326/L15-5071-2

Szanton, S. L., Thorpe, R. J., & Gitlin, L. N. (2014). Beat the Blues decreases depression in financially strained older African American adults. *The American Journal of Geriatric Psychiatry, 22*(7), 692–697. doi:10.1016/j.jagp.2013.05.008

Wilson, K. M., Brady, T. J., & Lesesne, C. (2011). An organizing framework for translation in public health: The knowledge to action framework. *Preventing Chronic Disease, 8*(2), A46.

TWENTY ONE

DISSEMINATING PROVEN BEHAVIORAL INTERVENTIONS: WHAT DOES IT TAKE?

JOHN BEILENSON, LAURA N. GITLIN, AND SARA J. CZAJA

> *In health care, invention is hard, but dissemination is even harder. . . . Even*
> *when innovations are implemented successfully in one location, they often*
> *[spread] slowly—if at all.*
> —Berwick (2003)

Developing an evidence-based behavioral intervention is hard, complex work, often requiring years of research and testing. However, this effort is just the beginning of a similarly difficult process of enabling large numbers of people to benefit from a behavioral intervention that has proven effectiveness. Too often, investigators falter at the dissemination phase or moving proven interventions from testing sites to real-world settings. Thus, understanding the specific activities involved in dissemination is important to distill.

What is "dissemination"? Although variably defined, dissemination refers to the active spread of an innovation such as a proven behavioral intervention, usually through specific plans and targeted distribution channels. The National Institutes of Health (NIH) formally defines dissemination as

> . . . *the purposive distribution of information and intervention materials to a specific*
> *public health or clinical practice audience. The intent is to spread information and the*
> *associated evidence-based interventions. Research on dissemination addresses how in-*
> *formation about health promotion and care interventions is created, packaged, trans-*
> *mitted, and interpreted among a variety of important stakeholder groups.* (NIH, 2011)

As shown in Table 21.1, Rogers's definition also emphasizes the planned nature of dissemination processes. Dissemination of a proven intervention is the phase along the elongated pipeline, as described in Chapter 2 (Figure 2.2), that is specifically focused on not only "getting the word out," so to speak, but also supporting adoption by organizations, systems of care, community groups, agencies, and/or end users including interventionists and recipients of an intervention. Of importance, however, is to recognize that there is a dynamic relationship between dissemination and implementation. We refer to "implementation" as the fit between a proven intervention and a real-world public health, clinical, and community service

TABLE 21.1 Key Terms Related to the Process of Dissemination

Term	Definition
Implementation	"The use of strategies to adopt and integrate evidence-based health interventions and change practice patterns within specific settings" (Schillinger, 2010).
Diffusion	"The process by which an innovation is communicated through certain channels and adopted over time among members of a social system" (Rogers, 2003).
Dissemination	"Planned, systematic efforts designed to make a program or innovation more widely available to a target audience or members of a social system" (Rogers, 2003).
Implementation science	"The study of methods to promote the integration of research findings and evidence into healthcare policy and practice" (Fogarty International Center of NIH, n.d.).
Social marketing	"The design, implementation, and control of programs calculated to influence the acceptability of social ideas and involving considerations of product planning, pricing, communication, distribution, and marketing research" (Kotler & Zaltman, 1971).
Scalability/going to scale	"The capacity of a practice to replicate design or strategic elements in a magnified, sustainable form" (Bondi, 2000).
Value proposition	"A clear, simple statement of the benefits, both tangible and intangible, that [a] company will provide, along with the approximate price it will charge each customer segment for those benefits" (Golub et al., 2000).

systems. As discussed in Chapter 2, we suggest that there needs to be some proof that an intervention can be implemented in a particular setting prior to investing in its dissemination for widespread adoption. While dissemination, adoption, and implementation are highly interrelated activities, we find it helpful, for heuristic purposes, to view dissemination as supporting adoption of an intervention by various settings following some proof of the implementation potential of an intervention (as previously illustrated in Chapters 19 and 20).

The dissemination of evidence is challenging in any industry, but the challenges are particularly pronounced for behavioral interventions where the knowledge–practice gaps exist across all areas of medical, public health, and human service practices (Institute of Medicine, 2001). While academic researchers are skilled in generating scientific reports that systematically relay findings of intervention studies, merely reporting the evidence to largely academic audiences has been shown to be an insufficient form of dissemination and one that does not lead to adoption of interventions. McCannon, Berwick, and Massoud (2007, p. 1937) observe that "good ideas, even when their value is thoroughly demonstrated in one place, will not reliably spread into action through normal communication channels at a pace truly responsive to enormous health care challenges . . ." Therefore, disseminating effective behavioral interventions is a significant challenge requiring thoughtful and purposeful thinking, planning, and actions by an investigator and/or investigative team.

This chapter focuses on what it takes to disseminate a proven intervention. We first discuss the key reasons why dissemination and subsequent adoption or uptake of an intervention may be challenging. Next, we consider ways to determine if a proven intervention is ready to be disseminated. Finally, we describe the core elements of a robust plan for dissemination. Even if an investigator does not want to personally disseminate his or her or another proven intervention, knowledge of the thinking and action processes involved for doing so can help inform how an intervention is developed early on in the pipeline. In this respect, understanding dissemination considerations is important to all behavioral intervention researchers seeking to advance programs that eventually can be used by communities, practice settings, and end user beneficiaries. As there are various terms related specifically to the process of dissemination, these are summarized in Table 21.1 and are referred to throughout this chapter. Although there is no consensus as to the meaning and usage of terms, Table 21.1 provides working definitions that can serve as a guide to this particular phase along the intervention pipeline.

WHY IS DISSEMINATION DIFFICULT?

Dissemination is hard work for several reasons. First, investigators may not have the skill set and/or time needed for engaging in dissemination activities. The skills used to create and rigorously test an intervention are distinct from those needed to disseminate a proven intervention. For example, understanding market conditions, developing key messages, naming and framing the value of an intervention for different stakeholders, and building a business plan are a few of the key activities conducted in a dissemination phase. Most investigators have not had formal training in these areas or ways of thinking or been exposed to what it takes to disseminate a proven intervention.

Moreover, dissemination requires dedicated time that an investigator may not have owing to other professional commitments and responsibilities. Dissemination may deter an investigator from pursuing other important activities such as conducting further research on the intervention or investigating new related scientific questions. In this regard, participating in the dissemination of a proven program needs to be a conscious decision on the part of an investigator and investigative team that is linked to professional and career goals.

A second factor contributing to the challenge of dissemination is that investigators may find it difficult to raise the funds or capital needed for this phase. Developing and carrying out a dissemination plan can be costly. Unlike other industries such as pharmaceuticals, there is not a dedicated channel or industry for disseminating a behavioral intervention; thus, investigators are on their own to figure out appropriate mechanisms for moving their programs forward from a testing environment to the public and into practice settings. In the United States, traditional funding mechanisms such as the NIH have demonstrated some interest in researching the relative effectiveness of different dissemination approaches, although few funds are allocated for research in this area, and there is no support for ongoing dissemination efforts of any one particular intervention.

A third issue in dissemination is that agencies, stakeholders, and individuals may not be ready to accept a particular intervention even when its benefits are proven and of interest (see the examples discussed in Chapter 20). Market conditions, including economic considerations and other programs competing for limited organizational resources, community readiness, or the lack of an apparent fit of the program with perceived community needs may hamper dissemination. Furthermore, agencies may not have the right staffing or resources for delivering a program or the sustained funding to train staff, implement a program, and sustain it as is discussed in previous chapters. There may not be funding or reimbursement mechanisms to support and sustain the adoption of an intervention making dissemination ineffective or unrealistic (see discussion in Chapter 20 of the Get Busy Get Better intervention [Gitlin et al., 2012] and also the initial reaction to Hospital at Home [Leff et al., 2005]).

Yet another reason why dissemination is challenging is that investigators may not be aware of, and consequently use, evidence-based approaches for this activity. Kerner, Rimer, and Emmons (2005) note that "Efforts to move effective preventive strategies into widespread use too often have been unsystematic, uncoordinated, and insufficiently capitalized, and little is known about the best strategies to facilitate active dissemination and rapid implementation of evidence-based practices." (p. 443). The science of dissemination, an aspect of implementation science, is emerging; however, as of yet, dissemination activities are not well studied or understood. Knowledge of best practices and what works or not for specific types of interventions, organizations, communities, stakeholders, and individuals is only in an incipient stage.

DETERMINING AN INTERVENTION'S DISSEMINATION POTENTIAL

Prior to engaging in dissemination, one must first evaluate whether a proven intervention has the potential to be effectively distributed and subsequently adopted by individuals, communities, and/or clinical settings. However, this is not a straightforward calculus. Existing but limited literature suggests that a proven intervention can be evaluated for its dissemination and ultimately its implementation potential based upon five considerations: the characteristics of the intervention, environmental context in which it would be delivered, fit between the intervention and the context or practice setting, leadership capacity, and access to communication channels. Each of these is discussed in the sections that follow.

Assessing Intervention Characteristics

The first consideration when evaluating the dissemination potential of an intervention concerns its delivery characteristics. Rogers (2003) identified five important characteristics of interventions: relative advantage, compatibility, complexity, trialability, and observability. Each characteristic, defined in Table 21.2, is not necessarily intrinsic to an intervention, but reflects how the intervention may be perceived or experienced by the organization, interventionist, and/or end beneficiary of an intervention.

There is not an agreed-upon understanding of the set of intervention characteristics that enhance its dissemination potential. Characteristics of an intervention have to be evaluated in relationship to the particular goals and outcomes being sought, the target population, and the particular location and context in which it

TABLE 21.2 Characteristics Influencing Dissemination and Adoption of an Intervention

Characteristic	Description
Relative advantage	The degree to which the innovation is perceived superior to existing models or products
Compatibility	How the innovation is perceived consistent with existing values and needs of potential adopters
Complexity	How an innovation is perceived as difficult (or easy) to use or implement
Trialability	Whether or how an offering may be experimented with on a limited basis
Observability	The degree to which the benefits of the innovation are visible to others

will be deployed. However, behavioral intervention researchers should critically examine the delivery characteristics of their interventions in the formative phases of developing an intervention (see Chapters 3 and 5) in order to understand whether the intervention may scale easily in the future or require a lot of effort such as hiring specialized staff, a prolonged or extensive training period to deliver the program, and/or resources such as special equipment, technology, space, or supplies.

An investigator must balance between developing a potent intervention and the real-world exigencies imposed by practice environments where it might be implemented. For example, an intervention that requires a specific skill set for its delivery may not be able to be adopted by settings that do not have access to the specialized staff (see further discussion of this matter in Chapter 20). This is illustrated by the Collaborative Care program, a primary care model for depression in older adults. Collaborative Care, originally known as IMPACT (Improving Mood—Promoting Access to Collaborative Treatment), was initially tested in an eight-site, randomized clinical trial and found to be twice as effective in reducing depression as usual care with significant cost savings (Unützer et al., 2002, 2008). Collaborative Care, however, was (and is) not immediately compatible with most primary care practices. The model requires a care manager, psychologist or social worker who is integrated into the practice. However, most primary care practices do not have easy access to such staff, and many do not have sufficient numbers of older patients to make Collaborative Care a priority. Furthermore, the program's resulting cost benefits do not accrue directly to practices in fee-for-service environments. Since 2002, with the primary publication of trial outcomes (Unützer et al, 2002), more than 6,000 clinicians have received training in Collaborative Care, and the interventionists have provided resources, training, coaching, and psychiatric consultation to more than 1,000 clinics around the world (Powers, 2015). This objectively impressive number, however, is modest when compared to the more than 200,000 primary practices in the country (Agency for Healthcare Research and Quality, 2011). That said, the rise of Accountable Care Organizations (ACO), interest in patient-centered medical homes, and new Medicare reimbursements for care coordination suggest that Collaborative Care may be more financially attractive for health systems in the future. This illustrates how a variety of contextual considerations (e.g., availability of staff, census of practices, financial incentives, and health policies) influence uptake of a needed intervention.

Understanding Context

Researchers need to be acutely aware of the elements in the organization in which an intervention will be embedded, as discussed in detail in Chapter 20. The characteristics of the environmental context of a practice setting, organization, and agency can influence the likelihood or speed of dissemination and eventual adoption of an intervention (Simpson & Dansereau, 2007). In addition to specific organization or agency characteristics for an intervention, the larger context of policy and societal trends and values also influence dissemination and wide-scale adoption as suggested in Chapter 1, Figure 1.2.

Certain characteristics of practice settings may yield differential outcomes for dissemination. For example, it has been found that a high level of environmental uncertainty may actually increase an organization's willingness to embrace change (O'Neill, Pouder, & Bucholtz, 1998). If a proven intervention can enable an organization to respond directly to a perceived threat, it may be taken up quickly (Bradley et al., 2004). Proven interventions that reflect novel ideas that are in fashion or are promoted by well-respected leaders may also be more likely to be adopted than those that do not (Abrahamson, 1996; Carlile, 2004). Alternately, the more radical or disruptive an intervention is to an organization and its workflow, staffing, and/or budgeting, the more value (e.g., cost savings, significant health benefits to individuals) it will need to generate and the more difficult it may be to find support for its adoption.

In some cases, an intervention may be too innovative, and may be adopted only with the passage of time or evolution of a particular practice or health policy environment. For example, years after they were first tested, interdisciplinary care coordination models in primary care, such as patient-centered medical homes and transitional care programs from hospital to home (including Coleman's Care Transition Program® [www.caretransitions.org/] and Naylor's Transitional Care Model [www.caretransitions.org/]), are receiving favorable attention in health care and community settings. Affordable Care Act programs (e.g., ACOs) and reimbursement changes that favor these approaches are making these evidence-based and well-tested models more attractive to organizations.

Another characteristic that influences dissemination potential involves whether an organization or setting has previously been an "early adopter" of an intervention (Rogers, 2003), or has a track record of taking on new programs. Organizations that have a track record of being early adopters may be more "receptive to change" than those that do not (Greenhalgh, Robert, Macfarlane, Bate, & Kyriakidou, 2004). Conversely, dissemination may falter when organizations with limited financial and staff resources are unable to take on new programs without significant external support. For example, Get Busy Get Better (originally known as Beat the Blues) is a community-based depression intervention designed for delivery within senior centers (Gitlin et al., 2012, 2013). However, better resourced mental health departments and state societies of geriatric care managers are more interested in the program as they have resources, including staff and allocations for staff training, to more easily support the program's training requirements than senior centers.

Evaluating Fit Between the Intervention and a Practice Setting

Another aspect that influences the potential of, and approach to, dissemination is the fit of a context and an intervention (again, discussed in more detail in Chapter 20). Here, several key attributes need to be considered: centrality of the intervention to the day-to-day work of an organization, agency, or individual; pervasiveness or behaviors expected to be affected by the intervention; and the degree to which the intervention challenges or changes accepted behaviors, cultural norms, or daily routines (Wolfe, 1994; also see Chapter 20 for other contextual elements). The perceived feasibility and ease of implementation of an intervention will influence how the intervention needs to be disseminated (Bradley et al., 2004). It is important to clearly describe how an organization can integrate a new program. For example, Care Management Plus (caremanagementplus.org/impsteps.html), a patient-centered medical home model developed at the Oregon Health & Science University, provides a clear step-by-step approach to integrating the intervention in a primary care clinic.

Determining Leadership Capacity

A fourth dimension that influences whether an intervention has dissemination potential is the person and/or group or team that will drive the process. An effective dissemination approach requires a charismatic and credible "champion" who can demonstrate the relevance and importance of an intervention to a variety of key decision makers and potential stakeholders. This person may be different from the lead investigator/researcher who developed/evaluated the intervention. The ability to create and nurture collaborative relationships with various settings, communities, or organizations is crucial (Gladwell, 2000) to successful dissemination. This champion must build awareness about an intervention and rally opinion leaders who influence decision making for the targeted setting.

Access to Communications Channels

The fifth dimension that influences dissemination potential is whether the investigator/ team has access to appropriate "communications channels" (Rogers, 2003), or ways to reach potential adopting agencies, settings, and interventionists and individuals who may benefit from the intervention. At the heart of a dissemination plan is identifying different forums for communicating about the intervention. This may include but is not limited to identifying local meetings, organizations, or settings where one can provide talks or demonstrations of the intervention in one-on-one or group meetings with key stakeholders such as agency or community leaders, Grand Rounds in health organizations, or other venues such as professional association meetings. For example, program leaders of the Chronic Disease Self-Management Program (CDSMP), a 6-week, six-class patient activation and peer-led model (Lorig et al., 1999), create a "drumbeat of touchpoints," including person-to-person marketing, in addition to more traditional flyers, brochures, and media outreach to disseminate the program in a particular locale (Compton, 2014).

For regional or national dissemination, researchers need access to professional journals and meetings, media (e.g., radio, television, print), social media, and/or other public relations vehicles to spread the word. Conduits that matter are the ones that provide access to the key decision makers of a practice setting and those individuals who may want to be interventionists as well as end users such as the consumers or ultimate beneficiaries of an intervention. This may mean publishing and presenting in settings other than traditional professional meetings. For example, in seeking to disseminate Guided Care, a patient-centered medical home model for older adults (Boult et al., 2011), the Johns Hopkins University team purposely sought out policy gatherings and meetings that involved clinicians and administrators of primary care practices and health systems (e.g., Case Management Society of America and TransforMED conferences), which the team had not attended previously.

Finding ways to partner with others who have access to key stakeholders and decision makers of organizations and settings is also important (Bradley et al., 2004). Identifying potential relationships and channels for broad dissemination early on in the pipeline when developing an intervention can be helpful.

To summarize, when advancing an intervention, it is important to determine its dissemination potential along five dimensions: intervention characteristics; the environmental context in which it might be embedded; the fit between the intervention and a particular context and perceived ease of implementation; capacity to lead a dissemination effort; and access to communication outlets. Helpful self-reflective questions to evaluate the dissemination potential of an intervention include the following:

- Does the intervention have characteristics that make it likely to be adopted?
- Is the broader environment or more local organizational context ripe for the innovation?
- Is the intervention team sufficiently credible and connected to the range of stakeholders necessary for adoption?
- Does the team have access to the right communication channels so that it can sufficiently communicate to and persuade potential adopters to implement the new program, intervention, service, or model?

BUILDING A ROBUST DISSEMINATION PLAN

If an intervention has dissemination potential, then the next step is to build a comprehensive dissemination plan. An effective dissemination plan has four key elements: knowledge of stakeholders and the potential environment in which an intervention will be implemented; persuasive value propositions for the intervention; an infrastructure to support dissemination activities; and a social marketing plan.

Knowledge of the Environment and Its Stakeholders

The first step in developing a dissemination plan is to conduct what is referred to as a "scan." This involves carefully identifying environments that may be conducive to implementing the intervention and deriving an understanding of what stakeholders in those environments (e.g., administrators, directors of agencies, community groups, organizations) need and want. Understanding the opportunities and potential challenges for implementing an intervention via scans is critical for efficiently moving an intervention into practice.

Typically, environmental and stakeholder scans are conducted following the publication of the trial outcomes for an intervention. However, scans can also be conducted early on in the pipeline as one is developing and evaluating an intervention at the pilot, efficacy, and/or effectiveness study phases (see Curran, Bauer, Mittman, Pyne, & Stetler, 2012). Similarly, in these early and evaluative phases, participants and/or their family members can be asked about their willingness to pay (Jutkowitz, Gitlin & Pizzi, 2010) for an intervention or the best way to promote the program among their peers as part of the battery of questions. Mixed methodologies (see Chapter 11) or community participatory research methods can also be used throughout the research process to understand the perceptions of interventionists, stakeholders, and participants concerning the acceptability and potential value of an intervention (Cornwall & Jewkes, 1995). For example, in the Personalized Reminder Information and Social Management System (PRISM) study (Czaja et al., 2015), individuals who participated in the pilot testing of the PRISM system were asked about the potential value of the system and how the system might enhance their ability to engage in everyday activities.

An environmental scan typically involves examining a combination of sources including conducting a systematic literature review, Internet research, focus group–type discussions with interventionists, and interviews with key informants who have an understanding of current relevant practices and/or community settings that may impact the implementation of an intervention (Berkowitz, 2010). Gathering information about perceptions of the intervention from stakeholders including interventionists and targeted populations also provides relevant information to the dissemination process. Table 21.3 outlines five key elements and related questions for an environmental scan in order to advance a dissemination plan for a proven program.

TABLE 21.3   Elements of, and Questions to Ask in, Environmental and Stakeholder Scans

Element	Relevant Research Questions
Current practice	How is a particular condition or problem currently addressed? What are strengths and limitations of current practices?
Competitive models and other market "threats"	How entrenched is the current way of addressing a problem? Is the environment stable or has it been involved with other successful or failed approaches? Are there new or developing interventions that represent future threats to the proposed new intervention that will need to be addressed? (Kotler, 1999)
Funding and reimbursement opportunities and challenges	How will the intervention be paid for? What are the most common reimbursement or other funding streams available?
Federal, state, and local policy opportunities and challenges	What is the current policy environment that might help or hinder the adoption of an intervention?
Health system or hospital policy opportunities and challenges	What is happening in the system or organization that may provide support for, or hinder the use of, an intervention? (Flood, 2013)

As noted earlier, a scan of stakeholders also typically involves key informant interviews. As Brugha and Varvasovszky (2000) explain, these types of interviews "generate knowledge about the relevant actors so as to understand their behaviors, intentions, interrelations, agendas, interests, and the influence or resources they can bring to bear on decision making" (p. 239). It is important to identify how stakeholders prefer to receive information to learn about evidence-based practices.

There are numerous ways to conduct this analysis depending upon the stakeholders, one's access to groups, and available budget and resources. One-on-one interviews with stakeholder representatives, such as organizational leaders, policy makers, agency heads, regulators, busy clinicians, or individuals targeted for the intervention are perhaps the easiest and most cost-effective way to obtain an initial sense of how an intervention is viewed. These qualitative conversations can reveal helpful insights concerning the level of engagement and the breadth and representativeness of the respondents' viewpoints toward an intervention. These interviews also provide an introduction to the intervention to potential decision makers and an opportunity to gauge their initial reactions, concerns, and the nature of their queries.

"Convenience" focus groups are another way to capture stakeholder viewpoints. Using existing monthly meetings, say of hospital nurses or long-term care facility's social workers, can provide rich information about the perceptions of frontline staff concerning an intervention. This approach requires an able facilitator and a systematic process for transcribing and identifying key issues that emerge from the group discussions. If budget allows, outsourcing this activity and using professionally run focus groups can be helpful. However, this may cost $5,000 per focus group or more (Lee, 2002). Finally, Internet services such as SurveyMonkey, Zoomerang, or Survey Gizmo provide inexpensive and accessible platforms for online surveys that can explore stakeholder attitudes and preferences. Even Facebook can be used to obtain quick feedback from select communities concerning an intervention. Use of these strategies can be helpful with larger groups, particularly later in the process to help determine pricing and even test messaging and other marketing approaches with consumers (e.g., patients, participants, families) before making significant investments in dissemination.

Value Propositions: Describing What Is in It for "Them"

With an understanding of the environmental/organizational context and the needs, attitudes, and values of key stakeholders, an investigator/team needs to create compelling messages or "value propositions" for these respective groups. A value proposition is a brief statement of the worth, potential benefits/costs, significance, or importance of an intervention. The concept derives from management consulting where it was formally defined as "a clear, simple statement of the benefits, both tangible and intangible, that [a] company will provide, along with the approximate price it will charge each customer segment for those benefits" (Golub et al., 2000). In the context of disseminating behavioral interventions, this statement or rationale should include both incremental benefits of the intervention for various stakeholders over usual practice (e.g., better outcomes, savings) and an acknowledgment of the costs involved (e.g., staff training costs) (Barnes, Blake, & Pinder, 2009). It is helpful to examine benefits and costs of an intervention for potential end users as early as possible.

A value proposition statement may vary according to the targeted stakeholder. For example, an intervention that provides respite and more time to self might be perceived as valuable to a family caregiver; whereas the low cost for delivery of a particular intervention and brief time for training interventionists may be what is valued most by an agency director who is considering integrating the intervention into its service offerings. Thus, a value statement targeting the caregivers would need to emphasize the respite benefits, whereas the value statement targeting agency directors would need to emphasize the low cost and minimal training requirements. The Hospital at Home program, noted earlier (and described in Chapter 20), improved a variety of health outcomes and lowered the cost of care per patient. However, for fee-for-service-driven hospitals with open beds, which depended on filling those beds and providing services for revenues, this benefit was initially viewed as a negative and a potential "cost" of the intervention (Dr. Bruce Leff, personal communication, January 25, 2015). With the change from fee-for-service to value-based health care, the Hospital at Home program is now more attractive to hospital systems.

An effective value proposition must describe the benefits of an intervention and acknowledge the potential costs. Potential intervention costs include financial (e.g., new salaries, materials, licensing, and/or training fees), marketing, staff time and effort for program implementation, and the psychological costs associated with having to give up (or deimplement) previously held ideas, favorite programs, services, or practices, even if they were not effective, in order to implement a new intervention (Barnes et al., 2009). An effective value proposition must persuasively frame the benefits of adopting the intervention such that the benefits outweigh perceived and real costs.

Take the example of Skills$_2$Care^R, a home-based occupational therapy intervention (originally called the Environmental Skills Program) developed and tested by Dr. Gitlin and her team at Thomas Jefferson University as part of the NIH REACH I (Resources for Enhancing Alzheimer's Caregiver Health) initiative. This program, delivered by occupational therapists, provides education and skill building including environmental modifications, and communication and task simplification strategies to help family caregivers provide better care for persons with dementia. In trying to persuade home health agencies to implement the intervention and train their occupational therapists, Skills$_2$Care^R staff first identified a fee structure similar to that of other professional development activities and within the average training budgets of agencies identified through interviews and Web-based research. This cost was then compared to the increased revenue that trained occupational therapists could generate by delivering Skills$_2$Care^R for an agency. By integrating the program within the traditional home care treatment of persons with dementia, the family training is reimbursable under Medicare Parts A and B. Despite the initial outlay for training their therapists, adopting agencies could effectively recoup their training costs by taking on 80 new Skills$_2$Care^R clients in a year (Gitlin, Jacobs, & Vause-Earland, 2010; Jefferson Elder Care, 2009). As a result, home care agencies could clearly perceive both the value of the program for their clients and understand the investment needed on their part and were thus willing to have their staff trained in this approach. As the training costs fit within an agency's typical allocation to support continuing education activities of therapists, the program was perceived as a win for therapists, a win for clients and their families, and a win for the agency.

However, a value proposition is not just about its cost savings or financial benefits. Other potential gains may be equally important. For example, demonstrating clinician satisfaction with an intervention either through a formal study or testimonials gathered at the testing phase may be important for convincing doctors, nurses, occupational therapists, social workers, or other health and human service professionals about the value of an intervention. Connecting an intervention to the larger strategic goals of an institution, care system, agency, or community organization can be an important part of the value proposition for administrators and leaders. Similarly, providing national or local recognition for an institution (e.g., positive publicity with a key patient segment or magnet or other meaningful designations) can be a critical part of the value proposition for a hospital, clinical facility, or system leadership.

In developing a value proposition, it is important to consider the following questions:

- What would it take to convince a particular stakeholder (e.g., agency director) to support the intervention or invest funds to have staff trained?
- What will convince a busy clinician to devote limited time and energy to become trained in an intervention?
- What will convince a participant or patient to sign up for, or even pay to receive, an intervention?
- What strategies can be used to help offset any perceived costs or barriers?

When creating value propositions, the investigative team may discover that the intervention does not yield enough compelling value for stakeholders. By understanding the values of stakeholders early on in the pipeline, investigators can shape or reshape the intervention accordingly or proceed as planned but with the knowledge of the potential dissemination challenges that will lie ahead. For example, although Skills$_2$Care^R created a strong financial value proposition for agencies, some potential adopters could not accommodate the 3 or more days of in-person training that the approach originally required. Agencies perceived it as too disruptive and expensive. The in-person training component was subsequently shortened to 1 day and was complemented by self-directed online lectures and ongoing technical assistance to provide interventionists varied approaches to obtain the needed knowledge and skills to implement the program (Gitlin et al., 2010).

As decisions to adopt a particular intervention are always local, value propositions may not be fully generalizable and will need to be adapted to meet local considerations of different systems, organizations, and communities, all of which have diverse values, cultures, and perceived needs.

Creating an Infrastructure and Plan for Dissemination

An infrastructure that includes resources, protocols, and staff is needed to support dissemination activities. This may include conducting environmental and stakeholder scans, creating value propositions, and identifying different ways of broadcasting or distributing information about the intervention. Some research institutions have, or are developing, an infrastructure to support this type of work; alternately, it is possible to engage professional consultants or staff to specifically take on the work of dissemination. In either case, there are six basic steps outlined in Table 21.4 that an investigator/team can pursue to get ready to disseminate an intervention.

One step is to develop a meaningful name for the intervention and to protect the rights to associated intellectual property (e.g., training materials or modules and technological tools). The name of an intervention should not be too long or difficult to use or remember, nor should it be used by others or previously trademarked. Some modest due diligence is important to ensure a name is useable. This can easily be done by conducting a Web search or a brief search on the Patent Office's website. When interviewing end users of an intervention (agency administrators, clinicians, participants), including questions about potential names can provide insight as to what name might be preferred.

When a program is ready (or almost ready) to be disseminated, contacting a university's Technology Transfer or similar office or an intellectual property lawyer can provide the investigative team with expert consultation on how to trademark a name, copyright materials, or patent the intervention. As trademarking a name typically requires a fee, assuring resources for this process is important. (LegalZoom. com., n.d.) Access to an attorney can be costly, as there may be costs involved for a professional trademark search, analysis, and associated applications of anywhere from a few hundred to a few thousand dollars (SecureYourTrademark.com, 2014). Universities may also charge for this service.

Registering a trademarked name is a way to ensure that others do not use the name for similar programs and create confusion in the marketplace. Conversely, it can protect an investigative team from trademark challenges from other, often private sector services that are seeking an exclusive use of that name. Ultimately, a trademark can serve as a brand asset if a program or service is sold to a private sector or other group interested in its broad dissemination.

Implementation and training manuals or supporting materials are also important to protect. These can easily be copyrighted to discourage use without proper attribution. In practice, many behavioral and other nonpharmacologic approaches do not try to generate significant revenues from their materials, either making them available for free or as part of licensing or training packages (Beilenson, 2012). However, the intervention and associated materials should still be legally protected.

A second step is to ensure that all intervention manuals and materials are finalized and ready to be disseminated. Materials should be written in clear,

---

TABLE 21.4 Checklist for Building a Dissemination Infrastructure

- Select a name for the intervention program that is not in use in similar programs and fields and may be trademarked or protected against improper use by others.
- Develop clear and easy-to-follow manuals and other training materials.
- Establish a protocol for training and technical assistance capacity.
- Consider developing a website (for marketing and to hold training and other materials).
- Develop a social marketing plan that includes a clear set of dissemination objectives, stakeholder analysis, value propositions, and strategies and tactics that deliver the value proposition to key stakeholders in the service of the objectives.
- Identify needed staff, consultants, expertise, and financial support to create the materials described above, as well as implement the social marketing plan.

nontechnical language and printed in formats that can be replicated easily or reside as PDFs on a website. Materials need to include step-by-step and easy-to-understand instructions concerning how to conduct the intervention and administer the assessments, and include sample forms, presentations, and other materials that staff or volunteers will need to use in delivering the intervention. These resources should be pilot tested to ensure their usability before broad dissemination.

The third step is to establish an approach to training interventionists to deliver the intervention on the basis of the best evidence whether it be face-to-face, an online platform, through webinars, or other media. The investigative team must consider who will deliver the training and whether a train-the-trainer program or other approach will enable wide-scale dissemination.

A fourth step is to consider creating a website that is dedicated to information about the intervention. A website can be a cost-effective approach for housing training materials, tutorials, and other support resources that agencies, interventionists, or others may need as they implement the intervention. A website, however, does have some costs, notably in terms of the staff resources required to keep it current.

The fifth step involves developing a social marketing plan and associated tactics that serve to build greater awareness about an intervention among key stakeholders, decision makers, and potential adopters (Kotler & Armstrong, 2010).

Finally, consideration must be given to staffing and the associated budget required to carry out the aforementioned activities. Developing a marketing plan and understanding the return on investment may be important as well as showing cost neutrality or revenue generation.

WHAT DOES DISSEMINATION COST?

Although there are no published guidelines, experience suggests that between $50,000 to $250,000 or even more in funding may be necessary to begin dissemination activities. Unlike pharmaceutical development, there is not an industry and associated infrastructure directed at promoting behavioral intervention research. In this respect, the drug development pipeline is significantly distinct from the dissemination activities necessary for behavioral interventions.

Finding access to sufficient capital for broad national or even international dissemination can be a challenge. Select private foundations can provide significant seed funding, sometimes ranging into the millions of dollars. For example, the Robert Wood Johnson Foundation and several other private funders provided significant seed money to establish the Center to Advance Palliative Care and the dissemination infrastructure that has ultimately established palliative care programs in hundreds of hospitals and more broadly (Center to Advance Palliative Care, 2014). The John A. Hartford Foundation and other funders provided more than $11 million to conduct a multisite trial of the IMPACT depression intervention. Following the positive results from this trial, the Foundation granted the University of Washington $2.4 million to start a dissemination effort and ultimately helped to establish the Advancing Integrated Mental Health Services (AIMS) Center, which now generates revenue sources from other private sources as well as grants and training fees (John A. Hartford Foundation, 2013). Between 2003 and 2012, the federal Administration on Aging, as well as private funders including The Atlantic Philanthropies, invested more than $50 million to help the National Council on Aging and 45 states build a national infrastructure to disseminate to community groups and help them implement evidence-based health promotion programs for older people, notably the Stanford CDSMP. This dissemination and implementation effort resulted in more than 100,000 participants in these programs between 2010 and 2012 alone and supported efforts sustained by many states to continue to make the program available to older people. Throughout this period and subsequently, Stanford has maintained its own dissemination system that has been fostered by this federal effort (National Council on Aging, 2012). Whatever the source of capital, resources are needed to pay for staff, materials, websites, meetings, and other necessary resources to launch, establish, and sustain an effective dissemination effort. Dissemination activities must be sustained, often through a combination of sources of funding including but not limited to some kind of government funding, in-kind university support, outside grants, and/or ongoing training and licensing revenue.

Efforts directed toward advocating for policy and reimbursement changes are related to this search for capital. This can be labor-intensive, requiring time, relationships, and resources. Seeking legislative or administrative support for a new program's distribution through a state or nationally is dependent on both the research team's capacity and the opportunities that may be (and are often not) available in the prevailing political environment. Seeking reimbursement adjustments to make an intervention more financially attractive to clinical providers can be a similarly challenging (though completely necessary) aspect of a dissemination effort. In all cases, it is better to know early on whether an intervention can be easily reimbursed, or know the payment mechanism that can support its implementation. If current payment structures are a barrier, then it may be very challenging for a proven intervention to be adopted by organizations. Alternately, the investigator needs to adjust his or her expectations accordingly, or seek modifications to the intervention to make it a more natural fit in a dynamic reimbursement environment.

CONCLUSION

In summary, dissemination may seem remote to researchers just beginning to develop an innovative behavioral intervention, when efficacy still needs to be proven. However, it is never too early to start thinking about dissemination. Consideration of dissemination at the beginning of the pipeline is helpful as the work of dissemination is long term and resource intensive. Environmental and stakeholder scans as well as identifying value propositions can be conducted early on in the pipeline and subsequently shape the choice of delivery characteristics of an intervention in addition to informing dissemination approaches. Also, clearly articulating a goal for dissemination is important. For example, is the goal for the intervention to be integrated in all primary care practices, churches, and hospitals or can individuals obtain the intervention off the shelf (e.g., a Web-based program or application for purchase)? Knowing what one wants to achieve with an intervention is critical. Given the dynamic nature of health and human service and community organizations and population needs, the investigator/team must remain agile and ready to modify dissemination plans to address developing challenges and emerging opportunities as they arise.

REFERENCES

Abrahamson, E. (1996). Management fashion. *Academy of Management Review, 21*(1), 254–285.

Agency for Healthcare Research and Quality. (2011, October). *The number of practicing primary care physicians in the United States: Primary care workforce facts and stats no. 1.* Rockville, MD: Author. Retrieved from http://www.ahrq.gov/research/findings/factsheets/primary/pcwork1/index.html

Barnes, C., Blake, H., & Pinder, D. (2009). *Creating and delivering your value proposition: Managing customer experience for profit.* London, England: Kogan Page.

Beilenson, J. (2012). *Field brief: Characteristics of successful diffusion efforts of geriatrics innovations.* Wayne, PA: Strategic, Communications & Planning (SCP).

Berkowitz, E. N. (2010). *Essentials of health care marketing* (3rd ed.). Burlington, MA: Jones & Bartlett Learning.

Berwick, D. M. (2003). Disseminating innovations in health care. *Journal of the American Medical Association, 289*(15), 1969–1975. doi:10.1001/jama.289.15.1969

Bondi, A. (2000). *Characteristics of scalability and their impact on performance.* Retrieved from http://www.win.tue.nl/~johanl/educ/2II45/2010/Lit/Scalability-bondi%202000.pdf

Boult, C., Reider, L., Leff, B., Frick, K. D., Boyd, C. M., Wolff, J. L., . . . Scharfstein, D. O. (2011). The effect of guided care teams on the use of health services: Results from a cluster-randomized controlled trial. *Archives of Internal Medicine, 171*(5), 460–466. doi:10.1001/archinternmed.2010.540

Bradley, E., Webster, T., Baker, D., Schlesinger, M., Inouye, S. K., Barth, M. C., . . . Koren, M. J. (2004). *Translating research into practice: Speeding the adoption of innovative health care programs.* Retrieved from http://www.commonwealthfund.org/programs/elders/bradley_translating_research_724.pdf

Brugha, R., & Varvasovszky, Z. (2000). Stakeholder analysis: A review. *Health Policy and Planning, 15*(3), 239–246. doi:10.1093/heapol/15.3.239

Carlile, P. R. (2004). Transferring, translating, and transforming: An integrative framework for managing knowledge across boundaries. *Organizational Science, 15*(5), 555–568.

Center to Advance Palliative Care. (2014). Retrieved from https://www.capc.org/

Compton, T. (2014). *Marketing your workshops.* Retrieved from National Council on Aging webinar slideset, https://www.ncoa.org/wp-content/uploads/BCBHMarketing-1.pdf

Cornwall, A., & Jewkes, R. (1995). What is participatory research? *Social Science & Medicine, 41,* 1667–1676.

Curran, G. M., Bauer, M., Mittman, B., Pyne, J. M., & Stetler, C. (2012). Effectiveness-implementation hybrid designs: Combining elements of clinical effectiveness and implementation research to enhance public health impact. *Medical Care, 50*(3), 217–226.

Czaja, S. J., Boot, W. R., Carness, N., Rogers, W. A., Sharit, J., Fisk, A. D., . . . Nair, S. N. (2015). The personalized reminder information and social management system (PRISM) trial: Rationale, methods and baseline characteristics. *Contemporary Clinical Trials, 40,* 35–46.

Flood, K. (2013, May). *Making the (business) case for acute care for elders programs in hospitals.* Presented at 2013 annual meeting of the American Geriatrics Society, Orlando, FL.

Fogarty International Center NIH. (n.d.). *Implementation science information and resources.* Retrieved from http://www.fic.nih.gov/researchtopics/pages/implementationscience.aspx

Gitlin, L. N., Harris, L. F., McCoy, M. C., Chernett, N. L., Pizzi, L. T., Jutkowitz, E., Hess, E., & Hauck, W. W. (2013). A home-based intervention to reduce depressive symptoms and improve quality of life in older African Americans. *Annals of Internal Medicine, 159*(4), 243-252.

Gitlin, L. N., Harris, L. F., McCoy, M., Chernett, N. L., Jutkowitz, E., Pizzi, L. T., & The Beat The Blues Team. (2012). A community-integrated home-based depression intervention for older African Americans: Description of the Beat the Blues randomized trial and intervention costs. *BMC Geriatrics, 12*, 4. doi:10.1186/1471-2318-12-4.

Gitlin, L. N., Jacobs, M., & Vause-Earland, T. (2010). Translation of a dementia caregiver intervention for delivery in homecare as a reimbursable Medicare service: Outcomes and lessons learned. *The Gerontologist, 50*(6), 847–854. doi:10.1093/geront/gnq057

Gladwell, M. (2000). *The tipping point: How little things can make a big difference.* New York, NY: Little Brown.

Golub, H., Henry, J, Forbis P. L., Mehta, N. T., Lanning, M. J., Michaels, E. J., & Ohmae, K. (2000, September). Delivering value to customer. *McKinsey Quarterly.* Retrieved from http://www.mckinsey.com/insights/strategy/delivering_value_to_customers

Greenhalgh, T., Robert, G., Macfarlane, F., Bate, P., & Kyriakidou, O. (2004). Diffusion of innovations in service organizations: Systematic review and recommendations, *MilbankQuarterly, 82*(4), 581–629.

Institute of Medicine. (2001). *Crossing the quality chasm: A new health system for the 21st century.* Washington, DC: National Academy Press.

Jefferson Elder Care. (2009). *Environmental skill-building program (ESP) business plan.* Prepared by SCP. Wayne, PA: SCP.

John A. Hartford Foundation. (2013). *2012 annual report: Spreading innovation through collaboration.* Retrieved from: http://www.jhartfound.org/ar2013/index.html

Jutkowitz, E., Gitlin, L. N., & Pizzi, L. T. (2010). Evaluating willingness to pay thresholds for dementia caregiving interventions: Application to the tailored activity program. *Value in Health, 13*(6), 720–725. doi:10.1111/j.1524-4733.2010.00739.x

Kerner, J., Rimer, B., & Emmons, K. (2005). Introduction to the special section on dissemination: Dissemination research and research dissemination: How can we close the gap? *Health Psychology, 24*(5), 443–446.

Kotler, P. (1999). *Kotler on marketing: How to create, win and dominate markets.* New York, NY: The Free Press.

Kotler, P., & Armstrong, G. M. (2010). *Principles of marketing.* New York, NY: Prentice-Hall.

Kotler, P., & Zaltman, G. (1971). Social marketing: A planned approach to social change, *Journal of Marketing, 35,* 3–12.

Lee, M. Y. (2002). Conducting surveys and focus groups. *Entrepreneur.* Retrieved from http://www.entrepreneur.com/article/55680

Leff, B., Burton, L., Mader, S. L., Naughton, B., Burl, J., Inouye, S. K., . . . Burton, J. R. (2005). Hospital at home: feasibility and outcomes of a program to provide hospital-level care at home for acutely ill older patients. *Annals of Internal Medicine, 143*(11), 798–808.

LegalZoom.com. (n.d.). *Cost to trademark—Trademark application prices and fees.* Retrieved from http://www.legalzoom.com/trademarks/trademarks-pricing.html

Lorig, K., Sobel, D. S., Stewart, A. L., Brown, B. W., Bandura, A., Ritter, P., . . . Holman, H. R. (1999). Evidence suggesting that a chronic disease self-management program can improve health status while reducing hospitalization: A randomized trial. *Medical Care, 37*(1), 5–14.

McCannon, C. J., Berwick, D. M., & Massoud, M. R. (2007). The science of large-scale change in global health. *Journal of the American Medical Association, 298*(16), 1937–1939.

National Council on Aging. (2012). *American recovery and reinvestment act communities putting prevention to work: Chronic disease self-management program (CDSMP) capping report.*

Retrieved from http://www.ncoa.org/improve-health/center-for-healthy-aging/content-library/ARRA-GRANTEE-Capping-eport-Final-6-25-1.pdf

National Institutes of Health. (2011). Retrieved 4th Annual NIH Conference on the Science of Dissemination and Implementation: Policy and Practice from http://obssr.od.nih.gov/scientific_areas/translation/dissemination_and_implementation/DI2011/abstracts.html

O'Neill, H., Pouder, R. W., & Bucholtz, A. K. (1998). Patterns in the diffusion of strategies across organizations: Insights from the innovation diffusion literature. *Academy of Management Review, 23*(1), 98–114.

Powers, D. (2015, April 30). *Partnership advances a revolution in mental health care.* Retrieved from http://www.jhartfound.org/blog/partnership-advances-a-revolution-in-mental-health-care/#sthash.ZO0w6F8o.dpuf

Rogers, E. (2003). *Diffusion of innovations* (5th ed.) New York, NY: Free Press.

Schillinger, D. (2010). *An introduction to effectiveness, dissemination and implementation research* (P. Fleisher & E. Goldstein, Eds.). From the series: UCSF Clinical and Translational Science Institute (CTSI) Resource manuals and guides to community-engaged research (P. Fleisher, Series Ed.). San Francisco, CA: Clinical Translational Science Institute Community Engagement Program, University of California, San Francisco. Retrieved from https://accelerate.ucsf.edu/files/CE/edi_introguide.pdf

SecureYourTrademark.com. (2014). *How much does it cost to trademark a name?* Retrieved from https://secureyourtrademark.com/blog/

Simpson, D., & Dansereau, D. (2007, September 26). Assessing organizational functioning as a step toward innovation. *Science & Practice Perspectives, 3*(2), 20–28. National Center for Biotechnology Information. Retrieved from http://www.ncbi.nlm.nih.gov/pmc/articles/PMC2851070/

Unützer, J., Katon, W., Callahan, C. M., Williams, J. W., Jr., Hunkeler, E., Harpole, L., . . . Langston, C. (2002). Collaborative care management of late-life depression in the primary care setting: A randomized controlled trial. *Journal of the American Medical Association, 288*(22), 2836–2845. doi:10.1001/jama.288.22.2836.

Unützer, J., Katon, W. J., Fan, M. Y., Schoenbaum, M. C., Lin, E. H., Della Penna, R. D., & Powers, D. (2008). Long-term cost effects of collaborative care for late-life depression. *The American Journal of Managed Care, 14*(2), 95–100.

Wolfe, B. (1994). Organizational innovation: Review, critique and suggested research directions. *Journal of Management Studies, 31,* 405–431. doi:10.1111/j.1467-6486.1994.tb00624.x

PART V

PROFESSIONAL CONSIDERATIONS AND REFLECTIONS

In this concluding section, we consider a range of professional activities important to behavioral intervention researchers. Given that behavioral intervention research is a complex form of inquiry requiring different skill sets, in Chapter 22 we explore what it takes to become a behavioral intervention researcher. Furthermore, as advancing a behavioral intervention requires resources, writing competitive grant applications is essential to intervention research. Thus, general grant-writing considerations and those specific to advancing behavioral interventions are explored in Chapter 23. In Chapter 24, we examine publication possibilities throughout the stages of the pipeline—for example, as one develops and evaluates an intervention and when waiting for the main outcomes of an efficacy or effectiveness trial. Finally, in Chapter 25, we offer a concise review and reflection of the significant points addressed in each chapter and offer suggestions for future directions for behavioral intervention research.

The key "take home" points of Part V include the following:

- Behavioral intervention researchers must possess various skills including how to develop and lead teams, how to involve individuals from diverse disciplines, and how to engage, train, and support team members.
- Writing competitive grant applications is necessary and important to support intervention development across the pipeline.
- Publishing is an important professional activity, and there are multiple opportunities for reporting about an intervention even before the main outcomes of a trial are available.

TWENTY TWO

BECOMING AND BEING A BEHAVIORAL INTERVENTION RESEARCHER: WHAT DOES IT TAKE?

What we find changes who we become.
—Peter Morville

As we have discussed in previous chapters, conducting behavioral intervention research can be challenging, involving complex decision making. Intervention development takes time, limited funds may be available, and multiple roles and skills are needed for success as one advances an intervention along a pipeline. Consequently, participating in this form of inquiry is not for everyone. It requires a wide range of skills and a particular disposition to become and be a behavioral intervention researcher.

The skills required to be a behavioral intervention researcher are manifold and differ as one proceeds with advancing an intervention. Besides envisioning an intervention and having sound research training, an intervention researcher needs to possess critical-thinking and action skills that include but are not necessarily limited to knowing how to (a) hire and effectively manage staff; (b) build and nurture teams; (c) communicate with and effectively involve multiple and different stakeholders; (d) write competitive grant applications to support intervention design and testing; (e) budget, rebudget, and monitor expenditures; (f) problem solve recruitment and retention challenges; (g) troubleshoot protocol violations; (h) address potentially serious adverse events that may or may not be related to the intervention or study; (i) publish and present findings to diverse audiences; and (j) either be responsible for or work with others who lead the efforts to translate, implement, and disseminate a proven intervention. Additionally, along the way, a researcher may need to develop new measures that are sensitive to the impact of the proposed intervention; be involved in cost analyses to determine intervention feasibility; and/or work with statisticians to identify different statistical analytic strategies for identifying who benefits and why, and all areas for which little to no previous exposure or training may have been formally obtained.

Unlike cross-sectional or epidemiologic studies that are typically time limited, involve secondary data sets, or require a well-defined and prescribed skill set, intervention research is much more dynamic in terms of its demands and continuous need for on-the-spot troubleshooting and learning of new techniques and strategies.

As it involves engagement in dynamic and changing contexts (e.g., diverse populations, clinical settings, communities, agencies, policies; see Chapter 1, Figure 1.2) and interactions with real people and end users of an intervention, participation in this line of work requires a particular disposition that includes persistence, tenacity, and flexibility, as well as being a proactive problem solver and team leader and having a high level of energy and dedication. Paramount, of course, is holding a firm belief in the value of an intervention—that the intervention can make a real difference in a person's life or a community—and then having the patience and, above all else, the passion for its advancement.

This chapter is about the real work of being a behavioral intervention researcher. We discuss a range of common challenges and professional considerations in the conduct of behavioral intervention research, and offer guidance where possible. Specifically, we examine "hot button" issues related to staffing, collaborating with others, leading teams, and career development and intellectual property considerations. As these aspects of behavioral intervention research are rarely written about, discussed, or formally presented and there is no consensus on, or documented, best practices, our discussion necessarily builds upon our many years of field experience. Our discussion encapsulates considerations that arise in, or are relevant to, any stage of an intervention's development, although some issues may dominate one phase along the pipeline versus another. However, understanding the considerations we present is helpful regardless of whether one is a novice or expert, at the beginning phases of developing an intervention, or seeking to translate, implement, or disseminate it.

STAFF-RELATED CONSIDERATIONS

Most behavioral intervention studies, regardless of phase of development or where they are situated along the pipeline, will require some type of staffing. A principal investigator of a behavioral intervention study simply cannot do it all or alone. This is an important difference between this form of research and other research endeavors such as the analyses of secondary data sets, in which the staffing needs are specific to analytic and related research techniques and skills. The type of staffing needed for a behavioral intervention study will, of course, depend upon the study phase, the level of complexity of the study design, the characteristics, scope, and nature of the intervention as well as control groups involved and the characteristics of the targeted population. For example, important questions include: Do staff need to be bilingual? Do they need specific clinical expertise or knowledge of a targeted population? A Phase III efficacy trial with two treatment arms and a targeted sample of 300 study participants will require more staffing and oversight than a Phase I pilot phase in which a single component intervention is initially being constructed and evaluated for feasibility with 25 individuals. Whereas the former may require hiring upwards of 20 staff with diverse skill sets and roles and responsibilities, the latter may necessitate employing only a part-time research assistant. An intervention involving face-to-face sessions will require hiring two or more personnel to serve as interventionists whereas the test of a computer-automated telephone information intervention may require an instructional design expert to develop content and its presentation and a technician to assist with technical difficulties if they should occur in the field.

Regardless of study design and evaluative phase, there is a host of issues to consider related to staffing. These include learning about the hiring process in one's institutional setting, securing space, specifying roles and responsibilities, designing a backup plan, and providing adequate training, ongoing support, and oversight.

Hiring Process

As each institution has different hiring practices and processes, prior to staffing a project it is important to know institutional requirements. Specifically, it is helpful to have an understanding of specific job titles and classifications and their associated salary ranges, available employment options (e.g., casual, part-time, or full-time) and associated benefits, hiring processes including who can hire and interview, titles for position descriptions and templates for posting positions, the typical length of time for the hiring process, onboarding practices, and yearly performance evaluations and firing guidelines. Knowing about and then navigating institutional policies, particularly as it concerns the hiring process, is essential. Hiring processes can take a long time (upwards of 6 months or more) and hence impact study time lines, what is possible to achieve, and the appropriate spending of one's grant budget within allocated time lines. The length of time to identify and bring a staff member on board can vary widely depending upon the candidate pool, institutional policies and practices, whether an internal or external candidate is hired, and availability of funding, space, and other needed resources. Allowing sufficient time for the hiring process is important as it may vary vastly from 1 to 9 months or more and, in turn, delay rapid start-up of a study and entering the field.

Space Considerations

A second consideration concerns staff needs with respect to space and equipment (e.g., telephone, computer, tablets). Availability of space and other needed resources vary tremendously among research environments. Space is always tricky as research staff are typically hired for a relatively brief period (1–5 years) to carry out particular research-related tasks supported through external grant funds. Thus, many institutions develop makeshift spaces or identify ad hoc locations for persons. If possible, however, it is preferable to negotiate space in which all project-related staff are in relative proximity (same floor, same office suite) as opposed to being dispersed across different buildings, wings, or floors. Dispersion of staff may result in the need to duplicate study materials and lead to inefficiencies and difficulties in supervising and smoothly performing daily research operations. Similarly, securing the right type of space is important. Staff responsible for screening or interviewing study participants by telephone will need quiet and private space, whereas those who need to remain masked to group allocation must be physically separated from those who need to be aware of group assignments. Thus, the location of staff offices can have methodological implications with some office space configurations presenting a challenge for maintaining confidentiality and concealment of group assignments. Furthermore, staff who spend most of their time in the "field" for interviewing or providing interventions in participants' homes or at community settings or agencies may not require dedicated office space; however, they will still need a touchdown space to complete computer or paperwork associated with their research tasks. Also, having ready access to adequate locked storage capacity for keeping informed consents and other data forms are important space considerations with methodological import.

Roles and Responsibilities

A third consideration is identifying and differentiating the roles and responsibilities of each staff member by breaking down each study-related task and identifying the associated activities for implementing the intervention study. As there is a high level of interdependency in the roles of staff members on an intervention study, clearly articulating how each staff member communicates and relates to another is also important.

Table 22.1 presents 10 common staff positions and their associated key roles and skill sets. Although this list is not exhaustive and is most relevant to a Phase III efficacy trial, it provides guidance to the potential staffing needs for other types and phases of intervention development work.

One key role in intervention research is that of the project coordinator/ manager or director. In early intervention development phases, the primary investigator may serve in this capacity. However, even for pilot efforts, or in testing and implementation phases, it is typically necessary to hire a part- to full-time coordinator or project manager. The role of this person will vary on the basis of the scope and

TABLE 22.1 Ten Key Roles on a Study Designed to Test a Behavioral Intervention

Role	Key Responsibilities	Key Skill Set Needed
Principal investigator	■ Oversees scientific integrity of study ■ Contributes content expertise ■ Establishes project structure	■ Content expertise ■ Skill developing and running project staff ■ Ability to oversee budget
Coinvestigator(s)	■ Contributes discrete area of content expertise	■ Content expertise
Project coordinator/ manager	■ Day-to-day coordination ■ Trains and supervises staff ■ Meets with investigative team ■ Organizes reports ■ Generates study updates (tables, charts, narrative summaries) ■ Coordinates recruitment efforts	■ Detail oriented ■ Problem solver ■ Good writing skills ■ Good communicator ■ Organized ■ Knowledgeable about Institutional Review Board (IRB) ■ Knowledgeable about data entry
Recruitment coordinator	■ Establishes recruitment strategy ■ Outreach and tracking ■ Assists with enrollment ■ Provides recruitment and enrollment accrual reports/ charts	■ Detail oriented ■ Good communicator ■ Organized ■ Able to provide brief talks to stakeholders/ recruitment sites

(Continued)

TABLE 22.1 Ten Key Roles on a Study Designed to Test a Behavioral Intervention (*Continued*)

Role	Key Responsibilities	Key Skill Set Needed
Interviewer(s)	▪ Obtains informed consent ▪ Interviews in-person, telephone, or online ▪ Checks code work for accuracy ▪ Reports adverse events	▪ Good problem-solving skills ▪ Able to follow a protocol ▪ Able to build rapport with study participants ▪ Organized ▪ Attention to detail ▪ Able to keep project coordinator informed in a timely way ▪ Comfortable with being observed or monitored and obtaining feedback for fidelity purposes ▪ Some knowledge of working with targeted study population
Interventionist(s)	▪ Implements experimental and/or control group protocols ▪ Completes study documentation ▪ Reports adverse events ▪ Balances protocol with clinical prerogatives	▪ Able to follow a protocol ▪ Able to build rapport with study participants ▪ Organized ▪ Comfortable with being observed or monitored and obtaining feedback for fidelity purposes ▪ Some knowledge of working with targeted study population
Data entry/ coders/ cleaners	▪ Cleans data ▪ Enters data ▪ Checks for accuracy of data entry	▪ Attentive to detail ▪ Knowledge of software program used ▪ Organized
Statistician	▪ Assists in determining statistical analyses and interpretation	▪ Working knowledge of clinical trial methodology, intention to treat, case modeling, moderator and mediation analyses
Database manager	▪ Establishes and maintains data files	▪ Working knowledge of statistical programs, setting up data collected over time at multiple testing occasions (if relevant)
Research assistant	▪ Helps with daily research-related activities such as duplicating materials, entering data	▪ Ability to work independently ▪ Organized ▪ Detail oriented

nature of the study. Roles may include but are not limited to coordination of and involvement in day-to-day operations; recruitment strategies; assigning interviewer and intervention schedules; data entry procedures; fidelity activities; training and supervising interviewers; and institutional review board submissions and required yearly reports to funders.

Persons with previous research experience and who are prepared at a master's or, preferably, a doctoral level who can excel at this position may be preferred. Having some research experience can be helpful as there are many moving pieces in an intervention study and field conditions often change and need to be efficiently managed. Nevertheless, individuals with a bachelor's degree with previous research experience and who are savvy, detail oriented, and organized may also perform effectively in this position.

Another key position is the interviewer/assessor. The needed level of expertise for this role will depend upon the nature and scope of the data being collected. If clinical testing is necessary, then persons with specific clinical training may be required. For vulnerable populations such as persons with cognitive impairments, or those with significant hearing loss, an understanding of some of the associated challenges is needed. Bilingualism and bicultural understandings may be critical as well depending upon, of course, the targeted populations. For most studies, however, individuals who are bachelor or master's prepared in any of the social sciences (sociology, anthropology, psychology) or who have a social work or public health background can serve as excellent interviewers. In all cases, personnel need to have training to orient them to the cultural nuances, needs, and preferences of the target population in addition to, of course, the study protocols and interview battery.

The skill set needed by interventionists is obviously dependent upon the content of the intervention and control groups. Careful thought should be given to who can deliver the intervention or an active control group condition (See Chapter 8 on attention control condition). The decision as to the skill set needed for an interventionist has important implications for the potential of implementation and scalability of that intervention if it is proven to be effective. For example, use of highly skilled and paid clinicians or health professionals as interventionists may be appropriate for the testing phase of an intervention. However, their involvement may in turn limit the future implementation potential of the intervention if real-world settings do not have access to the same level of trained personnel. At the efficacy trial phase, traditionally, interventionists are carefully selected such that only the most skilled individuals are selected to serve in this role. As the emphasis at this phase is on maximizing internal validity so that positive results may be attributable to the intervention, the goal is to minimize threats of possible confounding external factors such as an interventionist's poor skill level, style, or personality. Nevertheless, this overemphasis on specially selected interventionists may be limiting and not reflect the real-world circumstances in which the intervention ultimately will be embedded. Thus, achieving a balanced approach (e.g., adequately trained interventionists but possibly not trained specialists unless necessary) can be an important goal early on in the development of an intervention. This point is discussed more fully in Chapter 20.

Unique to behavioral intervention research is the high level of interdependency in roles and responsibilities among staff members. For example, in an efficacy trial, one person may be responsible for screening and enrolling study participants, another person may be responsible for randomization, another may be responsible for assigning interviews, and yet another for conducting the interviews. As each staff member is dependent upon the other sharing key information that may be needed by others, establishing a communication and work flow among team members (e.g., who does what and when) is essential.

A related point is that a backup plan is important to put into place in which the key roles and responsibilities of each staff member can be carried out by another. Study milestones must be met regardless of staff turnover, personal crisis, or other issues. Thus, cross-training of staff to potentially fill each other's roles is critical and must be factored in when designing the study and identifying staffing requirements. A project, at whatever stage of the pipeline, should not be dependent upon one staff member. If possible, hiring more than one interviewer and interventionist is critical to account for days off for vacation, sick days, and leaves of absence or for dismissals or individuals who choos to leave the position.

Training Staff

Given the complexity, multisteps, and nuanced considerations as well as the interdependency of staff in the conduct of an intervention study, staff training is critical to all intervention studies irrespective of the phase along the pipeline. There are three basic areas of training to consider for staff, regardless of role or prior experience. First, all staff must have knowledge of, and a clear understanding of, the study goals, research questions, and study protocol and study procedures. However, in single- and double-blinded studies, some staff may not be privy to specific hypotheses, participant group assignment, or intervention specifics. Nevertheless, understanding the study and its design and the intent of blinding is important to ensure that staff are able to perform their roles adequately. Also, staff (e.g., interviewers, interventionists) who interact with study participants will need to field questions and adequately and accurately respond to queries about the study posed by participants.

A second area of training is for staff to learn how to strike the right balance between working independently and keeping a project coordinator/investigator and others on the research team adequately informed about field conditions, coding decisions, adverse events, and related matters. For example, an interviewer may learn information that may impact other staff who will be interacting with a study participant. In the interview process, it may be revealed that a participant will be traveling in the near future, which will affect subsequent data collection efforts. A participant might reveal a recent hospitalization that would be important to document and that may affect outcomes. For interviews that occur in the home, a wide range of noteworthy conditions may be observed such as unsafe environmental conditions (e.g., a hole in the roof), infestation, or presence of smokers or unfriendly pets. This type of information needs to be passed along to other staff members in a systematic way. Using electronic tracking and project management programs can facilitate information sharing. In all cases, tracking contacts with study participants and sharing important information about participants are critical.

When interviewing or conducting an intervention in the home, various challenges can emerge that require independent problem solving: a study participant may become ill and need help; the environment may be uncomfortable or pose a risk to the participant and staff member; the staff member may be invited to eat or drink with the participant; and so forth. The point is that it is not possible to foresee every issue that will emerge in the course of implementing an intervention study. Staff must be armed with knowledge of the study, its purpose, and general guidelines regarding independent problem solving to address issues as they emerge in the field and which are typically not possible to identify a priori. When interacting with people and particularly in their living environments, anything can and will happen (Gitlin, 2003).

A third general area of training is the tracking systems that will be used in the study and instilling an understanding that every action taken by any staff member can have a methodological impact. Even what might appear as simple office work, such as duplicating an interview or consent form or filing study participant information in a locked cabinet, can be a source of measurement error or present as a methodological challenge if not carried out correctly. For example, misfiling consents, duplicating materials incorrectly such that an interview or consent form page is missing, using an outdated informed consent form, or failing to inform another staff member of an unsafe interviewing condition can lead to missing data, breaches in human subject–consenting ethics and procedures, placing others in harm's way, and analytic difficulties.

A related point is that all data must be considered confidential and locked in stored cabinets and offices. Personnel should have access only to the data they need to perform their particular role. Any information that can identify a study participant (e.g., signed consent form) must be separated from data-coded questionnaires. Team members must be trained to uphold subject confidentiality in every step and process of any study. Losing data by leaving behind a questionnaire in a person's home or a clinic area is a serious breach of confidentiality.

Thus far we have discussed general staff training. However, there are specific training considerations for assessors/interviewers and interventionists. If the study design involves data capture through face-to-face interviewing, at a minimum, the training of interviewers should cover but may not be limited to the following: (a) study design and study procedures; (b) the interview battery; (c) stopping rules; (d) consenting processes, confidentiality, and human subject ethics; (e) coding and/or scoring data; (f) procedures for reporting adverse events; and (g) personal safety.

We recommend developing a "certification" process that establishes what needs to be done and the specific competencies needed for a study interviewer. Certification requirements might include, for example, completion of readings and participation in face-to-face trainings in study procedures; the completion of three to five practice interviews with project coordinator/investigator and others and demonstration of competencies in explaining the study; obtaining consent; administering an interview battery; handling an adverse event; and problem solving common challenges in the field (e.g., quickly building rapport, redirecting study participants, active listening, accuracy in recording information).

Interventionists also need systematic training. They must be able to juggle protocol requirements with potentially challenging clinical and unpredictable circumstances and remain nimble in their thinking and actions. For example, let's say a participant expresses suicidal ideation in a treatment session of an intervention that is unrelated to mood disorders (e.g., a physical exercise or chronic disease self-management program). Although depression and suicidal ideation are not the focus of the intervention, this expression cannot be ignored. Interventionists will require training as to how to address this and other matters and also be given the flexibility to make a judgment as to how best to proceed (e.g., call 911 if participant indicates a plan, provide suicide prevention hotline crisis telephone numbers, refer for mental health counseling). Chapter 6 on standardization and Chapter 13 on ethics examine some of these issues as well.

Also, similar to interviewers, interventionists must have knowledge about the study design, when to stop the intervention owing to an adverse condition or event, and how to report adverse events. This is all in addition to the heart of the matter—training in the intervention protocol and documentation of its delivery. A certification process by which interventionists must demonstrate competencies in the delivery of the intervention and handling field conditions can help to promote uniformity and ensure fidelity in intervention delivery. Certification requirements will be specific to the intervention but may include the successful completion of selected readings, participation in face-to-face trainings, role-playing, demonstration of competencies in building rapport, and delivering each treatment component.

Another important consideration is that interventionists must possess confidence in the intervention protocol and firmly believe in its importance and potential to have a positive effect on study participants. If not, their lack of passion or enthusiasm for the intervention may be directly or subtlety conveyed to study participants and have unintended, negative consequences including attrition, poor treatment adherence, and/or the realization of limited treatment benefit. As the strength of the therapeutic alliance is critical to intervention success, the relationship formed with a study participant in effect becomes part of the intervention (Chee, Gitlin, Dennis, & Hauck, 2007). Also, lack of belief in the value of an intervention may lead to independent decision making. Interventionists who do not value the intervention protocol may choose to emphasize one treatment component over another on the basis of their personal preferences or what they think is best, resulting in omissions or commissions in treatment delivery. Chapter 12 discusses fidelity issues in more detail.

ONGOING SUPPORT AND OVERSIGHT

Ongoing support and oversight of staff are necessary throughout the duration of an intervention study and are an important quality control feature of behavioral intervention studies at any phase along the pipeline to ensure fidelity. The fidelity monitoring required in intervention research may involve direct observation of performance of staff and/or rating audiotaped sessions. Staff may not have had previous exposure to this level and type of oversight, so it is important that they be informed of its methodological importance and that they become comfortable with such approaches. Interventionists and interviewers in particular must be willing to receive direction, feedback, and redirection if drift or deviations from protocols occur.

For interviewers and interventionists (active treatment or control group conditions), ongoing oversight may be accomplished by listening to approximately 10% to 20% of randomly selected audiotapes, and directly observing interview or intervention sessions, case presentations at staff meetings, or one-on-one or group supervision sessions, or a combination thereof. Regular project meetings for the entire team are also important to ensure cohesiveness and ensure that the study remains on track. Clearly articulating the need for this level of oversight during the hire/interview process can help to avoid any misunderstandings or surprises down the road.

The organization and frequency of staff meetings will vary by project and its needs. Separate meetings with interviewers and interventionists may be necessary when keeping interviewers masked to the group allocation of participants. Any team meetings, however, should cover issues related to coding questions, review of completed assignments and scheduled interviews, troubleshooting, and case presentations. Also, team meetings present an opportunity to nurture essential team values such as mutual respect and a shared mission/goal and can be used to validate the hard work being done by individuals and recognize individual and group successes (e.g., meeting enrollment targets). As staff members themselves will reflect diverse skill levels, cultures, values, and beliefs, using meetings to model respect and to demonstrate how the contributions of each member are valued and important can go a long way to strengthen buy-in and build an effective team.

Finally, investing in the well-being and professional development of each team member is always important even when staff are hired for brief or time-limited periods. Interviewing or interacting with vulnerable populations and very ill, distressed or depressed study participants can be stressful. Attending to the staff's emotional reactions, encouraging the sharing of experiences in the study, and assuring their personal safety can help alleviate the stress, sadness, and attachment that may form with study participants (Lawton et al., 2015). This is typically an undervalued activity, yet one that is critical. It not only promotes the well-being of staff but also serves to strengthen commitment to the quality of the study.

Similarly, meeting with each staff member to identify reasonable professional goals within the scope of his or her study roles and responsibilities and offering opportunities for professional growth not only contribute to retention but also help to build an effective work force for behavioral intervention research. An interviewer may aspire to help train new interviewers and take on a study-monitoring or public-speaking role; a project coordinator may want to improve his or her public-speaking and writing abilities and participate in dissemination of findings. Staff development should be valued as a generative activity (e.g., preparing the next generation in research activity) and part of our ethical practices as behavioral researchers.

As an investment needs to be made in identifying, training, and supporting staff, it is of interest to an investigator and the team to keep people employed. However, this is often challenging if funding is not available beyond the scope of the specific project for which a staff member is hired. Moving staff from one study or phase of the intervention's development to the next is desirable, but this can be difficult to always achieve. Challenges for doing so involve securing funding and having seamless transitions from study to study or finding "gap" or bridge funding (e.g., internal funding from one's institution for a brief period until external funding is obtained) to support key personnel.

COLLABORATING AND LEADING TEAMS

Building and evaluating an intervention requires interactions and collaborations with different stakeholders, professionals, and staff from diverse areas of expertise and backgrounds. Thus, at some point along the pathway of developing an intervention, investigators will find themselves involved with establishing a team and refining their team leadership skills. As group work is typically a dynamic process, drawing upon and applying team principles and learning how to manage team dynamics go a long way to strengthen intervention work. Understanding potential and common emergent challenges in managing individual staff members and the group dynamics can be helpful (Bennett, Gadlin, & Levine-Finley, 2010; Gitlin & Lyons, 2013).

There are many critical aspects of working on, and leading, teams. One key consideration for behavioral intervention research is instilling and maintaining a sense of shared purpose, mission, and clearly articulated goals among staff and key stakeholders. In behavioral intervention research, we see this as the responsibility of the primary investigator who must set the right tone and energize staff and stakeholders concerning the potential importance of the work to which they are contributing. Helping staff understand the background, significance, and potential contributions of the study toward the betterment of the public overall, and their specific role in the process, fosters a strong sense of mission, purpose, and team work.

When directing intervention work, having staff work as a team is paramount. Fourteen indicators outlined in Table 22.2 can serve as a guide to fostering positive team work (Gitlin & Lyons, 2013). These indicators and the associated self-reflective questions shown in Table 22.2 capture the essential ingredients of effective team functioning. Applied to intervention studies, reinforcing mutual respect, valuing each team member's role and his or her contributions, fostering a safe environment for conveying issues as they arise, and troubleshooting are all critical for several reasons. They assure that, as problems develop in the field (which they will!), staff will feel empowered and comfortable expressing such events as they occur. As staff are on the front line, so to speak, of implementing a study and an intervention, its knowledge of field conditions and what is working or not is invaluable and can inform meaningful course corrections before it is too late. Given staff's direct experiences with the actual implementation of a study protocol and knowledge of field conditions, its involvement in troubleshooting is significant and key.

The value of team work is important to instill in the hiring process, and then it needs to be continually reinforced in staff training, supervision, and staff meetings. Setting the right tone in each of these situations is up to the primary investigator or leader of the intervention work, but also should be modeled and reinforced by the project manager and others who provide oversight in the field.

Developing a team for intervention work is not limited just to staff development. Team principles can be applied to any intervention phase and work activity involving community partners, stakeholders, and/or national leaders to advance an understanding and testing of an intervention. Effective involvement of stakeholders early on in the intervention development process to shape intervention delivery characteristics (or when translating, implementing, or disseminating an intervention within a practice context) will depend upon the extent to which the 14

TABLE 22.2 Indicators of Effective Team Work

Domain	Key Self-Reflective Questions
1. Clear statement of goals, expectations, and procedures	Are project team members aware of and endorse the goals of the project?
2. Role differentiation	Do team members understand their respective roles and responsibilities and procedures?
3. Open communication	Do team members listen and pay attention to each other and are ideas expressed openly and honestly?
4. Open, honest negotiation	Do team members feel free to suggest ideas for the direction of a project? Are differences of opinion sought out and clarified? Do team members feel free to disagree openly with each other's ideas?
5. Mutual goals	Do all team members share the group's goals and are they committed to carrying out the group's task?
6. Climate of trust	Do team members engage in active listening, disclose their ideas, feelings, and reactions, and demonstrate respect, confidence, and trust in one another?
7. Cooperation	Do team members seek out opportunities to work with one another on tasks?
8. Shared decision making	Do team members take responsibility for providing input into group decisions?
9. Conflict resolution	Are disagreements brought out into the open and faced directly?
10. Equality of participation	Does each individual, in light of his or her experience and skills, feel free to provide input to team deliberations?
11. Group cohesion	Do team members try to make sure others enjoy being members of the team?
12. Decision by consensus	Do team members listen to and consider other members' points of view before pressing their ideas?
13. Shared leadership	Do team members assume responsibility for making decisions for the group related to task accomplishment?
14. Shared responsibility for participation	Do all members of the team participate in discussions about important issues?

indicators are achieved. Of utmost importance is identifying, nurturing, and supporting mutual goals, respect, and expectations.

It is an unfair expectation that a single investigator have all of the requisite knowledge and skills to develop, evaluate, translate/implement, and disseminate any type of intervention. Intervention researchers, therefore, necessarily need to reach out to other experts and involve individuals, groups, and/or organizations in the work of building, evaluating, and implementing interventions. For example, although the investigators may have the content expertise, they may not know the clinical nuances or strategies for achieving a desired impact; thus, collaborating with clinicians can enhance treatment development. Similarly, an investigator may need to develop new items for measuring impact; collaborating with a psychometrician can improve measurement development and testing. As new statistical techniques emerge to tease out treatment effects, examine dose–response relationships, or identify who benefits and why, collaborating with statistical experts and methodologists becomes essential. Furthermore, as disseminating a proven intervention involves advancing value propositions (see Chapter 21) and understanding stakeholder interests in addition to developing a marketing plan, outsourcing these activities or collaborating with dissemination experts may be preferred.

An investigator for a behavioral intervention study is similar to a conductor of an orchestra—bringing together, coordinating and synthesizing varied nuances, components, and knowledge to the intervention research enterprise. As noted earlier, an investigator needs to develop a level of comfort with this orchestration process, which includes organizing and running meetings and facilitating a team spirit to assure all partners and their unique contributions are valued equally.

CAREER-RELATED CONSIDERATIONS

Yet another important consideration in the conduct of behavioral intervention research is career-related. As we have discussed throughout this book, developing an intervention takes time and upwards of 20 years from idea inception to its potential and actual use in real-world settings. A classically trained researcher may have the methodological background for developing and evaluating an intervention but as noted, not necessarily the know-how for conducting implementation studies, developing a comprehensive dissemination plan, or scaling up a proven intervention for widespread adoption. Intervention researchers have to decide whether to see an intervention through its inception and development to its evaluation and then implementation and dissemination (if effective), or whether to focus only on one particular phase and enable others (on one's team or others) to move the intervention forward for implementation or backward for additional modification and testing. The decision can affect other aspects of professional life including choice of publication outlets and grant applications that are pursued. The choice is challenging because one may have ideas for many different interventions; yet, investing energies in the pursuit of widespread implementation of a proven intervention requires dedicated time and energy.

A related consideration is that a tested intervention and its associated manuals and training programs represent a "product" or intellectual property that may warrant protection and that may also have market bearing. As mentioned also in Chapter 21, seeking a trademark for the name of the intervention/program, enacting copyright protections for manuals, forms, and other materials, and possibly obtaining a patent for unique aspects of an intervention (e.g., a device, algorithm, or procedure) are all important considerations. The rules guiding trademark and copywriting require consultation with experts in this area such as lawyers and/or technology transfer departments in universities. Collaboratively derived projects require special consideration and determination as to who has rights to what, how partners will be recognized and compensated, and the relative contributions of each partner. Submitting to technology transfer offices what is referred to as "disclosure" statements that describe the "invention" (e.g., intervention) and potential products (e.g., manuals, training programs) should occur once the intervention is shown to be effective. Technology transfer offices are essential for developing and overseeing joint agreements with collaborators who may be within or outside of one's institution.

CONCLUSION

To summarize, in this chapter, we have reviewed common but rarely discussed aspects of behavioral intervention work. The need to hire and train staff and form a team is common to any behavioral intervention study, and the practices pursued in these endeavors can have significant methodological bearing. Nevertheless, best practices and effective approaches remain hidden and are typically learned through trial and error or, if one is fortunate, by having an apprenticeship opportunity with a more experienced intervention researcher and his or her team.

One of the essential skills that investigators need to pursue in this line of work is an interest in, and ability to develop, coordinate, and lead, interprofessional teams. This is especially true today with the increasing emphasis on team science. Formation of a team spirit and team approach with staff, stakeholders, and interventionists is critical at almost every study phase but particularly when examining efficacy and effectiveness, and then when moving forward with an intervention's translation, implementation, and dissemination.

Engaging in behavioral intervention work also necessitates making key career decisions as one advances along the pipeline. For example, if an intervention is proven to be effective, a decision has to be made as to whether one will invest time in its dissemination or pursue its scientific advancement, or develop and test another intervention. An investigator cannot do it all! A handoff of a proven intervention to a dissemination team, for example, may be more appropriate than trying to engage in this phase. Alternately, it may be prudent to take a proven intervention and adapt it for a particular context or population rather than develop an intervention from scratch if resources are not available to do so.

The work of designing, evaluating, and implementing interventions involves a combination of passion and science; it is a long and arduous road full of challenges, excitement, learning, and "aha!" moments—all of these aspects need to be embraced to be an effective behavioral intervention researcher!

REFERENCES

Bennett, L. M., Gadlin, H., & Levine-Finley, S. (2010). *Collaboration & team science: A field guide*. Bethesda, MD: National Institutes of Health. Retrieved from https://ccrod .cancer.gov/confluence/download/attachments/47284665/TeamScience_FieldGuide .pdf?version=2&modificationDate=1285330231523&api=v2

Chee, Y. K., Gitlin, L. N., Dennis, M. P., & Hauck, W. W. (2007). Predictors of caregiver adherence to a skill-building intervention among dementia caregivers. *Journal of Gerontology Medical Sciences, 62*(6), 673–678.

Gitlin, L. N. (2003). Conducting research on home environments: Lessons learned and new directions. *The Gerontologist, 43*(5), 628–637. doi:10.1093/geront/43.5.628

Gitlin, L. N., & Lyons, K. J. (2013). *Successful grant writing: Strategies for health and human service professionals* (5th ed.). New York, NY: Springer.

Lawton, J., Kirkham, J., White, D., Rankin, D., Cooper, C., & Heller, S. (2015). Uncovering the emotional aspects of working on a clinical trial: A qualitative study of the experiences and views of staff involved in a type 1 diabetes trial. *Trials, 16*(3), 1–11. doi:10.1186/1745-6215-16-3

TWENTY THREE

GRANT WRITING CONSIDERATIONS FOR ADVANCING BEHAVIORAL INTERVENTIONS

If at first you don't succeed, try, try, try again.
—Titelman (1996)

Advancing behavioral interventions requires resources and financial support at each phase along the pipeline. As intervention work spans many years, different forms of resources and levels of funding are necessary depending upon the developmental phase, study design, and complexity of the intervention. The total cost to move an intervention forward from its initial inception as an idea to its test as an efficacious program and then to its implementation is unclear. However, there is no doubt that moving an intervention along the pipeline is a very costly enterprise, typically requiring many millions of dollars. Costs may include funding for the investigator and staff effort, space, software and equipment, statistical or other specialized consultations, honorariums for study participants and stakeholder meetings, materials or supplies, recruitment activities, and travel for data collection, intervention delivery, and dissemination activities. As such, writing grant proposals to support each developmental phase is a critical aspect of behavioral intervention research.

In this chapter, we provide an overview of essential considerations in grantsmanship—general tips as well as key challenges unique to writing proposals to support behavioral intervention research. We first consider basic strategies fundamental to grant writing irrespective of a particular funding mechanism, agency, or type of application. We then explore issues specific to intervention research. Also described are funding mechanisms to consider along the intervention pipeline and key challenges unique to intervention proposals.

Much has been written about grant writing in general and numerous helpful resources are available including videos and grant writing tips provided by various agencies (e.g., in the United States, see National Institutes of Health [NIH] grant writing tips at grants.nih.gov/grants/grant_tips.htm; and grant writing books, Gitlin & Lyons, 2013). However, there is little discussion and no consensus as to the best approaches, strategies, or practices in grant writing to support behavioral intervention research. This is in some respects uncharted territory, and our discussion necessarily draws upon our collective grant writing experiences.

At the outset, it is important to stress that the funding landscape is highly dynamic and agency and institutional requirements, priorities, funding levels, and review processes and criteria fluctuate and can change quickly. Thus, we present general principles for grant writing that transcend such variations and the specifications or guidelines that are provided by any one funding source or agency. The specifics for preparing a grant proposal *must* always be garnered from the most current sources of information such as a funder's website, active funding announcements, or through discussions with program officers of funding agencies. It is also a good idea to work with the development and research administration offices of one's organization as they may be in a position to identify a wide range of funding opportunities and their respective requirements.

GENERAL GRANT WRITING TIPS

Writing a competitive grant application to support the development, evaluation, translation/implementation, and dissemination of an intervention is similar in many respects to guidelines for writing a grant application to support any other type of research. Similar rules apply such as: assure the relevance of the proposal to the funding initiative; carefully follow instructions and submission rules; write using a clear, concise, and technical writing style; demonstrate having the necessary skills, staff, technical resources, and access to study populations; and make a solid case for the significance, innovation, and impact of the proposed work.

What Is a Grant Proposal?

The purpose of grant writing in general is obviously to seek money from a funding agency. Although it is typically a highly competitive process, a little recognized fact is that the goal of funders is actually to dispense with their funds. Agencies seek to provide funding to the best possible proposals that will also help to move their strategic mission and vision forward. Thus, the main purpose of a proposal is to convince reviewers and funders that monies should be granted to support the proposed idea and plan of implementation and that they fit within their purview of interest.

Specifically, a grant proposal is a carefully crafted document that describes the "who, what, where, when, how, and why" aspects of a research study. Each section of a proposal provides answers to a series of critical questions: What is the project about? Why is it significant or important? How is it novel or innovative? What is its potential impact? What specifically is planned for? How will the plan be carried out? Who is the investigative team and why are they the best to carry out the plan? Why is the research environment well suited for the proposed work and how will it support the proposed work? What will it cost and why? Furthermore, a proposal must convince reviewers and a funding organization of the significance, need, and novelty of the proposed research, and the ability of the team to carry out the planned activities. In this respect, a proposal can be thought of as a marketing tool in which one must package the science in such a way as to convince reviewers and funders of its significance, public health impact, novelty, and feasibility.

Understanding Agency Priorities

To be successful in obtaining a grant, it is essential to understand the funding priorities of an agency and its particular funding opportunities. As the funding environment is constantly changing, it is helpful to develop a plan for monitoring emerging research priorities and funding opportunities. This may include Web-based searches, setting up e-mail alert notifications of funding opportunities, following blogs and e-reports of funding agencies, and determining whether there are internal institutional activities for identifying and notifying researchers as to funding streams. Additionally, talking to colleagues at professional meetings regarding their funding sources and paying attention to the funding sources listed as part of the acknowledgment section of a published research article are helpful avenues for tracking possible funding outlets.

Each agency has a defined strategic mission and broad vision in terms of what it wants to impact and hence fund. For example, in the United States, the mission of the Agency for Healthcare Research and Quality (AHRQ) is to "improve quality, safety, efficiency, and effectiveness of health care," whereas the many institutes and centers composing the NIH fund intervention research specific to diseases and conditions. The relatively new Patient-Centered Outcomes Research Institute (PCORI) authorized by Congress as part of the Patient Protection and Affordable Care Act of 2010 funds comparative clinical effectiveness research and research to develop methods in this area. Foundations also have key missions. For example, the mission of the Robert Wood Johnson Foundation is to improve the health and health care of all Americans.

For a grant proposal to be competitive, the proposed idea must match an agency's mission and the intent of a particular funding opportunity. Additionally, a match must be made in terms of the level of funding offered by the funding mechanism and what is needed for the proposed idea. For example, novice researchers should start by submitting proposals that are commensurate with their level of experience and publication record in order to build and demonstrate a successful funding track record. Within the NIH, this might be an RO3 (Small Research Grant) or an R21 (Exploratory/Developmental Research Grant). In contrast, a seasoned intervention researcher may be able to seek funds through mechanisms that garner more funds and propose more complex design strategies (e.g., multisite, large efficacy trials) corresponding to their level of experience and track record. Again, within the NIH, this is typically an RO1 (Research Project Grant).

Agencies seek to fund proposals that will have significant impact on the health of the public. In addition to the strategic mission of an agency, it is important to align one's work with key reports. Examples of such in the United States include the Institute of Medicine Reports (www.iom.edu/Reports.aspx), Healthy People 2010/2020 (www.healthypeople.gov/HP2020/), or the NIH Roadmap for Medical Research (http://nihroadmap.nih.gov/). Reports generated by international organizations such as the World Health Organization are also important to review and reference.

In searching for funding opportunities, it is wise to initially cast a wide net and examine a range of funding sources. This should include federal agencies as well as foundations, industry, donors, professional organizations, crowdsourcing, and pilot funding mechanisms through one's own institution. There may be surprises by doing so. For example, in the United States, the Department of Defense has an interest in breast cancer research and dementia from traumatic brain injury, and, in recent years, has sought intervention development in these areas. Also, having a diversified funding portfolio such that funding support is not dependent upon a singular source can help assure continued funding successes over time. In addition, most research-intensive institutions offer internal competitive mechanisms to support pilot research efforts and the early developmental phases of an intervention through their Clinical and Translational Science Awards (CTSA) programs funded by the NIH, and these should always be pursued.

As a general rule, it is important to make contact with a program officer of any agency that may be of potential interest. Contact can be made at a professional association meeting as some program officers attend such conferences if their budgets permit. Alternately, more commonly, contact can be initiated by e-mail in which a project idea can be shared in the form of a brief abstract, a draft of an aims page or a short concept paper that outlines the key ideas for a grant proposal, and a request for a follow-up telephone call to review. Most program officers will agree to read a brief statement of the proposed effort prior to a telephone discussion. On a telephone call appointment, which may last from 15 minutes to 1 hour, the following information should be clearly articulated: name, institutional affiliation, statement of area of study and particular research aims, and well-framed questions. Such a call can help clarify whether the agency and a particular funding opportunity fit a proposed idea, and the agency's priorities, level of interest in the proposed topic, backgrounds of likely reviewers, the review process, and other related considerations including budgeting. Contact with a program officer can be invaluable. One's grantsmanship can be enhanced by reading funded grants and reviewers' comments, serving as a grant reviewer, attending grant writing workshops offered by one's institution or professional meetings, and obviously, staying on top of one's professional literature. For those applying to the NIH, it is helpful to identify previously funded studies relevant to one's own area by consulting the NIH RePORT (Research Portfolio Online Reporting Tools) website, which lists funded research and can be searched by investigator(s), substantive areas, or institutes.

Preparing a Grant Application

The preparation of any type of grant application requires a great deal of thoughtful planning and time. First, in preparing an application, it is important to understand the rules for developing and submitting it within one's institution. Each institution has its own set of procedures, internal deadlines, and rules for overseeing budget preparation and compliances as well as uploading and electronically submitting an application. Internal rules for submission may also vary depending upon whether the proposal is to a federal agency or a foundation. Key institutional considerations include identifying who must be notified of a potential proposal submission; the administrator responsible for budget preparation; and the official "signing" officer who is permitted to officially apply his or her signature on an application for its submission. It is also a good idea to identify a few individuals within the institution who might be willing to provide a review of the application prior to submission to the funding agency. Some institutions have an internal review as a required part of the grant submission process. If this is the case, it must be planned for and built into the grant preparation timeline. Finally, it is critical to identify all internal institutional deadlines for submission of proposal materials as soon as possible as they are necessarily earlier than those imposed by an agency.

Second, once a particular funding source and program announcement are identified, reading the application guidelines very carefully (and supplemental instructions if provided) is an imperative. To structure a proposal, it is recommended to use the suggested outline provided in a funding announcement or the specific criteria that will be used to evaluate the proposal. This makes it easier for reviewers to follow the ideas and methods presented and evaluate the proposal accordingly. Some applications have very strict guidelines and requirements, which if not followed may disqualify the proposal from being considered. It is also important to identify institutional resources that might be required as part of the application requirements such as letters of support from institutional officials, statements of institutional facilities such as laboratory or equipment facilities, or the need for matching funds. In addition, it is important to identify collaborators and any potential consultants early on and what materials or information they will need to provide for the application. Again, you must allow sufficient time for your collaborators to prepare what is needed such as a strong letter of support, outline of scope of work, budget, or biographical information.

Third, well-written proposals use a technical writing style, the active tense, and are clear, concise, and logical. Disorganized proposals or those that use jargon, or specialized terminology without providing a clear definition, are less likely to receive positive reviews. A proposal marred with grammatical and typographical errors bring into question the merit of the ideas and the ability of the investigative team to carry out the proposed activities and can significantly lower reviewers' scores. It is not just about the science, but also how it is packaged and visually presented. Writing the application is an iterative process. Whereas the study aims dictate the methodologies to be used, each is tied as well to budgetary considerations. Thus, while one starts with a study purpose and specific aims, the methodological and budgetary considerations may lead to multiple refinements to the aims.

Fourth, it is important to understand the review process of the agency to which a proposal will be submitted prior to developing the application. Discuss with a program officer the backgrounds of those who may review the grant application, the review processes followed including whether a grant can be resubmitted if not funded on the initial attempt, and the scoring procedures that are used. Also inquire about the evaluation criteria and what aspects of an application are most important to highlight (e.g., impact, innovation).

Most grant applications are critically reviewed along five basic areas: significance or the public health import of the idea; innovation; an investigator's/team's abilities and whether an appropriate team has been assembled; adequacy of the approach or research methods proposed; and whether the environment is adequate and supportive for the effective conduct of the proposed research. Common critiques from reviewers of any type of proposal include but are not limited to: lack of new or original ideas; unfocused research plan or research plan that does not match the proposed specific aims; poorly developed or insufficient theoretical base

---

TABLE 23.1 Common Reasons Why Intervention Proposals Fail

1. Lack of sufficient details (e.g., of intervention, recruitment plan, cost analyses, training staff)
2. Insufficient pilot support for the intervention and its components
3. Lack of attention to mechanisms of change
4. Replication and sustainability of intervention not clear
5. Lack of an appropriate control group
6. Poor or missing fidelity plan
7. Intervention too costly
8. Appears beyond capacity of principal investigator and/or team and environment
9. Outcome measures not linked to intervention, research aims, or not sensitive to detect change
10. Analytic plan inadequate, insufficient power
11. Insufficient power for primary or secondary aims
12. Intervention, methods not innovative

---

or link between project (e.g., measures) and theory not clear; inadequate review of published relevant work; lack of details concerning recruitment approaches; insufficient power; lack of experience in the proposed methodology or questionable experimental approach; or lack of sufficient experimental detail (Gitlin & Lyons, 2013). Key weaknesses noted by reviewers specific to intervention proposals are listed in Table 23.1.

FUNDING MECHANISMS ALONG THE ELONGATED PIPELINE

As developing, evaluating and translating, and implementing and disseminating interventions occur incrementally and over time, funds are needed for each phase along the pipeline. Figure 23.1 summarizes key funding sources organized by phase of the elongated pipeline (see Chapter 2) for systematically building a behavioral intervention. In the United States, federal agencies are the primary funders of intervention development and evaluation work, whereas foundations are more likely to fund pilot studies, translation, implementation, and dissemination efforts. As noted, some research-intensive institutions also provide funds for the early phases (developing and pilot testing) of an intervention, and more recently, there has been a funding appetite for translational efforts, although few dedicated funds are still available for this research activity.

When developing a proposal involving an intervention, first consider the level of development of the intervention, what is needed to advance the intervention, and the amount of funds required to conduct the proposed project activities. As to the latter, for example, funding requirements to support research activity will vary widely; efficacy trials (Phase III) will require greater funds to execute than Phase I pilot studies.

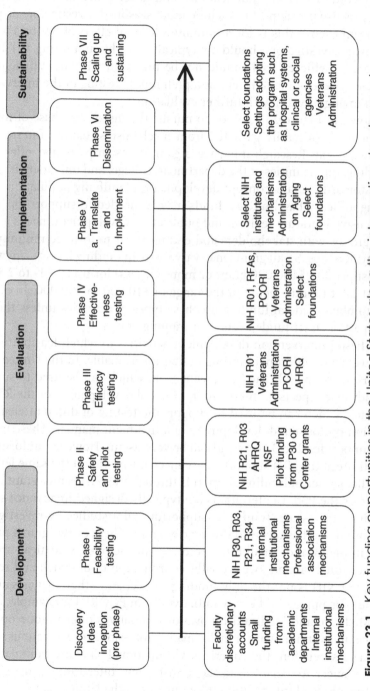

Figure 23.1 Key funding opportunities in the United States along the intervention development pipeline.

Another consideration is the level of experience of the investigator and investigative team. Investigators new to behavioral intervention research will have to prove their ability to conduct this complex form of research by demonstrating a previous record of funding, publications, and developmental work in the area. In this case, it is usually helpful to include more seasoned investigators as part of the research team even if this is for a minimum level of effort of 3% to 5%. As noted earlier, novice investigators should not typically start by submitting an efficacy trial; furthermore, an efficacy trial should not be proposed without sufficient evidence from previous developmental steps and preliminary testing of the intervention that supports moving forward with further evaluation.

As shown in Figure 23.1, funds to pursue the discovery phase of intervention development are primarily garnered from mechanisms that are internal to an academic institution. Research-intensive organizations in particular offer a range of pilot funding opportunities at the department, college, and university levels. As this phase customarily entails concept development, identifying population needs, and examining a theory base, modest funds may be needed to support the conduct of comprehensive literature reviews and publication development, needs assessments or focus groups with stakeholders and end users, or to form community or stakeholder partnerships. Small grants may vary vastly in funding levels—anywhere from a $1,000 stipend to $100,000 grant or more (or less) for up to a 1- to 2-year effort, with most pilot funding being in the range of $10,000 to $50,000. In general, it is difficult to obtain federal funding for these types of activities unless they are proposed as part of larger funded center or training grants.

For Phase I intervention development activities in which feasibility is the primary focus, a few additional funding outlets are available. In the United States and at the NIH, these include the R03 mechanism, which can be used to support pilot work to advance aspects of intervention protocol development, or the R34 and R21 mechanisms, which can be used to support the testing of different elements of an intervention protocol and development of a treatment manual. These mechanisms provide support for 2 to 3 years and can be very useful. However, unfortunately, not every institute at the NIH supports these mechanisms nor at the same level of funding. Another source of funding support is through the NIH center grant mechanism referred to as the P30. Center grants are typically designed to advance science in a focused area (e.g., sleep, frailty) by supporting pilot studies by investigators from the institution that has received this type of grant. These center grants provide core supports in the form of small funds to carry out the pilot, statistical, and methodological consultation and, occasionally, coordination of outreach and recruitment. However, the NIH is not the only funding source, and other agencies and foundations should be pursued. The new initiatives from PCORI, for example, or the Centers for Medicare and Medicaid Innovations initiatives offer unique opportunities to advance intervention work. Finally, many professional organizations, such as the Alzheimer's Association, the American Occupational Therapy Foundation, or the American Cancer Association, to name just a few, offer funding opportunities to support this phase of intervention development in the United States.

As is true for any type of proposal or testing phase, proposals for pilot studies or manual development must be novel and propose a systematic methodology to be competitive. It is not sufficient to simply ask for funds to develop an intervention or its manual without proposing a specific methodology for doing so. For example, one could propose to test an initial protocol in an open label trial with 10 participants from which needed modifications to the protocol are subsequently documented and used to inform refinements to a treatment manual or the components of an intervention. The refined treatment manual or a modified treatment component may then be tested with another 10 participants and so forth using a coding system and theory base to understand adaptations (Stirman, Miller, Toder, & Calloway, 2012).

For Phase II intervention activities, in addition to the funding mechanisms thus far mentioned earlier, the NIH R21 mechanism can potentially be a good fit to evaluate intervention safety, preliminary effect sizes, and other design elements such as use of different control groups, spacing of testing occasions, or underlying explanatory mechanisms.

There are more funding opportunities to support Phase III efficacy trials or Phase IV effectiveness trials. In the United States, the primary source of funding, however, remains through the NIH and its R01 Research Project Grant mechanism. As mentioned earlier, consideration should also be given to PCORI whose mission, in part, is to fund comparative effectiveness trials. This is an excellent source of funding if the desire is to compare two or more clinical interventions that have been shown to be efficacious previously.

Although funding levels in general for intervention development and testing are sparse, as mentioned earlier, there is even less funding available for the implementation phases (Phase V—translation/implementation; Phase VI—dissemination; and Phase VII—sustainability/maintenance). Only a few institutes of the NIH (e.g., see the Dissemination and Implementation division of the National Institute of Mental Health or the National Cancer Institute) specifically allocate resources, albeit limited, to these phases. The NIH also continues to support a multimillion-dollar initiative to universities; the CTSA in turn offers a range of research services to investigators of awarded institutions including pilot funding for translational research studies. Additionally, special funding opportunities such as one-time requests for applications (RFA) have also been a source of funding support for translation and implementation efforts. Additionally, some agencies and foundations do target this phase in specific areas such as caregiving (Veterans Administration, Rosalynn Carter Institute on Caregiving), dementia care (Administration on Aging's [AoA] Alzheimer's Disease Supportive Services Program [ADSSP]), bringing evidence to geriatric care services (Hartford Change AGEnts Initiative), or translating evidence for delivery in social services and area agencies (National Institute on Aging and AoA [*Translational Research to Help Older Adults Maintain Their Health and Independence in the Community*]).

Finally, it is worth mentioning the Centers for Medicare and Medicaid Services Innovations Awards, which, with health care reform in the United States, has provided funding for large demonstration projects that propose to evaluate novel interventions designed to lower costs and improve care. It is unclear how long this funding mechanism will be available, but currently funded projects demonstrating improvements and cost savings may have the chance of being scaled up, diffused nationally, and be recognized as reimbursable.

It is not certain if any of the initiatives or funding sources mentioned here will continue to support any aspect of intervention work. Funding mechanisms tend to come and go. Thus, it is best to continuously investigate potential sources for supporting intervention work and, as discussed earlier, cast a wide net.

GRANT WRITING CHALLENGES UNIQUE TO INTERVENTION RESEARCH

Writing any type of grant application can be challenging. However, writing a competitive grant application for intervention research presents its own unique set of issues. Here we discuss ten challenges specific to intervention research: naming and framing the phase of intervention development; specifying aims; the importance of pilot data; Research methods; describing the intervention; page limitations and need for intervention details; proof that the proposed methods are feasible such as recruitment plans; human subject considerations; appendices; and budgeting.

Naming and Framing the Phase of Intervention Development

In writing a grant proposal, it is important to specify the stage of development of the intervention and therefore the purpose of the request for funding (e.g., to develop an intervention, test its safety and feasibility or efficacy, effectiveness). As agencies conceptualize the intervention pipeline somewhat differently, understanding the terminology specific to the funder and providing a well-articulated statement as to the phase are important. Similarly, reviewers may disagree as to what constitutes an efficacy trial versus an effectiveness trial and they may be unfamiliar with emerging hybrid designs that combine developmental phases (Curran, Bauer, Mittman, Pyne, & Stetler, 2012; Riley, Glasgow, Etheredge, & Abernethy, 2013). Thus, describing, naming, and framing the phase of development and testing that is being proposed as well as citing a source to support one's statements can enable reviewers to respond appropriately. Furthermore, as some agencies have an interest in funding one phase versus another, speaking to a program officer about these matters is essential.

Aims Specific to Each Phase

Most grant applications require a clearly articulated set of research aims. For NIH proposals, the "aims page" is a single-spaced, one-page narrative that serves as a roadmap to the proposal. Although there is no single way to approach this one critical page, it is typically composed of four major components: an opening paragraph that describes the current state of and gaps in knowledge, and significance of the targeted problem area; a second paragraph that describes the specific purpose of the proposed study and short- and long-term goals, central hypotheses, and the investigative team and environment (e.g., if study builds on previous pilot data, expertise of the team); a third paragraph that outlines the specific study design and the primary aims, and if appropriate, secondary and exploratory aims and associated hypotheses; finally, a fourth paragraph that briefly highlights the innovation of the study, outcomes and expectations, and potential impact on the health of the public. Each paragraph must be written concisely and clearly so that it can be understood by reviewers from diverse backgrounds and disciplines. In essence, this page sets the tone for the reviewers.

The specific aims of a proposed study must reflect testable and measurable statements, each of which are associated with a particular methodology that will be subsequently explained in the proposal narrative. Specific aims will differ depending upon the level of intervention development and specific study purpose. For a grant seeking support for discovery and development of the components or characteristics of an intervention, an example of study aims may be to (a) identify treatment elements leading to a treatment manual that integrates empirically supported treatment and a content review by a panel of experts; (b) conduct an open trial (in which both researcher and participant are aware that a treatment is being provided) with 15 study participants from which to modify the manual through feedback from participants, their caregivers (if relevant), interventionists, and an expert panel; and (c) estimate rates of enrollment and retention and effect sizes through a small trial of 40 study participants.

For a proposal seeking to evaluate an intervention at Phase II, exemplar aims may include (but are not limited to) (a) evaluating acceptance of and engagement in the treatment; (b) testing the reliability and validity of a measure of treatment adherence; and (c) establishing a preliminary effect size for the impact of the intervention through the conduct of a small randomized trial.

For a proposal seeking to evaluate an intervention at the Phase III efficacy phase, aims and associated hypotheses may include (but are not be limited to) (a) testing the effect of the intervention on depression severity (primary outcome) (*Hypothesis*: Participants in the intervention group will report clinically meaningful and statistically significant reductions in depression severity at 4 months in comparison to participation in an attention control group); (b) testing the long-term effects of the intervention on depression severity and overall well-being at 12 months (*Hypothesis*: Participants in the intervention group will maintain reductions in depression severity and report improved well-being at 12 months in comparison to participation in an attention control group); and (c) evaluating the cost and cost-effectiveness of the intervention expressed as an incremental cost outcome achieved in the form of depression severity reductions at 4 and 12 months (*Hypothesis*: The intervention will be cost-effective compared to the control intervention at each test occasion).

Efficacy trials are typically powered to examine one to three primary aims. Secondary or exploratory aims might also be proposed to examine long-term impact, moderator and mediator effects, implementation processes, economic analyses, treatment adherence, and so forth.

The aforementioned exemplars highlight the differences in the scope and nature of aims at different phases of intervention development. However, despite the study phase or the funding agency, the aims of a proposal must be clear, concise, and feasible. It is not prudent to propose a large number of aims in a single application as this may raise questions as to the feasibility of the proposed research.

Importance of Pilot Data

It may seem ironic that pilot data are always needed to garner funding even when one is requesting funding to conduct a pilot study. The point is that some proof of concept is needed to show that the request for funds, whether for a small- or large-scale complex study, is reasonable, can be conducted in the proposed time line, and has potential to yield important outcomes. The type of pilot data required will depend upon the phase of development of the intervention. For example, even when requesting funds for manual development and protocol advancement, providing pilot data demonstrating the feasibility of the approach is necessary. This may take the form of focus groups or a needs assessment in which the outcomes demonstrate support for the significance of the proposed intervention. When requesting funds for a Phase III efficacy trial, each primary aim should be supported by pilot data that show positive outcomes and support an investment in the proposed trial. For proposed interventions that are multicomponent, it is necessary to demonstrate the feasibility of each component through pilot testing.

Pilot testing of some sort is important at every phase including translation and implementation. As discussed previously, obtaining even small funds from one's department or university can thus be extremely helpful in building an intervention and should be sought after and utilized to pilot test different elements or protocols of an intervention. In addition, pilot data to support other elements of a proposal are important. These include but are not limited to demonstrating that the recruitment plan (see Chapter 10) is feasible and will yield the targeted sample size (see Chapter 9), and that the interview battery does not cause undo participant burden. Also important are data supporting the projected attrition rate, the adequacy of measures, and approaches to data capturing.

Research Methods Section

The research methods section for an intervention study, particularly at the efficacy or effectiveness trial phases, must contain sufficient detail concerning every aspect of the design. Subsections and their organization will vary depending upon the nature and scope of the study and design and the requirements of the funding agency, but typically include eight basic sections: (a) brief overview of research design; (b) general procedures including data collection; (c) sample description, recruitment procedures, eligibility and ineligibility criteria, expected attrition; (d) retention considerations; (e) description of measures and specific treatment outcomes; (f) description of interventions; (g) statistical analytic considerations and plan of analysis for each aim including how clinical significance will be established; and (h) time line, project organization, and quality control procedures.

Describing the Intervention

As the heart of the matter is the intervention, describing it accurately and clearly in a proposal is of utmost importance. Reviewers must understand the importance of the intervention for addressing an identified problem area, why the intervention may be effective for a particular target population, and its potential benefits.

We recommend that six aspects of the intervention itself be described in proposals. As summarized in Table 23.2, these include: (a) the theory base or conceptual frameworks informing the intervention (see Chapter 4); (b) its delivery characteristics including dosage, mode of delivery, location of delivery, and what constitutes

TABLE 23.2   Elements to Include in a Description of an Intervention

Elements	Description
Theory base or conceptual framework	Describe how one or more theories or frameworks specifically inform the intervention. Use the theory to explain what is being targeted by the intervention (e.g., behavior, social relationships, cognition, environment) and why the intervention should achieve its desired outcomes.
Delivery characteristics	This includes dose, intensity, duration, setting, and form of intervention delivery (e.g., Web, telephone, face-to-face or technology).
Flow of intervention	Describe the specific activities, composition of sessions or flow. If possible, include a brief description of each session.
Interventionists	Describe skill set and background of the persons who will be delivering the intervention.
Training	Describe length of time and extent of training needed for interventionists and certification process.
Fidelity	Describe a fidelity plan including what enhancements will be used to assure implementation integrity and measures used.
Implementation potential	Describe potential context for delivery, organizational framework, future potential payment mechanism(s) for sustainability, and cost of intervention (if known).

a "completer" (see Chapter 5); (c) the intervention flow or what transpires in each treatment session (see Chapter 3); (d) the skill set and background of individuals who will provide the intervention (see Chapter 22); (e) the content of and approach to training interventionists (see Chapter 22); and (f) a treatment fidelity plan (see Chapter 12). The extent to which each of these elements is described will depend upon the phase of development of the intervention. For example, in proposing a pilot study (Phase I or II) to evaluate dosing, one might not have an extensive fidelity plan; whereas in an efficacy trial (Phase III), this would need to be fully explicated.

There is no right or wrong way to describe an intervention in a grant proposal. The goal is to enable reviewers to have a concrete understanding of the intervention and its importance upon reading an application. Providing a case example that summarizes the intervention components and expected benefits and using a table to outline the specific steps of the intervention or describe the activities of each treatment session are potentially useful illustrative tools. One must weigh the relative merits of any one of these approaches or use of graphics given page limitations to determine the best way to convey a compelling story about the intervention.

Page Limitations

As behavioral intervention research is complex, the page limitations frequently imposed by funders can be painful. There are many different components to explain in an intervention study as discussed earlier, particularly at the efficacy and effectiveness phases, and page limitations imposed by funders can be a challenge.

Unfortunately, behavioral intervention researchers are caught between needing to provide details and lack of space to do so. A common critique by grant reviewers is that a proposal lacks sufficient details to fully understand the proposed study particularly as it concerns a recruitment plan, the intervention, the measures, and/or the data analytic approach. Thus, despite page limitations, the narrative of a proposal must contain the essential details for reviewers to fully comprehend the applicant's plan of action. Therefore, every word and sentence in a proposal must be contributory. There is no room for superfluous statements.

It can be challenging to decide which detail to include in a proposal narrative. Using tables to summarize information such as proposed measures, their psychometric properties and testing occasion, or session-by-session (see Chapter 3) description of the intervention may save space and allow a lot of information to be displayed. As figures and tables can often be inserted in a proposal using small font sizes (e.g., Arial 9), they can save space yet provide important details; however, always check first as to whether the funding agency allows this type of approach and smaller font. While all grant proposals do have a certain level of redundancy, in an intervention proposal this has to be minimized given space constraints.

Page limitations are particularly challenging when proposing efficacy or effectiveness trials as study designs for these trials often have multiple components that must be explained. For example, when proposing a randomized trial, each of the following elements of the study design must be explained: the testing occasions, measures, each of the interventions to be tested (treatment and control groups), recruitment and retention plans, fidelity strategies, theory bases, pilot work justifying the trial, power and sample size considerations, and analytic plan. To maximize space, a flow chart to illustrate the proposed study design or conceptual model can help to illustrate the variables of interest and their hypothetical linkages. As stated previously, a table of measures can outline each measure being proposed, its purpose (e.g., covariate, baseline descriptor, primary or secondary outcome), psychometric properties, and other relevant details; and a table outlining the content of intervention sessions can efficiently relay what will be tested.

Proof of Feasibility

In writing a proposal to support intervention development or testing, an important aspect is providing evidence that each aspect of the proposed study is feasible including one's recruitment plans, approach to interviewing and acceptability of measures, and, as discussed earlier, delivery of the intervention. Recruiting study participants for intervention research is a frequently overlooked task that is critical, of course, to the success of any type of trial or testing phase. Having a well-developed recruitment and retention plan that is adequately budgeted for is paramount (see Chapter 10). Demonstrating some proof that the expected number of participants can be enrolled (and retained) in the trial is essential at any phase of the pipeline. Some agencies will require upon funding a quarterly or yearly accounting of enrollment progress, and funds may be adjusted if accrual goals are not met.

If one is proposing an innovative approach to data capture or treatment delivery (e.g., through the Internet or a technology), demonstrating proof of its feasibility is important as reviewers will evaluate the proposal on this basis.

Human Subject Considerations

Any study or research proposal involving human subjects must be concerned with establishing and maintaining ethical practices in the recruitment, enrollment, consenting, interviewing, and intervention delivery processes (see Chapter 13). However, in intervention research, there are additional concerns including the possibility of an adverse event from proposed treatments and participant burden. Thus, human subject considerations must take into account potential adverse events from a treatment (including for the control group conditions), and how the investigative team will handle such possibilities. Although most behavioral intervention studies do not report the occurrences of adverse events, precautions must be put into place in case they do occur. Also, as behavioral intervention research involves interacting with people over multiple occasions, it is possible for the research team to encounter any number of issues that are not due to the study itself but that may require action. These issues may include but are not limited to participant hospitalization, falls, death, unsafe home environmental conditions (e.g., home infestations, lack of heat or air conditioning), and financial, emotional, or physical abuse or neglect, to name a few of the common events that may occur. Having a plan in place to ethically respond to each of these challenges (e.g., contacting adult protective services or linking participants to needed home repair services) must be detailed in a human subjects plan. Furthermore, all staff must be trained in how to address or respond to, report, and record such events.

Appendices

Although appendices are permitted in most grant mechanisms, it is best to inquire if this is the case and if so, how many appendices and types of materials can be included. The materials included in an appendix should be helpful to understand the proposed study but not include critical study details to circumvent page limitations of the grant narrative. Appendices should be used only to offer supplemental information or information that supports the narrative. Appendices might include but are not limited to letters from stakeholders, screening and interview batteries, intervention manuals, intervention training agenda, fidelity measures, and recruitment brochures.

Budgetary Considerations

Developing a budget and a justification for each line item for an intervention study is not unlike budget development for any other type of study proposal. It takes time, careful thought, knowledge of technical budget terms, an understanding of the requirements of the targeted funding agency and one's own institution, and, of course, the specific needs of the proposed study.

It is helpful to sketch out a budget early on when developing a proposal. As intervention studies can be costly, an initial determination of what it will cost to recruit and enroll, deliver the intervention, assure fidelity, and evaluate outcomes can indicate its feasibility early on in the grant writing process and whether the potential budget is in keeping with the targeted funding mechanism. If the funds required to carry out the proposed set of activities exceed the limits imposed by an agency or specific program announcement, then a different funding mechanism needs to be identified or the approach must be modified to conform to the budgetary constraints of the funding announcement.

Each funding agency has its own rules about allowable and nonallowable expenses and the level of F&A (facility and administrative costs, formerly known as "indirect costs") permitted. This information should guide the development of a budget. Also, each institution has specific procedures for developing a grant budget including allowable yearly salary increases, fringe benefit rates, allowable in-kind contributions, and the F&A cost-recovery rate. Knowing these rules prior to developing a grant application will save considerable time and energy.

In developing a budget, it is important to be as realistic as possible and not to under- or overinflate budgetary needs. Budgets typically contain three sections: direct costs or the costs directly associated with specific grant activity (e.g., recruitment, interviewing, delivery of interventions, data capture, and analyses); F&A costs or the allowable indirect costs that are over and above direct costs to offset costs such as lighting, administrative financial oversight, and so forth; and institutional commitments. As to the latter, some agencies require or strongly encourage in-kind contributions whereas others do not. When an in-kind contribution is mandatory or encouraged, it is important to discuss this first with one's institution (e.g., department chair, dean, research administrator) to determine what would be allowed from an institutional perspective. Not every institution will agree or be able to provide an in-kind contribution and thus a grant submission may or may not be encouraged.

To determine direct costs, consider the activities that will need to be carried out to address each proposed study aim. Considerations include personnel and their level of effort, supplies, equipment, travel, costs associated with the delivery of the intervention and the comparison group, costs associated with carrying out a fidelity plan and staff training, and costs associated with recruitment such as advertisement, travel costs, brochures and staff effort, study participant honorariums, and time for consultants. Oftentimes, the real costs associated with recruitment (see Chapter 10) are underestimated or overlooked in grant applications, but this is a critical activity in intervention studies that is very time consuming and that requires resources (staffing and funds to support advertisements, media announcements, etc.).

CONCLUSION

As intervention development occurs over time and involves a wide range of activities requiring resources and funding, grant writing to obtain funding support is an essential part of this form of research for each phase along the pipeline. Grant writing to support intervention development is not dissimilar to grant writing for any other type of research effort. However, as discussed, there are specific challenges unique to advancing an intervention. One of the biggest challenges that the field confronts is that funding levels for behavioral intervention research are rather modest compared to funding levels for biomedical and drug development research. Nevertheless, some funds are available. Thus, learning how to write a competitive application is a necessary skill for being a successful behavioral intervention researcher.

REFERENCES

Curran, G. M., Bauer, M. Mittman, B., Pyne, J. M., & Stetler, C. (2012). Effectiveness imple-mentation hybrid designs: Combining elements of clinical effectiveness and implementa-tion research to enhance public health impact. *Medical Care, 50*(3), 217–226.

Gitlin, L. N., & Lyons, K. J. (2013) *Successful grant writing: Strategies for health and human service professionals* (4th ed.). New York, NY: Springer.

Riley, W. T., Glasgow, R. E., Etheredge, L., & Abernethy, A. P. (2013). Rapid, responsive, relevant (R3) research: A call for a rapid learning health research enterprise. *Clinical and Translational Medicine, 2,* 10. doi:10.1186/2001-1326-2-10

Stirman, S.W., Miller, C. J., Toder, K., & Calloway, A. (2012). Development of a framework and coding system for modifications and adaptations of evidence-based interventions. *Implementation Science, 8,* 65. doi:10.1186/1748-5908-8-65

WHAT TO PUBLISH AND WHEN: BEING PRODUCTIVE WHILE AWAITING MAIN OUTCOMES AND OTHER CONSIDERATIONS

Either write something worth reading or do something worth writing.
—Benjamin Franklin

Sharing knowledge generated from research is fundamental to the research enterprise and an ethical obligation of investigators. Publishing results is an essential action of research such that an investigation cannot be considered complete without engaging in a dissemination activity of some form (DePoy & Gitlin, 2015). Communicating the results of scholarly research is important across all disciplines and research designs whether qualitative, quantitative, or integrated mixed methods. While these points may appear obvious, it is important to recognize and honor this obligatory and contributory expectation when conducting behavioral intervention research.

Knowledge gained from a research study can be shared in multiple formats (e.g., video, oral presentations, blog posts, editorials, final reports). However, the most esteemed and respected approach in academia is the dissemination of evidence through peer-reviewed journal publications. Publications in peer-reviewed outlets are an explicit demand of academia and funders of research such as the National Institutes of Health (NIH). Evidence reported in peer-reviewed publications can garner important attention in news outlets and by stakeholders. In turn this helps to support and legitimize moving forward with the translation and implementation of a proven program.

It can take an extraordinary amount of time for the outcomes of an intervention study to be available for analyses, interpretation, and manuscript preparation. This is particularly the case when conducting Phase II (proof of concept), III (efficacy), or IV (effectiveness) trials. Main trial outcomes may not be available until upwards of 1 to 5 years from initiation of a study. Treatment outcomes from traditional research designs, such as the randomized clinical trial, can typically not be reported until data from all follow-up time points have been collected. Consequently, the question arises as to how to fulfill the need to maintain productivity while waiting for the final outcome data to be ready for analyses and write-up.

The delay in publishing main study outcomes until the completion of a planned trial can serve as an unnecessary deterrent to engaging in behavioral intervention research. Unfortunately, doctoral, postdoctoral, and early-stage faculty members are often dissuaded by their mentors to participate in this form of inquiry because of its complexity, and what appears to be an elongated time frame for generating manuscripts. However, there are many important opportunities for developing meaningful and contributory publications related to a trial that do not require waiting years for primary outcome results to be available. Thus, the need to publish should not serve as a barrier to participating in behavioral intervention research.

The purpose of this chapter is to offer guidance as to what to publish and when in behavioral intervention research. In particular, we focus our discussion on the efficacy trial phase as it poses the most challenges to publishing. We also discuss writing guidelines and key elements of a main outcomes paper. Our main message is twofold: developing contributory and meaningful publications is important and possible prior to waiting for main trial outcomes to be accessible; and selecting a journal outlet and developing a main outcome publication is a thoughtful process entailing the identification of key stakeholders one wishes to impact.

WHAT TO PUBLISH WHEN WAITING FOR MAIN OUTCOMES

Being productive while awaiting main trial outcomes may appear daunting; however, it is very feasible. There are multiple important opportunities for publishing prior to developing a main trial outcome paper. This is particularly the case if a trial is initially designed with the explicit goal of generating meaningful papers that are complimentary to, but independent of, reporting main trial outcomes.

Figure 24.1 outlines five key possibilities for generating meaningful publications when conducting a behavioral intervention trial. These include manuscripts that: (a) describe the study protocol; (b) involve systematic reviews or meta-analyses of research relevant to the intervention being tested; (c) describe an innovative collaborative partnership or model of care; (d) present novel recruitment, enrollment, and/or screening approaches; and (e) report baseline data collection efforts, such as the psychometric properties of a new measure being used in the study, or research questions of a correlational nature.

Protocol Manuscripts

Prior to actually launching a behavioral intervention, an important and initial manuscript can be generated by providing a description of the study's protocol. A protocol paper describes in detail the intervention protocol and trial design. These types of papers are gaining recognition and importance as evidenced by the increasing number of outlets for these types of manuscripts as shown in Table 24.1.

To publish a protocol paper requires prior formal approval of the study protocol by a funding source and/or institutional review board. Furthermore, the study should also be registered with at least one clinical trial registry, examples of which

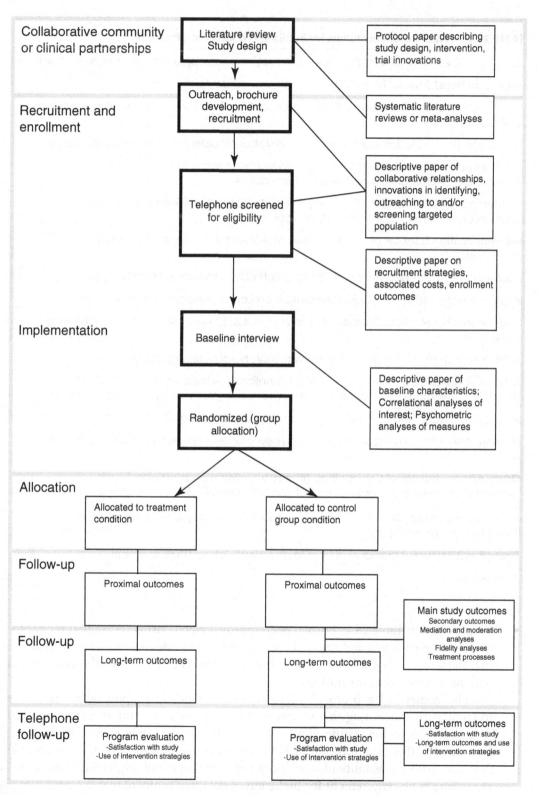

Figure 24.1 Study flow of a typical randomized trial and opportunities for manuscript development.

TABLE 24.1   Select Potential Outlets for Publishing a Research Protocol

Addiction Science & Clinical Practice (IF = n/a): www.ascpjournal.org/authors/instructions

American Heart Journal (IF = 4.50): www.ahjonline.com/authorinfo

BioMed Central (BMC, including *BMC Geriatrics* [IF = 1.97]): www.biomedcentral.com/authors/protocols

BMJ Open (IF = 1.58): bmjopen.bmj.com/site/about/guidelines.xhtml#studyprotocols

Clinical Interventions in Aging (IF = 2.65): www.dovepress.com/call-for-papers-clinical-interventions-in-aging-d57-j4

Contemporary Clinical Trials (IF = 1.60) (formerly *Controlled Clinical Trials*): www.journals.elsevier.com/contemporary-clinical-trials/

Implementation Science (IF = 2.37): www.implementationscience.com/authors/instructions

International Psychogeriatrics (IF = 2.19): assets.cambridge.org/IPG/IPG_ifc.pdf

Injury Prevention (IF = 1.76): injuryprevention.bmj.com/site/about/guidelines.xhtml

JMIR: Journal of Medical Internet Research (IF = 4.66): www.jmir.org/announcement/view/55

JMIR Research Protocols (IF = n/a): www.researchprotocols.org/about

Journal of Advanced Nursing (IF = 1.57): onlinelibrary.wiley.com/journal/10.1111/(ISSN)1365-2648/homepage/protocol_for_a_research_study_or_systematic_review.htm

Journal of Clinical Trials (IF = n/a): www.omicsgroup.org/journals/clinical-trials.php

Neurosurgery (IF = 3.01): journals.lww.com/neurosurgery/Pages/InformationforAuthors.aspx

Open Access Journal of Clinical Trials (IF = n/a): www.dovepress.com/aims-and-scope-open-access-journal-of-clinical-trials-d43-j51

Reproductive Health (IF = 1.31): www.reproductive-health-journal.com/authors/instructions/studyprotocol

Trials (IF = 2.21): www.trialsjournal.com/authors/instructions/studyprotocol

IF, impact factor.

---

are provided in Table 24.2. Formal peer-approval mechanisms assure that the protocol has been reviewed and deemed meritorious. It provides a measure of confidence that the study is not a fleeting idea, but a worthy endeavor, with the potential of making a scientific contribution.

The content of a protocol paper will vary depending upon what one seeks to emphasize concerning the novelty and importance of the intervention and trial (see examples such as Gitlin et al., 2012; Gitlin, Winter, Dennis, & Hauck, 2007; Gross et al., 2014; Szanton et al., 2014). On occasion, a protocol paper may include data concerning feasibility of recruitment or some aspect of implementation. However, there is no requirement for inclusion of data in a protocol manuscript.

Table 24.3 provides an outline of common, basic elements of a protocol paper. Sections can be informed by the original grant proposal or institutional review

TABLE 24.2   Sample of Clinical Trial Registries

Name	Description	Website Address
ClinicalTrials.gov	ClinicalTrials.gov is an international, Web-based registry and results database that provides patients, their family members, health care professionals, researchers, and the public with easy access to information on publicly and privately supported clinical studies on a wide range of diseases and conditions. The website is maintained by the National Library of Medicine (NLM) at the National Institutes of Health (NIH). Information on ClinicalTrials.gov is provided and updated by the sponsor or principal investigator of the clinical study. Studies are generally submitted to the website (i.e., registered) when they begin, and the information on the site is updated throughout the study. In some cases, results of the study are submitted after the study ends.	clinicaltrials.gov/
Alzheimer's Disease Education and Referral (ADEAR) Center—Clinical Trials	ADEAR's purpose is to "compile, archive, and disseminate information concerning Alzheimer's disease" for health professionals, people with Alzheimer's disease and their families, and the public. Information on current clinical trials in the United States is available through the website. Alzheimer's disease and related clinical trials are searchable through the ADEAR Center, a service of the National Institute on Aging (NIA), one of the federal government's NIH and part of the U.S. Department of Health and Human Services. The NIA conducts and supports research about health issues for older people, and is the primary federal agency for Alzheimer's disease research. ADEAR Center strives to be a current, comprehensive, unbiased source of information about Alzheimer's disease. All information and materials about the search for causes, treatment, cures, and better diagnostic tools are carefully researched and thoroughly reviewed by NIA scientists and health communicators for accuracy and integrity.	www.nia.nih.gov/alzheimers/clinical-trials
International Clinical Trials Registry Platform (ICTRP)	ICTRP Search Portal aims to provide a single point of access to information about ongoing and completed clinical trials. It provides a searchable database containing the trial registration data sets made available by data providers around the world meeting control. The mission of the WHO ICTRP is to ensure that a complete view of research is accessible to all those involved in health care decision making.	apps.who.int/trialsearch/

(Continued)

TABLE 24.2 Sample of Clinical Trial Registries   (Continued)

Name	Description	Website Address
UK Clinical Trials Gateway (UKCTG)	The UKCTG provides easy-to-understand information about clinical research trials running in the United Kingdom providing access to a large range of information about these trials. The UKCTG is established by the National Institute for Health Research on behalf of all the UK Health Departments and with the assistance of a number of clinical research charities, research professionals, and patient representatives. It fulfills the government's commitment in the "Plan for Growth," published by HM Treasury in March 2011 that the government will open up information about clinical trials to enable the public to get involved so that patients can find out about clinical trials that may be relevant to their condition.	www.ukctg.nihr.ac.uk/default.aspx
European Union Clinical Trials Register	The European Union Clinical Trials Register contains information on interventional clinical trials on medicines conducted in the European Union, or the European Economic Area (EEA), which started after May 1, 2004.	www.clinical trialsregister.eu
Australian New Zealand Clinical Trials Registry (ANZCTR)	The ANZCTR is an online register of clinical trials being undertaken in Australia, New Zealand, and elsewhere. The ANZCTR includes trials from the full spectrum of therapeutic areas of pharmaceuticals, surgical procedures, preventive measures, lifestyle, devices, treatment and rehabilitation strategies, and complementary therapies. In 2007, the ANZCTR was one of the first three trial registries to be recognized by the WHO ICTRP as a Primary Registry. WHO recognizes registries as Primary Registries if they fulfill certain criteria with respect to data content, quality and validity, accessibility, unique identification, technical capacity, and administration. The ANZCTR contributes data to the WHO ICTRP, which was developed in 2007.	http://www.anzctr.org.au/TrialSearch.aspx
International Standard Randomized Controlled Trial Number (ISRCTN)	The ISRCTN is a simple numeric system for the unique identification of randomized controlled trials worldwide. The ISRCTN Register also accepts registration of other forms of studies designed to assess the efficacy of health care interventions.	isrctn.org/

(Continued)

TABLE 24.2 Sample of Clinical Trial Registries (Continued)

Name	Description	Website Address
Japan Medical Association—Center for Clinical Trials (JMACCT)	The JMA has been conducting Clinical Trial Promotion Research Project subsidized by the Ministry of Health, Labor, and Welfare since 2003 to facilitate improvement of the clinical trial infrastructure through the model research of investigator-initiated trials and formation of regional clinical trial networks, and various advocacy efforts as well.	dbcentre3.jmacct .med.or.jp/jmactr/ Default_Eng.aspx
University Hospital Medical Information Network (UMIN)	UMIN was established in 1989 as a cooperative organization for national medical schools in Japan, sponsored by the Ministry of Education, Culture, Science, Sports, and Technology (MEXT), Japan. UMIN's purposes are as follows: ■ To provide up-to-date information to health care professionals ■ To promote communications between health care professionals ■ To support collaborative work among university hospitals ■ To support collaborative medical research ■ To standardize medical data and collect hospital statistics UMIN is now the largest and most versatile academic network information center for biomedical sciences in the world, and it is now considered an indispensable information infrastructure for the Japanese medical community.	www.umin.ac.jp/ctr/ new-registration/
Brazilian Clinical Trials Registry (Registro Brasileiro de Ensaios Clinicos [ReBec])	The ReBEC is an open-access virtual platform for registration of ongoing experimental and nonexperimental studies on humans performed in Brazil. ReBEC is a joint Project of Brazilian Ministry of Health, The Pan American Health Organization (PAHO), and The Oswaldo Cruz Foundation (FIOCRUZ). The Executive Committee of ReBEC is composed of the aforementioned institutions and also The National Health Surveillance Agency (ANVISA).	www.ensaiosclinicos .gov.br/
Chinese Clinical Trial Register (ChiCTR)	ChiCTR is hosted on Chinese Evidence-Based Medicine Center, West China Hospital, Sichuan University. The ChiCTR is a nonprofit organization, is established according to both the WHO International Clinical Trials Register Platform Standard and Ottawa Group Standard. ChiCTR provides the services that include register for trials, consultation for trial design, central randomization for an allocation sequence, peer review for draft articles, and training for peer reviewers.	http://www.chictr .org.cn

(Continued)

TABLE 24.2 Sample of Clinical Trial Registries (Continued)

Name	Description	Website Address
Clinical Research Information Service (CRIS)	The CRIS is a nonprofit online registration system for clinical trials (researches) to be conducted in Korea. It has been established at the Korea Centers for Disease Control and Prevention (KCDC) with support from the Ministry of Health and Welfare (MOHW). It joined the WHO ICTRP as 11th member of Primary Registry. The CRIS includes any clinical trial or research that will be prospectively conducted with human participants aiming to prevent, detect, diagnose, or treat diseases. The clinical trial or research should be approved by the Institutional Review Board (IRB) prior to the registration on the CRIS. For multinational clinical trials or researches, the principal investigator should register the trial or research to prevent inadequate information or double registration. The information registered into the CRIS is open to the public on a real-time basis, domestically and internationally, from the time when the system administrator approves the trial or research.	https://cris.nih.go.kr/cris/en/use_guide/cris_introduce.jsp
Clinical Trials Registry—India (CTRI)	The CTRI, hosted at the Indian Council of Medical Research (ICMR) National Institute of Medical Statistics (nims-icmr.nic.in), is a free and online public record system for registration of clinical trials being conducted in India that was launched on July 20, 2007 (www.ctri.nic.in). Initiated as a voluntary measure, since June 15, 2009, trial registration in the CTRI has been made mandatory by the Drugs Controller General of India (DCGI) (www.cdsco.nic.in). Moreover, editors of biomedical journals of 11 major journals of India declared that only registered trials would be considered for publication.	ctri.nic.in/Clinicaltrials/login.php
Internet Portal of the German Clinical Trials Register [Deutsches Register Klinischer Studien [DRKS]]	The DRKS is an open-access online register for clinical trials conducted in Germany that allows all users to search, register, and share information on clinical trials. The DRKS is funded by the Federal Ministry of Education and Research (BMBF) and implemented at the Center for Medical Biometry and Medical Informatics at the University Medical Center Freiburg as a common project of the Clinical Trial Unit of the University Medical Center Freiburg and the German Cochrane Center. The DRKS was implemented and is further developed in collaboration with the WHO, especially with the ICTRP. It is an approved WHO Primary Register since October 2008 and thus meets the requirements of the International Committee of Medical Journal Editors (ICMJE), whose members decided in September 2004 already that the prospective registration of clinical trials was a necessary requirement for later publications in the leading medical journals.	https://drks-neu.uniklinik-freiburg.de/drks_web/

(Continued)

TABLE 24.2 Sample of Clinical Trial Registries (Continued)

Name	Description	Website Address
Iranian Registry of Clinical Trials (IRCT)	IRCT is a nonprofit website set up with the help from the Ministry of Health and Medical Education. The three main objectives of this site are the following: ■ Informing the public of the ongoing trials ■ Increasing public awareness of their importance ■ Implementing the ICMJE's initiative for mandatory registration of trials before the enrollment of the first patient	www.irct.ir/
The Thai Clinical Trials Registry (TCTR)	The TCTR is an online register of clinical researches established in Thailand since 2009. The website has been operated by Clinical Research Collaboration Network (CRCN), an organization under the Medical Research Foundation, which is a nonprofit organization, and financially supported by Thailand Center of Excellence for Life Sciences (TCELS). CRCN has been retitled the Medical Research Network (MedResNet) since June 15, 2012. The mission of the TCTR is to encourage all clinical trials conducted in Thailand to be prospectively registered before the subject recruitment. This is to promote research transparency, to reduce redundancy, and to minimize publication bias or selective reporting. Registrants who wish to register clinical trials in TCTR are obliged to disclose details of the 20 mandatory items of the WHO ICTRP dataset. TCTR also aims to be a research database for clinical researches in Thailand, thus it welcomes the registration of all kinds of clinical researches including clinical trials and observational studies.	www.clinicaltrials.in.th
Netherlands Trial Register	Dutch Trial Register is part of the Dutch Cochrane Centre, one of the centers of the international Cochrane Collaboration. This international nonprofit organization of volunteers collects and analyzes mainly all possible information about clinical trials, compiling them into systematic reviews. For now, the Cochrane researchers are dependent on official publications, or manually sleuthing in conference reports. A public prospective trial registry will not only make it easier to review work but also make it more complete. In collaboration with other stakeholders, the Dutch Cochrane Centre was established. This is a prospective Dutch Trial Register in the Netherlands involving research into the effectiveness of interventions in health care. The Central Committee for Research Involving Human Subjects (CCMO) plays the role of advisor.	www.trialregister.nl/trialreg/index.asp

(Continued)

TABLE 24.2 Sample of Clinical Trial Registries (Continued)

Name	Description	Website Address
Pan African Clinical Trials Registry (PACTR)	The PACTR is a regional register of clinical trials conducted in Africa. The registry is an African initiative serving the needs of Africans. It provides an open-access platform where clinical trials can be registered free of charge. The PACTR aims to increase clinical trial registration in Africa by developing awareness of the need to register trials and by supporting trialists during registration.	www.pactr.org/
The Sri Lanka Clinical Trials Registry (SLCTR)	The SLCTR is an Internet-based, not-for-profit clinical trials registry providing free access to researchers, clinicians, funding agencies, and the public. It welcomes registration of trials conducted in Sri Lanka and overseas. The SLCTR has been operational from November 2006, and was the first functioning clinical trials registry in South Asia. It was recognized as a Primary Registry of the Registry Network of the WHO ICTRP in March 2008. The SLCTR currently accepts only clinical trials with a health-related intervention and does not register observational studies. It encourages prospective registration of all clinical trials, and does not accept trials for retrospective registration. It meets all the requirements specified by the WHO ICTRP and the ICMJE. The SLCTR is managed by the SLCTR Committee, an advisory group appointed by the Sri Lanka Medical Association (SLMA). The SLMA is the premiere professional medical association in Sri Lanka, and is the oldest medical organization in Australasia with a proud history dating back to 1887.	slctr.lk/

TABLE 24.3   Basic Contents of a Protocol Paper

Front matter
  Title page
  Abstract
  Trial registration: ClinicalTrials.gov #NCT00511680
  Acknowledgments
Background/significance
Methods/design
  Aims and study hypotheses
  Recruitment, eligibility, and randomization
  Measures
  Intervention
    Theory base
    Delivery characteristics
    Session content
  Control group
  Analytic plan
    Sample size and power
    Primary analyses
    Secondary analyses
    Exploratory analyses
    Determination of clinical significance
    Cost analysis (if relevant)
  Evidence of feasibility (if relevant and data available)
    Recruitment and enrollment outcomes
    Baseline characteristics of sample
    Program costs
Discussion
Tables (examples)
  Session-by-session content of intervention
  Recruitment results
  Baseline characteristics
  Intervention cost categories
Figure of study design

board protocol submission. As a result, there is efficiency in writing a manuscript of this type in that the materials that have been previously prepared can be repurposed and updated. Furthermore, a published protocol can also be referred to in subsequent publications that evaluate outcomes so that readers can refer to a more detailed explication of study design and protocols.

As with any journal submission, it is important to first carefully read author instructions in order to appropriately prepare the manuscript. In addition, it is helpful to read other protocol papers that have been published by the targeted journal, which can serve as a guide for observing conventions and providing the expected range of content included in these types of publications.

Publishing a protocol paper is important for several reasons.

First, reading protocol papers in general is an excellent way of learning about forthcoming intervention studies and study designs that are employed by others. This can help to advance one's own knowledge base and intervention work.

Second, a protocol paper serves as a foundational publication that provides the details of the intervention and study design, which can then be referred to in future manuscripts about the study. Because most data-driven journals impose word limitations on content, it is often difficult to provide study design and intervention details in manuscripts. Unfortunately, most interventions are not well described in publications. This is particularly the case for complex, multicomponent interventions and those directed at behavior change (Michie, Fixsen, Grimshaw & Eccles, 2009). Hence, referring readers to a protocol or methods paper that goes into depth with the important nuances of the trial design and the intervention delivery characteristics can be invaluable.

Third, it is a way to disseminate information about the ongoing trial. This provides others who are working in the field with an understanding of works-in-progress and forthcoming intervention developments and outcomes. This is helpful to the scientific community and in turn to authors themselves as others working in a similar area may seek out professional exchanges.

Fourth, a protocol paper reflects the established and approved methodologies of a study. As such, it can serve as a reference source for the investigative team concerning study details and key citations for future papers and presentations.

Finally, a published protocol paper reflects productivity of the investigative team and can be cited in progress reports to funders.

Systematic Reviews or Meta-Analyses Manuscripts

The development of an intervention typically requires conducting some type of literature review of previous related studies. Such a review informs the development of an intervention and also locates the intervention within a trajectory of knowledge building an incremental scientific advancement. There are many different approaches to conducting a literature review, but following a systematic process is of utmost importance, particularly if the end goal is to publish the results.

One approach is to conduct a systematic review. As White and Schmidt (2005) describe, "systematic reviews retrieve, appraise and summarize all the available evidence on a specific health question" (p. 54). Systematic reviews follow a particular protocol to avoid the researcher's own biases and to assure that a full and adequate appraisal of the existing literature is provided. The Agency for Health Research and Quality (AHRQ) is at the forefront of advancing this approach for health-related reviews and offers models and tutorials (see tectutorials.com/SRAHRQProcess.html). AHRQ also developed a Systematic Review Data Repository (see ahrq-srdr-prod-347362009.us-east-1.elb.amazonaws.com/) that serves as a searchable archive of systematic reviews of health-related issues. It may be helpful to review the repository to identify areas for which evaluations exist and the methodologies used.

Although not all journals publish systematic reviews, there is increased interest in these types of manuscripts. A few journals are expressly dedicated to publishing this type of study (see the journal *Systematic Reviews* at www.systematic reviewsjournal.com/).

Another form of a systematic review is the meta-analysis. A meta-analysis is considered the most rigorous form of a literature review: It uses statistical methodologies to examine the effect sizes of findings from a defined body of research. A meta-analysis equally informs future directions for intervention development and can be used to support a proposed intervention or study. The specific methodologies for conducting systematic and meta-analyses are beyond the scope of this chapter. However, it is important to recognize meta-analyses as a viable systematic approach for summarizing studies related to a behavioral intervention. This approach can be used to produce an important and contributory publication while developing and testing an intervention protocol.

Describing Innovative Models or Partnerships

Another consideration is to develop a publication concerning an innovative feature that is being evaluated in the design or model. Some journals have specific sections devoted to innovative models. Exemplars include but are not limited to Practice Concepts, a section of *The Gerontologist* that focuses on applying evidence to practice or intervention model; or Models of Geriatric Care, Quality Improvement, and Program Dissemination, a dedicated section in the *Journal of the American Geriatrics Society* (JAGS).

Describing novel partnerships between academic and community-based settings, for example, or collaborative arrangements designed to advance an intervention, warrant a rich description of what works, lessons learned, steps or processes followed, and recommendations for future efforts. Exemplars of innovative models worthy of reporting include but are not limited to use of community health workers to deliver health promotion interventions or a community–academic partnership to deliver an intervention (Counsell, Callahan, Buttar, Clark, & Frank, 2006; Gitlin et al., 2012; Samus et al., 2014).

Describing Novel Recruitment, Enrollment, or Screening Processes

Most, if not all, behavioral intervention studies confront a myriad of challenges in recruiting and enrolling study participants (see Chapter 10 on recruitment). Although there is a large corpus of literature on recruitment and enrollment techniques, there is always room for more publications in this area. This is particularly the case for articles that report on the recruitment, enrollment, or screening of a specific clinical or minority population. Also, reporting on the use of novel strategies for outreach and results of these approaches, and/or the costs associated with specific approaches employed, are potentially important contributions (Morrison, Winter, & Gitlin, 2014). Recruiting and enrolling participants from within specific practice or clinical settings (e.g., primary care, hospital, senior centers) versus recruiting and enrolling participants through the community-at-large pose very different challenges and require different strategies worthy of description and evaluation in publications (Gross et al., 2014). Describing strategies, models, approaches, or costs can all form the basis of meaningful publications.

Baseline Data Collection

Data collected at baseline and prior to randomization and group allocation can inform specific research questions that lead to meaningful publications. One type of publication is the evaluation of the psychometric properties of a new measure if a sufficient sample size is available. Gitlin and colleagues' (2005) publication on the psychometric properties of the Caregiver Assessment of Function and Upset (CAFU) is an example of such an approach. The data presented was from the baseline data collection effort of the NIH Resources for Enhancing Alzheimer's Caregiver Health (REACH I) multisite initiative involving an evaluation of six distinct caregiver interventions in diverse geographic locations (Gitlin et al., 2003). The CAFU, a 17-item measure of caregiver report of functional dependence of the person with dementia and the caregiver's own level of upset with dependency, was developed by REACH investigators and utilized by three of six sites. Once baseline data collection was completed, an evaluation of the psychometric properties of this measure was possible. The psychometric properties were important to report as the CAFU was subsequently used as an outcome measure.

Similarly, a psychometric evaluation may be warranted if the population included in the trial represents a new group of individuals for whom validation of a previously developed scale has not occurred. For example, Roth and colleagues (2003) used the NIH REACH I baseline data set involving over 1,200 dyads (family caregivers and persons with dementia) to evaluate the psychometric properties of the Revised Memory and Problem Checklist (Teri et al., 1992). The analyses extended an understanding of its psychometric properties by confirming its factor structure with White/Caucasians, examining its properties for Hispanic/Latino and African American/Black, not previously considered, and evaluating its subscale, caregiver upset with behaviors, that had also not previously been examined.

In addition, there is always a need to develop and advance appropriate measures for intervention studies. Therefore, introducing items at baseline relevant to the study purpose and testing their psychometric properties as part of a trial can advance measurement in important ways (Gitlin, Winter, Dennis, & Hauck, 2006; Gitlin et al., 2002).

Although the main goal of a trial is to evaluate intervention benefits, there is a multitude of research questions of a correlational nature that can be posed using cross-sectional data collected at the baseline of a trial. For example, the Maximizing Independence at Home (MIND at Home) Trial examined the effects of an 18-month intervention helping 308 individuals with cognitive impairment to remain at home (Samus et al., 2014). Although main study outcomes of most interest were gathered at 18 months, important questions were also posed using cross-sectional analyses with the data collected at the baseline interview. These have included a description of unmet needs of persons with cognitive impairment (Black et al., 2013), how needs differ by cognitive impairment level (Hodgson, Black, Johnston,

Lyketsos, & Samus, 2014), and the relationship between level and type of need and caregiver burden (Hughes et al., 2014).

Structure of Evaluations

Reporting the evaluation of an intervention must contain: sufficient details about the study design and intervention to enable an understanding of potential study biases; support replication, and translation of findings into practice; and facilitate cross-study comparisons (Curry, Grossman, Whitlock, & Cantu, 2014; Glasziou, Chalmers, Green, & Michie, 2014; Grant, Mayo-Wilson, Melendez-Torres, & Montgomery, 2013; Mayo-Wilson et al., 2013). The structure of a report and the details that should be included vary considerably across journals.

In response to the persistent, inconsistent, and inadequate detailing of interventions in scientific journals across all areas of inquiry, reporting guidelines have emerged over the past two decades. The purpose of such guidelines is to improve transparency and quality and assure comprehensiveness of reports. There is no comprehensive and appropriate published guideline for behavioral intervention research. In fact, Grant and colleagues (2013) identified 19 different reporting guidelines that involve a total of 147 reporting standards relevant to behavioral intervention research. Evidence suggests that using reporting guidelines enhances the quality and consistency of reporting and can potentially advance a field of inquiry (Moher, Jones, Lepage, & CONSORT Group, 2001). Unfortunately, however, many journals currently do not require or endorse particular guidelines, and researchers do not systematically abide by them. Poor adherence to published guidelines continues to plague publications of behavioral interventions. Samaan and colleagues (2013) found in a review of 50 studies that 86% did not adequately adhere to reporting guidelines.

Nevertheless, guidelines are important and provide a roadmap for reporting a study. As such, various checklists are being advanced to address specific forms of evaluative designs and categories of behavioral interventions. Examples include the Transparent Reporting of Evaluations with Nonrandomized Designs (TREND) to guide reporting of nonrandomized studies that include evaluation of an intervention (Des Jarlais, Lyles, Crepaz, & TREND Group, 2004), and the Complex Interventions in Healthcare (CReDECI) for reporting complex behavioral interventions (Möhler, Bartoszek, Köpke, & Meyer, 2012).

One guideline in particular, the Consolidated Standards of Reporting Trials (CONSORT; 2010), is the most consistently used. It has been adopted by over 100 major journals, most of which are biomedical. The CONSORT checklist consists of 25 items for reporting a randomized trial of a nonpharmacological intervention including, for example, but not limited to, randomization procedures, blinding, statistical methods, and harms. Although its limitations are discussed later, we recommend using the CONSORT (see www.consort-statement.org/ for all items) checklist to help structure manuscripts for journals, even for those journals that do not require it. The checklist can also help guide the preparation of a grant application that proposes to evaluate a behavioral intervention (see Chapter 23 on grant writing for intervention research). Our purpose in this chapter is not to provide a comprehensive review and evaluation of the relative merits of existing guidelines, but to highlight their necessity and utility. As the most widely used is the CONSORT checklist, this is a good place to start when seeking guidance for structuring a main trial outcome paper.

Describing Behavioral Interventions

Despite the proliferation of reporting guidelines, there is no consensus as to what should be included in the actual description of an intervention that is evaluated. The elements of behavioral interventions that are reported tend to vary widely. Report details tend to be inconsistent across and even within journals. Michie and colleagues (2009) indicate that, in their review of over 1,000 behavioral change intervention outcome studies, from 5% to 30% provided sufficient details of actual interventions. Correspondingly, Grant and colleagues (2013) in a review of 239 trials found that less than half provided sufficient details about the experimental (43%) and control group (34%) conditions.

There are numerous significant consequences of inadequately reporting details of an intervention. These include the lack of ability to understand an intervention's treatment components and the relationship between components, and the specific delivery characteristics that may contribute the most to changes observed in outcome measures. Additionally, an inadequate description of an intervention can hinder its replication potential. Ioannidis (2005) found that, of 45 studies demonstrating intervention effectiveness, only 20 (44%) had findings that were subsequently replicated in further investigations. It is unclear whether failures were due to poor replication of an intervention, a possible Type II error of subsequent studies; or whether an intervention was not effective in the original trial, a Type I error. Difficulties in replication may contribute in part to the "17+" lag between idea inception of an intervention to its testing and implementation (Institute of Medicine [IOM], 2001).

Inconsistencies in reporting interventions are due to a range of causes. These may include the lack of scientific reporting guidelines specific to describing behavioral interventions; absence of a uniform and agreed-upon language to categorize and understand interventions and their delivery characteristics and treatment elements; restrictions imposed by scientific journals concerning page and/or word counts; lack of investigator understanding of the theory base and underlying mechanisms of an intervention; and, in some cases, proprietary considerations in which the commercialization of an intervention is the goal such that providing intervention details would interfere with marking and purchase potential. The lack of a uniform language to describe behavioral interventions is particularly disconcerting. For instance, terms such as "multimodal" and "multicomponent" are inconsistently defined and utilized in the literature. Also, in any one area, behavioral interventions are categorized and defined variably. Take for example, nonpharmacological interventions for persons with dementia and their caregivers. There is no consensus as to what constitutes a psychoeducational intervention versus a counseling intervention. Cognitive stimulation interventions vary widely, and there is no agreement as to the key elements of this approach. Care management and care coordination interventions remain "black boxes" such that the specific elements that constitute and distinguish these interventions from others are unclear. Similarly, the suboptimal reporting of behavior change interventions in preventing and treating HIV has resulted in poor uptake and replication. Abraham and colleagues (2014) identify four such inadequacies in this area: inadequate descriptions of interventions, variation in the content and reporting of active control groups, inadequate examination and reporting of underlying mechanisms by which the intervention has its effects and who benefits the most, and lack of replication limiting generalizability.

Despite the importance of the CONSORT statement, two critical aspects of intervention research are not clearly articulated. First, the CONSORT checklist does not include any mention of fidelity. One consequence of this may be that few publications on randomized trials include fidelity information (see Chapter 12 on fidelity concerning the consequences of not reporting fidelity).

Second, the CONSORT checklist does not provide sufficient guidance on the specific elements to include when describing an intervention. Schulz and colleagues (2010) suggest that "sufficient details [of each intervention] to allow replication including how and when they [interventions] were actually administered" (p. 2) be given.

To address the aforementioned shortcomings, many researchers and editors have developed extensions of the CONSORT checklist. Davidson and colleagues (2003) recommend that, at a minimum, details be provided about an intervention that address the "who, what, where, when, and how" aspects of delivery. The Workgroup for Intervention Development and Evaluation Research (WIDER) has advanced recommendations specific to behavior change interventions that have been adopted by several journals including *Implementation Science* (Michie et al., 2009) and *Addiction* (West, 2008). WIDER recommendations focus on four areas: "detailed description of interventions," "clarification of assumed change process and design principles," "access to intervention manuals/protocols," and "detailed description of active control conditions" (Albrecht, Archibald, Arseneau, & Scott, 2013, p. 3). Mayo-Wilson and colleagues (2013) are currently developing standards specific to social and psychological intervention trials (CONSORT-SPI) that complement, extend, and update CONSORT guidelines.

Building on these previous efforts and on the basis of our collective experiences, we recommend that seven elements of interventions be described as listed in Table 24.4.

The first element is a description of the theory base or underlying conceptual framework that guided intervention development, which can explain connections between treatment components. This should offer an understanding of why the intervention may have an impact on desired outcomes. Next is a description of seven aspects of the intervention's delivery including the dose, intensity and duration, target of intervention, mode and location of delivery, and format. If the intervention is complex, then describing each of its components is important. Providing a sense of the content of each session and the way in which the intervention unfolds are also helpful. There should also be a discussion about the interventionists including their level of skill and professional backgrounds, and the training required for the intervention. Certification procedures or how competence in intervention delivery is assessed should also be stated. Finally, a fidelity plan and associated measures should be described.

In addition to following reporting guidelines and adequately describing the intervention, there are other considerations in developing a main trial outcome paper.

TABLE 24.4 Basic Reporting Details of a Behavioral Intervention

Domain	Description
Theory base or conceptual framework	Specify theory base(s) or guiding conceptual framework(s) that are used to explain why or how the intervention may have benefits
Seven delivery characteristics	Describe (a) dose (number of sessions); (b) intensity (length of sessions); (c) duration (length of time of intervention); (d) mode of delivery (e.g., technology, telephone, face-to-face, combinations); (e) location or context of delivery; (f) target of intervention (e.g., who receives intervention); and (g) format (e.g., group, one-on-one, self-directed)
Treatment components	State components, modules, or elements that compose the intervention
Content of sessions	Specify range of content delivered
Interventionists	Describe who can administer the intervention and their characteristics
Training of interventionists	Describe length of time and basic content of training
Fidelity plan and measures	Describe plan, measures, and how used analytically

Foremost is what to include. Reporting on primary endpoints is of course paramount, but other research questions may also be included depending upon the data and the story it imparts. As suggested in Figure 24.1, these may include secondary outcomes, long-term outcomes, moderation analyses concerning which groups benefit, mediation analyses, why or how the intervention achieved its effects, long-term use of intervention strategies, satisfaction and acceptability of the intervention, and so forth. Although all of these elements would not be appropriate to include in one report, it suggests that, for any one trial, there are multiple potential outcome papers that can and should be generated.

WHERE TO PUBLISH

Choosing a publication outlet for presenting the primary outcomes of a behavioral intervention takes some thought. There are three key considerations: (a) the audience one wants to impact, (b) journal characteristics, and (c) strength of the evidence and study design.

The underlying purpose or ultimate goal of developing and evaluating behavioral interventions is to change practice and improve health care or health outcomes for a specified population. Thus, one consideration is determining the stakeholders one wishes to impact and the journal that effectively targets that group. For instance, let's say one is interested in changing the way in which family caregivers of frail older adults are integrated into the medical encounter with physicians (Wolff et al., 2014). Identifying and submitting the manuscript to a journal that is widely read by primary care physicians, geriatricians, and other health professionals in geriatrics would be appropriate and a preferred approach. A related consideration is whether to publish in a discipline-specific journal or one that has a broader readership. An evaluation of a social work–based intervention published in a journal that is read mostly by social workers may bring needed evidence to that professional group, but other health professionals might not have access to a discipline-specific journal or become aware of what might be a potentially beneficial program to their practice setting.

Another consideration concerns the characteristics of a journal. Factors such as its reach or breadth of distribution, whether its focus is general or disease- or topic-specific, its impact score, word limitations, and turnaround time from acceptance of the manuscript to its publication are considerations in decision making as to the relative benefits of publishing in a journal. As to word limitations, most medical journals, such as the *Journal of the American Medical Association* (JAMA), *Annals of Internal Medicine*, or the *Journal of the American Geriatrics Society*, impose word limitations that can hinder the inclusion of important details of an intervention such as its theory base or fidelity plan. Further, some journals may have a 1-year or more delay between accepting a manuscript and its actual publication. This delay significantly slows down dissemination processes. Thus, selecting a journal outlet entails balancing all of these factors with the underlying message and impact one seeks.

A helpful Internet-based tool for selecting a journal by inputting the manuscript title is JANE (journal/author, name estimator; biosemantics.org/jane/index. php). Upon identifying a journal, the first course of action is to carefully read the instructions for authors, as they will vastly differ from one journal to the other. Also, it is important to understand the rules for presenting findings in other outlets. Most medical journals will embargo the presentation or reporting of outcomes prior and up to the publication release date. It is essential that an embargo be strictly followed; otherwise, the journal may refuse publication. Finally, some journals refuse to publish a manuscript in which the data has previously been displayed on a website as it has already been released for public consumption. Thus, knowing the rules of the targeted journal is critical for a successful publication outcome.

A final consideration is the strength of the design of a study and its outcomes. It can be difficult to find a publication outlet for very weak or negative results unless the null findings are groundbreaking, contradict previously reported highly touted findings, or disprove a prevailing popular theory. Reports of studies using quasi-experimental designs or a pilot may best be classified as a brief report or titled "preliminary findings," in recognition of the need to build the evidence for the intervention. Reports of randomized controlled trials with statistically significant and clinically meaningful outcomes have a better chance of being published in a high-impact journal.

DISSEMINATING RESULTS AFTER PUBLICATION

Disseminating the knowledge gained from a trial is always a challenge, and developing a plan of action can be helpful. Publishing in a peer-reviewed journal is only the first step in disseminating results regardless of the journal's impact factor and reach. There are other important steps that can be taken to disseminate an effective intervention with the intent of positively impacting practice. Chapter 21 discussed the concept of having a dissemination plan. Here we consider media and publication outlets.

If the outcomes reported are considered a significant contribution or groundbreaking, then developing a press release would be important. Occasionally, the journal itself will develop a press release and coordinate with the primary author's institution. Press releases of articles reporting critical findings serve as an important mechanism for disseminating results. A press release may result in radio or television spots, blogs by newspapers, or access to other publicly available interviews.

If one's study outcomes change the paradigm of treatment and/or are topical (e.g., there is national debate on the topic or new related legislation), then it is worthwhile considering writing an op-ed piece or submitting a letter to an editor of a national and/or local newspaper. This approach allows one to provide an accessible, consumer-friendly version of the findings to maximize dissemination and outreach.

Presenting already published results in the form of blogs can also be part of a dissemination plan. Finally, it is important to provide key results to former participants of the study. Sending a letter to participants that explains in lay language the primary findings of the study is an ethical practice. Finally, speaking at professional association meetings and consumer-oriented conferences also helps with dissemination.

CONCLUSION

As in all steps and processes related to developing, evaluating, and implementing behavioral interventions, advancing publication entails a thoughtful process and set of actions geared toward cumulative knowledge building and changing practice. There are multiple and important opportunities in the form of publications to contribute scientifically prior to obtaining the main outcomes in an intervention study. This is particularly the case if a thoughtful stance is assumed in the initial design of the study. Identifying relevant research questions secondary to the primary trial outcome–oriented questions and including associated measures at baseline data collection can yield critical publications. For any manuscript, but particularly one reporting the main trial outcomes, selecting an appropriate journal is a strategic process. It entails balancing multiple factors with the primary goal of reaching key stakeholders who can act upon the evidence in a meaningful way to ultimately effect some type of change in practice. Publishing is not only a professional expectation but an ethical responsibility to use allocated resources for the advancement of knowledge and improvement of the public's health.

REFERENCES

Abraham, C., Johnson, B. T., de Bruin, M., & Luszczynska, A. (2014). Enhancing reporting of behavior change intervention evaluations. *Journal of Acquired Immune Deficiency Syndrome, 66,* S293–S299.

Albrecht, L., Archibald, M., Arseneau, D., & Scott, S. D. (2013). Development of a check-list to assess the quality of reporting of knowledge translation interventions using the workgroup for intervention development and evaluation research (WIDER) recommendations. *Implementation Science, 8*(52), 1–5.

Black, B. S., Johnston, D., Rabins, P. V., Morrison, A., Lyketsos, C., & Samus, Q. M. (2013). Unmet needs of community-residing persons with dementia and their informal caregivers: Findings from the maximizing independence at home study. *Journal of the American Geriatrics Society, 61*(12), 2087–2095.

Counsell, S. R., Callahan, C. M., Buttar, A. B., Clark, D. O., & Frank, K. I. (2006). Geriatric resources for assessment and care of elders (GRACE): A new model of primary care for low-income seniors. *Journal of the American Geriatrics Society, 54*(7), 1136–1141.

Curry, S. J., Grossman, D. C., Whitlock, E. P., & Cantu, A. (2014). Behavioral counseling research and evidence-based practice recommendations: US preventive services task force perspectives. *Annals of Internal Medicine, 160*(6), 407–413.

Davidson, K. W., Goldstein, M., Kaplan, R. M., Kaufmann, P. G., Knatterud, G. L., Orleans, C. T., . . . Whitlock, E. P. (2003). Evidence-based behavioral medicine: What is it and how do we achieve it? *Annals of Behavioral Medicine, 26*(3), 161–171.

DePoy, E., & Gitlin, L. N. (2015). *Introduction to research: Understanding and applying multiple strategies* (5th ed.). London, England: Elsevier Mosby.

Des Jarlais, D. C., Lyles, C., Crepaz, N., & TREND Group. (2004). Improving the reporting quality of nonrandomized evaluations of behavioral and public health interventions: The TREND statement. *American Journal of Public Health, 94*(3), 361–366.

Gitlin, L. N., Schinfeld, S., Winter, L., Corcoran, M., Boyce, A. A., & Hauck, W. (2002). Evaluating home environments of person with dementia: Interrater reliability and validity of the home environmental assessment protocol (HEAP). *Disability and Rehabilitation, 24*, 59–71. doi:10.1080/09638280110066325

Gitlin, L. N., Belle, S. H., Burgio, L. D., Czaja, S. J., Mahoney, D., Gallagher-Thompson, D., . . . Ory, M. G. (2003). Effect of multi-component interventions on caregiver burden and depression: The REACH multi-site initiative at six months follow-up. *Psychology and Aging, 18*(3), 361–374.

Gitlin, L. N., Harris, L. F., McCoy, M., Chernett, N. L., Jutkowitz, E., Pizzi, L. T., & Beat the Blues Team. (2012). A community-integrated home-based depression intervention for older African Americans: Description of the beat the blues randomized trial and intervention costs. *BMC Geriatrics, 12*(4), 1–11.doi:10.1186/1471-2318-12-4

Gitlin, L. N., Roth, D. L., Burgio, L. D., Loewenstein, D. A., Winter, L., Nichols, L., . . . Martindale, J. (2005). Caregiver appraisals of functional dependence in individuals with dementia and associated caregiver upset: Psychometric properties of a new scale and response patterns by caregiver and care recipient characteristics. *Journal of Aging and Health, 17*(2), 148–171. doi:10.1177/0898264304274184

Gitlin, L. N., Winter, L., Dennis, M. P., & Hauck, W. W. (2006). Assessing perceived change in the well-being of family caregivers: Psychometric properties of the perceived change index and response patterns. *American Journal of Alzheimer's Disease and Other Dementias, 21*(5), 304–311.

Gitlin, L. N., Winter, L., Dennis, M. P., & Hauck, W. W. (2007). A non-pharmacological intervention to manage behavioral and psychological symptoms of dementia and reduce caregiver distress: Design and methods of project ACT3. *Clinical Interventions in Aging, 2*(4), 695–703.

Glasziou, P. P., Chalmers, I., Green, S., & Michie, S. (2014). Intervention synthesis: A missing link between a systematic review and practical treatment(s). *PLoS Medicine, 11*(8), 1–7. doi:10.1371/journal.pmed.1001690

Grant, S. P., Mayo-Wilson, E., Melendez-Torres, G., & Montgomery, P. (2013). Reporting quality of social and psychological intervention trials: A systematic review of reporting guidelines and trial publications. *PloS One, 8*(5), 1–11. doi:10.1371/journal.pone.0065442

Gross, D. A., Belcher, H. M., Ofonedu, M. E., Breitenstein, S., Frick, K. D., & Chakra, B. (2014). Study protocol for a comparative effectiveness trial of two parent training programs in a fee-for-service mental health clinic: Can we improve mental health services to low-income families? *Trials, 15*(70), 1–10.

Hodgson, N. A., Black, B. S., Johnston, D., Lyketsos, C., & Samus, Q. M. (2014). Comparison of unmet care needs across the dementia trajectory: Findings from the maximizing independence at home study. *Journal of Geriatrics and Palliative Care, 2*(2), 5.

Hughes, T. B., Black, B. S., Albert, M., Gitlin, L. N., Johnson, D. M., Lyketsos, C. G., & Samus, Q. M. (2014). Correlates of objective and subjective measures of caregiver burden among dementia caregivers: Influence of unmet patient and caregiver dementia-related care needs. *International Psychogeriatrics, 26*(11), 1875–1883.

Institute of Medicine (US), & Committee on Quality of Health Care in America. (2001). *Crossing the quality chasm: A new health system for the 21st century.* Washington, DC: National Academies Press.

Ioannidis, J. P. (2005). Why most published research findings are false. *PLoS Medicine, 2*(8), e124.

Mayo-Wilson, E., Grant, S., Hopewell, S., Macdonald, G., Moher, D., & Montgomery, P. (2013). Developing a reporting guideline for social and psychological intervention trials. *Trials, 14*(242), 1–7. doi:10.1186/1745-6215-14-242

Michie, S., Fixsen, D., Grimshaw, J. M., & Eccles, M. P. (2009). Specifying and reporting complex behaviour change interventions: The need for a scientific method. *Implementation Science, 4*(40), 1–6.

Moher, D., Jones, A., Lepage, L., & CONSORT Group. (2001). Use of the CONSORT statement and quality of reports of randomized trials: A comparative before-and-after evaluation. *JAMA, 285*(15), 1992–1995.

Möhler, R., Bartoszek, G., Köpke, S., & Meyer, G. (2012). Proposed criteria for reporting the development and evaluation of complex interventions in healthcare (CReDECI): Guideline development. *International Journal of Nursing Studies, 49*(1), 40–46.

Morrison, K., Winter, L., & Gitlin, L. N. (2014). Recruiting community-based dementia patients and caregivers in a nonpharmacologic randomized trial: What works and how much does it cost? *Journal of Applied Gerontology.* Advance online publication. doi:10.1177/0733464814532012

Roth, D. R., Burgio, L. D., Gitlin, L. N., Gallagher-Thompson, D., Coon, D. W., Belle, S. H., ... Burns, R. (2003). Psychometric analysis of the revised memory and behavior problems checklist: Factor structure of occurrence and reaction ratings. *Psychology and Aging, 18*(4), 906–915.

Samaan, Z., Mbuagbaw, L., Kosa, D., Debono, V. B., Dillenburg, R., Zhang, S., ... Thabane, L. (2013). A systematic scoping review of adherence to reporting guidelines in health care literature. *Journal of Multidisciplinary Healthcare, 6*, 169–188.

Samus, Q. M., Johnston, D. J., Black, B. S., Hess, E., Lyman, C., Vavilikolanu, A., ... Lyketsos, C. G. (2014). A multidimensional home-based care coordination intervention for elders with memory disorders: The maximizing independence at home (MIND) pilot randomized trial. *American Journal of Geriatric Psychiatry, 22*(4), 398–414.

Schulz, K. F., Altman, D. G., & Moher, D. (2010). CONSORT 2010 statement: Updated guidelines for reporting parallel group randomised trials. *BMC Medicine, 8*(18), 1–9.

Szanton, S. L., Wolff, J., Leff, B., Thorpe, R., Tanner, E., Boyd, C., ... Gitlin, L. (2014). CAPABLE trial: A randomized controlled trial of nurse, occupational therapist and handyman to reduce disability among older adults: Rationale and design. *Contemporary Clinical Trials, 38*(1), 102–112.

Teri, L., Truax, P., Logsdon, R., Uomoto, J., Zarit, S., & Vitaliano, P. P. (1992). Assessment of behavioral problems in dementia: The revised memory and behavior problems checklist. *Psychology and Aging, 7*, 622–631.

West, R. (2008). Providing full manuals and intervention descriptions: Addiction policy. *Addiction, 103*, 1411.

White, A., & Schmidt, K. (2005). Systematic literature reviews. *Complementary Therapies in Medicine, 13*(1), 54–60.

Wolff, J. L., Roter, D. L., Barron, J., Boyd, C. M., Leff, B., Finucane, T., . . . Gitlin, L. N. (2014). A tool to strengthen the older patient-companion partnership in primary care: Results from a pilot study forthcoming. *Journal of the American Geriatrics Society, 62*(2), 312–319.

TWENTY FIVE

SYNTHESIS AND FUTURE DIRECTIONS

This book addresses the complex considerations in developing, evaluating, and implementing behavioral interventions. We highlight the major issues in the conduct of this form of inquiry, summarize what is known, and highlight areas where more research is needed to advance best practices. A broad range of topics are covered including strategies for developing an intervention, study design considerations, strategies for evaluating an intervention, lessons learned from the implementation of proven interventions, and professional issues associated with being behavioral intervention researchers. Our goal is to provide important insights into the critical issues for advancing interventions to enhance the likelihood that they will be implemented and that their impact will be optimized.

One of the overarching themes of this book that underscores its unique and important perspective is the need for new models and strategies to develop and evaluate behavioral interventions that foster successful implementation of proven interventions in real-world settings. In this regard, we propose that a systems and user-centered perspective can propel behavioral intervention research forward and lead to a better fit between our interventions and targeted contexts (clinical, social service, and community settings) and populations.

The evidence is overwhelming that behavioral interventions directed at changing behavioral, health, psychosocial, and environmental outcomes can make a significant difference (statistically, clinically, and from a cost perspective) in preventing, mitigating, or reducing pressing public health issues such as chronic disease management, health disparities, mental health, or cognitive and physical functioning. Yet novel strategies are needed for moving interventions more rapidly from inception to implementation. In this final chapter, we provide a summary of the major points discussed in this book, emergent themes, and key directions for future research.

In Part I, we focused on what we refer to as the "heart of the matter," that is, designing behavioral interventions. Taken as a whole, all five chapters discuss different but interrelated considerations in the design of interventions. We began in Chapter 1 with a justification for behavioral interventions showing that social, emotional, cognitive, and behavioral health changes are more powerful than genetics in shaping key behavioral and health outcomes. That chapter also provides an important overarching social ecological framework that locates behavioral interventions within interactive layers of influence including the immediate environment in which an intervention is embedded as well as within communities and social policies. This social ecological framework is referred to throughout the book as it provides the broad context in which interventions are designed, evaluated, and implemented and identifies the many interrelated factors that need to be considered in behavioral intervention research. By focusing on the ecological context in which we develop our interventions, we may be able to make wiser decisions regarding an intervention's delivery characteristics and the approaches used to evaluate an intervention to advance the evidence base more rapidly. This is our essential premise and a key theme throughout this book, although we recognize that this point needs empirical verification.

In Chapter 2, we examine in some specificity what has been referred to as the "pipeline" for developing the evidence for an intervention. Whereas drug discovery and biomedical research follow a prescribed set of research steps moving from bench to bed to public health impact, for behavioral intervention research there is no consensus, agreed-upon approach, or recipe for advancing interventions and then implementing and sustaining them in real-world settings. Here we suggest that the four-phase traditional pathway (Phase I—proof of concept; Phase II—feasibility, safety, pilot testing; Phase III—efficacy; and Phase IV—effectiveness) imposed on behavioral intervention research from the experience with drug discovery is inadequate. We postulate, as others, that additional phases must be considered that reflect the specific activities or work related to implementation. We thus suggest that the pipeline be elongated or extended to include a Phase VI (translation/implementation activities), a Phase VII (dissemination activities), and a Phase VIII (sustainability or maintenance activities). We also group these phases into four larger domains of interconnected activities: development, evaluation, implementation, and sustainability. Chunking phases in this manner may better promote and reflect the iterative process of intervention development and enable a more fluid approach within each domain such that implementation processes may shape developmental steps and so forth. Although we refer to the elongated seven-phase pipeline throughout this book, we also highlight a more iterative style for intervention development that integrates various strategies such as a more user-centered perspective (see Chapter 2, Figure 2.3). We also identify various innovative strategies to help move intervention work forward more rapidly. We recognize that evidence is needed that supports the use of any of these strategies or their combination for shortening the pipeline for advancing interventions.

In Chapter 3, we take a deep dive into intervention development and identify eight essential tasks for designing an intervention. Obviously, interventions are designed to address problem areas, so one of the first tasks in intervention development is to clearly articulate a problem area, the population most at risk or affected, the pathways contributing to the problem area, specification as to what can be modified, the outcomes of interest, and current practices for addressing the problem. While there is not an agreed-upon formulaic approach to intervention development, we provide guidance as to how to systematically move forward with a viable intervention. A critical theme is assuring that the context and user perspective is identified early on and integrated into the developmental process of evolving an intervention.

Theory remains a neglected stepchild of intervention development although ample evidence shows that, without a theory or conceptual framework, interventions are not as effective. In Chapter 4, we discuss the roles of theory in behavioral intervention work at each phase of the pipeline and also highlight some of the issues in using theories. For example, one issue is that there may not be an adequate theory that addresses the particular problem area and/or intervention idea. Another issue is that it is often necessary to use more than one theory or conceptual framework, particularly for multimodal (interventions directed at changing different pathways by which a problem area occurs) and multicomponent (interventions that involve different elements to address a complex problem) interventions. How theories are combined or how one theory relates to another can be challenging. Many theories do not adequately account for the role of cultural influences on behavior and also lack specificity as to how behavior change occurs. Thus, although theory is critical to behavioral intervention research, future research is needed to attend to developing new and refining existing theories.

In Chapter 5, we discuss delivery characteristics of behavioral interventions, which are the backbone of any intervention. Delivery characteristics include the content of the intervention, dose and intensity, the mode of delivery (e.g., face-to-face, group, through videoconferencing), and staffing requirements. Behavioral interventions address a wide range of issues and populations and can target individuals, communities, organizations, or the social, physical, or policy environments. Interventions can thus involve many different approaches such as counseling, training, psychotherapy, education, skill building, stress management techniques, environmental modifications, or some combination thereof. They may also target different aspects of behavior such as coping skills, knowledge, or affect, and/or involve modifications to the physical and social environment. That chapter offers an overview of the range of issues/factors that need to be considered in the design of behavioral interventions such as what should be delivered, how it should be delivered, and by whom, at what intensity, and for how long.

An important issue in behavioral intervention research is validity: both internal validity, which refers to the accuracy and reliability of the outcomes of a study, and external validity or the generalizability of the study findings. Ensuring internal and external validity requires a systematic approach to the design, evaluation, and implementation of behavioral interventions. Thus, in Chapter 6, we discuss the topic of standardization. We identify the aspects of an intervention that need to be standardized as well as strategies to help foster standardization such as developing manuals of operation and training team members in intervention protocols. We also touch on the topic of tailoring. Our intent is to highlight the importance of taking steps to ensure that research activities at all stages of the pipeline are of the highest scientific quality so that potential benefits of the intervention are maximized and potential threats to validity are minimized.

Given the ubiquitous and important role of technology in health care and other settings, technology is increasingly being used in behavioral intervention research as a vehicle for intervention delivery, as a data collection tool, and as an aid to data analyses. Clearly, the use of technology within behavioral intervention research holds promise in terms of enhancing the outreach, efficiency, and cost-effectiveness of behavioral interventions. In Chapter 7, we provide examples of technology applications in intervention delivery and data collection. We also discuss the advantages and challenges associated with technology-based approaches and highlight issues such as privacy, usability, and the informed consent process that warrant further investigation.

Part II examines strategies for evaluating interventions. Highlighted are essential considerations in evaluation and issues specific to behavioral intervention research. We begin the discussion in Chapter 8 (invited contributor, Dr. Rebok) by providing a thorough examination of the role of control groups in evaluating behavioral interventions. As interventions are often compared to control groups in terms of their impact, attention to what type of control group should be used is critical. Unfortunately, in many studies, little attention is given to the selection of a control group. This chapter carefully describes the range of options available to investigators. Clearly, there is not one type of control group that can be applied uniformly across intervention studies; selecting a control group should be based on the scientific question posed, the resources available, and ethical considerations.

In most cases, it is not feasible to evaluate a behavioral intervention with populations, as populations are typically large and geographically diverse. Thus, a critical issue in behavioral intervention research, at all phases of the pipeline, is the selection of the study sample. Biases in sample selection can lead to errors in the interpretation of results and limitations in the ability to generalize findings from the study to other groups of people. In Chapter 9, we discuss two important considerations in sampling: sample size and sample composition. We also discuss approaches to sampling and provide some guidelines to help optimize the selection of samples for behavioral intervention research studies. A critical point is that the composition of the sample must reflect the targeted group and problem area that an intervention is designed to address. Although this point may seem obvious, historically, behavioral intervention research has been plagued with studies in which there is a mismatch between the intent of the intervention and composition of the study sample such that it is not possible to demonstrate treatment effects. For example, clearly, an intervention designed to address chronic pain must include a study sample that possesses a certain level of pain.

In Chapter 10 (invited contributor, Dr. Jimenez), we move on to a discussion of participant recruitment and retention. A carefully developed, implemented, and evaluated recruitment plan ensures adequate representation in intervention studies from diverse groups of individuals (e.g., age, gender, ethnicity) and is essential to developing interventions that are generalizable and that will ultimately positively impact on the health and well-being of populations. Yet recruitment and retention of study participants remain a central challenge to many investigators. We hope to provide guidance on this issue and describe general strategies to enhance recruitment-specific recommendations for the recruitment process. We also discuss issues that impact on participant retention.

Next, Chapter 11 (invited contributors, Drs. Gallo and Lee) provides a solid introduction to the use of mixed methodologies in behavioral intervention research. Mixed methods afford important insights concerning how interventions work, why they have a desired benefit, what aspects of interventions are more acceptable than others, and what are some facilitators and barriers to implementation of an intervention. There are numerous mixed methodologies that can be employed at any phase of intervention development and can be considered by investigators. Mixed methods promise to propel intervention development forward by enabling the distillation of complex processes in one study design.

Chapter 12 (invited contributor, Dr. Parisi) tackles the issue of treatment fidelity. That chapter offers a comprehensive understanding of this evolving construct and considers three of its dimensions—delivery, receipt, and enactment—and how treatment fidelity can be enhanced, monitored, and measured. Although fidelity has been considered in various fields such as psychology and education, it is not always integrated into study designs for behavioral interventions. Nevertheless, this is a critical consideration—we do not really know if our treatment effects are real if we do not monitor fidelity.

Behavioral intervention research by its nature involves human participants; thus, ethical considerations with respect to the involvement and treatment of research participants is a critical issue at all stages of the pipeline and throughout the research process. In Chapter 13, we provide an overview of the topic of research ethics and discuss some of the guidelines/requirements surrounding the ethical conduct of research. We also highlight issues related to the informed consent process, institutional review boards, and the role of data- and safety-monitoring boards. The topic of research ethics is complex, evolving, and a subject of much discussion.

Part III focuses on considerations related to measurement, outcomes, and analytics. We begin this discussion in Chapter 14 (invited contributor, Dr. Loewenstein), which focuses on the selection of measures, one of the most important and challenging aspects of behavioral intervention research. A common source of misleading results from intervention trials often stems from inadequate attention to the choice of measures—a mismatch between the intent of the intervention and the measurement strategy. Different measures can relay different stories about the impact of an intervention, so measures need to be carefully aligned with the research questions of interest. To address this issue, we discuss the types of measures available, provide general criteria for measure selection, and discuss the emerging role of technology in measurement.

We continue with the discussion of measurement in Chapter 15 (invited contributor, Dr. Harvey) and focus on performance-based measures. The primary reason for using objective performance-based measures, rather than other types of measurement strategies such as self-report or informant-report, is that these types of measures are purported to provide less biased assessments of performance and can identify specific areas of needed intervention. In addition, objective measurement approaches often include a selection of tasks or behaviors that can be assessed, and thus, they can be adapted to the unique needs of a population and task/behavior of interest.

The design of a study and data analysis are fundamental aspects of behavioral intervention research as they provide investigators the means by which to determine whether the obtained results show reliable differences between one or more treatment or control groups, or are merely obtained as a matter of chance. Chapter 16 (invited contributors, Drs. Savia and Loewenstein) highlights some of the key issues to consider when designing a research study to evaluate a behavioral intervention. Also discussed are key analytic strategies including mediating and moderating effects that can provide understanding for whom an intervention is most effective and the mechanisms by which an intervention affects targeted outcomes.

In behavioral intervention research, the outcomes of a study or evidence for a treatment can be evaluated according to different criteria: effectiveness with respect to important outcomes, relevance, feasibility, cost versus benefit, and sustainability potential. Traditionally, the focus has been on identifying the efficacy of an intervention on the basis of a randomized trial with respect to specific outcomes.

However, with an increased emphasis on the importance of evidence-based treatments, a higher bar must also be met and that is identifying the clinical significance of an intervention. Thus, in Chapter 17, we discuss the topic of clinical significance. We define what is meant by "clinical significance" within the realm of behavioral intervention research and review methods for measuring clinical significance. We also provide guidance on how to maximize clinical significance within a behavioral intervention trial.

Yet another analytic consideration is an economic evaluation of our interventions. Chapter 18 (invited contributors, Dr. Pizzi, Mr. Jutkowitz, and Dr. Nyman) provides a comprehensive overview of economic evaluations and their application in behavioral intervention research. Until recently, understanding the costs of interventions has received limited attention. However, with the current emphasis on cost-effectiveness, there is a sea change and greater appreciation for the importance of systematically evaluating the economic value of behavioral interventions and comparing their costs and cost-effectiveness to traditional practices. While economic evaluation may be foreign to many behavioral interventionists, this chapter provides a clear and methodologically sound presentation of its essential aspects and a basic foray into key considerations of this approach.

In Part IV, we turn our attention to considerations related to implementation and dissemination. Chapter 19 (invited contributor, Dr. Hodgson) provides foundational knowledge concerning the emerging science of implementation and the relevant theories that have emerged to help understand the implementation of evidence-based programs. The premise, in keeping with the major theme of this book, is that theories can also inform intervention development by alerting investigators to considerations or factors early on in the pipeline that may impact implementation of an intervention.

Next, Chapter 20 (invited contributor, Dr. Leff) provides an interesting discussion on lessons learned from implementing evidence-based programs. Using three evidence-based programs as exemplars, the importance of context (settings, organizations, or agencies), interventionist characteristics, and value alignment (e.g., between intervention outcomes and stakeholder values and needs) are illustrated. The lessons derived from the implementation experience with these three cases can inform decision making when developing a behavioral intervention.

Chapter 21 (invited contributor, Mr. Beilenson) takes a focused look at the dissemination phase and asks the essential question: What does it take to get an evidence-based program widely distributed? Dissemination is typically viewed as a simple act of either publishing an outcomes paper or providing a presentation. However, highlighted by this chapter, this phase of the pipeline has its own unique processes that require considerable time, commitment, and resources on the part of an investigative team. An innovative concept is the notion of a dissemination infrastructure, particularly in the absence of an industry base for behavioral intervention research such as exists in pharmacological development.

Finally, in Part V, key professional issues are examined. As behavioral intervention research is unlike other forms of inquiry, Chapter 22 examines some of the most pressing and challenging aspects including staffing, hiring, management and support, and building and leading teams. We also emphasize the importance of collaboration and discuss career development paths. For example, it may be that an investigator does not have the desire, resources, or know-how to move his or her proven intervention forward for implementation and dissemination. Rather, an investigator may choose to work on enhancing the evidence base of the intervention or other related scientific questions or develop a new intervention. These become critical personal, professional, and ethical questions that behavioral intervention researchers must grapple with and that we raise in this chapter.

Chapter 23 focuses on grant writing as it is an essential responsibility of behavioral intervention researchers that must occur throughout the pipeline. We emphasize basic grant writing strategies as well as considerations specific to intervention proposals. The primary challenge for all behavioral intervention researchers is the lack of available funding to address the many scientific questions concerning an intervention. Despite the difficulties in obtaining money, proposing a novel intervention and strong science, as well as having the skill to package one's ideas, are all critical for successful grant writing.

Finally, we look at the important role of publishing in Chapter 24. We debunk the myth that intervention work delays publication productivity and highlight the many opportunities to publish even when main outcomes from a trial are not available.

Overall, this book illustrates the many challenges in behavioral intervention research and the complex decisions that need to be made within any one particular intervention study while one advances the evidence base for an intervention across the pipeline. Each chapter has offered best practices, identified methodological gaps, and has sought to push the field forward to adopt new ways of advancing novel behavioral interventions.

INDEX